HANDBOOK OF VETERINARY PROCEDURES AND EMERGENCY TREATMENT

2nd Edition

ROBERT W. KIRK, B.S., D.V.M.

Professor of Small Animal Medicine,
New York State Veterinary College,
Ithaca, New York

STEPHEN I. BISTNER, B.S., D.V.M.

Associate Professor, Small Animal Medicine and
Ophthalmology, New York State Veterinary
College, Ithaca, New York

W. B. SAUNDERS COMPANY   Philadelphia/London/Toronto

W. B. Saunders Company: West Washington Square
Philadelphia, Pa.   19105

1 St. Anne's Road
Eastbourne, East Sussex BN21 3UN, England

833 Oxford Street
Toronto, M8Z 5T9, Canada

Listed here is the latest translated edition of this book together with the name of the publisher.

Japanese *(1st edition)*—Ishiyaku Publishers, Inc., Tokyo, Japan

Library of Congress Cataloging in Publication Data

Kirk, Robert Warren, 1922–

Handbook of veterinary procedures and emergency treatment.

Includes bibliographies and index.

1. Veterinary medicine—Handbooks, manuals, etc.

2. First aid for animals—Handbooks, manuals, etc. I. Bistner,
Stephen, I., joint author. II. Title.

[DNLM: 1. Emergencies—Veterinary. 2. Veterinary medicine.
SF745 K59h]

SF745.K5 1975   636.089   74–4574

ISBN 0–7216–5473–8

Handbook of Veterinary Procedures   ISBN   0–7216–5473–8
and Emergency Treatment

Last digit is the print number: 9   8   7   6   5   4   3

PREFACE

This Second Edition of the HANDBOOK OF VETERINARY PROCEDURES AND EMERGENCY TREATMENT has been greatly expanded and completely updated. We have made every effort to embrace the tremendous explosion of knowledge that has taken place in our profession since 1969 while maintaining the essential character of this book as an "action reference." The original sections, each emphasizing a facet of early examination, clinical methods, or emergency care, have been retained, but you will notice that the revision process has been a highly selective one and that significant changes have occurred throughout. Emphasis has, of course, been placed on those areas of most direct importance to the clinician, be he student, intern, or full-time practitioner.

Completely new information has been added on the evaluation of gastrointestinal function, the diagnosis and management of heartworm disease, and shock. Many of the charts and tables have been revised, and some of them, such as those dealing with growth curves and poison control centers, have been deleted. Those charts concerned with immunization procedures in exotic pets and immunization recommendations for the dog and cat have been expanded. The section on drug dosages has, of course, been completely revised and updated.

The extremely warm reception accorded the first edition was indeed gratifying, and we sincerely hope that readers will continue to find this a convenient action book that provides easily accessible data and key references to more detailed information.

ACKNOWLEDGMENTS

We are indebted to many colleagues who have shared their ideas and methods.

Gary Bolton authored the sections on cardiac emergencies, cardiovascular examinations and dirofilariasis.

Michael Lorenz wrote on endocrine and metabolic emergencies, endocrine function tests, skin scrapings, biopsies and allergy tests and the section on fecal examination.

Alexander deLahunta has again authored the section on neurologic examination, and examination of the cerebrospinal fluids, and collaborated with Eric Trotter on neurologic emergencies. Dan Scott wrote on blood parasites and organized the drug dosage and worming charts.

Wilbur Amand organized the section on immunization of exotic animals.

We are indebted to Donald Patterson for allowing us to modify his publication on genetic defects to produce the chart Breed Incidence of Hereditary Defects.

Lennart Krook, Jack Geary, William Roenigk, Richard Hoffer, John Tasker, Robert Habel, Tass Dueland and Ingemar Settergren have been especially helpful in examining and modifying manuscript. Their help is gratefully acknowledged.

George Batik produced many of the line drawings, Robert Smith and John Lauber did the photographic illustrations and Judy McPherson masterfully deciphered our writings and produced the typescript. It has been a pleasure to work with so many helpful colleagues.

ROBERT W. KIRK
STEPHEN I. BISTNER

CONTENTS

SECTION I. EMERGENCY CARE

SECTION II.   INTERPRETING SIGNS OF DISEASE

SECTION III.   SPECIAL SYSTEMS EXAMINATION

SECTION IV.   CLINICAL PROCEDURES

SECTION V.   INTERPRETATION OF LABORATORY TESTS

SECTION VI. CHARTS AND TABLES

NOTICE

Extraordinary efforts have been made by the authors, the editors and the publisher of this book to insure that dosage recommendations are precise and in agreement with standards officially accepted at the time of publication.

It does happen, however, that dosage schedules are changed from time to time in the light of accumulating clinical experience and continuing laboratory studies. This is most likely to occur in the case of recently introduced products.

It is urged, therefore, that you check the manufacturer's recommendations for dosage, especially if the drug to be administered or prescribed is one that you use only infrequently or have not used for some time.

THE AUTHORS

I

EMERGENCY CARE

I-1. PRIORITY OF EVALUATION AND TREATMENT

The following conditions are serious and require immediate attention:

Respiratory embarrassment
Cardiac arrest
Massive hemorrhage
Profound shock from any cause
Anaphylaxis
Penetrating wounds of the thorax or abdomen
Coma and loss of consciousness
Rapid-acting poisons (Tables 1 and 2)
Massive musculoskeletal injuries
Acute, overwhelming bacteremia and toxemia

I-2. EMERGENCY INFORMATION, EQUIPMENT, AND DRUGS

The supplies needed will vary with the practice, but have the following items in the office and readily available.

EMERGENCY INFORMATION

Keep a copy of this book and other information pertaining to methods of emergency care in a single file cabinet or drawer.

Know the location and telephone number of the nearest Poison Control Center.

Get to know a local exterminator and find out the poisons he uses routinely in his work. Make a list of these together with counteracting agents and antidotes and keep it readily available (Table 1).

ESSENTIAL EQUIPMENT

Aspirator bulbs or 50 ml. syringes for gastric lavage.

Bandages, 1, 2 and 3 inch widths.

Blood specimen tubes, clean.

Catheters, urinary, canine male and female.

Catheters, urinary, feline male and female.

Colon Tubes, 1/4, 3/8, and 1/2 inch O.D., 5 ft. rubber.

Culture tubes, sterile.

Endotracheal tubes (cuffed), 16, 18, 22, 28, 34, 40, 46, French scale.

Enema can and tubing.

Finger cots.

Forceps, for removal of foreign objects.

Forceps, obstetrical, clam shell.

Forceps, sponge, rongeur.

Hypodermic needles.

Intravenous catheters and stylets.

Lubricating jelly.

Mechanical respirator (e.g., Bird respirator).

Minor surgical pack, sterile—

    Cat gut, plain and chromic

    Eye spud, 1

    Forceps, splinter, small, 1

    Forceps, thumb, plain tip, 1

    Forceps, thumb, rat-tooth, 1

    Hemostat, Carmalt, 2

    Hemostat, Kelly, 4

    Needle holder, 1

    Rubber gloves, sterile

    Scalpel blades, assorted sizes

    Scalpel handle, 1

    Scissors, Mayo, sharp-blunt points, 1

    Suture material, Dermalon, assorted sizes

Oxygen tank.
Pliers, side-cutting, for removal of foreign objects.
Rubber gloves, nonsterile.
Specimen collecting bottles, plastic, wide mouth, 4 ounce to 1 pint.
Stethoscope.
Stomach tubes, 1/4, 3/8, and 1/2 inch O.D., clear polyethylene.
Syringes, assorted sizes.
Tape, adhesive, 1 inch width.
Thermometer, clinical.
Venostomy set, regular I.V.
Venostomy set, scalp vein infusion.

DRUGS AND SOLUTIONS (See also Cardiovascular Emergency Tray, Section I-8-A.)

Acetic acid, 0.5 per cent
Activated charcoal
Ammonia water, 0.2 per cent
Apomorphine
Atropine sulfate, parenteral
Caffeine sodium benzoate, parenteral
Calcium disodium versenate (EDTA)
Calcium gluconate, parenteral, 10 per cent
Chlorpromazine
Dexamethasone
Dextran, regular and low molecular weight
Dextrose in water, 5 per cent
Dimercaprol (BAL)
Diphenhydramine hydrochloride (Benadryl), parenteral
Doxapram hydrochloride
Epinephrine hydrochloride
Ethanol, 50 per cent
Heparin, parenteral
Hydrocortisone sodium succinate, ampules
Hydrogen peroxide, 3 per cent
Mannitol ampules, 30 per cent
Meperidine hydrochloride
Metaraminol bitartrate (Aramine bitartrate), parenteral
Methylene blue, parenteral, 1 per cent
Milk of magnesia
Morphine hydrochloride
Nalorphine hydrochloride

Olive oil
Pentobarbital sodium, parenteral
Phenobarbital sodium, parenteral
Phenylephrine hydrochloride, parenteral
Pitocin (posterior pituitary extract)
Potassium chloride
Potassium permanganate
Pyridine-2-aldoxime (2-PAM)
Prussian blue
Ringer's solution, lactated
Sodium bicarbonate, 1.5 per cent
Sodium chloride, 0.9 per cent
Sodium sulfate
Sodium thiosulfate, parenteral, 25 per cent
Starch
Thiamylal sodium
Vitamin K₁ (Aquamephyton injection)

I–3. INITIAL EMERGENCY EXAMINATION AND MANAGEMENT

The examination of the acutely injured animal, i.e., unconscious, in shock, or suffering from acute hemorrhage or respiratory distress, must proceed simultaneously with lifesaving treatment. There is no time for a detailed history taking. Diagnosis is based on physical examination and simple diagnostic aids, and must be carried out quickly. The examination and rapid classification of emergency cases by the urgency with which treatment is required is known as triage. The immediate recognition and prompt treatment of the following conditions are lifesaving.

Emergency Measures

1. Relieve asphyxiation:
a. Clear air passage by rolling the tongue forward and remove any mucous debris obstructing the passageway.
b. Perform a tracheotomy or tracheal intubation, if indicated.
c. Close any open wounds of the throat.
d. Institute artificial respiration, if necessary.
e. Administer oxygen, if necessary.
2. Stop hemorrhage by pressure or tourniquet.

TABLE 1. SUMMARY OF DRUGS USEFUL IN THE TREATMENT OF CHEMICAL POISONING*

Purpose	Drug	Dosage and Route
Absorption of poison	Activated charcoal	5 heaping teaspoonfuls in 200 ml. tap water orally for a 30 lb. dog.
Emesis	Apomorphine	20 µg./lb. by rapid intravenous injection.
	Hydrogen peroxide	5 ml. orally.
Lavage fluid	Tap water at body temperature	200 ml./cycle orally and 1 l./cycle rectally for a 30 lb. dog. Repeat until the washings are clear.
Catharsis	Sodium sulfate	0.3 to 0.4 gm./lb. orally.
Sedation	Diazepam (Valium)	I.V. 5 to 20 mg.
	Thiobarbiturates followed by an inhalation anesthetic	To effect.
Analgesia	Phenobarbital	2 mg./lb. every 12 hours, for dogs and cats.
	Meperidine	5 mg./lb. subcutaneously, for dogs and cats.
	Morphine	1 mg./lb. subcutaneously, for dogs only.
Forced diuresis	Mannitol (20 per cent) in isotonic sodium chloride.	0.5 gm./lb.
Dehydration and acid-base imbalance	See section on fluid therapy.	
Hypotension and cardio-vascular shock	See section on shock.	

*Modified from Aronson, A. L.: Emergency and general treatment of poisonings. *In* Kirk, R. W. (ed.): Current Veterinary Therapy V. Philadelphia, W. B. Saunders Co., 1974.

TABLE 2. EQUIPMENT USEFUL IN THE TREATMENT OF CHEMICAL POISONING§§

1. Mechanical respirator. The Bird Respirator is recommended.
2. Tube sizes for toxicologic procedures.*

Weight of animal	Endotracheal tubes†	Stomach tubes‡	Colon tubes§
5 lbs.	22 French	⅛ to ¼ in. O.D.	⅛ in. O.D.
5 to 10 lbs.	28 French	¼ in. O.D.	¼ in. O.D.
10 to 20 lbs.	34 French	⅜ in. O.D.	⅜ in. O.D.
20 to 45 lbs.	40 French	½ in. O.D.	⅜ in. O.D.
45 to 65 lbs.	46 French	⅝ in. O.D.	½ in. O.D.

3. Aspirator bulbs. Assorted sizes commensurate with the stomach capacity of various animals should be on hand. Large syringes also can be used for gastric lavage.
4. Venostomy (scalp vein infusion) sets. A wide variety of kits are available, which contain instruments suitable for dissecting veins that may be difficult to locate.
5. Intravenous catheters and stylets. A plastic catheter is left in the vein. This procedure is useful for prolonged intravenous administration of fluids of repetitive intravenous injections.
6. Miscellaneous equipment: syringes, needles, clinical thermometers, stethoscope, urinary catheters, and adhesive tape.
7. Collection of tissues for toxicologic analysis: An assortment of unused wide-mouth plastic bottles and plastic bags having capacities of 4 oz. (100 ml.) to 1 qt. (1 l.).

*The largest tube diameter possible should always be used. The tube diameters given for dogs and cats of various weights are presented only as a guide. In conversion of the French scale to the metric, 1 French = 3 mm.

†Cuffed endotracheal tubes are recommended.

‡Clear polyethylene tubing or rubber is satisfactory.

§Soft rubber tubes are recommended.

§§From Aronson, A. L.: Emergency and general treatment of poisonings. *In* Kirk, R. W. (ed.): Current Veterinary Therapy V. Philadelphia, W. B. Saunders Co., 1974.

3. Administer whole blood, plasma, plasma expanders, or fluids in conjunction with other forms of treatment for shock.

4. Temporarily immobilize fractures. Animals who are suspected of having spinal cord injuries should be placed on boards to be moved.

5. Relieve pain by the judicious use of analgesics.

THE INITIAL RAPID SURVEY EXAMINATION IN THE EMERGENCY CASE

General Examination

The animal should be examined to detect any obvious abnormalities in body conformation, evidence of external bleeding, skin color, rate and quality of pulse and respirations, temperature, state of consciousness, and unusual odors.

Head and Neck

The animal should be examined for injuries of the face and skull, neck rigidity and pain, the appearance of the pupils and their response to light, fluid or blood coming from the nose or ears, color of the mucous membranes of the mouth, position of the tongue, and displacement of the teeth.

Throat and Thorax

The animal should be examined for external evidence of injury, sucking wounds, and rib fractures. Percussion and auscultation should be performed for the presence of fluid or air in the thoracic cavity, kind of breathing present, cardiac arrhythmias or murmurs, and areas of thoracic dullness.

Abdomen

The animal should be examined for external evidence of injury, presence of tenseness and pain, absence or presence of peristaltic sounds, and palpation of bladder and kidney areas.

Extremities

The animal should be examined to assess the color and position of the extremities. The extremities should be palpated in order to demonstrate possible fractures or dislocations. The wings of the ilium and prominences of the tuber ischii should be compressed to check for pelvic fractures; a rectal exam should be performed to check for pelvic fractures.

Neurologic Examination

The animal should be examined to assess the deep and superficial reflexes, presence of flaccidity or rigidity of the limbs, and the presence of paralysis, coma, or paresis.

Emergency Treatment of Specific Conditions

I-4. ACUTE ABDOMEN

The diagnosis of the acute abdomen is one that often confronts the veterinarian. The syndrome may have many different causes but is commonly characterized by the sudden onset of acute abdominal pain, vomiting, diarrhea, negative or marked peristaltic activity, fever, dyspnea, anorexia, depression, shock, coma, and death. Occasionally, onset of acute abdominal pain may be insidious, as with rupture of the bile duct or slow necrosis of a strangulated loop of bowel. It may be difficult to distinguish between the acute surgical abdomen and other less fulminating conditions. In a high percentage of cases, a tentative diagnosis can be based upon an adequate history, physical examination, and the judicious use of radiographs and laboratory tests.

GENERAL DIAGNOSTIC PROCEDURES

History

Obtaining an adequate history is important. The owner of the young animal should be carefully questioned about the signs of acute infection, the ingestion of foreign bodies or poisons, or the possibility of a traumatic incident. For the older animal a careful history may reveal the possibility of a chronic infection, a slowly progressive neoplasm, or a vascular disorder. Question the owner with regard to his pet and:

Any previous infectious disease or trauma.

Any previous abdominal surgery.

Any exposure to foreign bodies or toxins.

Any excessive weight change.

The activity status of the animal and the time of its latest feeding.

How quickly the present signs have developed.

General Physical Examination (See Section III-3-A)

1. The abdomen should be inspected for size and symmetry.

2. The abdomen should be auscultated for normal or abnormal peristaltic sounds. For example, in advanced peritonitis peristalsis is absent, and in acute gastritis peristalsis is hyperactive.

3. The abdomen should be percussed for tympany (the sound associated with accumulation of gas in a hollow organ, e.g., gastric distention).

4. The abdomen should be carefully palpated. Splinting and rigidity of the abdominal musculature may indicate severe abdominal pain; however, spinal trauma, spinal disc protrusions, and acute soft tissue injuries of muscle and skin may produce signs of referred abdominal pain. Palpation may reveal an enlarged liver, spleen, kidneys, foreign body, intussusception, cystic calculi, enlarged uterus, abdominal masses, or abdominal fluid. During palpation, it is advisable to try to locate one specific area of pain since it may be a clue to the organ that is primarily affected.

5. Rectal examination should be performed and the color and consistency of the stool should be noted. In a male the prostate should be palpated.

Clinical Laboratory Procedures (See Sections V-3, V-4, V-9, and V-11)

The following tests are not meant to be run on every patient. Rather, a careful history taking and physical examination will enable the clinician to select those tests that will provide the most valuable information.

Laboratory Screening Tests

1. Blood tests including blood chemistries:

Hematocrit—used in determining the state of hydration and blood volume.

Total white count and differential count—used in determining acute and chronic infections.

Erythrocyte sedimentation rate—used in determining the change in blood proteins and immunoglobulin levels.

Bilirubin test—used in diagnosing liver diseases, acute breakdown of erythrocytes, and biliary obstruction.

Serum glutamic-oxaloacetic (aspartate) transaminase (SGOT)—aids in diagnosis of acute myocardial infarction and acute hepatic necrosis.

Serum glutamic-pyruvic (alanine) transaminase—applicable in the specific determination of hepatic disease, viral hepatitis, and hepatic necrosis.

Blood urea nitrogen (BUN)—reflects impairment of the excretory function of the kidneys.

Serum amylase, serum lipase levels—increased levels are observed in acute pancreatitis, intestinal obstruction, peritonitis, acute stress, and anemia.

Blood clotting time—used in diagnosis of hepatic disease.

Prothrombin time—provides an indication of the total quantity of prothrombin in the blood; also useful in diagnosis of hepatic disorders.

Alkaline phosphatase—also used in diagnosing hepatic disease and biliary obstruction.

2. Urinalysis—complete urinalysis should be performed, including bilirubin and urobilinogen determinations. Urine sediment should be stained and examined.

3. Stool analysis—color and consistency should be noted. Microscopic examination may reveal the presence of starch granules, fat droplets (steatorrhea), undigested meat fibers (creatorrhea), blood or blood pigment (melena), or parasite ova. Pancreatic digestion tests for trypsin may be performed (see Section V-8).

4. Abdominal paracentesis (see Section IV-6)—a valuable aid in selected cases provided adequate abdominal fluid is present and the clinician is familiar with basic cytology or can have a cytologic examination competently carried out. The examination of the abdominal fluid for odor, color, specific gravity, protein content, and cellular composition provides a basis for identifying the fluid as a transudate or exudate, blood or urine.

Radiographic Examination of the Abdomen
(See Section IV-14)

Survey radiographs of the abdomen may permit confirmation of a tentative diagnosis without extensive manipulation of the patient.

However, more specific radiologic procedures may be required to confirm a diagnosis. If indicated, the alimentary tract should be evacuated by mild enema (soap and water) or Fleet enema (2 to 4 ounces diluted 1:2 for a 30 pound dog). Enemas are contraindicated in acute intestinal obstructions, intussusceptions, or other conditions in which normal bowel vitality has been impaired. Two radiographic views of the abdomen, lateral and dorsal, should be taken. Standing lateral radiographs are suggested for demonstrating air-fluid interfaces as seen, for for example, in obstruction. The entire abdomen should be visible on the radiograph and all the organ systems should be systematically examined for any abnormalities. Additionally, the diaphragm, caudal lung fields, spine, inguinal area, external genitalia, and pelvis should be examined since lesions involving these organs may produce referred pain.

In the initial screening radiographs of the abdomen, careful attention should be paid to the overall relationship of abdominal structures to each other, the overall abdominal density patterns, and the distribution of the intestinal loops within the abdomen.

Determine if the appearance of the intestinal canal correlates with the history and findings on physical examination. Determine if any ileus is evident (see chart on page 12).

If the first films fail to clearly reveal the normal pattern of intestinal loops, and if the patient's condition permits it, a contrast study can be performed (see Section IV-18). Examine the outlines, densities and size of all solid abdominal organs.

1. Examine the normal outline of the kidneys (see Section III-3-A). Look for densities within the kidneys indicating calculi formation. An increase in the size of a kidney may be associated with hydronephrosis, tumor formation, or subcapsular accumulation of blood, transudates or urine. An irregular outline of the kidney with free gas or increased soft tissue density in the sublumbar area may indicate renal trauma.

2. Examine the posterior abdomen for presence of a bladder shadow. The absence of bladder shadow may indicate a rupture of the bladder (see Section I-5). Examine the prostatic shadow in the male. Increased densities or blurring of the prostatic shadow may indicate presence of a prostatic cyst or abscess. In the female, masses in the caudal abdomen may be indicative of pyometra, mucometra, torsion of a gravid uterus, or pregnancy.

3. If the patient's condition permits, a barium contrast study, a pneumocystogram, a pneumoperitoneum, or an excretory pyelogram may be of value.

Differential Diagnosis of Intestinal Gas Pattern*

A. *Ileus confined to one or several small segments of intestinal loops.*

1. Mechanical ileus—obstruction by a foreign body, neoplasm, intussusception, or pressure from the outside exerted by incarceration, adhesion or neoplasms.
2. Spastic ileus—persistent contraction or spastic contractions of the intestines. String-like foreign bodies, bowel ruptures forming adhesions, inflammatory changes within and outside a segment of the intestines.
3. Irritation of intestinal wall—causing persistent abnormal patterns without signs of gaseous distention. "Beading" in cats; stiffened, unpliable or asymmetrical intestinal wall in tumors (lymphosarcomas); or inflammation within or adjacent to the intestinal wall (pancreatitis, abscesses).

B. *Ileus generalized, involving all or large sections of the intestinal canal: few, but long, gas levels can be seen:*

1. Adynamic or paralytic ileus (reflex inhibition) superimposed on a prolonged obstruction of the mechanical or spastic type, or following impairment of blood supply. Volvulus, torsion of the stomach, peritonitis, abdominal hemorrhage, intestinal inflammation, acute renal diseases, bladder rupture, abdominal and spinal trauma, rupture of the pyometra, abdominal surgery, diabetic crisis, cholecystitis, hepatitis, neoplasia, constipation, toxemias, intoxications, thrombosis.
2. Transient ileus and generalized abdominal distention may follow simple procedures such as enemas, rectal examinations, intravenous urograms. Excitation, swallowing of gas, or dyspnea result in a "pseudo-ileus."

Exploratory Celiotomy (See Section I-5)

DIFFERENTIAL DIAGNOSIS

There are three general groups of acute abdominal disorders:

1. Those requiring immediate surgical intervention. Specific disorders of this type include:

---

*Adapted from Suter, P. F.: Acute Abdominal Diseases: Possibilities and Limitations at Radiographic Examination in Small Animals. Proc. Amer. Animal Hosp. Assoc., Thirty-ninth meeting, 1972.

    a. Acute intestinal, urinary, and biliary obstructions (see Section I-15-I).
    b. Foreign bodies with or without perforations (see Section I-15-A).
    c. Rupture of a hollow viscus (see Section I-5).
    d. Torsion of the intestine, spleen, testis, or stomach (see Section I-15-B).
    e. Vascular occlusion (see Sections I-15-B and I-23).
    f. Incarcerated hernia (see Section I-15-G).
    g. Acute abscess (see Section I-22).
    h. Aortic and portal thrombosis.
  2. Those requiring immediate medical treatment. Disorders of this type include:
    a. Pancreatitis
    b. Cystitis
    c. Hepatitis
    d. Nephritis
    e. Prostatitis
    f. Peritonitis
    g. Lymphadenitis
    h. Ileus
    i. Trauma (see Section I-5)
  3. Those causing referred abdominal pain that may require medical or surgical treatment. Included in this group are:
    a. Pericarditis
    b. Passive congestion of liver or spleen
    c. Pleuritis
    d. Diaphragmatic hernia
    e. Abdominal tumors
    f. Lesions of the spinal cord or central nervous system
    g. Metritis
    h. Abdominal adhesions
    i. Lead poisoning.
    j. Neoplasms of visceral or mesenteric nodes.

I–4–A. Acute Peritonitis

    Peritonitis, localized or general, is the most important complication of a wide variety of acute abdominal disorders. Peritonitis can be caused by: infection or chemical irritants, direct contamination of the abdomen from septic abdominal surgery, bowel puncture from trauma, damage to the renal or biliary system with escape of free bile or urine into the abdominal cavity, extension of inflammation from other areas, or chemical or foreign bodies within the peritoneal cavity producing an intense inflammatory response. Regardless of etiology, certain signs and symptoms are usually present. Systemic reactions include nausea, vomiting, leukocytosis, electrolyte imbalances, toxemia, shock, and increased temperature, pulse and respiration rates.

Abdominal signs include:

a. Pain and tenderness, which may be variable in degree.

b. Muscle rigidity (splinting), which may be absent in subsequent stages when toxemia develops.

c. Paralytic ileus, resulting in a decrease or absence of peristalsis and progressive abdominal distortion.

d. Fluid accumulation (ascites), the amount depending on the degree of inflammation and its duration. When the peritonitis is associated with bile or urine accumulation in the abdomen, aspiration of this material is indicated.

Radiographic Findings

Peritonitis may be seen as a localized or diffuse soft tissue density which permits only poor visual delineation of the loops of the bowel and organs. Suter* reports, "if peritonitis is suspected from the radiographs, the foremost problem is to decide whether it resulted from a perforated inflammatory disease or rupture of a hollow viscus, or whether it is due to a nonperforating inflammatory disease such as pancreatitis. It is still all too often assumed that free gas should be present in the abdomen following intestinal ruptures. Unfortunately, this is not so. Significant amounts of free gas can sometimes be found after gastric, colonic and rectal ruptures. The small amount of gas normally found in the small intestine, the rapid absorption of gas by the peritoneal surfaces and the sealing of a perforated area by adhesions to the mesentery or omentum make the presence of free gas a very unreliable sign of bowel rupture." The wall of the bowel may appear thicker than normal owing to edema and inflammation, and loops of bowel may be fixed in place because of adhesions.

---

*From Suter, P. F.: Acute abdominal disease possibilities and limitations of radiographic examination in small animals. Proc. Amer. Animal Hosp. Assoc., Thirty-ninth meeting, 1972.

Abdominal Paracentesis

Abdominal paracentesis is a valuable diagnostic measure in those subjects in whom an inflammatory exudate can be demonstrated. (See Section IV-6.)

Treatment of Acute Peritonitis

The measures used in the treatment of acute peritonitis are, in general, applicable to most acute abdominal disorders. The basic aims of treatment are:

1. To treat the specific cause (remove foreign bodies, correct torsions, and repair ruptured hollow viscera).

2. To control infection. Acute abscesses should be surgically drained. Infection by the mixed intestinal flora should be treated with broad spectrum antibiotics. When cultures and sensitivity patterns are available, the appropriate antibiotics should be administered. Cultures may be taken from material obtained by abdominal paracentesis. While culture and sensitivity pattern tests are being performed, broad spectrum antibiotics should be administered. The use of intermittent peritoneal lavage has proved valuable in the treatment of diffuse peritonitis (Hoffer).

3. To correct fluid, electrolyte, and nutritional disorders. Avoid giving solid food and medication by mouth; substitute fluids and electrolytes as needed (see Section IV-16). If septic shock develops, treat as indicated (see Section I-9).

4. To provide adequate ancillary care. The patient should be hospitalized and kept as comfortable as possible. Pain relievers and sedatives should be used judiciously. Excessive buildup of gas in the intestines and the stomach can be relieved by oral and rectal intubation. Caution should be exercised, however, especially when the bowel is suspected to be necrotic or gangrenous.

I-5. ABDOMINAL INJURIES

NONPENETRATING ABDOMINAL INJURIES

Nonpenetrating injuries are very common, especially following automobile accidents, and may be accompanied by various degrees of shock, hemorrhage, or peritonitis. They present a diagnostic challenge because (1) they are often consequences of other serious trauma, like fractures and coma, (2) relatively minor abdominal trauma may produce rupture of a hollow viscus, and (3) the absence of any external wounds on the abdomen may be deceptive. When an animal has suffered from nonpenetrating abdominal injury, the presenting signs often reflect multiple organ damage. The signs and symptoms of blunt abdominal trauma are associated with blood loss, bruising and tearing of solid organs and leaking of irritating juices from hollow abdominal organs.

Careful and gentle palpation of the injured abdomen may be helpful. Abdominal masses following blunt trauma occur late in the course of the clinical signs, and such a mass may represent a hematoma of the liver, spleen, mesentery or kidney. Auscultation may be of value; despite extensive intra-abdominal injury and bleeding, peristaltic sounds may be heard. Peristaltic sounds heard in the chest may aid in the diagnosis of a traumatic diaphragmatic hernia.

Abdominal paracentesis may be a valuable diagnostic aid in nonpenetrating abdominal injury. Multiple diagnostic needle aspiration should be performed. A negative diagnostic abdominal tap may have no significance; however, the finding of blood, bile, urine or free gas has definite diagnostic significance and indicates that an exploratory celiotomy should be performed.

The spleen, liver, stomach, intestines and pancreas are vulnerable to blunt injury. Injury may result when the viscous is crushed against the vertebral column or is suddenly displaced from its normal mesenteric attachments. Patients with nonpenetrating abdominal injuries often require prolonged observation because the onset of acute signs may be delayed three or four days.

Ruptured Solid Viscus

Rupture of the Kidney

Renal injuries may range from mild ecchymosis, bruises, or contusions to lacerations or rupture. Rupture of large renal arteries or veins or avulsion of the renal artery and vein from the renal hilus may result in hemorrhage and sudden death from shock. A rent in the renal parenchyma may extend into the collecting system with blood clots obstructing urine flow. Comminution of the collecting system with the abdominal cavity or retroperitoneal tissue may be associated with inflammation caused by the extravasation of urine. The most frequent type of renal injury in dogs and cats appears to be contusions with the formation of subcapsular hematomas.

Signs. Clinical signs are variable and depend partly on the extent of damage. The animal may feel pain in the kidney, but it may be obscured by pain from other lesions. Hematuria is usually present and may be accompanied by shock, oliguria, or anuria. A mass palpated in the sublumbar area may represent either a hematoma or an infiltration of urine into surrounding soft tissues.

Laboratory Findings. Abnormalities associated with primary renal failure will not develop if only one kidney is affected. Urinalysis will reveal gross or microscopic hematuria and proteinuria. There is not good correlation between the degree of hematuria and kidney damage. Abdominal paracentesis may reveal blood or extravasated urine. A negative tap does not eliminate the possibility of severe renal damage.

X-Ray Findings. Striated sublumbar density obliterating the kidney shadow and depressing the colon is typical of sublumbar hematoma and renal or ureteral rupture. As soon as shock has been treated, an excretory urogram (IVP) should be taken. Because there frequently is associated nephron damage and poor renal perfusion in injury, the standard method of performing an IVP may not provide sufficient dye in the collecting system. High dosage excretory urograms (2 to 3 ml./15 lbs. 50 per cent Hypaque) may be helpful in these situations. If the urogram shows evidence of injury to one kidney, it is important to note whether the other kidney is normal, since an emergency nephrectomy may have to be performed.

Differential Diagnosis. Trauma to the lumbar region and rib and spinal fractures may cause local signs that suggest renal injury; however, hematuria is usually absent and urograms are normal.

Treatment. 1. Treat shock and hemorrhage.

2. Follow progress of patient carefully for 48 hours. Measure urine volume for the first 24 hours. If renal trauma is associated with gross hematuria, institute appropriate fluid therapy to induce a marked diuresis to minimize blood clot formation in excretory pathways. Subcapsular and perirenal hematomas usually undergo spontaneous resorption in seven to 10 days. Surgical intervention is indicated during the first 24 hours if (a) intravenous pyelograms reveal a ruptured kidney, kidney laceration, or ruptured ureter or (b) the patient continues to decline despite intensive treatment, as evidenced by a falling hematocrit, rising temperature, and signs of deepening shock.

3. Nephrectomy can be considered only if the contralateral kidney appears normal. Some kidney lacerations can be sutured; however, swelling and loss of normal kidney parenchyma may make this very difficult. Excessively tight sutures through the kidney parenchyma may

result in further kidney laceration and necrosis. If severe injury is confined to one pole of the kidney, partial nephrectomy utilizing the transverse technique of amputation could be utilized.

4. Nephritic infections and abscesses may follow initial kidney damage. Peritonitis resulting from extravasation of urine into the peritoneum may also follow kidney trauma. These complications usually develop two to four days after the initial trauma.

Rupture of the Ureter

This is not a common condition, but some of the signs may resemble those of kidney trauma. Unless both ureters are involved, signs of uremia will not develop. Leakage of urine results in inflammation. Obstruction of the ureter may result in the development of hydronephrosis. Common results are abdominal pain, oliguria, anuria, hematuria, shock, progressive signs of uremia, and toxemia.

Laboratory Findings. Laboratory findings are of little value.

X-Ray Findings. A plane film of the abdomen may reveal loss of soft tissue detail if urinary extravasation and peritonitis have occurred. Sublumbar densities may indicate concurrent kidney trauma. Conclusive diagnosis can be reached only by the use of excretory urograms (IVP).

Treatment. 1. Treat for hemorrhage and shock. Control secondary infections.

2. If contralateral kidney is normal, nephrectomy may be considered.

3. Reanastomosis of the ureter over a splinting catheter may be attempted. Ruptures of the distal end of the ureter may permit reimplantation of the proximal end into the bladder.

Complications. Ureteral stenosis, hydronephrosis, renal infection, peritonitis, and ureteral abscess are frequent complications.

Rupture of the Spleen

A rupture of the spleen may follow any sudden, severe blow to the abdomen or may be associated with splenic tumors such as hemangioma or hemangiosarcoma. Small tears in the spleen may cause continuous or recurrent bleeding.

Additionally, the gastric torsion-dilatation complex may result in twisting of the splenic pedicle, causing acute venous obstruction and thrombosis with massive splenic infarction.

Signs. Pain may center over the anterior quadrant of the abdomen, or it may be restricted to the left anterior quadrant. There may be signs of blood loss and shock, palpable swelling in left anterior quadrant of abdomen, fluid—free blood, possibly—within the abdomen, mild peritoneal irritation and ileus.

It is important to remember that subcapsular splenic hemorrhage may occur without extravasating into the free peritoneal cavity. Also, delayed or intermittent splenic hemorrhage may occur some 10 to 30 days following the initial insult. Multiple abdominal paracentesis (see Section IV-7) should be performed and can be helpful in making a diagnosis.

In the case of ruptured hemangiomas or hemangiosarcomas, there is usually no history of trauma; however, evidence of debilitated, chronic anemia, abdominal distention and dyspnea may have been developing over a protracted period of time.

Laboratory Findings. Hematocrit (HCT) and hemoglobin (Hb) levels fall. Because of blood loss, a mild leukocytosis or anemia may develop. If blood loss is prolonged there may be evidence of bone marrow hyperplasia. Diagnostic abdominal paracentesis may be helpful when free, unclotted blood is present within the peritoneal cavity (see Section IV-7); however, a negative tap does not rule out a ruptured spleen.

Treatment. 1. Treat shock and control secondary infections. Stabilize the patient.

2. In cases of tumor, radiographically evaluate the thorax, and if surgery is performed, carefully evaluate the entire abdomen for any indication of metastasis.

3. Perform a splenectomy.

Rupture of the Liver

Rupture of the liver is characterized by a history of trauma followed either immediately or after several hours by anterior abdominal pain and tenderness, signs of hemorrhage, shock, coma, and death. Bile peritonitis may develop 24 to 72 hours following the initial injury. In some cases free blood may be aspirated from the abdomen by abdominal paracentesis. Rupture of the liver involving the biliary ducts produces a characteristic ''motor oil'' type of exudate. Rupture of the liver should be suspected in all cases of abdominal trauma.

Laboratory Findings. HCT and Hb levels drop as hemodilution occurs. The white blood count (WBC) is elevated. Transient relief of shock and hypotension may occur following the intravenous administration of fluids and electrolytes; however, with continued hepatic bleeding, hypovolemia and shock again develop.

Treatment. Treatment of hepatic rupture varies with the degree of injury. Simple hepatic lacerations that do not continue to bleed may be treated by drainage alone. Hepatic lacerations that continue to bleed require exploratory surgery, suturing and abdominal drainage. Rupture or extensive damage to a large portion of the liver may require excision of a portion of or the entire lobe of the liver.

Injuries to the Gallbladder

Traumatic rupture of the gallbladder and bile ducts are usually associated with other hepatic trauma. Damage to the gallbladder may be indicated on paracentesis by the finding of a heavy, greenish-brown fluid in the abdomen or may only be found at the time of exploratory laparotomy. Additionally, the gallbladder may rupture following obstruction caused by calculi or abscessation.

Treatment depends on the location and the extent of the damage to the biliary system. If one of the divisional bile ducts is damaged, repair may be attempted. If repair is not possible, the duct may be ligated, and bile will flow through the other ducts in the system. Small tears in the gallbladder can be treated by suturing. Large tears usually require a cholecystectomy.

In all cases where bile escapes into the abdominal cavity, peritonitis will develop. Thorough irrigation of the abdomen with warm Ringer's solution, adequate abdominal drainage, and intensive treatment for peritonitis are very important.

Pancreatic Injuries

Traumatic damage to the pancreas may be associated with blunt abdominal trauma. Damage to the pancreas may result in intra-abdominal hemorrhage, and frequently in the delayed development of focal peritonitis associated with the escape of digestive enzymes. Radiographically, a dense, mottled area appears between the stomach and distended gas-filled loops of the small intestine. There is dorsal or dorsomedial displacement of the duodenum, and corrugation and spasticity of the duodenal wall. Laboratory tests utilizing serum lipase and amylase values can be very helpful (see Sections V-3-L-2 and V-3-L-21).

The diagnosis of traumatic or hemorrhagic pancreatitis is confirmed on exploratory laparotomy. Surgical correction of this condition is described by DeHoff.

Diaphragmatic Hernias (see Section I—20—G).

Ruptured Hollow Viscus

If signs of peritonitis develop within 24 to 48 hours following blunt abdominal trauma, perforation of a hollow viscus should be suspected. The signs usually consist of increasing abdominal pain, muscle spasm, ileus, elevated temperature, increased pulse and respiration rates, pallor, vomiting, shock, toxemia, and collapse, and may result in death.

Laboratory Findings. If concurrent hemorrhage is present, there may be a decrease in the HCT and Hb levels. Peritonitis causes leukocytosis. A prognostic abdominal tap may reveal an exudate and the presence of intestinal contents within the peritoneal cavity.

Radiographs. Peritonitis or pneumoperitoneum may be revealed. Free fluid may also be seen in the peritoneal cavity.

Rupture of the Bladder

Rupture of the bladder associated with trauma is most often seen in the male dog and may be associated with the inability of the urethra in the male to dilate rapidly subsequent to trauma-induced increased bladder pressure. Rupture of the bladder is also more frequently seen in obstructed male tomcats. Because of the anatomical location of the bladder in dogs and cats, rupture of the bladder wall usually communicates with the peritoneal cavity. Traumatic rupture of the bladder does not always cause acute abdominal pain. Pain is more severe if there is associated cystitis and peritonitis because of bladder rupture.

Signs. Signs are abdominal pain, tenseness, and in severe cases, increased temperature, pulse and respiration; vomiting; and progressive uremia and toxemia. There may follow anuria or oliguria, possibly incipient hematuria followed by collapse, coma, and death. Large amounts of hypertonic urine collecting in the peritoneal cavity lead to the development of severe hemoconcentration and electrolyte abnormalities. Additionally, hypertonic urine in the peritoneal cavity produces a peritonitis. Some animals with a ruptured bladder may be completely anuric; others may continue to pass small quantities of blood-tinged urine.

Laboratory Findings. There may be leukocytosis and, if uremia is present, an elevated BUN. The PCV may be markedly elevated because of the hemoconcentration present when urine accumulates in the peritoneal cavity. A scanty amount of urine may be obtained. Urinalysis reveals the presence of red blood cells. Abdominal paracentesis should reveal the presence of fluid with a high content of urea.

Radiographic Findings. Survey radiographs usually fail to reveal outline of a normal bladder. Perform a pneumocystogram and take a standing lateral. If the bladder is ruptured, this would show air in the peritoneal cavity just ventral to the vertebral column. Positive retrograde contrast cystography can also be performed, utilizing a dilute solution (2.5 to 5.0 per cent) of Hypaque. The bladder must be fully distended with the contrast agent in order to visualize and focalize the site of rupture. The lack of development of back pressure within the bladder following injection of air or contrast material into the bladder can also be indicative of bladder rupture.

General Treatment of Nonpenetrating Abdominal Wounds

A period of close observation may be necessary before the diagnosis of an intra-abdominal lesion can be made. During this observation period, the following procedures may be carried out:

1. Hospitalize animal, watch all vital signs carefully, and observe for increasing abdominal findings or development of deepening shock. Do not dose too heavily with pain relievers or abdominal signs will be masked.

2. Administer no food orally, and maintain patient on parenteral fluids.

3. Treat shock, if indicated (see Section I-9).

4. Perform serial hematocrit, white blood count, and differential tests (see Section V-3).

5. Failure to respond to treatment for shock and blood loss, or relapse into shock after an initial treatment period, usually indicate continuing major blood loss, or the development of a fulminating infection. In either event surgical intervention is warranted.

6. Indications for an exploratory celiotomy in any nonpenetrating abdominal injury are as follows: (a) the presence of pneumoperitoneum, as evidenced by radiographs; (b) abdominal paracentesis yielding blood (not by puncture of the spleen), or evidence of contamination from contents of a hollow viscus (stomach contents, bile, feces, or urine); (c) secondary collapse, following recovery from post-traumatic shock, if associated with suggestive abdominal signs; (d) the presence of an enlarging mass within the abdomen; (e) when radiographs show free air to be present within the abdomen; or (f) when abdominal signs are obscure, and there is a continuation or recurrence of signs with an increase in severity or frequency. An unnecessary exploratory celiotomy is often far less dangerous than is the failure to intervene surgically in the case of a ruptured hollow or solid viscus.

Penetrating Abdominal Wounds

Any sharp, pointed object or projectile that could have penetrated the free peritoneal cavity must be assumed to have lacerated a hollow viscus. Thus, exploratory celiotomy is indicated in all penetrating abdominal wounds. The probing of a penetrating wound is not a reliable means of assessing the extent of the injury. All patients with rupture of a hollow viscus should be treated for peritonitis.

References

DeHoff, W., Greene, R., and Greiner, T.: Surgical management of abdominal emergencies. Vet. Clin. North Amer., Vol. 2, No. 2, pp. 301–330, May, 1972.

Hoffer, R.: Peritonitis. Vet. Clin. North Amer., Vol. 2, No. 1, pp. 189–194, 1972.

Olsson, S. E.: Radiological diagnosis of some acute abdominal disorders in the dog. J. Amer. Vet. Rad. Soc., 5:5, 1964.

Suter, P. F., and Olsson, S. E.: Traumatic hemorrhagic pancreatitis in the cat: a report with emphasis on radiological diagnosis. J. Amer. Vet. Rad. Soc., 10:4–11, 1969.

Suter, P. F.: Acute abdominal diseases: possibilities and limitations of radiographic examination in small animals. Proc. Amer. Anim. Hos. Assoc., 39th Meeting, 1972, pp. 262–270.

Suter, P. F., and Olsson, S. E.: The diagnosis of injuries to the intestines, gallbladder and bile ducts in the dog. J. Small Animal Prac., 11:575, 1970.

I–6. ALLERGIC REACTIONS

Allergic reactions requiring emergency care may be divided into two main categories.

ANAPHYLACTIC SHOCK

This is an immediate type of hypersensitivity reaction in which death may occur rapidly owing to respiratory and circulatory collapse. In animals, anaphylactic shock hardly ever develops without the interference of man. An exception is the condition that results from the stings of bees or wasps.

The main signs are attributable to the effect of histamine, slow reacting substance (SRS), serotonin, heparin, acetylcholine, and bradykinin on smooth muscle. In the dog, the signs are restlessness, diarrhea, vomiting, circulatory collapse, epileptiform seizures, coma, and death.

Agents which may cause anaphylaxis are penicillin, streptomycin, tetracyclines, chloramphenicol, erythromycin, vancomycin, foreign serums (antitoxins), adrenocorticotropic hormone (ACTH), insulin, Pitocin, vaccines, penicillinase, procaine, benzocaine, tetracaine, lidocaine, salicylates, antihistamines, tranquilizers, iodinated contrast media, vitamins, heparin, stinging insects, food, and allergens (hypersensitization and skin testing).

Treatment

1. Administer immediately an intravenous injection of 1:1,000 epinephrine hydrochloride (Adrenalin), 0.5 to 1.0 ml. If indicated, repeat in 20 to 30 minutes. Infiltrate subcutaneously the entrance site of the allergen (insect bites) with 1:10,000 epinephrine, 0.3 ml.

2. Insure a clear air passage and administer oxygen by endotracheal tube or face mask.

3. Administer an intravenous injection of a rapidly acting steroid, such as hydrocortisone sodium succinate (Cortef sterile solution), 100 to 500 mg., or prednisolone sodium hemisuccinate, 50 to 200 mg. Repeat injection in three to four hours, if necessary.

4. Give an intravenous injection of an antihistamine like diphenhydramine hydrochloride (Benadryl), 0.5 to 1.0 mg./pound.

5. Hospitalize and observe patient closely following the above procedures. If recovery occurs within five to ten minutes following this intensive treatment the prognosis is good.

6. In cases of atopy in the dog, the use of potential sensitizing drugs should be avoided.

ANGIONEUROTIC EDEMA OR URTICARIA

Angioneurotic edema or urticaria is characterized by swelling of the soft tissues of the head, especially around the eyes, mouth, and ears. An ocular discharge may develop and the animal frequently rubs its mouth and eyes with its paws or on the ground. This type of allergic reaction may develop within 20 minutes after contact with the inciting allergen and is very alarming to the owner although it seldom causes serious damage to the animal.

Etiology

Food allergies, ingestion of spoiled protein material, blood transfusions, insect bites, and contact with certain chemicals are the primary causes.

Treatment

1. Try to ascertain the cause and remove the irritating substance if possible (laxatives and high colonic enemas are indicated in food allergies). Stop blood transfusions. Wash the animal free of any known chemical residues.

2. Administer high doses of rapidly acting steroids and antihistamines. Administer Adrenalin only if angioneurotic edema is very severe, i.e., if swelling interferes with normal respirations.

3. Less serious allergic conditions may be manifested as gastroenteritis or skin problems. Acute hemorrhagic gastroenteritis may be associated with the ingestion of proteins such as horse meat, milk, or garbage. It is characterized by the sudden onset of acute vomiting, diarrhea which may be bloody, anorexia, and depression. This condition usually responds well to symptomatic treatment. Skin allergies may present an emergency situation because of self-mutilation; however, they usually require a protracted course of diagnostic work-up and therapy once the emergency treatment has been instituted.

TREATMENT OF SKIN ALLERGIES

1. If possible, separate the animal from its allergen.
2. Sedate the animal with tranquilizers.
3. Clip and clean area of skin which has been traumatized.
4. Compresses using aluminum acetate (Burow's solution, Domboro tablets) in a 1:20 dilution, or potassium permanganate, diluted 1:10,000, may be helpful in reducing inflammation.
5. Apply topical antibiotic-steroid preparations.
6. Administer steroids and antihistamines systemically with prednisolone, 1.0 mg./pound intramuscularly or intravenously, or diphenhydramine hydrochloride, 0.5 to 1.0 mg./pound, intramuscularly or intravenously.
7. Control secondary infections by systemic administration of antibiotics.

I-7. BURNS (See Sections I-8, I-9, I-16 and I-19-C)

Causes

Most burns result from the patient's contact with hot water, grease, hot tar, or other liquids (scalds), from chewing wires (electrical burns), or from entrapment in burning buildings (smoke inhalation).

Severity

The most severe burns are those involving very young and very old subjects, and those that involve the head and joints and result in the formation of scar tissue.

Prognosis

Burns causing extensive damage to less than 15 per cent of the body have a reasonable prognosis. Those in which 15 to 50 per cent of the body is involved cause severe complications and the prognosis is only fair to poor. Burns that involve more than 50 per cent of the body have a very poor prognosis; nearly all patients in this group die within two weeks, and attendant suffering is great. Serious consideration should be given to prompt euthanasia without treatment unless compelling circumstances to the contrary are present.

Classification

Depth of Burn

Group I: Superficial. Group I burns involve the entire epidermis with variable damage to the dermis and accessory structures. The lesion is painful and erythematous and vesicles *may* be present. The hair may be singed but still firmly attached. Healing is rapid once epithelial desquamation has occurred.

Group II: Partial Thickness. Loss of skin substance is greater than I but less than III. The lesion is painful but the hair may be intact. Severe subcutaneous edema subsequently develops followed by the appearance of a dry, tan crust. Healing occurs slowly after sloughing but without grafting.

Group III: Full Thickness. The entire skin is destroyed. The lesion is painless, hair falls out, and the eschar may be black or pearly white. Healing is slow unless grafting is performed. A full thickness burn is four times as serious as Group II lesions of similar size.

Extent of Burned Area

Use a metric ruler to measure the area of burned tissue (Table 3):

$$\frac{\text{Area burned (in sq. cm.)}}{\text{Total body area (in sq. cm.)}} \times 100 = \text{Percentage of body burned}$$

TABLE 3. CONVERSION OF BODY WEIGHT TO SURFACE AREA*

| Body Weight | | Surface Area | |
Kilograms	Pounds	Sq. Meters	Sq. Centimeters
2	4.4	0.16	1600
4	8.8	0.25	2500
6	13.2	0.33	3300
8	17.6	0.40	4000
10	22.0	0.46	4600
12	26.5	0.52	5200
14	30.9	0.58	5800
16	35.3	0.64	6400
18	39.7	0.69	6900
20	44.1	0.74	7400
22	48.5	0.79	7900
24	52.9	0.83	8300
26	57.3	0.88	8800
28	61.7	0.92	9200
30	66.1	0.97	9700
32	70.6	1.01	10100
34	75.0	1.05	10500
36	79.4	1.09	10900
38	83.8	1.13	11300
40	88.2	1.17	11700
42	92.6	1.21	12100
44	97.0	1.25	12500
46	101.4	1.28	12800

*From Davis, L. E.: Treatment and management of burns. Veterinary Scope, 8:7–11, April, 1963.

Principles of Treatment

1. Make a rapid evaluation of the other systems.

2. Elicit vital signs: note especially respiratory involvement (type of respirations, history of steam or smoke inhalations), degree of shock, and the length of time between the burn and treatment. Determine urine output, hematocrit, and examine for hemoglobinuria.

3. Decide prognosis early: perform euthanasia if the case is hopeless.

4. For group I burns:

a. Use pain relievers such as morphine or Demerol p.r.n.

b. Clip and cleanse area gently.

c. If burn is very recent, apply cold water or ice compresses for 20 minutes.

d. Blot gently and apply thin film of topical, antibacterial, and steroid medication (Furacin or Panalog).

e. Bandage and use systemic antibiotics only if lesions are extensive.

5. For Group II burns and less than 50 per cent involvement:

a. Treat shock (see Section I–9).

b. Administer pain relievers (morphine) intravenously p.r.n. only if absolutely necessary.

c. Large amounts of fluid will be needed. A 14 to 16 gauge jugular catheter is advisable. Chlorpromazine may be used as an alpha blocker and to control patient.

d. Use the following formula to determine the volume of Ringer's solution required: body weight (in pounds) × percentage of body burned × 2 = Volume (in ml.) of lactated Ringer's solution required in 24 hours. Give 50 per cent of the solution during the first eight hours, and 25 per cent apiece during the second and third eight-hour periods.

e. If burns are extensive, fresh, whole blood equal to the amount lost will be required. (Follow hematocrit.) Plasma or dextran may be used in some cases. Fluids will also be required to replace current losses. Use dextrose in water, 5 per cent, at the rate of 20 ml./lb./24 hours. For the next two days, ¼ strength lactated Ringer's solution may be given orally.

f. Begin administering antibiotics systemically (penicillin or streptomycin) in fluids, followed, once shock is controlled, by intramuscular injection. If sepsis develops (in five to seven days), use chloramphenicol systemically injected beneath the eschar or use gentamicin systemically. It may be necessary to culture the burn wound every few days to guide therapy accurately. Isolation of *Pseudomonas* is particularly ominous. Local wound treatment is similar to that used for Group I burns. Always bandage. Keep patient in ambient temperature of 75° F. and on soft clean blanket bedding. Provide adequate nutritional support during convalescence.

6. For Group III burns: treat as Group II, except:

a. If burned area is extensive, explain to the owner that prognosis is very poor and prolonged treatment and grafting are necessary.

b. If small area is involved, excision and suture, or early surgical or enzymatic debridement may be helpful. Surgical excision of those portions of the eschar which are no longer adherent is performed without sharp dissection. Sulfamylon acetate cream, 10 per cent, should be applied twice daily.

c. If sepsis develops, use chloramphenicol, 1 per cent, injected locally beneath the eschar. Repeat every eight to 12 hours. The daily total dose should not exceed the 24 hour systemic dose.

d. Hydrotherapy daily in warm water containing Betadine solution is helpful. It stimulates healing, it is gently cleansing, and it accomplishes debridement. It also facilitates initial mobilization of the patient.

7. For smoke and steam inhalation:

a. Observe subject carefully; severe lung edema often develops after 24 hours.

b. Vigorous therapy is needed in cases of severe edema of the larynx and respiratory epithelium. Perform tracheostomy if needed. Use positive pressure oxygen therapy and nebulization, if possible.

c. If infection is severe, administer systemically a combination of prostaphlin, kanamycin, and coly-mycin, or gentamicin alone.

d. Use high levels of corticosteroids systemically. Prognosis is poor for four to five days.

References

Additional information may be found in the following sources:

Ballinger, W. F., Rutherford, R. B., and Zuidema, G. D.: The Management of Trauma, 2nd ed. Philadelphia, W. B. Saunders Co., 1973.

Burns Symposium, Stanford University School of Medicine, 1967.

Davis, L. E.: Treatment and management of burns. *In* Kirk. R. W. (ed.): Current Veterinary Therapy III. Philadelphia, W. B. Saunders Co., 1968.

I-8. CARDIAC EMERGENCIES (Bolton)

The treatment of diseases of the heart naturally depends on the type of pathologic process involved. Most heart disease requires extensive, long-term treatment. There are, however, several conditions in which the most immediate and intensive treatment will save the life of the patient (see Table 4).

I-8-A. *Cardiac Arrest*

This is the acute stoppage of all effective heart action. Cardiac arrest may be due to complete asystole or ventricular fibrillation. Cardiac arrest occurs suddenly and unexpectedly, usually during a surgical procedure.

Causes

1. Obstruction of the respiratory tract leading to hypoxia and asphyxia.
2. Too rapid, careless, or excessive administration of any anesthetic.
3. Existing cardiac disease, pulmonary edema, or shock.
4. Extensive surgical manipulation of the heart or abdominal mesentery.

(Text continued on page 32.)

TABLE 4. CARDIOVASCULAR EMERGENCY TRAY*

1. *Levarterenol bitartrate (norepinephrine)*—(Levophed)
   Winthrop Labs—2 mg./ml. in ampules. Given in an intravenous drip to effect. Dilute 1 to 2 ml. in 250 ml. of drip. Used as a potent vasopressor to increase blood pressure. Does have some chronotropic and inotropic effects on the heart.
2. *Epinephrine HCl*—1:10,000
   Give 1 to 5 ml. intracardially. Used primarily in an attempt to convert cardiac standstill to either ventricular fibrillation or a normal heart beat. Epinephrine causes coarse ventricular fibrillation which can be more successfully converted to sinus rhythm by direct current electric shock. Fine fibrillations may be converted to coarse fibrillations by the intracardiac administration of epinephrine.
3. *Isoproterenol*—(Isuprel)
   Winthrop Labs—1 or 5 ml. ampules, 0.2 mg./ml. Given intravenously in a drip. Dilute 1 mg. in 250 ml. of solution, and give as needed to maintain

TABLE 4. CARDIOVASCULAR EMERGENCY TRAY *(Continued)*

heart rate between 80 and 140 beats per minute. Isuprel is used for its positive inotropic and chronotropic effects. It also causes peripheral vasodilatation.

4. *Phenylephrine HCl*—(NeoSynephrine)
Winthrop Labs—1 ml. ampules, 2 mg./ml. Give 0.8 mg. intravenously. Phenylephrine is used to raise blood pressure because of its potent vasopressive action. It has no direct effect on the heart.

5. *Doxapram HCl*—(Dopram)
Robins Co.—20 mg./ml. Give 0.5 mg./lb. intravenously as a potent analeptic to reverse respiratory depression. May need to be repeated frequently.

6. *Atropine sulfate*—0.5 mg./cc.
Give 1 ml. per 20 lbs. of body weight intravenously to block vagal reflexes and prevent severe bradycardias.

7. a. *Calcium gluconate*—10 per cent solution
Give 5 to 10 ml. intravenously or intracardially.
b. *Calcium chloride*—10 per cent solution
Give 1 to 2 ml. intravenously or intracardially.
Calcium solutions strengthen myocardial contraction. They also increase myocardial contraction. They also increase myocardial excitability, which may be helpful during cardiac arrest.

8. *Lidocaine HCl*—(Xylocaine)—WITHOUT EPINEPHRINE!
Astra Pharmaceutical—20 mg./ml. Give 2 to 4 mg./lb. by slow intravenous bolus and follow with a 2 mg./ml. intravenous drip if needed. Xylocaine is used as an antiarrhythmic drug to control ventricular arrhythmias. It may be used if ventricular fibrillation tends to recur.

9. *Ouabain*—0.25 mg./ml.
Eli Lilly—Initial dose is one-quarter of calculated total dose, given intravenously. Total dose is 0.02 mg./lb. Repeat in 30 minutes if necessary. Digitalis strengthens myocardial contraction, increases cardiac output, and thus controls congestive heart failure. It controls supraventricular tachycardias by delaying conduction through the atrioventricular node and by vagal effects on the sinoatrial node.

10. *Sodium bicarbonate*
Abbott Labs—44.6 mEq./50 ml. Given in an intravenous drip. Dilute 25 to 50 ml. in 250 ml. of drip. May give 10 to 20 mEq. intracardially. The administration of sodium bicarbonate helps alleviate acidosis during cardiac arrest.

11. *Aminophylline*
Searle—250 mg./ml., ampules of 2 ml. Give 2 to 4 mg./lb. intravenously. Aminophylline causes bronchodilation for effective exchange of gases, and has a myocardial stimulatory effect.

---

*From Bolton, G.: Cardiovascular emergencies. Vet. Clin. North Amer., Vol. 2, No. 2, p. 414, May, 1972.

5. Vasovagal reflex.
6. Postoperative pulmonary embolization.
7. Ventricular asystole or ventricular fibrillation. The former is more common.

Premonitory Signs

1. The presence of dark blood, indicating cyanosis.
2. Increased rate and shallowness of respirations.
3. Pulse irregularities and a precipitous drop in blood pressure.
4. Absence of bleeding, dilation of pupils, and coldness of skin.

Management

It is important to remember that the time between the onset of cardiac arrest and the start of irreversible brain damage is only about 3½ minutes. *Act immediately.*

1. Verify cardiac arrest at once:
   a. Take pulse in major vessels.
   b. Note the presence or absence of heart sounds.
   c. Stop administration of all anesthetics. Raise subject's hindquarters and lower its head.
   d. Adequate ventilation must be established immediately. All surgical patients should be routinely intubated. With an adequate artificial airway in place, optimum ventilation can be established at rates of 20 to 40/minute with a ratio of 1:1 between inspiratory and expiratory times. Inspiratory pressures in automatic respirators (Bird respirator) should be between 20 to 25 cm. water. Adequate ventilation must be maintained to ensure normal blood pH.

2. External cardiac massage should be instituted. Subject is placed in dorsal recumbency and ventrodorsal pressure over the sternum is applied (60 to 70 pounds pressure for a large, 30 to 40 pounds pressure for a medium-size, subject). Compression of the thorax should be held for a count of 2 and released for a count of 1 with 60 cycles/minute. An assistant should palpate the femoral pulse while cardiac massage is being performed to make sure that an effective pulse wave is being produced.

3. Use the electrocardiograph to differentiate between cardiac standstill and ventricular fibrillation.

4. If cardiac asystole is present and external cardiac massage does not restore a beat:

a. Inject 1:10,000 epinephrine 0.1 to 5 ml. intracardially and continue massage.

b. Begin rapid intravenous drip of lactated Ringer's solution with sodium bicarbonate.

c. If pulse and heartbeat are not restored following epinephrine, inject calcium chloride solution or calcium gluconate 10 per cent, 1 ml./20 lbs. intracardially, and continue massage.

d. If a heartbeat returns, begin intravenous drip of isoproterenol. Maintain drip to keep heart rate between 80 and 140 beats per minute. Continue cardiac massage if femoral pulse is weak or absent.

e. If heart begins to fibrillate, see Section I-8-B for treatment.

f. If cardiac standstill persists, continue massage and repeat epinephrine and calcium; also inject 10 to 20 mEq of sodium bicarbonate intracardially. Continue massage.

5. Open chest cardiac massage is only indicated if no distal pulse can be produced with external cardiac massage, or if defibrillation must be attempted internally. Properly performed, closed chest cardiac massage can be effective. Open chest massage should not be performed unless absolutely necessary, especially when the chest would be contaminated by this procedure. To perform internal cardiac massage:

a. Make an emergency thoracotomy incision at the left sixth intercostal space. Do not waste time preparing the surgical site. Do not incise the phrenic nerve.

b. Cup heart in hand with fingers on one side and thumb on the other and compress and release ventricular walls. Continue massage until normal rhythm occurs. Stop at intervals to observe if normal cardiac function is returning. Pressure applied 70 to 90 times per minute should be adequate to maintain effective peripheral perfusion (however, the rate should not exceed the ability of the heart to fill adequately with blood during diastole).

I-8-B. *Ventricular Fibrillation*

External Defibrillation

1. Initial management:

a. Maintain adequate respiration.

b. Get heart oxygenated by external cardiac massage.

c. Defibrillate heart using a D.C. defibrillator at maximum strength impulses. In most instances the defibrillation electrodes should be placed on the chest transversely. Make sure that adequate electrode paste has been used on the skin. If defibrillation fails, inject epinephrine intracardially, massage briefly, and repeat defibrillation attempt. If heartbeat returns, begin an isoproterenol drip and maintain heart rate at between 80 and 140 beats/minute. If fibrillation persists after the second defibrillation attempt, repeat the epinephrine injection and inject 10 to 20 mEq. of sodium bicarbonate intracardially. Repeat attempt at defibrillation.

2. The indications for an emergency thoracotomy and internal cardiac massage are:

   a. Inability to obtain a distal pulse with external cardiac massage.
   b. The inability to convert a fibrillation through external defibrillation.

3. The care given to the patient following initial treatment for cardiac arrest is very important in maintaining normal blood pressure and circulation.

   a. Blood pressure must be maintained (see Section I-9).
   b. Maintain adequate respiration.
   c. Avoid metabolic acidosis. A blood pH and bicarbonate combining power should be obtained. If acidosis is suspected, administer fluids containing sodium bicarbonate.
   d. Combat the possibility of intravascular thrombosis by intravenous injection of heparin, 0.5 mg. (100 units = 1 mg.)/pound every two to four hours to increase clotting time to 30 minutes.
   e. If an adequate peripheral pulse was not obtained within three and a half to five minutes following cardiac arrest, treatment for cerebral edema should be instituted (mannitol, 20 per cent, 1.5 gm./pound). After treatment the body temperature should be reduced to 90° F. for several hours.

4. Lidocaine hydrochloride has been used in the treatment of ventricular fibrillation when an electric defibrillator is not available. It may be very difficult to start normal heart contractions following the use of procaine even though the ventricular fibrillations are abolished.

   a. Begin heart massage.
   b. Give 2 to 4 mg./lb. of lidocaine hydrochloride by slow intravenous bolus and follow with a 2 mg./ml. intravenous drip if needed. Continuous EKG monitoring should be available. Duration of action of lidocaine bolus is 20 minutes.
   c. Once ventricular contractions begin, a vasopressor such as levarterenol bitartrate, 0.02 mg./lb., is injected into the left ventricle and an infusion of levarterenol, 0.004 mg./ml., is administered in the form of a continuous intravenous drip.

OTHER CARDIAC ARRHYTHMIAS REQUIRING EMERGENCY TREATMENT

Ventricular Ectopic Arrhythmias

Ventricular arrhythmias (ventricular premature beats, ventricular tachycardia) occur and cause clinical signs fairly frequently in the dog. They signify that the dog has myocarditis. Myocarditis is usually a sequela of another disease process. It has been associated with most of the bacterial, viral, mycotic, and protozoan infections. It may occur with toxemias caused by such diseases as pyometra, uremia, pancreatitis, intestinal foreign bodies, and poisoning. It may be secondary to advanced congestive heart failure. Tumors at the base of the heart, hemangiosarcomas, or other tumors that invade the myocardium can cause myocarditis, as can digitalis overdose. It may be secondary to severe chest trauma with myocardial bruising. It has known association with chronic mitral valvular fibrosis, congenital aortic stenosis, and idiopathic cardiomyopathy.

An occasional animal may have severe myocarditis with no known origin. These are referred to as having primary or idiopathic myocarditis. A thorough evaluation of the entire patient should be done. Likewise, auscultation of the heart for arrhythmias should be done in any animal that has a severe disease, or a disease that causes unexplained weakness, fatigue, or collapse.

Symptoms vary from weakness and fatigue to collapse and sudden death, depending on the severity of the arrhythmia. The diagnosis is made by auscultating an arrhythmia. The EKG diagnoses the type of arrhythmia present. It is essential to do an EKG to determine the type of arrhythmia, because treatment is critical.

Treatment. The urgency of the treatment depends on the status of the patient.

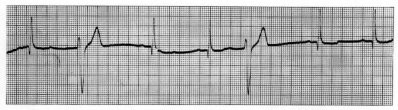

Figure 1. Two ventricular premature beats break the normal rhythm. They are bizarre in conformation.

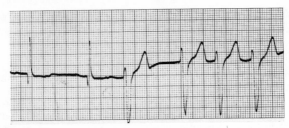

Figure 2. Four or more ventricular premature beats in succession constitute a ventricular tachycardia.

1. Emergency: patient collapsed or comatose with ventricular tachycardia or frequent ventricular premature beats. Treatment should consist of:

    a. Lidocaine (without epinephrine) given intravenously, 2 to 4 mg./lb. bolus to effect cardioversion, followed by 2 mg./cc. drip in 5 per cent dextrose and water to effect for maintenance.

    b. Begin on oral maintenance therapy when possible:

        (1) Quinidine sulfate tablets, 3 grain tablets 5 to 10 mg./lb. orally every six hours.

        (2) Quinidine polygalacturonate (Cardioquin—Purdue–Frederick), 5 to 10 mg./lb. orally every eight to 12 hours.

        (3) Quinidine gluconate (Quinaglut—Cooper), 5 to 10 mg./lb. orally every eight to 12 hours.

2. Urgent, but oral therapy adequate: patient showing moderate weakness or fatigue with ventricular premature beats.

    a. Begin quinidine sulfate, 5 mg./lb. orally, and repeat every two to four hours if necessary. Check EKG every hour.

    b. Keep dog on cage rest until conversion.

    c. Can switch to longer-acting quinidine preparations after conversion (same dosage as previously given).

3. Patient asymptomatic; few or many ventricular premature beats; may have ventricular tachycardia.

    a. Any ventricular arrhythmia must be regarded as potentially dangerous, even if only a few ventricular premature beats are seen.

    b. Oral therapy with long-acting quinidine preparations is adequate.

A paradoxical situation sometimes occurs and may cause a therapeutic dilemma. Severe congestive heart failure may cause severe myocarditis. On the other hand, a dog with severe myocarditis may develop ventricular tachycardia and then develop congestive heart failure secondary to the tachycardia. Therefore, if the clinician is presented with a dog who has both congestive heart failure and a severe ventricular arrhythmia, it is hard to determine which came first. If congestive heart failure is primary, the treatment is digitalis. Lidocaine or quinidine would further depress the heart and kill the dog. If the myocarditis is primary, then lidocaine or quinidine is the treatment. Digitalis would further aggravate the myocardial irritability and kill the dog. The correct treatment is essential.

There are several signs that are helpful in making the correct diagnosis. First, most dogs with severe myocarditis collapse and die suddenly without developing congestive heart failure. Chances are good that congestive heart failure is primary. Secondly, treatment can be used as a diagnosis. However, *do not use the following scheme if you do not have an EKG machine.* Give ouabain, 0.02 mg./lb., one-fourth of the total dose given intravenously. Give Lasix, 5 to 20 mg. intravenously, depending on the size of the dog. Give aminophylline, 5 mg./lb. intravenously. Stand by with lidocaine if needed. The principle is this: chances are good that congestive heart failure was primary. Ouabain peaks in 30 minutes and is essentially gone in an hour. The arrhythmia (and the animal) will be improved in 30 minutes if congestive heart failure was the cause. If we guessed wrong and ouabain makes the dog worse, we can control the arrhythmia with lidocaine until the ouabain wears off, and proceed with oral quinidine when possible. This procedure requires constant EKG and patient monitoring.

Atrioventricular Heart Block

Complete (3°) heart block occurs uncommonly. It may cause excessively slow heart rates. At rates below 60 beats per minute an animal may show clinical signs, ranging from weakness and fatigue to collapse and sudden death. Generally, the animal does well at rest, but experiences symptoms when he attempts to move about, because he cannot increase his heart rate to meet the increased demands on cardiac output. Heart rates may go as low as 15 or 20 per minute.

The etiology may not be found. Myocarditis may be a cause (see causes of myocarditis in previous section). Digitalis overdose can cause it. Occasionally, irritability of the vagus nerve may be causative. Regardless of the cause, when the arrhythmia carries a guarded prognosis the diagnosis is made by auscultating the bradycardia and recording an electrocardiogram (see Figure 3).

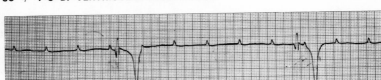

Figure 3. Three-degree atrioventricular heart block.

Treatment. 1. Hospitalize the animal and keep on cage rest.

2. Try atropine first to rule out vagal causes. Give 1/120 gr. (0.5 mg.) per 20 lbs. intravenously. This is usually unsuccessful.

3. Isoproterenol (Isuprel—Winthrop; Proternol tablets—Key).

a. Isuprel injection (0.2 mg./cc.), 0.1 to 0.2 mg. subcutaneously every six hours.

b. Proternol tabs (10 mg. or 30 mg.), 15 to 30 mg. orally every four to six hours.

Usually, medical therapy is not effective. The isoproterenol may at least increase the heart rate above 70 beats per minute so that the dog can have moderate exercise without symptoms.

The treatment of choice for complete heart block is the installation of a cardiac pacemaker.

If digitalis is the cause of the arrhythmia, the digitalis is withdrawn completely until the arrhythmia goes away. Serum potassium should be checked and potassium therapy given if needed. If the heart rate is excessively slow, or the symptoms are severe, treatment as outlined above may be needed until the digitalis wears off. When the arrhythmia abates, the digitalis is resumed at a lower dosage.

Atrial Standstill

This arrhythmia occurs when hyperkalemia develops. Hyperkalemia may result from adrenal insufficiency, severe uremia, or diabetic ketoacidosis. The excessive serum potassium causes very slow heart rates, which accounts for symptoms of weakness, fatigue, collapse, or death. The arrhythmia may be overlooked if the heart is not auscultated. The diagnosis is made by auscultating a bradycardia and recording an EKG (see Figures 4 and 5).

Treatment may be instituted even before a final diagnosis of the primary disease is made:

1. Begin rapid intravenous drip of 5 per cent dextrose in saline (buffered). If a urine sample contains dextrose and ketones, then plain

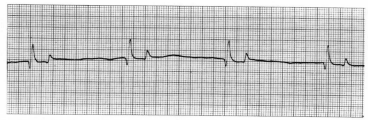

Figure 4. Atrial standstill. A slow heart rate (60 to 70 beats per minute) and a steady, quiet baseline with no P waves. This EKG is from a six-year-old standard poodle suffering from adrenal insufficiency. The serum potassium was 8.5 mg. per 100 ml.

sodium chloride may be given. Even if the patient is diabetic, a 5 per cent dextrose concentration in his fluids would not be harmful.

2. Give 100 mg. hydrocortisone intravenously and another 100 mg. in the intravenous drip. This will probably not harm even a diabetic.

3. Give 1 to 2 mg. DOCA acetate intramuscularly.

4. Begin insulin if animal is diabetic.

Regardless of the cause of the hyperkalemia, this treatment will improve the situation, usually within one or two hours. The hydrocortisone is repeated every two to four hours; the DOCA is given once a day. The fluids establish renal function for elimination of potassium from the body. The treatment of the primary disease must of course be continued beyond these emergency procedures.

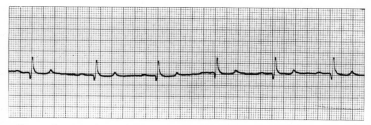

Figure 5. Atrial standstill following therapy for acute adrenocortical insufficiency. Treatment consisted of hydrocortisone, 100 mg. intravenously; DOCA acetate, 2 mg. intramuscularly; sodium chloride with 5 per cent dextrose fluids intravenously; and 10 units of regular insulin subcutaneously.

Ventricular Fibrillation in the Cat

Cardiac arrest due to ventricular fibrillation is less complicated to treat in the cat than it is in the dog. The patient will usually respond to cardiac massage for five to 10 minutes and to being well ventilated.

I–8–C. Acute Congestive Heart Failure

Acute congestive heart failure occurs when the patient no longer has cardiac reserves and the heart, failing to maintain adequate blood flow, cannot meet the requirements of the body for oxygen. The clinical manifestations are influenced by the nature of the etiologic defect and by its effects upon circulatory dynamics, and may show great variation from animal to animal. Signs that usually remain constant are dyspnea, tachycardia, cardiomegaly, circulatory collapse, pulmonary edema, cyanosis, ascites, hepatomegaly, decrease in systolic blood pressure, and collapse, leading ultimately to death.

Fortunately, chronic congestive heart failure is much more common than acute failure in small animals. The following are instances when acute congestive failure develops:

1. Dogs that develop congestive heart failure due to mitral insufficiency may do well for long periods of time on treatment with digitalis. They can have flare-ups of acute congestive heart failure. These flare-ups almost always occur at night during sleeping hours, and require emergency therapy.

2. Rupture of the chordae tendineae cordis usually occurs in a previously asymptomatic dog. Generally the dog is middle-aged or old, and of a smaller breed, and the congestive heart failure develops acutely.

3. Cardiac tamponade usually occurs due to a ruptured left atrium secondary to severe mitral insufficiency. The dog usually has shown symptoms of chronic congestive heart failure and suddenly gets worse. It is hard to distinguish this from a flare-up in a dog that has chronic mitral insufficiency. This condition is most commonly seen in Dachshunds and Cocker Spaniels. There are occasional traumatic episodes of cardiac tamponade that can also produce acute congestive heart disease.

4. Puppies that chew electric cords and receive a shock may have acute congestive heart failure.

5. Myocardial infarction is a very rare occurrence in small animals, and is usually diagnosed at necropsy.

The dog with acute congestive heart failure has severe dyspnea. He may sit on his haunches and support his weight on his forelegs. His head is extended as he breathes, and pulmonary edema fluid may bubble out of his mouth and nose. His eyes are glazed and he does not notice the activity around him. His breathing sounds are rattling and bubbling and moist rales can be auscultated. His heart rate is usually very rapid and murmurs may or may not be auscultated. He cannot move or tolerate being moved or restrained. He can't eat or drink. All his energies are consumed in breathing enough air to stay alive.

Treatment. Any unnecessary stress, such as attempts at oral medication, or restraint for radiography or blood sample collection, may lead to irreversible respiratory and cardiac arrest. Upon admission to the hospital the animal in acute congestive heart failure should receive the following medication and then be immediately placed in an oxygen unit. No additional stress should be placed on the animal.

1. Aminophylline, 5 to 10 mg./lb. intramuscularly.
2. Lasix, 5 to 20 mg. intramuscularly (depending on size of dog).
3. Morphine, 8 to 15 mg. intramuscularly.
4. Mercuhydrin (Lakeside), 1 cc./30 lbs. subcutaneously.

Place animal in oxygen cage. If he is going to survive he will show improvement within 30 minutes to an hour. The aminophylline and lasix may be repeated in two hours. If the dog continues to fail despite therapy, anesthetize and intubate the dog and provide positive pressure ventilation.

Digitalization may be accomplished intramuscularly or intravenously. If it is given intramuscularly: inject digoxin, one-fourth of total dose (total = 0.02 mg./lb.) every six to 12 hours until effect or toxicity (vomiting, diarrhea, arrhythmias). Maintenance dose is one-fourth of total amount that got effect or toxicity, given s.i.d.

Intravenous administration of ouabain (Lilly) should not be used without EKG. Dose equals one-fourth of total (total = 0.02 mg./lb.), given every 30 minutes to effect or toxicity (arrhythmias). Maintenance dose is one-fourth of total amount that produced effect or toxicity. Give every three hours or switch to digoxin intramuscularly. *Note:* Recommended dosages of digoxin do not apply to cats. Cats are very sensitive to digoxin and dosages are not well worked out.

To give digoxin intravenously, the dose should be one-fourth of total dose (total = 0.02 mg./lb.). Give every hour until effect or toxicity. Maintenance dose is one-fourth of what got effect or toxicity. Again, these dosages of digoxin do not apply to cats.

When possible, the dog should be switched to oral maintenance

TABLE 5. RAPID DIGITALIZATION—PARENTERAL FORMS§§

Therapeutic Indices	Ouabain Injection, U.S.P.	Digoxin Injection, U.S.P.
Size of vial	0.5 mg./2 cc.	0.5 mg./2 cc.
Method of administration	Intravenous only	Intravenous or intramuscular (intramuscular causes local pain; if used, preferred site is lumbar muscles)
Total dose	0.02 mg./lb.†	0.02 mg./lb.*
	0.01-0.015 mg./lb.†	0.02-0.03 mg./lb.†
Division of dosage	25% to 50% initially, then 25% every 30 min. until intoxication or desired effect is reached	25% to 50% initially, then 25% every 1 to 6 hr. until intoxication or desired effect is reached
Time from administration to onset of effect	3 to 10 min.‡§	5 to 30 min.‡
		10 to 30 min.§
Time from administration to maximum effect	30 min. to 2 hr.‡	1½ to 5 hr.‡
	30 min.§	1 to 2 hr.§
Maximum duration of intoxication	2 to 6 hr.§	12 to 36 hr.§
Maintenance therapy required	Longer acting glycosides required immediately after treatment to maintain the effect	25% of total dose required for digitalization is given once daily to maintain the effect

*Acetylstrophanthidin is not advised for clinical use because of the rapid onset of its effect (1 to 5 min.) and the danger of inducing fatal arrhythmias. Recommended by the authors.

†Detweiler, 1965.

‡Moe and Farah, 1965.

§Rubin, Gross, and Arbeit, 1968.

§§From Ettinger, S. J., and Suter, P. F.: Canine Cardiology. Philadelphia, W. B. Saunders Co., 1970, p. 236.

therapy with digoxin. Oral maintenance is 0.01 mg./lb. per day, half in the morning and half in the afternoon.

Adjunctive Therapy. 1. Venoclysis. Bleeding the animal may help by reducing blood volume and venous return. This will relieve some pressure from the failing heart. One may safely remove about 5 to 8 cc. of blood per pound of body weight. It is best to monitor central venous pressure during this procedure (see Section I V-20-E).

2. Rotating tourniquets. Placing a tourniquet on two of the legs effectively reduces blood volume by the amount that is in the legs. These tourniquets should be rotated every 20 minutes.

3. Paracentesis. By tapping and removing fluid from the chest if the animal has hydrothorax, we can increase the vital capacity of the lungs. Abdominocentesis may relieve the pressure of an overdistended abdomen. This increases vital capacity and lowers central venous pressure. Sometimes abdominocentesis is necessary before diuretics can be effective. These adjunctive procedures can only be done if the animal can tolerate manipulation.

I-8-D. Pericardial Effusion

Pericardial effusion generally presents as an emergency when the effusion develops rapidly. When the effusion develops slowly, the pericardial sac has time to stretch, and the circulatory system has time to adapt to the hemodynamic alteration. Clinical signs develop due to interference with venous return to the heart and impairment of cardiac function because of the pressure of the trapped effusion. Obstruction to venous inflow causes backup of pressure into the central and peripheral venous system, resulting in peripheral venous distention, prominent jugular pulse, hepatomegaly, ascites, and eventually generalized peripheral edema.

Pericardial effusions of rapid onset are almost always due to bleeding into the pericardial sac. This occurs with trauma, but most often it is caused by left atrial rupture, a condition seen in older dogs of smaller breeds who are suffering from severe mitral insufficiency. A chronic pericardial effusion that has gone undiagnosed may eventually present as an emergency.

An animal with pericardial effusion may show signs of weakness, ascites, dyspnea, muffled heart sounds, and low electrocardiographic potentials. There will be a greatly enlarged circular heart shadow on radiographic examination. Definitive diagnosis may be obtained by

TABLE 6. DIFFERENTIAL DIAGNOSIS OF PERICARDIAL EFFUSION*

Type of Pericardial Effusion	Etiology	Characteristic Features
Blood	1. Heart base tumors	Usually brachycephalic breeds over 8 years old, blood usually nonclotting.
	2. Other neoplasia (metastatic)	Usually occurs in male dogs of smaller breeds, over 8 years old.
	3. Left atrial rupture	
	4. Physical trauma	
	5. Iatrogenic trauma	Due to cardiac puncture or cardiac catheterization.
Transudate	1. Congestive heart failure	Effusion not commonly recognized by physical or radiographic examination.
	2. Hypoproteinemia	
	3. Secondary to peritoneopericardial diaphragmatic hernia	
Exudate (Pericarditis)	1. Benign idiopathic pericardial effusion	Fluid serosanguineous; port wine color, nonclotting, and sterile (Luginbühl and Detweiler, 1965).
	2. Infectious pericarditis	Serous exudate in distemper and leptospirosis; sanguinous exudate in tuberculosis (Labie, 1962); or in conjunction with pleuritis and coccidioidomycosis.

*From Ettinger, S. J., and Suter, P. F.: Canine Cardiology. Philadelphia, W. B. Saunders Co., 1970, p. 404.

coupling physical findings with examination of fluid obtained by pericardiocentesis (see Table 6).

Immediate treatment is aimed at reducing intrapericardial pressure by pericardicentesis (see Section IV-8). Following pericardicentesis, antibiotics administered systemically are indicated. A complete diagnostic work-up should be performed to arrive at a cause for the pericardial effusion.

References

The following were used as reference material and are available for further reading:

Bolton, G.: Cardiovascular emergencies. Vet. Clin. North Amer., Vol. 2, No. 2, pp. 411–417, May, 1972.
Ettinger, S. J., and Suter, P. F.: Canine Cardiology. Philadelphia, W. B. Saunders Co., 1970.

I-9. SHOCK

Shock is a clinical syndrome in which the cardiovascular system, unable to perfuse peripheral tissues adequately, fails to provide nourishment and remove waste products. Adequate perfusion is provided by a balance between blood pressure and blood flow. In retrospect, some cases of shock are called "irreversible" because the tissue changes were extensive enough to cause death.

CAUSES

Each cause merely initiates the shock syndrome, and once started the pathophysiology is similar.

1. Hypovolemia (hemorrhage, dehydration, or trauma). The patient is weak and comatose, and has a rapid, weak, and thready pulse and blanched, cool membranes. Peripheral vessels contract to shift functional circulation to the vital organs.

2. Inadequate peripheral resistance (drug-induced, central nervous system, anaphylaxis). The patient is weak and comatose, and has a rapid weak pulse and abnormally pink, warm membranes. Vascular resistance has collapsed and the vascular capacity is now three or four times normal.

3. Septicemia or bacteremia. Shock resulting from either of the previously mentioned causes may develop into septic or endotoxic shock. The patient is weak and comatose, has a rapid, weak pulse and slightly blanched or muddy membranes. The rectal temperature is usually subnormal, and the desquamating rectal mucosa appears as "raspberry jam" on the thermometer. The packed cell volume is often 65 to 75 per cent and the erythrocyte sedimentation rate is very rapid.

4. Cardiogenic causes. These are extremely rare in dogs and cats. They are best treated with isoproterenol.

EVALUATING SHOCK

Capillary Circulation
Determine capillary refill by pressing oral mucosa until blanching occurs. A rapid return to pink color indicates good capillary circulation; a slow return indicates poor circulation.

Vital Organ Circulation
Place indwelling catheter in urinary bladder. Rate of urine flow (normally, 0.5 to 1.0 ml./pound/hour) parallels rate of perfusion of kidneys (which normally receive 25 per cent of cardiac output).

Circulating Blood Volume
Determine circulating blood volume clinically. Firm, full, femoral pulse, rapid capillary refill, and filled veins are good signs.

Packed Cell Volume
Occasionally it may be desirable to attempt to keep the packed cell volume between 30 and 60 per cent by giving blood or plasma expanders as indicated. Red blood cells are rarely needed in burn and shock patients, but fluids always are! The PCV is helpful primarily to evaluate sludging.

Acid-Base Balance
Shock usually causes severe tissue acidosis. Although this can be managed by assisted ventilation and intravenous administration of sodium bicarbonate, it requires careful and complex monitoring. The degree of acidosis has an important bearing on shock. Additional injectible sodium bicarbonate is almost always needed in large amounts (see Section IV-20).

Rectal Temperature
Hypothermia is common in shock patients. Maintain temperature within normal range by conservation of heat, if possible. Do not allow temperature to go below 94° F. Be careful in using heat; serious burns occur easily.

TREATMENT OF SHOCK

Close supervision and frequent monitoring are essential in all the following types of shock.

Anaphylactic Shock (see Section I–6)

Mild Shock

1. Complete rest and quiet, subject blanketed unless body temperature rises.

2. Mild sedative (chlorpromazine 15 mg./lb. primarily for alpha blockade and vasodilator effect).

3. Antibiotics (penicillin, 20,000 units/lb. and streptomycin, 5 mg./lb.).

4. Administer buffered lactated Ringer's solution intravenously as needed. (Use capillary and vital organ circulation as guide to amount.)

5. Continuously monitor signs (evaluation) and change treatment to the following methods if indicated.

Hypovolemic Shock

1. Provide adequate airway. Use assisted ventilation and 40 per cent oxygen if needed.

2. Control external bleeding. (Control internal bleeding by surgical exploration later if needed.)

3. Place and secure 14 to 16 gauge jugular catheter.

4. Start rapid infusion of buffered lactated Ringer's solution (10 mEq. of $NaHCO_3$/liter). Total volume given in first hour may equal total blood volume, 40 ml./lb. of body weight. More is indicated in cases with severe blood loss.

5. Administer 2 mg./lb. dexamethasone intravenously at once. Repeat in four to six hours if needed.

6. Administer 0.25 mg./lb. chlorpromazine intravenously at once.

7. Administer one million units penicillin and 10 mg./lb. streptomycin intravenously at once.

8. Place urethral catheter and monitor urine output. Normal is 0.5 to 1.0 ml./lb./hr.

9. Blanket to maintain body temperature above 94° F. Heating pads and lights may cause local burns!

10. Monitor peripheral profusion, urine output, pulse pressure and rate, respiration and rectal temperature. Record every 20 to 30 minutes. Consider monitoring PCV, pH, pCO_2, and pO_2 if facilities permit.

11. Consider use of isoproterenol (see Table 4). This is especially indicated in cardiogenic shock. Use plasma expanders or whole blood if needed. PCV should not decrease below 20, nor rise above 60.

12. Maintain effects of dexamethasone, antibiotics and chlorpromazine by repeating medication appropriately. Sodium bicarbonate may be needed in large doses, and in severe shock 1 mEq./lb./hour can be given.

Septic Shock

This form of shock is often a late stage of other types. Particularly serious problems are the severe acidosis, low pO_2, high PCV, and disseminated intravascular coagulation (DIC).

1. Generally follow treatment outlined for hypovolemic shock, but emphasize the following points:

2. Lower blood viscosity (PCV). Blood is contraindicated. Low molecular weight dextran (Rheomacrodex, 10 ml./lb. intravenously) may be used *with* the buffered lactated Ringer's solution to reduce viscosity.

3. Correct the bacteremia and reduce endotoxin production. Emphasize antibiotic agents.

4. Compensate for the severe acidosis. Use assisted ventilation with 40 per cent oxygen. Give 0.4 per cent solution of $NaHCO_3$ in intravenous drip. Consider use of 0.3G THAM in intravenous drip if acidosis still persists.

5. Consider use of heparin, 0.5 mg./lb. intravenously, to prevent microemboli formation.

6. Sludging and capillary stasis facilitates DIC. Improved perfusion will help prevent this (see Sections IV-20 and V-3-J).

Reference

Additional information may be found in the following source:

Brasmer, T. H.: Shock, basic pathophysiology and treatment. Vet. Clin. North Amer. Vol. 2, May, 1972.

I-10. EAR EMERGENCIES

Foreign bodies within the ear canal, foxtails for example, may result in acute inflammation and pressure necrosis of the tissue of the external auditory meatus, causing severe pain and discomfort. Acute inflammation of the external auditory meatus or middle ear may result in sudden pain and discomfort for the animal.

Adequate examination and treatment of the ear in an animal in pain requires the use of a short-acting anesthetic, like thiamylal sodium, or a neuroleptanalgesic agent. Examine the ear canal as described in Section III-5-B. Visible foreign bodies may be carefully removed with alligator forceps. Pus or exudates in the ear canal should be cultured (see Sections IV-4 and V-5) and the external ear canal then gently irrigated, removing debris and exudates. When irrigating, do not allow excessive pressure (over 50 mm. of Hg) to build up since it may rupture an inflamed tympanic membrane. Once all detritus and exudate is removed and the ear canal dried, the tympanic membrane can be inspected. Inflammation of the ear canal requires instillation of antibiotic-steroid ointment such as Panalog and the use of narcotics if pain is severe.

Characteristics of otitis media involving the inner ear are head rotation with the affected ear down, circling to the affected side, falling or rolling to the affected side, nystagmus, fever, depression, and severe pain. Most cases of otitis media are accompanied by a severe otitis externa which must be treated simultaneously. In most cases of otitis media the tympanic membrane is ruptured. If the tympanic membrane is not ruptured but is swollen and hyperemic, perform a myringotomy. Debris and exudate in the tympanic cavity should be cultured and a sensitivity test performed. Clean the tympanic cavity and instill a liquid antibiotic like chloramphenicol solution. If otitis media persists despite initial treatment, radiographic examination of the bullae is of value in better defining the pathology involved. Surgical drainage of the tympanic bulla may be required.

Reference

Additional information may be found in the following source:

Spreull, J. S. A.: Otitis media of the dog. *In* Kirk, R. W. (ed.): Current Veterinary Therapy V. Philadelphia, W. B. Saunders Company, 1974.

I–11. MANAGEMENT OF OCULAR EMERGENCIES*

INTRODUCTION

An ocular emergency is any serious situation which threatens, or has already caused, loss of vision or severe pain and deformity. The practicing veterinarian is often faced with ocular emergencies most frequently seen secondarily to generalized trauma. Prompt recognition of ocular disorders is most important if effective treatment is to be accomplished. Chemical burns of the cornea must be treated immediately to achieve the greatest success. The following ocular emergencies should be treated within one to several hours following injury and are most commonly seen in practice:

1. Penetrating injuries of the globe.
2. Proptosis of the globe.
3. Acute corneal abrasion or ulcer.
4. Acute iritis.
5. Hyphema.
6. Descemetocele.
7. Lid laceration.
8. Pupillary block glaucoma (acute glaucoma).
9. Orbital cellulitis.
10. Corneal laceration.

ASSESSMENT OF OCULAR INJURIES

A carefully performed ocular examination is necessary to assess the degree of ocular injury. Many times adequate sedation or a short-acting general anesthetic will be required to permit a complete examination. Of course, the use of these agents depends on the general physical condition of the animal.

The following equipment has proved very helpful in performing an ocular examination in the emergency situation (Fig. 6):

1. Loupe.
2. Direct ophthalmoscope with rechargeable handle and Finoff transilluminator.

---

*This section is reprinted from Bistner, S. I., and Aguirre, G. D., in Vet. Clin. North Amer., Vol. 2, No. 2, pp. 359–378, May, 1972.

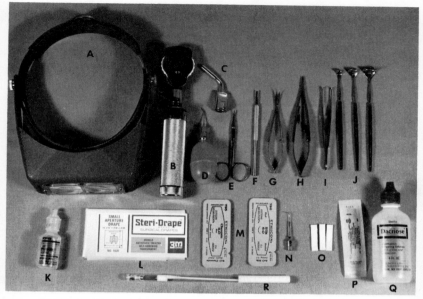

Figure 6. Equipment used to examine the eye in ocular emergencies: *A,* Loupe; *B,* hand ophthalmoscope; *C,* Finoff transilluminator; *D,* irrigator bulb and anterior chamber irrigating needle; *E,* Stevens tenotomy scissors; *F,* Beaver handle and No. 64 blade; *G,* Castroviejo corneal scissors; *H,* Castroviejo needle holder; *I,* Elschnig fixation forceps; *J,* various size lid retractors; *K,* topical anesthetic; *L,* steri-drapes for minor lid lacerations; *M,* 6-0 ophthalmic silk and 6-0 ophthalmic gut; *N,* lacrimal cannula; *O,* Weck-cel sponge; *P,* fluorescein sterile strip; *Q,* sterile ocular irrigating fluid; and *R,* culture swab.

3. Fine-toothed forceps.
4. Lid retractors.
5. Lacrimal probes.
6. Sterile eye wash solution in irrigating bottle.
7. Fluorescein-impregnated sterile strips.
8. "Weck-cel" sponges.
9. Topical anesthetic (proparacaine 0.5 per cent).
10. Culture swabs and culture media.
11. Schiötz tonometer (not pictured).
12. Short-acting mydriatic (tropicamide 1 per cent).

When examining the animal with an ocular emergency the following procedures may be of aid in obtaining a diagnosis and instituting effective therapy:

1. Obtain an adequate history from the owner. This may reveal the existence of previous eye disease, the instillation of some chemical irritant, or the occurrence of trauma. Try to determine when the injury occurred and if any medication or eye wash has been used.

2. Examine the eye for any discharge, blepharospasm, or photophobia. If discharge is present, note the type. If the animal is in extreme discomfort with the eye completely closed *do not* try to force open the lids.

3. Note the position of the globe within the orbit. Note whether exophthalmos or proptosis is present. If the eye is exophthalmic there is frequently strabismus and protrusion of the third eyelid, exposure keratitis, and, in cases of retrobulbar or zygomatic salivary gland inflammation, pain on opening the mouth. Note any displacement of the globe medially or temporally.

4. Note any swelling, contusions or lacerations of the lids. Are the lids able to cover the cornea? In cases of lid lacerations try to determine the depth of the laceration. Penetrating lid lacerations may be associated with secondary injury to the globe.

5. Palpate the orbital margins, feeling for fractures, crepitus, air, and cellulitis.

6. Examine the cornea and sclera for evidence of partially penetrating or completely penetrating injuries. The use of lid retractors in these cases can be very helpful. If the wound is completely penetrating, look for loss of uveal tissue, lens, or vitreous.

7. Examine the conjunctiva for hemorrhage, chemosis, lacerations, or foreign bodies. Examine the superior and inferior conjunctival cul-de-sacs for foreign bodies. On occasion, topical anesthesia and a sterile cotton swab can be used to "sweep" the conjunctival fornix in order to pick up foreign bodies. Use a small, fine-toothed forceps to pick up the third eyelid and examine its bulbar aspect for foreign bodies.

8. Examine the cornea for opacities, ulcers, foreign bodies, abrasions, or lacerations. A loupe and a good focal source of illumination are important in conducting this examination.

9. Record pupil size, shape, and response to light, both direct and consensual.

10. Examine the anterior chamber and note its depth and the presence of hyphema, iridodonesis, or iridodialysis.

11. If indicated, and if the cornea is undamaged, measure intraocular pressure.

12. Examine the posterior ocular segment using a short-acting dilating agent and a direct or indirect ophthalmoscope to look for intra-ocular hemorrhage, retinal hemorrhage or edema formation, and retinal detachment.

When examining an animal with an ocular emergency, the history may indicate sudden loss of vision occurring unilaterally or bilaterally. The following conditions can produce sudden loss of vision:

1. Hyphema or vitreous hemorrhage.
2. Traumatic lid swelling.
3. Extensive corneal edema or exposure keratitis.
4. Acute congestive glaucoma.
5. Retinal hemorrhage or extensive retinal edema.
6. Retinal detachment.
7. Extensive trauma to or avulsion of the optic nerve.
8. Intracranial damage secondary to hemorrhage, ischemia or anoxia, resulting in the interruption of visual pathways.
9. Proptosis of the globe.

In addition to having the aforementioned diagnostic equipment available, the following basic surgical instruments also should be at hand to treat periocular and ocular lacerations and other types of emergencies (Fig. 7):

1. Castroviejo or Barraquer lid speculum.
2. Bishop-Harmon tissue forceps.
3. Stevens tenotomy scissors—standard.
4. Castroviejo corneal scissors.
5. Castroviejo needle holder—standard jaws with lock.
6. Beaver knife handle and #64 blades.
7. Lacrimal cannula—straight 22 gauge.
8. Barraquer iris repositor.
9. Foreign body spud (not pictured).
10. Enucleation scissors—medium curve (not pictured).
11. Suture material—6-0 silk, 4-0 ethilon, 7-0 collagen or 6-0 ophthalmic gut.

Injuries of the Lids

Lid contusions and lacerations are not infrequently seen in veterinary medicine. They are most commonly associated with bite wounds or automobile trauma. Basic principles of surgical treatment of lid lacerations are similar to other areas of the body, except that very careful primary repair must be undertaken to ensure adequate physiologic

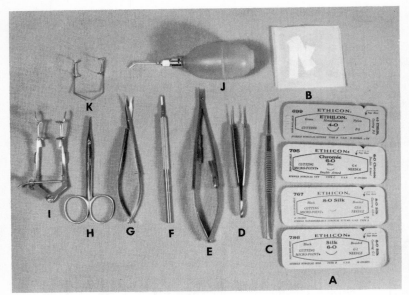

Figure 7. Minimal set of instruments for repair of ocular and periocular lacerations: A, Different types of suture material; B, Weck-cel sponge; C, iris repositor; D, Bishop-Harmon tissue forceps; E, Castroviejo needle holder; F, Beaver handle with No. 64 blade; G, Castroviejo corneal scissors; H, Stevens tenotomy scissors; I, eye speculum; J, irrigating bulb; and K, Barraquer wire lid speculum.

and cosmetic results. An accurate understanding of lid anatomy is necessary before attempting lid surgery.

The lids are covered externally by epidermis and internally by conjunctiva, and between these layers are contained muscular and adnexal structures. Eyelid cilia are present on the upper eyelids of dogs and cats. The cilia may be present in two to three rows, with each cilium emerging from an individual follicle. A clearly marked furrow is present in the margin of the upper and lower lids. Openings for the meibomian glands are located within this furrow. In the dog and cat the meibomian glands are situated in a poorly developed tarsal plate, permitting manipulation of the upper and lower lids.

The lid aperture in the dog varies widely (from 10 mm. to 35 mm.), depending on age and breed. The two eyelids converge to form medial and lateral angles. The extremities of the palpebral aperture are maintained in their normal position by virtue of the two palpebral ligaments. There are two main patterns of motility of the lids—closure and elevation. The eyelids are closed by the action of the orbicularis oculi supplied by the 7th nerve. The upper lid is elevated mainly by the *m. levator palpebrae superioris*. Elevation of the upper lid is helped by smooth muscle fibers that arise from among the fibers of the *levator palpebrae superioris*. These fibers (Muller's fibers) are supplied by the sympathetic nervous system.

The puncta lacrimale are located in the mucocutaneous junction, 2 to 4 mm. from the medial canthus of both upper and lower lids. In the dog and cat the puncta are slitlike openings frequently surrounded by a small amount of pigment. In correcting eyelid lacerations, the surgeon must keep in mind the location of the puncta, and all attempts should be directed toward maintaining their normal function.

The lids can be considered as a two-layered structure with the anterior layer composed of skin and orbicularis muscle and the posterior layer composed of tarsus and conjunctiva. The openings of the meibomian glands in the lid margin form the approximate line separating the lids into anterior and posterior segments. Splitting the lid into these two components facilitates the use of sliding skin flaps to close wound defects. Large defects in the conjunctiva and tarsus can be corrected by transposing the lid tissue with the same tissue from the opposing lid.

The conjunctiva is a mucous membrane which covers the posterior surface of the lids (palpebral conjunctiva) and reflects onto the globe (bulbar conjunctiva) at the fornix. The natural looseness of the conjunctiva permits extensive mobilization for surgical repairs.

Gentle cleansing and careful and thorough irrigation are necessary as preoperative routines before correcting lid lacerations. Sterile saline intravenous set is used to irrigate the wound. The conjunctival sac is also irrigated and foreign bodies removed. Application of tincture of iodine followed by isopropyl alcohol can be used on the skin. Draping of the wound is necessary to prevent further contamination. We have found that the small- and large-aperture disposable plastic eye drapes are excellent for this purpose.

Adequate lighting and magnification are necessary for proper surgical correction of lid lacerations. The surgeon should be sitting, and his forearms and elbows should be well supported.

In lid lacerations, ragged wound margins should be trimmed and necrotic tissue debrided. However, *as much tissue as possible should be saved* to minimize wound contracture and lid deformity. When correcting a ragged lid margin, trim the tarsus in a slightly curved fashion which will permit slight overcorrection and "pouting" of the suture incision when the lid is sutured vertically. This helps to insure tight lid closure and prevents excessive scarring.

Small wounds of the lid margin can be closed by a figure-of-eight suture using 4–0 or 5–0 silk. The lid margins must be tightly apposed to prevent postoperative lid notching.

In more extensive lacerations, splitting the lid along the margin just anterior to the meibomian gland openings permits mobilization of the skin, orbicularis muscle layer and a two-layered closure. The conjunctiva is sutured with 6–0 or 7–0 gut or collagen, and an interrupted pattern is used with the knots tied so as not to touch the cornea. The skin is sutured in a different plane, using 6–0 ophthalmic silk.

Ecchymosis of the Lids

Because of the excellent vascular supply to the eyelids, direct blows may cause ecchymosis. Associated ocular injury such as orbital hemorrhage, proptosis or corneal laceration may occur. In addition to trauma, allergic reactions and internal or external hordeolum may result in lid ecchymosis.

Eyelid hemorrhage following trauma may itself be of little consequence, but the globe should always be examined for any associated injury. Treatment of lid ecchymosis is initially by the use of cold compresses followed later by warm compresses. Resorption of blood may occur anywhere from three to ten days. Ocular allergies respond to topical and systemic administration of corticosteroids plus the application of cold compresses.

Conjunctival lacerations and contusions are not uncommon following trauma. A small conjunctival laceration may overlie and conceal a larger scleral laceration or rupture. Conjunctival hemorrhage can obscure from view vitreous or uveal tissue that has herniated through a scleral rupture. Therefore, it is important to carefully examine conjunctival lacerations for evidence of underlying pathologic conditions. The conjunctiva may have to be carefully dissected away from the underlying sclera to provide a better view of any abnormalities. Undue pressure should not be placed on the globe when performing this dissection in order to prevent herniation of intraocular contents through a scleral wound.

Repair of large conjunctival lacerations can be accomplished by the use of 6–0 gut or collagen using an interrupted or continuous suture pattern. The margins of the conjunctiva should be carefully approximated to prevent inclusion cysts from forming. Care should be taken to avoid suturing the conjunctiva of the membrana nictitans to the more laterally positioned bulbar conjunctiva, as this may result in the partial prolapse of the membrana nictitans.

When large areas of conjunctiva have been damaged, conjunctival advancement flaps may be used to close the defect. If grafts are required, conjunctiva from the superior fornix of the contralateral eye may be obtained. Buccal mucous membrane grafts have also been used and can be obtained by free-hand dissection using a scalpel.

Subconjunctival Hemorrhage

Subconjunctival hemorrhage is a common sequela to head trauma. In itself, subconjunctival hemorrhage is not a serious problem. However, it may indicate the presence of more severe intraocular damage, including traumatic iritis, retinal detachment, and luxation or subluxation of the lens. Therefore, a complete eye examination is indicated in all cases of subconjunctival hemorrhage. Subconjunctival hemorrhage also may be associated with various type of blood dyscrasias and systemic diseases, including thrombocytopenia, autoimmune hemolytic anemia, hemophilia, leptospirosis, severe systemic infections, and difficult or prolonged labor (dystocia).

Uncomplicated subconjunctival hemorrhage usually clears within 14 days. If the conjunctiva is exposed because of the hemorrhage, a protective ophthalmic antibiotic ointment (neomycin, polymyxin B, bacitracin) can be used. Methylcellulose drops or hydroxymethylcellulose drops also can be used until the chemosis is reduced.

Chemical Irritants

Occasionally, chemical irritants such as caustic soda (alkali) or acids may cause extensive conjunctival and corneal lesions in small animals. Acid burns tend immediately to precipitate tissue proteins, causing localized, nonprogressive necrosis of corneal epithelium. On the other hand, alkalies combine with the lipids of the cellular membranes, producing rapid and extensive destruction of the corneal stroma. The alkali may continue to penetrate the cornea for days following initial contact.

The degree of chemical damage to the eye is directly proportional to time lapse before neutralization of the chemical by irrigating the eye.

Irrigation of the eyes should be conducted as quickly as possible. Sterile saline or water from any source can be used. The lids must be held apart manually, or the animal may be anesthetized and the lids held apart with retractors. Any residual particulate matter should be removed from the conjunctival fornices. Following lavage, a cycloplegic (1 per cent atropine) should be administered to reduce the discomfort resulting from iridocyclitis. Topical antibiotic drops (neomycin, bacitracin, polymyxin B) should also be used (six times/day). It has recently been demonstrated that the ulcerated alkali-burned cornea releases the enzyme collagenase, which can lead to rapid stromal destruction and corneal perforation. *In vitro* inhibitors of collagenase are effective in neutralizing the effects of collagenase. We have used 10 per cent acetylcysteine (two drops in the affected eye five times a day) to neutralize the effects of corneal collagenase. Clinical impressions indicate that this form of treatment has been very effective in halting the progression of rapidly spreading deep corneal ulcers.

Corneal Abrasions

Corneal epithelial abrasions are exceedingly painful and are characterized by intense blepharospasm, lacrimation and photophobia. Movement of the eyelids or third eyelid seems to cause more discomfort. Animals in such discomfort can prove very difficult to examine until effective relief from pain is achieved. Topical use of 0.5 per cent proparacaine hydrochloride will, in most cases, permit relaxation of the lids so that the eye can be examined. Using a focal source of illumination and an eye loupe, the inferior and superior conjunctival fornices and medial aspect of the membrana nictitans should be examined for foreign bodies. Place a drop of sterile saline on a sterile paper strip impregnated with fluorescein and touch the superior conjunctiva. The fluorescein spreads rapidly in the tear film to cover the cornea. Irrigate the excess fluorescein from the eye with sterile saline. Areas of corneal epithelial damage will remain green.

Barring complications, minor corneal epithelial abrasions rapidly heal. A short-acting cycloplegic (tropicamide 1 per cent) is used every six hours during the first 24 hours to make the eye more comfortable and to reduce the effects of the secondary iridocyclitis which usually develops. A broad spectrum antibiotic drop is used six times a day to prevent secondary infections. The animal is kept out of bright light and an analgesic administered (Demerol 2 mg./lb.) if pain is severe. The eye is reexamined in 48 hours. Topical anesthetics or antibiotic-steroid-anesthetic combinations are not dispensed to owners. These products tend to retard healing, and may lead to superinfection.

Corneal lacerations may be nonpenetrating or may invade the anterior chamber. Penetrating corneal lacerations may result in prolapse of intraocular contents. Frequently, pieces of uveal tissue or fibrin effectively but temporarily seal the wound and permit the anterior chamber to reform. Manipulation of these wounds should be avoided until the animal has been anesthetized. Care should be used in anesthetizing an animal with a corneal laceration because struggling and/or excitement during administration of anesthesia may result in loss of the temporary seal in the corneal laceration and extrusion of intraocular contents.

Preparation for repair of a corneal laceration should be as meticulous as for any intraocular surgery. Superficial corneal lacerations need not be sutured. However, if the laceration extends through 50 per cent or more of the cornea, or if it is more than 3 to 4 mm. in length, sutures are required to close the wound.

Careful, accurate suturing is essential to maintain a watertight corneal wound and to minimize scar formation. Use of adequate magnification by the surgeon is advantageous in properly placing sutures in the cornea. Silk sutures, 7–0 or 8–0, collagen sutures 7–0 or 8–0, or fine 10–0 Dermalon sutures, all with micropoint spatula type needles, are effective in closing corneal wounds. Sutures are tied individually and are left in place for a minimum of three weeks. Many corneal wounds are jagged in appearance, or the cornea is edematous and tight closure is not possible. In these cases a thin conjunctival flap is pulled down (or up) over the corneal wound to help seal it and prevent aqueous loss. Sutures must never be placed through the entire full thickness of the cornea but should lie in the middle third of the stroma.

Having closed the corneal wound, the anterior chamber must be reformed to prevent synechia formation and the resulting secondary glaucoma. Taking care to avoid injury to the iris, a 25 or 26 gauge needle is inserted into the anterior chamber at the limbus. Sterile saline solution is gently instilled to reform the anterior chamber. Defects in the suture line will be recognized by leakage of fluid, and they should be repaired. The anterior chamber should not be overfilled for fear of inducing secondary glaucoma, nor should the eye be left hypotonic.

Incarceration of uveal tissue in corneal wounds presents a difficult surgical problem. Persistence of incarcerated uveal tissue predisposes to a chronic filtering wick in the cornea, shallow anterior chamber, chronic irritation, edema and vascularization of the cornea, and intraocular infection leading to panophthalmitis.

On occasion, the use of a mydriatic agent (e.g., 1 per cent atropine and/or 10 per cent phenylephrine) permits removal of a small tag of uveal tissue from a corneal wound. This is only possible soon after the injury, before synechiae have formed.

Incarcerated uveal tissue (usually iris) can be surgically removed from a corneal wound in several ways. The uveal tissue can be trimmed from the corneal wound using an electroscalpel and/or scissors and the wound swept with a blunt cyclodialysis spatula to free further adhesions. The corneal wound is repaired as previously described.

Conjunctival flaps can be used in the correction of large corneal lacerations and in deep stromal ulceration or perforation.

A second method of repair where uveal tissue is incarcerated into a corneal wound is to make a small limbal incision under a limbus-based conjunctival flap. A blunt cyclodialysis spatula is then introduced into the anterior chamber and the adhesions are carefully swept free. The anterior chamber is reformed by inserting a blunt cannula through the incision and injecting saline.

Ocular Foreign Bodies

Periorbital, scleral or corneal punctures or lacerations may be due to foreign bodies which can penetrate the eye. The most common foreign bodies associated with ocular injuries in small animals are birdshot, B-B pellets, and glass. The site of intraocular penetration of these foreign bodies may be obscured by the eyelids.

A foreign body entering the eye may take several trajectories depending on its velocity and angle of entry. It may penetrate the cornea and fall into the anterior chamber or become lodged in the iris. Foreign bodies may penetrate the anterior capsule of the lens, producing cataracts. Some metallic, high-speed foreign bodies may pass through the cornea, iris, and lens to lodge in the posterior wall of the eye or in the vitreous cavity. On occasion a foreign body may pass entirely through the eye and remain within the orbit.

There are numerous techniques available to determine the presence and location of ocular foreign bodies. Direct visualization of a foreign body is the best means of localization. Examination of the eye with the biomicroscope or indirect ophthalmoscope may prove invaluable in locating foreign bodies. The anterior chamber and anterior drainage angle can be directly viewed with the aid of a gonioprism. Careful ocular examination should be performed as early as possible before secondary ocular inflammation or cataract formation opacifies the ocular media.

Indirect demonstration of an intraocular foreign body may be achieved by radiographic techniques. After having demonstrated the presence of a radiopaque foreign body, the location of the foreign body must be determined. At least three radiographic views should be taken. These should include the anteroposterior, oblique, lateral, or dorsoventral projections. A Flieringa metallic fixation ring corresponding to the diameter of the cornea can be sutured in place at the limbus with 6–0 silk. This radiopaque metallic ring can then be used as a reference point for outlining the limits of the globe.

In addition to radiography, the more refined technique of ultrasonography may be employed to locate foreign bodies.

Intraocular penetration by a foreign body always results in a guarded prognosis, and the outcome depends largely on the foreign body's chemical nature and its position within the eye. Foreign bodies composed of iron or copper can produce extensive ocular inflammation.

Chalcosis is produced by the retention of copper or its alloys of bronze and brass. High levels of copper within an eye can result in rapid inflammation, hypopyon, and localized abscess formation. The slow release of copper results in the deposition of this metal on the limiting membranes within the eye, especially Descemet's membrane and the anterior lens capsule.

Retained foreign bodies of iron and steel may lead to repeated episodes of ocular inflammation and siderosis. In siderosis iron pigments are deposited in the cornea, iris, and lens, and degenerative changes occur in these areas as well as the retina. Repeated episodes of ocular inflammation may lead to secondary glaucoma or phthisis bulbi, resulting in eventual enucleation.

Other metals besides copper and iron may produce ocular inflammatory reactions. Agents such as mercury, aluminum, nickel, zinc, and lead (in decreasing order) may produce inflammation. Precious metals, stone, carbon, glass, building plaster, and rubber are usually inert in the eye; however, the mechanical trauma produced by these objects may produce serious sequelae.

When considering removing any foreign body from an eye, one must weigh the dangers of leaving the foreign body in the eye against surgically removing it. Foreign objects in the anterior chamber are much easier to remove than objects at the posterior pole. Magnetic foreign bodies are easier to remove than nonmagnetic ones. Attempted removal of foreign bodies from the vitreous cavity of animals has consistently produced poor results. In many cases the eye has been enucleated.

Ocular Traumatic Injuries

Blunt trauma to the eye can result in luxation or subluxation of the lens. The subluxated lens may move anteriorly, thus shallowing the anterior chamber. Trembling of the iris (iridodonesis) may be noticed when the lens is subluxated. In complete luxation, the lens may come to lie in the anterior chamber, thus causing obstruction to aqueous outflow, or may be lost in the vitreous cavity. Luxation of the lens is almost always associated with rupture of the hyaloid membrane and herniation of the vitreous through the pupillary space.

Emergency surgery for lens dislocation is required if the lens is entirely within the anterior chamber or incarcerated within the pupil, thus causing a secondary pupillary-block glaucoma. Incarceration of the vitreous in the pupil can also produce pupillary block glaucoma. Recognition of vitreous herniation into the anterior chamber prior to surgery is important. Complications of vitreous loss may then be minimized by administering systemic hyperosmotic agents or by aspiration of liquid vitreous at the pars plana. Intravitreal dislocation of the lens is a serious problem; however I do not routinely operate on these cases since postoperative results are uniformly poor.

Surgical management of dislocated lenses is a difficult problem with many complications, chief of which is loss of vitreous. Preoperative management is extremely important. If the lens is in the anterior chamber, one must take measures to prevent it from falling into the posterior chamber during surgery. Constriction of the pupil prior to surgery by the use of 2 per cent pilocarpine drops may help to ''trap'' the lens in the anterior chamber. A Calhoun needle can be inserted from pars plana to pars plana to prevent the luxated lens from moving backward. Intraocular tension should be reduced by the use of intravenous mannitol just prior to surgery. This also helps to shrink the vitreous body, aiding in the prevention of vitreous loss.

Further details on the different techniques used in extraction of subluxated and luxated lenses are beyond the scope of this paper.

Severe trauma to the globe or a direct blow to the head can result in retinal and/or vitreous hemorrhage. There may be large areas of subretinal or intraretinal hemorrhage. Subretinal hemorrhage usually assumes a discrete, globular form, and the blood appears reddish-blue in color. The retina is detached at the site of hemorrhage. Superficial retinal hemorrhage may assume a flame-shape appearance, and preretinal or vitreal hemorrhage assumes a bright red amorphous appearance, obliterating the underlying retinal architecture. Retinal and vitreous hemorrhage associated with trauma usually resorbs spontaneously over a two- to three-week period. Unfortunately, vitreous hemorrhage as it organizes can produce vitreous traction bands which may eventually produce retinal detachment.

Extensive retinal hemorrhage may be associated with scarring and glial proliferation as the blood resorbs.

Expulsive choroidal hemorrhage can occur at the time of injury and usually leads to retinal detachment, severe visual impairment and total visual loss.

Treatment of retinal and vitreous hemorrhage involves rest and the correction of factors which may predispose to intraocular hemorrhage. It is questionable whether any local measures are of value in aiding in the resorption of blood.

Hyphema refers to blood in the anterior chamber of the eye. Its most common cause is trauma resulting from automobile injuries. Hyphema also may be present secondary to penetrating intraocular wounds.

Blood within the eye may come from the anterior uveal tract, posterior uveal tract, or both. Trauma to the eye may result in iridodialysis or a tearing of the iris at its root, permitting excessive bleeding from the iris and ciliary body. Expulsive choroidal hemorrhage in the posterior pole may result in hyphema and secondary retinal detachment.

Usually, simple hyphema resolves spontaneously in seven to ten days and does not cause visual loss. Loss of vision following bleeding into the anterior chamber is associated with secondary ocular injuries including glaucoma, traumatic iritis, cataract, retinal detachment, endophthalmitis, or corneal scarring.

Treatment of hyphema must be individualized to the case in question. However, several general principles of treatment can be followed:

    a. Arrest continuing bleeding and control recurrent bleeding.

    b. Aid in the elimination of blood from anterior chamber.

    c. Control secondary glaucoma.

    d. Treat associated injuries, including traumatic iritis.

    e. Detect and treat late complications of hyphema.

Unfortunately, little can be done to arrest and prevent rebleeding in the eye. The iris stroma has marked fibrinolytic activity and this may be associated with the failure of fibrin clots to effectively occlude damaged ocular vessels. The role of movement by the iris and ciliary body in producing recurrent ocular bleeding is a controversial one. Despite the fact that parasympathomimetic drugs increase vessel permeability, there is still no good, controlled study indicating whether maintaining an immobile pupil by the use of mydriatics or miotics will alter the tendency of damaged ocular vessels to bleed.

In cases of early hyphema, it is advisable to keep the affected animal confined and to prohibit active exertion. If the hyphema is so extensive that it may produce a secondary glaucoma, the animal should be observed while hospitalized. The use of medications such as vitamin C, vitamin K, calcium, rutin, or estrogenic substances does not appear to accelerate an already functional clotting mechanism.

If possible, daily examination of the animal with hyphema should be conducted. Rebleeding within the first five days following injury may occur. The intraocular pressure should be closely observed.

After five to seven days, the blood in the anterior chamber changes from a bright red color to a bluish-black color (eight-ball hemorrhage). If the total hyphema persists and an elevation in ocular pressure is evident despite medical therapy, surgical intervention is indicated. Continued presence of blood in the anterior chamber under increased pressure may lead to blood staining of the cornea.

Primary escape of red blood cells from the anterior chamber is via the anterior drainage angle, with iris absorption and phagocytosis accounting for minor removal of blood elements. Theoretically, because a miotic agent increases the facility of outflow from the anterior chamber, it should accelerate the escape of red blood cells from the anterior chamber. In addition, miotics tend to expose more of the iris stroma and its associated fibrinolytic activity to blood in the anterior chamber. Experiments conducted in rabbits have confirmed these findings. On the other hand, hyphema in animals is almost always associated with a traumatic iritis that may be severe and lead to complications such as anterior or posterior synechiae and secondary glaucoma. If the traumatic iritis is mild, miotic treatment of the eye for several days will not worsen the iritis. In order to prevent posterior synechiae from occurring, the pupil can be dilated periodically (every two days) with a short-acting mydriatic such as 1 per cent tropicamide. Because of the associated traumatic iritis in hyphema, topical corticosteroids such as 0.1 per cent dexamethasone or 1 per cent prednisolone should be used to control anterior segment inflammation. In addition, if the anterior segment inflammation is severe, a cycloplegic agent such as atropine 1 per cent should be used.

The hyphemas secondary to retinal detachment (e.g., Collie Ectasia Syndrome) and end-stage glaucoma are extremely difficult to treat medically and have a poor prognosis.

One of the most serious complications of hyphema is secondary glaucoma. Glaucoma of this type is due to angle obstruction by blood clots. Large hyphemas producing eight-ball hemorrhage may effectively block the anterior drainage angle.

Control of glaucoma secondary to hyphema may prove extremely difficult. Carbonic anhydrase inhibitors such as acetazolamide or dichlorphenamide decrease aqueous secretion and may effectively reduce intraocular pressure if the trabecular outflow system is still functioning to 40 per cent of capacity. An eye with glaucoma and a completely blocked trabecular outflow system will respond poorly to a carbonic anhydrase inhibitor. Osmotic agents, such as oral glycerol, or intravenous mannitol may be helpful in controlling glaucoma secondary to hyphema. Reduction in vitreous volume deepens the anterior chamber and may increase aqueous fluid outflow.

Evacuation of blood or blood clots from the anterior chamber is not advisable unless there is secondary glaucoma which cannot be controlled medically or if there is no indication, over a prolonged period, that blood resorption is occurring. Experimentally, it has been shown that irrigation of the anterior chamber that contains fresh blood clots (one to two days old) with 1250 units/ml. of fibrinolysin will help to lyse the blood clots. This treatment is ineffective in treating older, organized blood clots.

It is important to emphasize that surgical intervention and blind probing of the anterior chamber in an attempt to remove blood or blood clots may cause serious surgical complications such as rebleeding, luxated lens, extensive iris damage, and damage to the corneal endothelium.

In most instances, blood in the anterior chamber has formed a large clot and cannot be aspirated through a small incision. A large formed clot should be extracted through a limbal incision under a conjunctival flap. The clot is removed by counter-pressure from the outside using Daviel lens spoons. Since the intraocular contents cannot be visualized, instruments are not placed in the anterior chamber, for fear of damaging the lens or inducing rebleeding. Once having removed the clot, the anterior chamber is not vigorously irrigated, but enough sterile saline is introduced to wash out remaining cellular elements and to reform the anterior chamber. If rebleeding occurs during surgery, 1/10,000 epinephrine can be introduced directly into the anterior chamber.

Proptosis Globe

Proptosis of the globe secondary to trauma is not uncommon, especially in brachycephalic breeds. Proptosis of the globe in the dolicocephalic breeds requires a greater degree of initiating contusion than in the brachycephalic breeds. Therefore secondary damage to the eye and central nervous system associated with proptosis of the globe may be far greater in the Collie than in the Pekingese.

When presented with a case of proptosis of the globe following trauma, the tendency is to replace the globe as quickly as possible. One should not disregard the general physical condition of the animal presented with a proptosed globe. Careful evaluation of the cardiovascular system for evidence of shock and examination of the respiratory and nervous system should be carried out. Treatment to establish an adequate airway, treat shock, control overt bleeding, etc., should be carried out before any attempt is made to replace the eye in the orbit. While this initial examination and treatment are being carried out, the proptosed globe should be protected against further exposure and drying. This can be accomplished by using sponges soaked in cold, hypertonic solution (hypertonic 10 per cent dextrose) to reduce ocular edema and prevent corneal drying.

Proptosis of the globe results in several pathologic phenomena which must be considered in establishing treatment and prognosis:

1. Occlusion of the vortex and ciliary veins of the eye by the lids produces venous stasis and a form of congestive glaucoma. The resulting venous stasis also limits accessibility of intravenous medication to the eye. The venous stasis is relieved once the eye is replaced in the orbit.

2. Proptosis results in marked exposure keratitis and corneal necrosis. Initial protection of the eye with moist gauze soaked in a hypertonic solution will prevent excessive drying.

3. Proptosis of the globe can be associated with severe intraocular problems such as iritis, chorioretinitis, retinal detachment, luxation of the lens, and avulsion of the optic nerve.

It is advisable to attempt to replace most of the proptosed globes encountered despite the severity of the condition. Exceptions to this are eyes in which the intraocular contents have been extruded, massive destruction of the intraocular contents has taken place, or the owner wishes to have the eye removed because of cosmetic or economic considerations.

Surgical replacement of the proptosed globe should be carried out under general anesthesia if possible. Careful evaluation of the patient should be made to determine whether general anesthesia can be tolerated. A lateral canthotomy incision is made to widen the palpebral fissure. The canthotomy incision can extend from the canthus to the orbital ligament. It is not a good policy to cut the canthal ligament; however, if the globe cannot be replaced by enlarging the palpebral fissure with a canthotomy, the canthal ligament can be partially severed. To facilitate identification, black 5–0 silk sutures should be placed at the ends of the severed canthal ligament. Following replacement of the globe, the ligament should be sutured.

Using gentle pressure applied to the globe with a moistened, sterile sponge, an attempt is made to replace the globe into the orbit. Swelling of the globe and retro-orbital hemorrhage and/or edema may make this difficult. The examining veterinarian may feel that if swelling of the globe can be reduced by paracentesis, the globe can more easily be replaced into the orbit. This type of procedure should be avoided, since the sudden release of intraocular pressure combined with tension on the globe by the lids can result in possible choroidal hemorrhage, retinal detachment, luxation of the lens, and a general displacement of all intraocular structures. In addition, probing of the retro-orbital space with a needle in an attempt to aspirate blood or fluid should be avoided because further damage to the globe and optic nerve may result.

Once it has been demonstrated that the globe can be replaced in the orbit, proptosis is allowed to recur while preparation for postoperative treatment and suture placement are made.

The implantation of a subpalpebral lavage apparatus can be very helpful in postoperatively medicating the eye which is protected by a temporary tarsorrhaphy. Once the subpalpebral tube has been positioned, a nictitating membrane flap suture is placed but not tied. The nictitating membrane flap aids in keeping the globe in the orbit and protects the cornea if the lid sutures become loose and the lids part too early. Following placement of the nictitating membrane sutures, three nonpenetrating mattress sutures are placed in the lid margins but not drawn taut. The eye is gently replaced in the orbit and the nictitating membrane and lid sutures tightened. Small pieces of rubber tubing are used under the sutures to prevent pressure necrosis of the skin overlying the lids. The nictitating membrane sutures are also tied over a piece of rubber tubing.

After replacing the eye in the orbit, 2 to 4 mg. of methylprednisolone acetate are injected into the retrobulbar space to aid in reducing inflammation.

Postoperative treatment must be aimed at controlling traumatic iritis and the extensive corneal damage that is associated with proptosis and exposure keratitis. Systemic broad spectrum antibiotics are indicated. Atropine 1 per cent is used t.i.d., and topical steroids and antibiotics are used five to six times a day. Although steroids are a "two-edged sword," the extensive vascularization, inflammation, and scar tissue which can form after ocular injury make them a very valuable aid in treating traumatic proptosis. The topical medication can be delivered as an ointment placed through the eyelid margins directly on the cornea or in liquid form delivered via the indwelling subpalpebral catheter. If we feel that trauma to an eye has been extensive, we will supplement out topical steroids with systemic steroids for a one-week period.

Sutures are left in place until intraorbital swelling is markedly reduced—usually ten days to two weeks. After this time the sutures are removed with the animal under anesthesia, and the globe is inspected. If proptosis recurs, the sutures are replaced and removed after an additional two weeks.

Extraocular muscle injury and resultant strabismus are very commonly seen following proptosis. The most frequent deviation observed is upward and outward, indicating possible paralysis or rupture of the medial rectus, superior oblique and inferior rectus muscle, or an overaction of the lateral superior rectus muscles. The strabismus is most noticeable immediately following removal of the lid sutures. Surprisingly, in most cases, return to a relatively normal visual axis occurs in three to four months following the initial injury.

Acute Glaucoma

Acute glaucoma (a rise in intraocular pressure not compatible with normal ocular function) is not uncommonly seen in practice. Unfortunately owners many times fail to recognize the cardinal signs of glaucoma: sudden onset of pain, photophobia, lacrimation, deep episcleral vascular engorgement, an edematous ("steamy") and insensitive cornea, shallowing of the anterior chamber depth, dilated and unresponsive pupil, and loss of visual acuity.

Most glaucomas in small animals are secondary and are associated with other ocular problems, such as luxated lenses, uveitis, hemorrhage, etc. It is beyond the scope of this paper to discuss, in depth, the differential diagnosis of secondary glaucoma or the concepts involved in primary glaucoma. We can, however, outline several steps which will help to reduce intraocular pressure during early acute glaucoma, thus preserving vision until a more complete diagnosis can be reached and controlled medical or surgical therapy instituted.

Intraocular pressure may be reduced by three medical methods: 1. Improve the facility of aqueous outflow; 2. Reduce ocular volume by the use of osmotic agents; 3. Reduce aqueous formation.

1. The filtration angle may be increased by the instillation of pilocarpine drops (two to four per cent) once an hour for three to four hours, then once every three hours. Excessive treatment with pilocarpine may lead to the development of toxic systemic side effects due to cholinergic stimulation. The dilated pupil in acute glaucoma associated with very high intraocular pressure (above 60 mm. Hg.) may be unresponsive to pilocarpine therapy because of paralysis of the sphincter muscle. Miotics instilled during this period will produce constriction of the pupil once intraocular pressure is lowered.

If angle-closure glaucoma is secondary to forward displacement of the lens, as occurs in lens subluxation, miotic therapy is contraindicated because it may worsen the glaucoma by increasing pupillary block and further narrowing the angle.

2. Osmotic agents can be used to reduce the size of the vitreous body and to reduce the amount of aqueous present. These agents create an osmotic gradient between intraocular fluids and the vascular bed, thus acting independently of the aqueous outflow and inflow system. Oral glycerol (50 per cent) can be used 0.3 ml./lb. every eight hours to effectively reduce intraocular pressure. Intravenous mannitol therapy (20 per cent) 1 gm./lb. will rapidly (within one hour) reduce intraocular pressure. If the filtration mechanism is open and working, pressure may be controlled medically. If increased intraocular pressure rapidly recurs following osmotic therapy, there is extensive obstruction to the aqueous drainage mechanism and filtering procedures or other types of glaucoma surgery are indicated.

3. The third method of glaucoma control utilizes carbonic anhydrase inhibitors to reduce aqueous secretion. This method of controlling greatly increased elevated levels of intraocular pressure in narrow angle glaucoma is not very effective because secretory inhibition by carbonic anhydrase inhibitors is incomplete, decreasing aqueous production by only 50 to 60 per cent. If the aqueous drainage apparatus is so severely damaged that it cannot handle 40 per cent of its normal drainage function, then the carbonic anhydrase inhibitors will not be able to control intraocular pressure effectively. Thus the use of carbonic anhydrase inhibitors alone in acute, narrow angle glaucoma will not effectively control and stabilize intraocular pressure.

Glycerol, 50 per cent, may be helpful in the evaluation of acute glaucoma when it is applied topically to the eye. Application of hypertonic glycerol does not have any effect on intraocular pressure; however, it may rapidly clear corneal edema, thus permitting greater visualization of the anterior chamber. Prior to the use of glycerol, several drops of topical anesthesia should be placed in the eye. Reduction in corneal edema will help in examining the anterior ocular segment and in performing gonioscopy so that an etiologic diagnosis can be made and effective medical or surgical therapy instituted.

References

Brown, S. I., and Weller, C. A.: Collagenase inhibitors in prevention of ulcers of alkali-burned cornea. Arch. Ophthalmol., *83*:352–353, 1970.

Havener, W. H.: Management of traumatic hyphema. In Symposium on Ocular Pharmacology and Therapeutics. St. Louis, C. V. Mosby Co., 1970, pp. 190–203.

Paton, D., and Goldberg, M. F.: Injuries of the Eye, the Lids and the Orbit. Philadelphia, W. B. Saunders Company, 1968.

I–12. ENDOCRINE EMERGENCIES

ACUTE ADRENOCORTICAL INSUFFICIENCY (Lorenz)

This is a severe shock syndrome resulting from the decreased production of adrenocortical hormones. Early clinical signs include vomiting, diarrhea and episodes of weakness. The more severe acute signs may be precipitated by stress or infection and include severe hypotension, oliguria, bradycardia, weak femoral pulse and coma. The cause of this disease in most cases is idiopathic adrenal cortical necrosis.

Diagnosis

1. Hyperkalemia. The serum potassium levels may be greatly elevated (6.0 to 9.5 mEq) and produce typical cardiovascular changes (see Section I-8-B).

2. Hyponatremia. The serum sodium levels are greatly reduced (115 to 130 mEq). A decrease in the sodium-potassium ratio from a normal of 33 : 1 to 25 : 1 or below is present.

3. Cardiovascular changes:

a. Bradycardia (less than 60/min.).

b. Weak pulse.

c. An elevated, spiked T wave.

d. Decreased amplitude of p waves and atrial arrest.

e. A widening of the QRS complex.

Treatment

1. Establish a patent intravenous catheter.
2. Begin a rapid intravenous infusion of 0.9 per cent NaCl or 2.5 per cent glucose in 0.45 per cent NaCl (see Section IV-16-C).
3. Inject 100 to 200 mg. hydrocortisone hemisuccinate intravenously. Repeat the dose every 30 minutes until diuresis occurs.
4. Continue therapy until blood pressure rises and urine output has returned to normal.
5. Administer the mineralocorticoid, desoxycorticosterone acetate in oil (DOCA), 1 to 2 mg. intramuscularly.
6. Continue DOCA injections daily and monitor serum sodium and potassium levels. Give 50 mg. hydrocortisone acetate intramuscularly every 12 hours. Salt the food heavily.
7. Once the crisis has been controlled and the serum electrolytes are normal, begin therapy for chronic adrenal insufficiency.

References

Lorenz, M. D.: Metabolic emergencies. Vet. Clin. North Amer., Vol. 2, No. 2, May, 1972.
Siegel, E. T.; Adrenal insufficiency. In Kirk, R. W. (ed.): Current Veterinary Therapy IV. Philadelphia, W. B. Saunders Co., 1971.

I-13. ENVIRONMENTAL EXPOSURE

I-13-A. Cold Injuries

FROSTBITE

Local freezing is most commonly experienced in peripheral tissue (ears, tail) which may be sparsely covered with hair, poorly vascularized, or previously traumatized by cold.

Immediate treatment includes rapid rewarming by moist heat applications (75° F.) Analgesics may be needed to alleviate pain and administration of prophylactic antibiotics must be considered. The injured areas should be gently dried and protected from trauma.

Do not rub or apply pressure dressings or ointments. Do not use corticosteroids, and do not be in a hurry to amputate or debride the frozen area. Many tissues recover which do not appear to be viable on first examination. Since intravascular coagulation is a common problem, dextran given (100 to 200 ml. intravenously) and repeated every 12 hours for two days may reduce the extent of tissue necrosis.

HYPOTHERMIA

Chilling of the entire body from exposure results in a decrease in physiologic processes which becomes irreversible at a body temperature of about 75° F. The duration of exposure and the animal's physical condition influence its ability to survive.

If the body temperature is low, rapid, careful rewarming by warm water baths, or careful heating by electric heaters may be necessary. The body temperature increases slowly no matter what warming procedure is used. The body's response to drugs is unpredictable, so medications should be avoided if possible until the body temperature approaches normal.

A urinary catheter should be inserted and fluids given intravenously only after renal function is reestablished.

The heart should be monitored for arrhythmias.

I-13-B. Heat Injuries

BURNS AND LOCAL HEAT INJURIES (See Section I-7)

HYPERTHERMIA

Since dogs and cats do not sweat, salt losses do not constitute a major problem. Most heat injuries are the result of heat retention (heat stroke) caused by confinement in closed cars exposed to the sun.

Immediate treatment is to lower the patient's temperature below 103° F. This is best accomplished by immersion in cold water, alcohol sprays, or cool water enemas. Fluids may be given intravenously after temperature has been lowered. As an alternative, the patient may be given 2 per cent sodium chloride solution by mouth. Corticosteroids and cardiac stimulants such as caffeine sodium benzoate (50 mg.) may be given intravenously. Occasionally, convulsions caused by hypo-calcemia may be observed. These may be controlled by intravenous injections of calcium gluconate, 10 per cent, 5 to 15 ml. Affected animals should always be maintained in a cool (70° F.) oxygen chamber for 24 hours after recovery.

Reference

Ballinger, W. F., Rutherford, R. B., and Zuidema, G. D.: The Management of Trauma, 2nd ed. Philadelphia, W. B. Saunders Co., 1973.

I–14. FRACTURES AND MUSCULOSKELETAL TRAUMA

The conditions at the site of fracture are very important in formulating general principles of fracture management. A simple greenstick fracture is handled differently from a compound, comminuted fracture. The treatment of a fracture will also depend on whether the animal is examined and treated immediately after injury, a few days after injury, during the peak of an inflammatory reaction, or a few weeks after the injury occurred.

IMMEDIATE CARE

1. Maintain an adequate, open airway for respiration and assist respiration, if necessary.
2. Control hemorrhage by pressure dressings over the bleeding area or, as a second choice, a tourniquet.
3. Treat the degree of shock (see Section I–9).

INITIAL TREATMENT OF MUSCULOSKELETAL INJURIES

1. The possibility of multiple fractures or of injury to the spinal column, head, thorax, and abdomen must be kept constantly in mind in musculoskeletal injuries.
2. Use care and gentleness when handling a broken limb and avoid handling the subject unnecessarily.
3. Splint the fractured limb first if subject is to be moved or radiographed.

INITIAL EXAMINATION

In addition to examining for a fracture, determine:

1. If the circulation at or distal to the site of injury has been seriously injured.

2. If there has been any associated nerve injury.

3. If there has been a dislocation at an associated joint. It is often very difficult to differentiate between fractures in or near joints and luxations.

4. The presence and extent of any injuries to adjacent tendons, muscles, and ligaments.

The presence or absence of a fracture can be diagnosed by an examination carried out in the following sequence:

Inspection

May reveal swelling, ecchymosis, deformity, and inability to use the injured part. In occasional fractures, however, there is no deformity and the animal may continue to have limited use of the affected part.

Palpation

Palpation may reveal a local point of tenderness, bony crepitus, false point of motion of a bone, and irregularity of bone contour. Crepitus and motion within a bone should not be deliberately tested for; it is exceedingly painful and may cause more injury.

Comparative Measurements

Comparative measurements of the length of extremities may be a valuable diagnostic aid.

Physical Changes

Swelling, an increase or loss of normal skin temperature, change in color of the skin, and changes in sensation of the skin may help to localize a point of fracture.

Radiographs

Radiographs are a necessary part of all complete examinations for fractures. In making the films, the injured part must not be moved excessively. A bone with a suspected fracture should be examined along its entire length including the associated proximal and distal joints. It may be of value to take radiographs of the opposite limb for comparison.

TREATMENT OF MUSCULOSKELETAL INJURIES

Fractures fall into three classifications, according to the need for repair.

1. Critical fractures require immediate repair to maintain life or normal physiological function of the structure involved. This category includes skull fractures, spinal fractures, compound fractures, and certain types of luxations.

2. Semicritical fractures may give rise to severe problems and abnormal function if not treated quickly. These would be fractures of joint surfaces or of epiphyseal growth plates and luxations of the femoral head, shoulder, and elbow.

3. Noncritical fractures do not require early reduction. Examples are scapular and pelvic fractures, green stick fractures, and closed fractures of the shafts of long bones.

Until definitive treatment is determined, a temporary dressing on the injury and immobilization of the part will: (1) prevent further comminution of fragments, (2) prevent additional trauma to nerves, blood vessels, and soft tissues, (3) decrease pain, (4) prevent further bacterial contamination, (5) decrease edema and circulatory impairment, and (6) prevent extension of a closed fracture into an open (compound) fracture.

The modified Robert Jones dressing is readily made of sterile material. It is a heavily padded splint with multiple layers of a wound dressing held on by cast padding, one or two pounds of rolled cotton uniformly wound around the entire extremity and compressed with several rolls of conforming gauze, and a final layer of elasticon, adhesive tape, or elastic bandage. With small dogs and cats, rolls of cast padding may be substituted for the cotton. Although this splint appears bulky, it gives support without interfering with the circulation.

Temporary immobilization may also be achieved with metasplints, inflatable pneumatic splints, Velpeau and Ehmer slings, and the Thomas splint.

Fractures with displacement should be reduced as soon after the injury as possible and before excessive swelling and muscle traction develop. Closed reductions should be carried out as gently as possible with the animal under general anesthesia. Manual traction is applied by a slow, steady pull on the long axis of the limb. If manipulation of the fractured bone is necessary, radiographs should be available while the bone fragments are manipulated. It is important to remember that a splint does not reduce a fracture but only maintains the reduction that has been previously attained.

Use open reduction if the expected results will be superior to those of closed reduction. The methods of reduction are beyond the scope of this discussion.

Open Fractures

1. All wounds associated with fractures should be regarded as contaminated.

2. Protect open fractures temporarily by a sterile dressing while the fracture is examined and radiographed and the animal is treated for shock.

3. Treat recent, open fractures in the operating room. Treatment of open fractures which are several days old and grossly contaminated may be limited to cleansing, debridement, and establishing temporary drainage and immobilization. This procedure can be carried out in a treatment room.

4. In treating open fractures of recent origin, take care not to recontaminate the wound. Protect the wound and exposed bone fragments by a sterile dressing while the skin is being clipped and washed. Control hemorrhage by a tourniquet if necessary. Irrigate the wound with sterile saline and enlarge it if necessary to expose all injured soft tissue. Devitalized and grossly contaminated soft tissue should be debrided.

Clean contaminated bone ends and remove avascular bone fragments. Preserve skin wherever possible. Repair lacerated tendons and joint capsules and reduce and immobilize the fracture by appropriate means. Close wounds except when the time between injury and treatment exceeds six hours, or when the presence of gross contamination makes it advisable not to. Bacterial cultures should be made at the time of debridement, and sensitivity tests performed. Until sensitivity results are known, give a broad spectrum antibiotic such as one of the tetracyclines.

In severely contaminated or old wounds, "delayed closure" is indicated. Pack the open wound with an antibiotic dressing and repeat debridement in three to 10 days as indicated.

TREATMENT OF SPECIFIC MUSCULOSKELETAL INJURIES

Coxofemoral (Hip) Luxations

Do not attempt reduction of a coxofemoral luxation until the relationship of the bones of the hip is established and the extent of the injury assessed. Radiographs are helpful. Closed reduction of the luxated joint may not be possible when soft tissue is interposed in the joint cavity or when coexisting fractures are present. Reduce luxations as soon as possible. A general anesthetic will be required to overcome pain and muscle spasm.

The animal is placed in lateral recumbency with the luxation uppermost. The pelvis must be restrained either manually by using an oversized Schroeder Thomas splint, or by passing a padded rope or heavy piece of gauze over the medial side of the thigh and anchoring it to the table. If the luxation is anterior or dorsal, the leg is grasped just below the stifle and flexed. The other hand palpates the trochanter major and acetabulum. The leg is abducted and rotated inward so that the femoral head will be dorsal to the acetabulum and the femoral neck and shaft anterior. By applying slow, steady traction at the stifle and guiding the femoral head with the opposite hand, the luxation should reduce. With a posterior luxation, the same procedure may be followed except that the leg is rotated outward. Confirm reductions by palpation and roentgenography. Temporary splintage such as an Ehmer sling can be used to maintain the reduction.

Another method used to reduce coxofemoral luxations is to manipulate the luxation to the anterior dorsal position, grasp the leg below the stifle joint, and rotate the limb outward to dislodge the femoral head. Pull downward and backward. Once the femoral head has reached the rim of the acetabulum, inward rotation of the leg and abduction should permit the femoral head to enter the acetabulum again.

Luxations of the Elbow

Supination of the elbow joint to any degree in the dog indicates a fracture or luxation in the elbow region. Luxation of the elbow joint frequently involves injury to the radius and ulna. A roentgenogram should be taken in the A-P position.

If the luxation is amenable to closed reduction, place the animal under surgical anesthesia and flex the affected limb. With the angle of the elbow less than 45 degrees, rotate the foot outward so that the semilunar notch faces medially. Apply traction at the olecranon to force it beyond the epicondyle of the humerus. At the same time the ulna and radius are forced medially. A full pin may have to be drilled through the olecranon to permit the application of sufficient traction to the radius and ulna.

References

Leonard, E. P.: Orthopedic Surgery of the Dog and Cat, 2nd ed. Philadelphia, W. B. Saunders Co., 1971.

Ross, G. E., Jr.: The initial management of skeletal injuries in the dog. Vet. Clin. North Amer., Vol. 2, No. 2. pp. 397–403, May, 1972.

Whittick, W. G.: Canine Orthopedics. Philadelphia, Lea and Febiger, 1974.

I-15. GASTROINTESTINAL EMERGENCIES

Treatments are listed here for emergencies involving foreign bodies, obstructions, perforations of the gastrointestinal tract, gastric distention, gastric torsion, fractured teeth, hemorrhage from the mouth and rectum, hernias, prolapse of the rectum, and severe diarrhea or vomiting.

I-15-A. Foreign Bodies

Foreign bodies are the most common cause of intestinal obstructions in dogs and cats and are far more prevalent in young animals. History can be very helpful in making a diagnosis. Not all foreign bodies are visible radiographically, especially the plastics which are commonly ingested.

The clinical signs that follow the ingestion of a foreign object depend upon the degree of gastrointestinal blockage. Foreign objects that produce only partial obstruction may result in intermittent episodes of vomiting and anorexia.

Foreign bodies in the mouth, esophagus, and stomach can often be removed without great difficulty. Those in the mouth should be removed, anesthetizing the patient if necessary, followed by thorough inspection of the mouth, and treatment of any local trauma. Although the oral mucosa is susceptible to infection, it heals rapidly and local debridement or suturing, together with antibacterial treatment, is advisable.

Foreign bodies in the esophagus and stomach should be accurately located by radiographs. Small objects (stones, buttons, needles and pins) may pass through the alimentary tract, although feeding the animal an indigestible substance (such as cotton wads) to surround the objects may facilitate their passage. Three days is usually an adequate time to wait for passage of the object. If the object stops, or if the patient shows signs of tenseness, vomiting, or fever, an exploratory operation should be done at once. With the patient anesthetized, some rounded, dull objects can be removed from the esophagus with gastric forceps or by utilizing endoscopy and biopsy forceps.

A common nonobstructive foreign body often found in the cat is string. The string, with perhaps a needle attached, becomes lodged in the mouth, especially around the base of the tongue. The end of the string is usually swallowed, and if it passes through the pylorus it may become lodged in the intestinal tract. Contractions of the intestine around the string may cause the intestines to become plicated and eventually the string may produce intestinal necrosis. If the string is found lodged in the mouth it should be cut, but it should *not* be pulled out, as this may produce further gastric or intestinal damage. The animal should then be carefully observed for the development of any signs associated with gastrointestinal obstruction and, additionally, the stool should be carefully examined to see if the string has been passed. If the string appears at the rectum it should *not* be pulled out. If a string cannot be passed, it must be removed by a series of enterotomy incisions.

Foreign objects in the rectum or colon may have become imbedded during passage, but are more likely the work of sadists. The object must be carefully removed with the patient anesthetized. Local infection by perianal fistulas is a common sequela; therefore, systemic antibiotics together with neomycin and Sulfathalidine should be administered orally for seven days. Foreign bodies often become lodged in the ileum and produce a characteristic syndrome. Early treatment by surgery is the only solution.

I–15–B.   Obstructions

An obstruction of the intestinal tract is any condition that produces interference with, or depresses the movement of, the gastrointestinal contents in an orderly physiologic manner. Causes include foreign bodies, tumors, torsion, intussusception, strangulated hernias, pyloric stenosis and fecal impactions. In general, high intestinal obstructions (pylorus, duodenum and proximal jejunum) cause a more acute problem than low intestinal problems (distal jejunum, ileum, colon, rectum). High intestinal obstructions are usually associated with persistent vomiting and severe fluid and electrolyte disturbances (see Section I-15-B).

If a foreign body is able to pass through the pylorus, it will usually pass through the duodenum and the first one-third of jejunum whence it will become lodged at the point where the intestinal lumen narrows. Occlusion of normal intestinal blood supply and local edema formation may lead to intestinal necrosis.

Signs associated with intestinal obstruction vary greatly, depending on the type and degree of obstruction. Signs frequently seen are vomiting, depression, dehydration, abdominal pain, abdominal distention, fever, restlessness and reduced production of feces.

Careful and thorough abdominal palpation (see Section III-3-A) will reveal evidence of a foreign body in many cases. Both scout films and contrast studies of the abdomen should be utilized when necessary (see Section IV-18). In general, if the diagnosis of a foreign body is uncertain and the animal's condition is becoming progressively worse, it is better to perform exploratory surgery on the abdomen at once, because delay may cause the patient's condition to deteriorate rapidly with a greatly added surgical risk.

Intussusception is an invagination of the proximal portion of the intestine into the area immediately distal. As the intussusception enlarges, the proximal portion is pushed further into the dilated distal portion. The condition is seen most frequently in young animals. Intussusception develops most frequently in the area of the ileocecal valve. Additionally, the intussuscepted bowel may protrude through the anus and the condition must be differentiated from a rectal prolapse (see Section I-15-G).

The signs associated with intussusception are variable and depend on whether or not a complete intestinal obstruction exists and how long the intussusception has been present. Signs frequently seen are abdominal pain, emesis, bloody diarrhea, and the presence of a palpable, sausage-shaped mass in the abdomen, possibly in the right sublumbar area.

Abdominal radiographs may reveal gas accumulation anterior to a cylindrical soft tissue mass.

The distal ensheathing layer of the intussusception is called the intussuscepiens and the enclosed proximal portion is called the intussusceptum.

Treatment for intussusception is exploratory laparotomy and surgical correction.

Fecal impactions commonly must be broken up by forceps and removed by colonic irrigations, a procedure that may require light anesthesia. Usually such cases should not be worked on for longer than 30 minutes at one time because of resultant trauma. Daily administration of sodium dioctyl sulfosuccinate orally and by enema helps water to penetrate and soften the fecal mass.

I-15-C. Perforations of the Gastrointestinal Tract

Perforations may result from internal causes, like foreign bodies, ulcers, and trauma, or from external causes, like penetrating wounds and other severe trauma.

External wounds that penetrate the abdomen must always be explored to determine the extent of damage and to repair any perforated organs. Antibiotic therapy should be instituted presurgically.

Internal perforations may present bizarre signs, but common signs are peritonitis, shock, and free air in the abdomen (radiographic evidence). Patients who manifest such signs require emergency surgical exploration and shock therapy (see Section I-9).

I-15-D. Gastric Distention

Gastric distention is usually caused by overeating, eating fermentable food, or swallowing air, which may be brought on by nervousness or throat inflammation. Additional causes of gastric distention may be anesthesia, traumatic injury, abdominal surgery and ingestion of foreign materials.

Gastric distention is characterized by an enlarged and painful abdomen, excessive salivation, non-productive vomiting and extreme restlessness.

Severe cases are extreme emergencies. A stomach tube should be passed to relieve gas and prevent gastric torsion. Emetics, such as apomorphine, will evacuate soft food but are contraindicated in extreme impactions, or in overloading with sharp objects, like bones. In the latter case, gastrotomy must be performed. Injury to the stomach should be allowed to heal by withholding food orally for 48 hours, followed by small feedings every four to six hours for seven days.

If gastric dilatation occurs repeatedly, a pharyngostomy can be performed and a flexible tube inserted into the stomach and left indwelling through the pharyngostomy incision. Repeated episodes of gastric distention require a complete diagnostic study, including radiographic studies and pyloric function studies (see Section IV-18).

I–15–E.   Gastric Torsion

Gastric torsion is seen in large, deep-chested breeds. Although the exact etiology is unknown, it is generally agreed that gastric distention precedes gastric torsion. A large number of cases have eaten a large, bulky meal two to six hours prior to admittance.

The signs of gastric torsion are much the same as in gastric distention, but they are complicated by shock, electrolyte imbalances and cardiorespiratory complications. Extensive gastric distention interferes with blood circulation through the portal vein and caudal vena cava; the spleen becomes severely engorged and the animal becomes hypotensive.

Treatment must be aimed at correcting cardiorespiratory problems, relieving the gastric distention, surgically correcting the malpositioned organs and medically treating metabolic alterations.

An attempt should be made to pass a stomach tube in order to relieve the gastric distention. If a tube cannot be passed into the stomach, the diagnosis of complete gastric torsion is confirmed and an exploratory laparotomy should be *immediately* performed.

Once torsion occurs, shock, coma, and death follow within a few hours.

FRACTURED TEETH

Transverse fractures leave razor-sharp tooth edges. Under anesthesia these edges can be filed down easily with a fine-tooth carpenter's file. Longitudinal fractures are in reality split teeth. If the line penetrates below the gumline the tooth should be extracted; otherwise filing is indicated.

I-15-F. Hemorrhage from the Mouth and Rectum

Fresh, frank blood from the mouth is usually the result of trauma. If there are no skin or mucosa petechiae, or bleeding from other body openings which might indicate systemic disease, look for local trauma. Esophagoscopy or bronchoscopy may be needed to find the source of bleeding. Cold packs, ice water lavage, sutures or transfusions, or shock therapy may be needed, depending on the cause and location of the bleeding.

Hemorrhage from the anus usually results from granulomatous colitis, neoplasia, poisonings, traumatic injury or shock, and pooling of blood in the splanchnic vessels, with resulting necrosis of the intestinal mucous membrane. Emergency treatment is usually conservative and confined to spasmolytics, antibiotics, or blood transfusions if blood loss is severe. Proctoscopy is subsequently indicated if the cause of hemorrhage is not evident.

I-15-G. Hernias

Hernias are emergencies only if structures like the intestines or uterus are incarcerated within the hernial ring. Immediate herniorrhaphy is indicated in such cases.

PROLAPSE OF THE RECTUM

This may occur in puppies. The condition may be associated with rectal foreign bodies, neoplasms, rectal diverticula, colitis, dystocia or sadism. The young, debilitated animal with persistent diarrhea seems more prone to develop this condition. It may be either a true prolapse, partial or complete, or the extra-anal protrusion of an intussusception of the bowel. To differentiate a true rectal prolapse from a protrusion of an intussuscepted piece of bowel, insert a blunt object such as a glass rod between the prolapsed mass and the anus. If the glass rod cannot be inserted, a true rectal prolapse exists. If the rectum is prolapsed, lubrication and immediate replacement may be effective. However, purse-string sutures should be placed in the anus for three to seven days. Colopexy is indicated if prolapse recurs. If intussusception is diagnosed, a laparotomy should be performed.

I–15–H. *Acute Gastritis*

Acute gastritis in small animals is usually associated with over-eating or the ingestion of garbage or spoiled foods. Various toxins, such as the heavy metals, arsenic, thallium or ethylene glycol, may also produce severe gastric irritation. Gastritis is characterized by pain in the anterior abdomen, vomiting, excessive water drinking, depression and dehydration.

A careful history and examination of the vomitus may be helpful in arriving at a differential diagnosis (see Section II-19). Persistent severe vomiting can be very debilitating and lead to severe dehydration and electrolyte imbalances. The following supportive steps are helpful until a more conclusive diagnosis can be reached.

1. Withhold oral fluids and solids for first 24 hrs.
2. Correct fluid and electrolyte imbalances (see Section IV-20).
3. Control vomiting with antiemetics such as Compazine.
4. Institute controlled cage rest.
5. Administer digestive protectants.

I–15–I. *Acute Pancreatitis*

Acute pancreatitis usually produces sudden and severe vomiting, abdominal pain, marked depression, hypotension and a shock-like syndrome. The exact etiology of acute pancreatic inflammation is unknown; however, the pathogenesis of the disease involves the activation of enzymatic activity in and around the pancreas and in the bloodstream.

Laboratory examination is essential for an accurate diagnosis (see Section V-3). Serum amylase levels rise to abnormal levels (two-fold increase above normal) early in the course of the disease. Serum lipase levels also become elevated, but this occurs later in the course of the inflammation. Hypotension and prerenal azotemia result in an elevated BUN. There is frequently serum hyperlipemia and there may be hyperglycemia.

Initial treatment in this disease state should include the following:

1. Withhold food and oral medication for 72 hours.
2. Correct dehydration and electrolyte imbalances (see Section IV-20).
3. Control pain.
4. Use antibiotics prophylactically.
5. Reduce gastric motility.

References

DeHoff, W. D., Greene, R. W., and Greiner, T. P.: Surgical management of abdominal emergencies. Vet. Clin. North Amer., Vol. 2., No. 2, pp. 301–330, May, 1972.

Geokas, M. C.: Acute pancreatitis. Calif. Medicine, *117*:25–39, August, 1972.

I-16. GENITOURINARY EMERGENCIES

Emergency treatments are listed here for retention of urine, paraphimosis, acute mastitis, acute metritis, prolapsed uterus, vaginal hyperplasia, mismating, and dystocias.

I-16-A. Uremic Crises

Death from uremia is due to retention of toxic levels of electrolytes and other metabolites and from pH and fluid abnormalities. The objectives of emergency treatment are as follows.

1. Correct the renal abnormality and improve renal function to its maximum capacity.

2. Apply supportive and symptomatic treatment to modify the lethal metabolic abnormalities.

PRERENAL UREMIA

Since the cause is decreased renal perfusion with normal kidneys, treatment is as follows.

1. Correct the extrarenal cause rapidly, before renal damage develops.

2. Place intravenous catheters and rehydrate rapidly (see Section IV-20-E).

3. Treat shock vigorously (see Section I-9).

RENAL UREMIA

Prognosis and type of treatment depend on whether the renal lesion is reversible and whether or not three-fourths of the nephrons have been completely destroyed. Emergency treatment should correct dehydration, reduce acidosis, correct hyperkalemia and provide caloric support.

1. Place intravenous catheter. Draw blood samples for base line laboratory studies and start 10 per cent dextrose in saline infusion.

2. Depending on evaluation of acidosis, add at least 10 to 20 mEq. of bicarbonate per liter of saline solution.

3. Obtain EKG tracing to evaluate serum potassium levels.

4. Uremic patients in this category may be oliguric or polyuric. Oliguria is a grave sign and volume of fluids given should be monitored carefully to avoid overtreatment. If dextrose does not show in the urine after 20 minutes, consider the use of mannitol intravenously (0.5 mg./lb. of body weight); or give test doses of furosemide intravenously (0.5 mg./lb. of body weight) to induce diuresis. If this fails, consider peritoneal dialysis (see Section IV-20-G).

5. If polyuria is present, administer large amounts of balanced electrolyte solutions (lactated Ringer's) intravenously to rehydrate the patient.

6. Continue therapy as indicated by results from base line laboratory results.

POSTRENAL UREMIA

Obstructions and ruptures of the urinary system may prevent excretion of urine from the body. This condition, if acute and complete, may cause death in three to five days due to the accumulation of metabolic wastes. Causes are trauma, calculi, neoplasia, stricture or congenital anomalies. In most cases, definitive treatment is surgery. Immediate treatment should reestablish urine flow, support, and correct metabolic imbalances.

I–16–B. *Retention of Urine*

CAUSES

Ruptured Bladder

1. Immediate surgical repair is imperative.

2. The utmost care in administering anesthesia and treatment of shock is crucial to a successful repair. Epidural or local block anesthesia may be best for toxic patients. Steroid, antibiotic, and adequate fluid or transfusion support is also essential.

3. The peritoneum should be thoroughly lavaged to remove all traces of residual urine.

4. Following repair, fluid intake should be promoted to encourage renal function and correct the uremia.

Urethral Occlusion

In male dogs, catheterization is often possible. If temporary relief is achieved, definitive surgery may be postponed 24 to 48 hours to prepare the patient with antibiotics and to use water diuresis to correct uremia. If a catheter cannot be passed, calculi in a male dog may be removed by dilation of the urethra with fluid under pressure. The dog is placed under sedation. A finger in the dog's rectum compresses the proximal urethra on the pelvic floor while saline is injected under pressure into the distal urethra; a catheter should be used and the distal urethra compressed around it. The catheter is withdrawn suddenly to release the pressure (the occlusion of the urethra in the pelvic canal is maintained) and saline and calculi commonly are ejected distally. This procedure may be repeated several times and often successfully removes the obstructing stones.

If this method fails, aseptic cystocentesis with a 22 gauge two-inch needle may be necessary for temporary relief. Corrective surgery often can be delayed to prepare the patient as a better surgical risk. If all of these steps fail, definitive surgical removal should be performed at once.

In male cats, urethral obstruction is a common emergency. If the occlusion is recent or is composed of cellular debris, gentle pressure on the bladder together with penile massage will often dislodge it. The bladder should be completely emptied and medical treatment instituted.

In obstruction of longer duration, some depression will be present but low doses of anesthetics or ketamine sedation may be needed to allow catheterization. An 18 or 20 gauge flexible plastic catheter is used to backflush the urethra. Walpole solution (buffer of pH 4.5) is an ideal flushing solution. It can be injected under pressure to wash debris back into the bladder, and several ounces can be placed in the bladder and removed to help dissolve crystalline particles. Alternate solutions of vinegar 50 per cent or saline may be used with less effect.

Intramedic tubing (PE60 or PE90) may be used as a catheter and taped and sutured to the prepuce to hold it in place. It also may be cut into a three-inch length and then flared at the distal end by holding it over a match. These short catheters are often self-retaining. This material can be left in place for several days to allow the urethra to heal, while the bladder can be kept empty or can be irrigated as needed.

If catheterization fails, a two-inch, 21 gauge needle can be used to enter the bladder through the abdominal wall to remove the urine. This must be done in a sterile manner, and is a temporary expedient to help overcome uremia, while the patient is being prepared for laparotomy or further treatment. It should be emphasized that all manipulations must be gentle in order to minimize urethral trauma.

Medical treatment to acidify urine (d-1 methionine, 200 mg. twice daily), increase urine flow (water and hydrochlorothiazide, 6.25 mg./day), and provide antibiotic urine levels (chloramphenicol 50 mg. three times daily) should be initiated.

The various salvage operations for exteriorizing the penile urethra are not emergency procedures.

Paralysis of Bladder Musculature

This causes retention of urine with overflow, and commonly occurs when a housebroken dog is confined for long periods. Urine may dribble and give the appearance of incontinence. It is imperative to catheterize or express urine from the greatly dilated bladder, and keep the bladder nearly empty for roughly two weeks by frequent emptying. Healing usually occurs. Smooth muscle stimulation with bethanechol chloride (5 to 25 mg. every 8 hours orally) may also be helpful. Paralysis of bladder musculature is also frequently seen with neurologic abnormalities, especially those of traumatic origin.

I–16–C. Renal Trauma

Because the kidneys are well protected and somewhat pendulous, they are not commonly injured. Trauma may be extreme and may rupture large renal vessels, with death occurring in minutes. Less severe trauma may produce intracapsular damage or hematomas, which usually heal spontaneously. In such cases hematuria may result and thrombosis of vessels may cause infarction and permanent loss of some renal tissue. In these cases, forced diuresis may be desirable to reduce the possibilities of clots and obstruction of urinary outflow.

If the renal capsule is torn, blood and urine may escape into the peritoneal cavity. Paracentesis and peritoneal lavage may be useful to check for urea and red blood cells. If in doubt, exploratory surgery may be necessary to detect the type of injury. Partial or complete nephrectomy or renal capsule repair with gelfoam or cellulose strips may be indicated.

I–16–D. Paraphimosis

Paraphimosis is invariably the result of coitus. Gentle cleaning with pHisoHex and water, thorough lubrication with K-Y jelly or Lubritine, and replacing the prepuce over the penis usually correct paraphimosis in the early stages. No further treatment is needed.

Severe edema, hemorrhage, or lacerations of the penis, may require cold packs or hypertonic solutions to reduce tumescence. A small incision in the dorsal commissure of the sheath may be needed to replace the sheath. In rare cases the penis may have to be amputated.

I–16–E. Genital Trauma

This usually involves male dogs, since the female genitalia are well protected. Contusions and lacerations of the sheath, penis and scrotum are common. Small injuries to the scrotum prompt the dog to lick them, which results in acute infection. In all cases, sedation and/or restraint to prevent this are important. Most areas are highly vascular, and careful ligature of vessels, tunics and fascia may be necessary to control hemorrhage. Urethral trauma may also be involved, so drains or catheters should be used to prevent tissue infiltration of extravasated blood and urine leakage. A Foley catheter works well in larger breeds. A more proximally located urethrotomy may bypass urine and allow the traumatized area to heal. Heavy sedation and avoidance of sexual stimulation are necessary to avoid penile erection. Most wounds are infected, so the use of topical and systemic antibacterial medications is desirable.

I–16–F. Acute Mastitis

In dogs and cats the common condition is an acute inflammation with localization (abscess formation) in one breast. The patient is febrile and septic. Antibiotic therapy (tetracycline or penicillin-streptomycin) plus cold compresses should be started at once. Incision and drainage of abscesses should be performed as soon as localization develops. Suckling animals should be removed and fed as orphans, or the affected breast taped so that it cannot be nursed. Recovery is usually uncomplicated.

I–16–G. Acute Metritis

Acute metritis is seen several days after whelping and is a febrile, highly fatal septicemia. Antibiotic therapy (tetracycline, administered intravenously first and orally, later) should be started at once. Culture and sensitivity of uterine discharge should be obtained.

The uterus should be drained of all fluids by inserting a catheter through the cervix and employing postural drainage, or irrigation. Furacin solution (15 to 30 ml.) should be left in utero and any suckling animals removed and raised as orphans.

I–16–H. Pyometra

Pyometra is a hormonal dysfunction often associated with bacterial toxins. This often produces glomerular damage and renal complications of considerable severity. There are an open cervix type and a closed cervix type of pyometra (no vaginal discharge in the latter, which may be more toxic).

In bitches with compelling reasons to try to save breeding capability, uterine drainage may be considered. In most cases, early ovariohysterectomy is preferred. Metabolic problems may be severe and the surgical risk will be great, so measures to counteract dehydration, acidosis and shock are imperative. Renal function should be stimulated and extreme care taken to use the safest anesthesia compatible with the needs of the case. The BUN is a good prognostic test. Patients that survive the stormy 4 to 5 day postoperative period usually recover.

I-16-I. Prolapsed Uterus

Prolapsed uterus occurs after whelping. It is an emergency of the utmost concern. Treatment requires anesthesia and replacement of the organ. In some cases this is done easily, but it is essential to be certain the entire organ has unfolded properly in the abdomen. If it has not, a laparotomy should be carried out to complete proper restoration of the uterus. Pitocin can then be given to cause contraction of the uterus. The lips of the vulva should be sutured to prevent recurrence. Administer antibiotics and treat shock if necessary.

If severe edema is present in the prolapsed uterus, application of hypertonic glucose or saline solution and kneading and massage will help remove the fluid. If the uterus cannot be effectively replaced or if it becomes necrotic and/or gangrenous, ovariohysterectomy is indicated.

I-16-J. Vaginal Hyperplasia

Vaginal hyperplasia occurs during estrus in large breeds of dogs. This is not a real emergency since commonly only a small amount of tissue protrudes from the vulva. Frequent application of ointments to keep the exposed tissue soft, protected and viable is recommended until surgical correction is carried out or hormonal (progesterone) effects are evident. The condition often recurs at subsequent estral cycles, so ovariohysterectomy is often performed for permanent cure.

I-16-K. Mismating

Since, at the completion of coitus in dogs, sperm are present at the fimbria, douching and local treatments are not effective. Giving repositol stilbestrol by intramuscular injection (1 mg./pound repeated in seven to ten days) usually prevents implantation and is effective in preventing conception. It should be given within 48 hours of breeding and will usually prolong the signs of external "heat" by at least one week. Caution the owner to keep the animal confined during this period. Continual confinement is necessary until signs of heat have disappeared, so that additional matings do not occur.

I–16–L. Dystocia

The normal onset of labor is marked by the following events:

24 hours before—bitch makes a nest and goes off to hide.

12 hours before—bitch refuses food and a white vaginal discharge may appear (cervical seal).

12 to eight hours before—bitch's rectal temperature drops at least 1°F.—often to 98°F.

Four hours before—cervix begins rapid dilatation.

One hour before—cervix dilates and labor pains begin.

The presence of a greenish-black discharge indicates placental separation.

If no puppy is delivered within four hours after the onset of labor, a pelvic examination is indicated. Two puppies are usually presented in close succession followed by a pause of one to two hours. Delivery of the entire litter may take 24 to 30 hours. Fetal membranes may be eaten by the bitch but they often produce a gastroenteritis lasting eight to 12 hours.

Primary uterine inertia is common in pampered toy bitches, especially the dachshund, Scottish terrier, and Chihuahua. It can be treated by giving calcium gluconate, 10 per cent, intravenously (2 to 10 ml.) followed by Pitocin (2 to 10 units). Pitocin, intramuscularly, can be repeated every 30 to 40 minutes, if needed. In nervous bitches, intramuscular injections of Demerol may promote labor by its analgesic and relaxing effect. If no results are obtained following these procedures, a cesarean section should be considered.

When only one or two puppies are to be delivered, medical attempts at stimulating uterine contractions or forceps manipulations are worth exploiting. However, if a large number of pups are involved, a cesarean section usually offers the best chance for successful delivery of viable offspring. This procedure tends to conserve the strength of the bitch (and her attendants).

Secondary uterine inertia results from fatigue due to obstruction of the pelvic canal. Fetal displacement or pelvic measurements less than 1½ inches D.V. by 1½ inches lateral are the usual causes.

References

Additional information may be found in the following sources.

Greiner, T. P.: Genital emergencies. *In* Kirk, R. W. (ed.): Current Veterinary Therapy V. Philadelphia, W. B. Saunders Co., 1974.

Mara, J. L.: Pyometra. *In* Kirk, R. W. (ed.): Current Veterinary Therapy IV. Philadelphia, W. B. Saunders Co., 1971.

Osborne, C. A.: Urinary tract emergencies. *In* Kirk, R. W. (ed.): Current Veterinary Therapy V. Philadelphia, W. B. Saunders Co., 1974.

Osborne, C. A., and Piermattei, D.: Non-surgical removal of urethral calculae. *In* Kirk, R. W. (ed.): Current Veterinary Therapy V. Philadelphia, W. B. Saunders Co., 1974.

Smith, K. W.: The female genital system. *In* Archibald, J. (ed.): Canine Surgery, 1st Archibald ed. Santa Barbara, Am. Vet. Pub., 1965.

I–17. METABOLIC EMERGENCIES

Emergency treatments are listed here for hyperglycemia (diabetic ketoacidosis), hypoglycemia, puerperal tetany (canine eclampsia), and acidosis.

I–17–A. Diabetic Ketoacidosis

This syndrome is the terminal result of insulin insufficiency. Early in the disease patients exhibit the typical signs of diabetes mellitus. Diabetic ketoacidosis is characterized by vomiting, dehydration, hypotension, oliguria, severe depression, and deep and forceful respirations.

Treatment

1. Draw blood for hemogram, glucose, BUN, and ketones. Blood pH, bicarbonate, sodium, potassium, and chloride should be monitored if possible. Collect urine for glucose, pH, and ketone determinations.

2. Start an intravenous infusion of 0.9 per cent NaCl, or 2.5 per cent fructose in 0.45 per cent NaCl. Add 10 to 20 mEq. of sodium bicarbonate per liter of fluid given. Do not overtreat with sodium bicarbonate.

3. Give 0.5 to 1 unit/lb. of regular insulin intravenously. Check blood glucose levels every two hours. If the blood glucose has not fallen in two hours, double the initial insulin dose and repeat the intravenous administration. Repeat this procedure every two hours until the blood glucose begins to fall.

4. Once the blood glucose begins to fall, do not administer more insulin until the full effect of the last dose is known (Table 125).

5. Measure blood glucose, urine volume, urine pH, glucose, and ketones every hour.

6. Perform EKG or take blood samples to assess potassium needs.

7. As urine volume increases, begin lactated Ringer's solution intravenously.

8. As the animal begins to respond to insulin, careful monitoring for hypoglycemia and hypokalemia is necessary. Insulin facilitates movement of potassium from the extracellular fluid compartment into the cell, and hypokalemia may result. Potassium supplementation will be needed, and in most cases the oral route, being safer, is preferred. Potassium gluconate, 40 mEq./oz., can be given orally every six hours if urine output is adequate. In severe cases of hypokalemia, 10 mEq. of K^+ can be added to each liter of intravenous fluids administered only if renal function is re-established (no more than 10 mEq./hr.).

9. Once the blood glucose has decreased to below 250 mg. per cent and urine ketones have decreased, subcutaneous regular insulin may be given at a dosage of 0.5 units/lb. every six hours.

10. Once the patient is stabilized, begin maintenance therapy for chronic diabetes mellitus.

I-17-B. Hypoglycemia

Decreased blood glucose values can result from the failure of glucose secretion or from accelerated glucose removal from the blood. Clinical signs include incoordination, restlessness, exercise intolerance, seizures and coma.

Treatment

1. Give 10 to 20 ml. of 50 per cent glucose intravenously. Ten cc./lb. of 10 per cent glucose may also be given.

2. Administer glucagon 0.03 mg./kgm. intravenously or IM, or give 0.5 ml. of 1:1000 epinephrine intramuscularly.

3. When patient recovers, begin frequent administration of food.

4. Watch closely for relapse.

5. Schedule patient for tests to determine the cause of hypoglycemia.

6. Causes of hypoglycemia:
    a. Accelerated glucose removal:
      1. Insulin overdose.
      2. Functional islet cell tumor.
      3. Toxicity of oral hypoglycemic drugs.
      4. Renal glycosuria.
    b. Failure of glucose secretion:
      1. Functional hypoglycemia.
      2. Glycogen storage diseases.
      3. Adrenal insufficiency.
      4. Hepatic insufficiency.
      5. Malabsorption and starvation.

I–17–C. Puerperal Tetany

1. History and clinical signs are usually diagnostic, and result from the reduction of serum calcium to levels below 7 mg./100 ml.
2. Other workers have reported cases in which hypoglycemia was present, and as the disease is seen primarily in small, excitable dogs, a stress factor may be involved in the etiology.

Treatment

1. Administer intravenously 2 to 15 ml. of calcium gluconate, 10 per cent. Administer calcium slowly and monitor the heart rate during administration.
2. If tetany persists, sedate the patient intravenously with barbiturates.
3. Administer prednisolone orally (¼ mg./pound every twelve hours) until puppies are weaned. It is better to wean them if possible, but with steroid therapy the bitch can nurse them with very little risk of relapse.

I–17–D. Acidosis

1. Acidosis is the accumulation of acid products in the body more rapidly than removal or neutralization can take place. It produces a depressed state of "toxemia" characterized by weakness, progressive stupor (and coma), tachycardia, fruity or uremic odor to the breath, and hyperpnea.

2. In small animals the usual causes are renal insufficiency, diabetes mellitus, deep narcosis or anesthesia, various toxemias, diarrhea, severe dehydration, and cardiac or respiratory insufficiencies.

3. Therapy must be directed at the causative agent. However, treatment to improve ventilation (a respirator) and renal function (fluid therapy) should be emphasized to help the body compensate more quickly.

Conserving body heat by blanketing, circulatory stimulants, and plasma or electrolyte solutions in large doses to improve circulation will often be of inestimable value in supporting cardiac and renal functions (see Sections I-9 and IV-20).

References

Kirk, R. W. (ed.): Current Veterinary Therapy V. Philadelphia, W. B. Saunders Co., 1974.

Lorenz, M. D.: Metabolic emergencies. Vet. Clin. North Amer., Vol. 2, No. 2, May, 1972.

Winegrad, A. I., and Clements, R. S.: Diabetic ketoacidosis. Med. Clin. North Amer., Vol. 55, No. 4, July, 1971.

I-18. NEUROLOGIC EMERGENCIES

Although infrequently seen, neurologic emergencies can seriously jeopardize an animal's life. This section is divided into four conditions that constitute neurologic emergencies: (1) head injuries; (2) injuries of the spinal cord and spinal column; (3) coma; and (4) convulsions.

I-18-A. Head Injuries

Head injuries may include skin and superficial lacerations, concussions, fractures including extracranial, linear, and depressed intracranial, and extra- and intracranial hemorrhage, including extradural, subdural, subarachnoid, and intracerebral.

Immediate Care

The animal must be handled carefully so that it does no harm to the handler or further injury to itself. Tranquilizers (in minimal dosages) and pain relievers may have to be administered. Morphine should be used in minimal amounts since it depresses respiration and vital signs in an animal that is already severely depressed because of injury to the central nervous system.

Hypoxia is one of the most common causes of death following severe head trauma. An adequate airway and exchange of air must therefore be maintained. In the comatose animal an endotracheal tube can be inserted and oxygen administered. An intermittent positive pressure apparatus like the Bird respirator may be necessary to assist respiration. Oxygen may also be administered by the use of a face mask or oxygen tent (see Section IV-20). The level of oxygenation of the brain may be reflected in the state of consciousness of the animal.

Control any bleeding and treat shock (see Section I-9).

Frequently examine and elicit vital signs such as pulse, respirations/minute, depth of respiration, and temperature, and evaluate the neurologic status, including the state of consciousness, size and response of pupils, pain perception, and voluntary motor activity. Progressively dilating pupils usually indicate cerebral anoxia. Any deterioration of the aforementioned neurologic data usually indicates progressing cerebral edema and anoxia. With an initial rapid rise in intracranial pressure the pulse and respirations become slowed and the temperature is elevated. If intracranial pressure continues to rise and reduced cerebral circulation leads to progressive hypoxia, vital signs may become reversed, producing a rapid pulse, rapid respirations, and an elevated temperature.

Initial Examination

In order to follow the patient's course, a baseline neurologic assessment must be made as soon as possible and the neurologic status must be continually re-evaluated.

Initial neurologic examination should include evaluation of the following parameters:

1. State of consciousness: Examine the animal's state of consciousness and elicit the response to commands, to painful stimuli such as a pinch on the toe, and to movement of people in the room. The various levels of consciousness may be described as: coma (unconscious with no response to painful stimuli); semicoma (unconscious but responsive to painful stimuli); delirium; confusion; depression; and alertness. Initial consciousness followed by unconsciousness generally indicates severe brainstem injury. In dogs, hemorrhages into the midbrain and pons are relatively frequent, pro-

ducing coma and decerebrate rigidity. Brainstem compression can be associated also with compressed skull fractures, extradural or subdural hematomas, or cerebral edema.

2. Pupil size and response: Bilateral miotic, bilateral mydriatic or asymmetrical pupils are all suggestive of midbrain contusion. A favorable prognosis is indicated by a change from pupillary abnormality to normality. Nystagmus (with quick phase away from the affected side of the labyrinths) may indicate petrous temporal bone fracture or a lateral cerebello-pontine contusion.

3. Posture and motor function: Decerebrate rigidity (extensor rigidity of all four limbs) may occur with severe brainstem lesions caudal to the red nucleus. Severe vestibular disturbance peripherally or centrally in the pons and medulla will cause a head tilt and/or neck and body flexion. Note any degree of paresis or ataxia that may be present.

4. Vision: Visual defects in patients with intracranial lesions are usually due to cerebral edema of the visual cortex. Pupillary response will be normal if there are no accompanying midbrain lesions.

Evaluation of cranial nerve function repeated at frequent intervals may reveal an initial nerve injury or the presence of a progressive, expanding lesion of the brain (see Section III-8). Signs of severe vestibular disorientation with rolling movements, marked head tilt and nystagmus occur with contusion of the membranous labyrinth, which is usually associated with a fracture of the petrosal bone. Hemorrhage may occur from the external ear canal.

Paralysis or weakness of one side of the body following head injury can result from laceration or contusion of the opposite side of the brain.

Convulsions following head injury may be associated with intracranial hemorrhage and an expanding intracranial mass. If the injury is not amenable to surgery, medical treatment to control the convulsive state should be instituted. If necessary, intravenous injections of diazepam (5 to 10 mg.) should be given or Dilantin sodium orally (1 mg./lb. at four- to six-hour intervals), supplemented by phenobarbital, 1 to 2 mg./lb. intravenously. If convulsions persist despite this treatment, intravenous pentobarbital should be administered to produce light general anesthesia (see also Section I-18-D).

Decerebrate rigidity may occur with contusion of the brain stem.

Special Studies

Special studies useful in the management of animals with head injuries include roentgenographic examination of the head. Roentgenographic studies of the skull should be taken only after all other emergency procedures have been initiated. If the animal is not cooperative and sedation and the use of a short-acting anesthetic are contraindicated, radiographs should be delayed until diagnostic films can be safely obtained. Roentgenograms of both skull and cervical vertebrae are indicated in traumatic injuries of the head.

Treatment of Specific Head Injuries

Generalized edema of the brain can be found in any traumatic injury of the head. The intravenous administration of a solution like mannitol (20 per cent, 1 gm./lb.) repeated at three-hour intervals for two or three doses, helps to control the developing edema and increased intracranial pressure. Glucocorticoids such as dexamethasone should be administered intravenously at high doses (1 to 2 mg./lb.) at six-hour intervals. Insert an indwelling catheter into the bladder to avoid bladder distention which may occur during unconsciousness. Animals with evidence of skull fractures should be given broad spectrum antibiotics. If hyperpyrexia occurs, cool the animal with cold water baths and cool enemas.

A common gross lesion in the dog and cat with severe intracranial injury is hemorrhage on the median plane of the midbrain tegmentum. Suprachoroid hemorrhage is rare. When present, it is usually associated with a focal cerebral laceration.

An animal may have an extradural hemorrhage if, after the initial unconsciousness, it regains consciousness and then, as intracranial pressure builds up (due to hemorrhage), develops weakness, vomiting, slowed heart and respiratory rates, dilated pupils, convulsions, and coma. Treatment involves decompression of the cranium over the site of the injury, removal of blood clots, and control of hemorrhage.

Subdural hemorrhage presents many of the same signs as extradural hemorrhage except that the signs of the former usually develop more rapidly. Surgery must be performed if coma is produced. However, symptomatic conservative treatment, as outlined previously, can be used if coma, paralysis, or convulsions are not present.

Skull fractures may be extracranial or intracranial. If intracranial, they may be either linear or depressed. The most severe fractures are intracranial depressed skull fractures, causing compression of brain substance. The skull may be visibly deformed and bone fragments in the damaged area may crepitate. It is important not to overpalpate the area of injury as it may cause further brain damage.

TABLE 7. DIFFERENTIAL FEATURES OF TENTORIAL HERNIATION AND BRAIN STEM HEMORRHAGE*

	Brain Stem Hemorrhage	Tentorial Herniation
Onset	Early	Delayed
Course	Static to progressive	Progressive
Pupils	Constricted early, dilated late	Unilateral dilation, progression to bilateral dilation
Consciousness	Stuporous to comatose	Alert or apathetic, progressing to coma
Muscle Tone	Decerebrate rigidity or flaccid paralysis	Normal or weak progressing to decerebrate rigidity or flaccid paralysis
Reflexes	Usually symmetrical	Often unilateral asymmetry

*From Oliver, J. E.: Neurologic emergencies in small animals. Vet. Clin. North Amer., Vol. 2, No. 2, May, 1972.

Immediate emergency surgery may be warranted in brain trauma if there is a skull fracture which is depressed more than the thickness of the skull, if bone fragments are present within the brain, in all compound skull fractures, and in cases where there are persistent C.S.F. leaks. Other indications for surgical intervention include (1) decreasing level of consciousness; (2) onset of unilateral pupillary dilation or progression from unilateral to bilateral dilation; (3) progressive hemiparesis; and (4) vomiting, slowed heart and respiratory rate, and convulsions.

Burr holes in the calvarium can be used to determine if there is extradural or subdural hemorrhage. Burr holes are placed in four corners of the temporal fossa in the frontoparietal and parietotemporal areas. Large blood clots can be removed and, if extensive brain swelling is noted, a bone flap may be cut out.

I-18-B. Spinal Cord Injuries

Spinal cord injuries are usually associated with disc ruptures, fractures, or dislocations of the vertebral column.

Initial Handling and Management

Animals suspected of having spinal injuries should be moved with extreme care and caution. They should be moved on a wide board or rolling cart, and flexion, extension, or torsion of the spinal cord should be rigorously avoided. The spinal cord should be kept as immobile as possible from the time of injury to the time of repair.

Sedation with tranquilizers and pain relievers may have to be induced before the animal can be moved safely. Narcotics should be used in amounts necessary only to relieve pain since, if more than minimal amounts are used, respiration and other vital signs may also be depressed.

Shock, respiratory embarrassment, and open wounds should be treated immediately.

Initial Examination

In the initial examination try to identify the location and evaluate the extent of the spinal lesion and establish an initial prognosis for the case.

The presence of pain, edema, hemorrhage, or a visible deformity may localize an area of spinal injury.

Identifying the location of spinal cord injuries may require a neurologic examination (see Section III-8-B). This examination should be carried out without excessive manipulation of the animal.

Good roentgenographic visualization of the area of spinal cord injury is essential to achieve an early diagnosis and institute treatment. In almost all cases, the animal must receive a short-acting anesthetic (thiamylal sodium) so that good radiographs can be taken without causing further injury. Myelography may be needed to delineate more clearly the area of spinal injury.

Prognosis in spinal cord injury depends on the extent of the injury and the reversibility of the damage. Perception of pain on the part of the animal when stimulus is applied caudal to the level of the lesion is a good sign. To give pain, firm pressure to a toe may be applied with hemostatic forceps. Flexion of the leg is a spinal reflex and is not a significant response unless the animal exhibits evidence of pain perception. Absence of pain response following recovery from spinal shock (one to two hours) is a very poor prognosis.

Focal lesions in one or more of the spinal cord segments from the third thoracic to the fourth lumbar may cause complete dysfunction of the injured tissue from concussion, contusion or laceration. They

TABLE 8. SIGNS OF COMPLETE SPINAL CORD TRANSECTION*

Spinal Cord Segments	Signs Caudal to Lesion		
	Motor	Sensory	Autonomic
C1-4†	Tetraplegic with hyperreflexia	Anesthesia	Apnea, no micturition
C5-6	Tetraplegia with hyperreflexia, LMN suprascapular nerve	Anesthesia, hyperesthesia mid-cervical	Apnea, phrenic nerve LMN, no micturition
C7-T1	Tetraplegia or paraplegia with hyperreflexia, LMN brachial plexus	Anesthesia, hyperesthesia brachial plexus	Diaphragmatic breathing only, no micturition
T2-L3	Paraplegia with hyperreflexia, Schiff-Sherrington syndrome	Anesthesia, hyperesthesia segmental	Diaphragmatic, some intercostal and abdominal respiration depending on level, no micturition
L4-S1	Paraplegia with LMN lumbosacral plexus	Anesthesia, hyperesthesia segmental	No micturition, S1-anal sphincter may be atonic
S1-S3	Knuckling hind foot, paralysis of tail	Anesthesia, hyperesthesia segmental	No micturition, sphincters atonic
Cy1-Cy	Paralysis of tail	Anesthesia, hyperesthesia segmental	None

*From Oliver, J. E.: Neurologic emergencies in small animals. Vet. Clin. North Amer., Vol. 2, No. 2, May, 1972.

†C=Cervical
T=Thoracic
L=Lumbar
S=Sacral
Cy=Coccygeal
LMN=Lower Motor Neuron

result in paraplegia with intact pelvic limb and spinal reflexes and analgesia of the body and limbs caudal to the lesion.

These lesions are usually associated with vertebral fractures and displacements of the vertebral canal. The most common site is the caudal thoracic and cranial lumbar region. Lesions here often result in the Schiff-Sherrington syndrome, which is characterized by rigidly extended hypertonic thoracic limbs and flaccid hypotonic paralyzed analgesic pelvic limbs with intact spinal reflexes. The thoracic limbs have normal voluntary motor function despite their marked hypertonia. They can perform all the postural reactions and spinal reflexes and have intact sensation.

Injuries to the spinal cord from the sixth cervical to the second thoracic segments will cause tetraparesis or tetraplegia with depressed spinal reflexes from the thoracic limbs and hyperactive spinal reflexes from the pelvic limbs. Horner's syndrome (miosis, protruded third eye-lid, smaller palpebral fissure, and enophthalmos) occurs with lesions in the first three thoracic segments. Injuries cranial to the sixth cervical segment will cause spastic tetraparesis or tetraplegia with hyperactive reflexes in all four limbs. If the injury is severe, death will occur from respiratory failure. The patient should be assessed for respiratory function and supplemented if necessary.

Initial Therapy

Contusions, concussions, hematomyelia, and injuries of the spinal cord which do not cause spinal cord compression may be handled medically. Intravenous injection of mannitol, 20 per cent, 1 gm./pound during an interval of one-half to one hour may reduce spinal cord edema resulting from injury. Glucocorticoids such as dexamethasone should be administered intravenously at high doses (1 to 2 mg./lb.).

Movement of the vertebral column should be restricted by using a padded back brace or splint taped around the body and over the vertebral column. The activity of the animal must be severely restricted.

An animal with severe spinal cord injury must receive special care with respect to bowel and bladder function. Retention of urine develops quickly after many spinal cord injuries and may not cause any distress to the animal because of associated loss of sensory innervation to the bladder. Urinary retention leads to bladder infections and loss of the normal tonicity of the bladder wall. Frequent manual expression of the urine and washing the hindquarters with warm water may be enough to keep the bladder empty. Repeated catheterizations (two to three times

TABLE 9. CENTRAL SYNDROME*

Level	Consciousness	Pupils	Eye Movements	Motor	Autonomic
Early diencephalic	Apathy	Small but reactive	Normal	Hemiparesis	Normal to irregular respiration
Late diencephalic	Stupor	Same	Same	Hemiparesis to tetraparesis	Cheyne-Stokes
Midbrain	Coma	Dilated bilaterally	Poor oculocephalic response	Decerebrate rigidity	Hyperventilation
Pons	Coma	Midposition unresponsive	Oculocephalic response absent	Flaccid paralysis	Rapid, shallow respiration
Medulla	Coma	Midposition, dilated terminally	Absent	Flaccid paralysis	Irregular to apnea; pulse slowing

*From Oliver, J. E.: Neurologic emergencies in small animals. Vet. Clin. North Amer., Vol. 2, No. 2, May, 1972.

daily), especially in males, may be necessary to prevent urinary retention. This often predisposes to infection and these animals should receive appropriate antibiotic and urinary antiseptic therapy. Indwelling catheters of the Foley type may be used in larger dogs but urine should be carefully collected in sealed, plastic bags placed on the end of the catheter. Many animals will not tolerate any type of indwelling catheter.

Paralytic ileus and fecal retention are also frequent complications of spinal cord injury. The correction of fluid and electrolyte imbalances, together with the ingestion of small amounts of highly digestible foods, will help to relieve the ileus. Mild enemas (Fleet enema) will help to control the fecal retention.

Special care of the skin is also required in spinal cord injuries. Areas of decubital ulceration may develop rapidly and lead to ischemic necrosis of dermal and muscle tissue. The injured animal should be placed on an air mattress or foam rubber pad and its body position changed frequently. Preventing excessive moisture like urine from accumulating on the skin over pressure points will also help to prevent decubital sores. Following bowel movement, enemas, expression of urine, or catheterization of the bladder, the perineum or preputial area should be cleaned and dried. The use of a warm whirlpool bath may be exceedingly valuable by providing hydromassage in paralytic animals and by keeping the skin clean.

The initial handling of fractures of the vertebral column or ruptures of the intervertebral discs is discussed in the earlier paragraphs of this section. Acute compression of the spinal cord is a surgical emergency. In this situation, permanent damage to the spinal cord can only be prevented if decompression is performed soon after the initial insult. If pain response persists after injury, the prognosis is improved.

If the vertebral canal is displaced at the site of the injury, realignment and/or laminectomy should be performed. If there is a complete discontinuity of the vertebral canal, nothing can be done for the patient to recover the lost neurologic function. Displacements of 50 to 100 per cent of the vertebral canal have a very poor prognosis.

References

Additional information may be found in the following sources:

Averill, D. R., Jr.: Intracranial injuries. *In* Kirk, R. W. (ed.): Current Veterinary Therapy V. Philadelphia, W. B. Saunders Co., 1974.

Ballinger, W. F., Rutherford, R. B., and Zuidema, G. D.: Management of Trauma, 2nd ed. Philadelphia, W. B. Saunders Co., 1973.

Breazile, J. E.: Convulsive disorders in dogs. *In* Kirk, R. W. (ed.): Current Veterinary Therapy IV. Philadelphia, W. B. Saunders Co., 1971.

deLahunta, A.: Diagnosis and evaluation of traumatic lesions of the nervous system. Notes from New York State Veterinary College, 1971.

Hoerlein, B. F.: Canine Neurology, 2nd ed. Philadelphia, W. B. Saunders Co., 1971.

Oliver, J. E.: Neurologic emergencies in small animals. Vet. Clin. North Amer., Vol. 2, No. 2, May, 1972.

Trotter, E.: Management of thoracolumbar disc disease. Proc. Conf. Veterinarians, N. Y. S. Veterinary College, 1972.

I–18–C. Coma

Coma is the complete loss of consciousness with no response to painful stimuli, and is a symptomatic expression of disease (see Section II-5). In some animals presented in a stuporous or comatose state the cause will be apparent. However, in most instances a careful diagnostic work-up must be performed.

Initial Treatment

1. Maintain a clear airway and provide respiratory assistance if needed; treat shock and control existing hemorrhage.

2. Take a history as complete as possible from the owner, especially noting the presence of trauma or previous convulsive or comatose episodes.

3. Begin the physical examination by taking the temperature, pulse, and respiration. An elevated temperature suggests a systemic infection like pneumonia or hepatitis, or a brain lesion with loss of normal temperature control. Very high temperatures associated with signs of shock are indicative of heat stroke. A lowered body temperature is seen in barbiturate intoxication and circulatory collapse. Slow breathing can be seen in barbiturate intoxication or with elevated intracranial pressure. A rapid respiratory rate may indicate pneumonia, and diabetic or uremic acidosis.

Examine the skin and note any bruises, ecchymoses, swellings, or lacerations which may signify a traumatic incident. Examine the mucous membranes, noting the presence of pallor indicative of possible internal hemorrhage, or the presence of icterus indicative of possible liver disease. Smell the breath for the odor of spoiled fruit indicative of diabetic acidosis, for uremic odor or for the musty odor associated with hepatic coma.

4. Following the initial examination a more complete physical examination including neurologic evaluation should be conducted.

5. The following laboratory tests may be of value:

a. A urinalysis which should include test for specific gravity, sugar, acetone, and albumin. Urine of high specific gravity, glycosuria, and acetonuria are indicative of diabetic coma. Urine of low specific gravity with an elevated protein content is found in uremia together with high fevers. Urine may be saved for specific tests such as determining barbiturate intoxication.

b. A venous blood sample should be obtained for a white blood cell count, differential, hematocrit, hemoglobin, glucose, sodium, potassium, and chloride (see Section V-3).

c. A sample of cerebrospinal fluid should be obtained (see Section IV-3), examined (see Section V-1), and the cerebrospinal pressure determined.

Care of the Comatose Animal

Therapy should be aimed at finding and eliminating the cause of coma; however, there may be no specific therapy for some disease processes. If direct, specific therapy is not possible, supportive measures must be instituted (see Sections I-8-B and IV-16).

Specific Forms of Therapy

Diabetic Coma. In the uncontrolled diabetic animal, disorientation, prostration, and coma can result from ketoacidosis, or severe hyperglycemia. Hypoglycemia may affect cells of the central nervous system that depend directly upon glucose for energy in metabolism. Excessive plasma concentrations of acetoacetate and hydrogen ion together with dehydration lead to decreased oxygen consumption by the brain.

Treatment of diabetic acidosis is accomplished by reducing ketoacid production, stimulating carbohydrate utilization, and impeding the peripheral release of fatty acids (see Section I-17-A). During ketosis a marked insulin resistance may be present. Intravenous rehydration with Ringer's solution or sodium chloride should be carried out. In severe acidosis, sodium bicarbonate, 7.5 per cent, may be added to the fluids.

I-18-D. Convulsions

A convulsion is a transient disturbance of cerebral function characterized by a violent, involuntary contraction or series of contractions of the voluntary muscles. It is usually accompanied by disturbances of consciousness and autonomic hyperactivity. See Section II-6 for diagnostic considerations.

Immediate Measures

Most seizures are of short duration and may have subsided by the time the animal is presented for treatment. It is important, however, to prevent the patient from injuring either itself or a bystander. Confinement in a blanket may be useful in this regard.

In beginning treatment of the animal that has seizures it is important to evaluate the possibility of coexisting systemic diseases that can predispose the animal to epileptic attacks. Among these we include: uremia, hepatic disorders, insulin-secreting tumors of the pancreas, electrolyte imbalances, hypoglycemia, lead poisoning, carbon monoxide poisoning, organophosphate poisoning, chlorinated hydrocarbon poisoning, cyanide poisoning, strychnine poisoning and thiamine deficiency in cats. Treatment of these disease entities will help to control the symptomatic seizures.

Status epilepticus, meaning continuous seizures, is an emergency situation in which there is usually no time for an extensive diagnostic work-up. The seizures must be controlled as quickly as possible.

To stop the seizures, give diazepam (Valium), 10 to 35 mg. intravenously, and phenobarbital, 60 to 120 mg. intravenously or intramuscularly. If this regimen fails to control the status epilepticus, anesthetize the patient with a gaseous anesthetic or intravenous barbiturate. Immediately begin supportive treatment with fluids and collect blood, urine and C.S.F. samples for diagnostic work-up. Careful attention should be given to blood sugar and calcium levels, and dextrose and/or calcium gluconate should be provided if needed.

Epilepsy in cats is not nearly as common as in the dog. It can be associated with systemic diseases such as infectious feline peritonitis, cryptococcosis, toxoplasmosis, lymphosarcoma, meningiomas, and thiamine deficiency.

Thiamine deficiency in the cat may present as a neurologic emergency characterized by dilated pupils, ataxic gait, cerebellar tremor, abnormal oculovestibular reflex and seizures. Treatment consists of administration of thiamine 50 mg. per day for three days.

Text continued on page 114.

TABLE 10. DIFFERENTIAL DIAGNOSIS OF SEIZURES*

Acquired Seizures

Viral encephalitis
History of previous symptoms suggestive of viral invasion (distemper complex). Hyperexcitability or depression. Electroencephalography is useful for diagnosis.

Toxoplasmosis
Previous chronic disease signs; i.e., anorexia, weakness, emaciation, pulmonary symptoms, ocular lesions, seizures progressively more frequent and occasionally of long duration. (Test: serum titer.) Electroencephalography is useful for diagnosis.

Cerebral neoplasia
Neurological examination usually suggestive of focal abnormality, abnormal reflexes, "Jacksonian" fit. Seizures progressively more frequent. Electroencephalography and radiography (plain and contrast) are useful for diagnosis.

Trauma
History of injury to skull, unconsciousness followed by incoordination. Seizures may start three to six months after injury. Electroencephalography and radiography are useful for diagnosis.

Cryptococcosis
Variable neurological signs, occasional seizures. Culture of cerebrospinal fluid.

Familial (Congenital) Seizures

Idiopathic epilepsy
Neurological examination negative in young animal six to 18 months old with no previous illness. Aura, short seizure period (20 to 90 seconds), rapid recovery after seizure. Seizures may occur at regular intervals. Electroencephalographic findings usually negative.

Hydrocephalus
Retarded intelligence, incoordination, lethargy. May or may not have increased head size and open fontanelles. Seizures start at three to nine months of age. Electroencephalography and radiography (plain and contrast) are useful for diagnosis.

Table continues on following page.

TABLE 10. DIFFERENTIAL DIAGNOSIS OF SEIZURES* *(Continued)*

Metabolic Seizures

Carbon monoxide poisoning	History of riding in truck or trunk of automobile prior to seizure, which occurs five to 15 minutes after muscular activity. Pink mucous membranes.
Parasitism	Very young puppies affected. Low blood calcium, low blood sugar, anemia. Frequent seizures of short duration.
Hypoglycemia	Muscular twitching, hunger, low blood sugar. Seizures occur 30 to 60 minutes after exercise and are related only to the exercise. (Exception: islet cell tumor.) Interseizural electroencephalogram nondiagnostic.
Hypocalcemia	Muscular twitching, anxious attitude, low blood calcium associated with pregnancy, whelping, and parasitism in puppies. Seizures of the tonic type.

Drug-Induced Seizures

Organophosphate poisoning	Gastrointestinal hypermotility, salivation, miosis, dyspnea. Muscular twitching followed by seizures of long duration.
Chlorinated hydrocarbon poisoning	Hyperexcitability, tremors followed by tonic-clonic seizures of long duration.
Cyanide poisoning	Weakness, tremors, rapid deep respirations, seizures tonic in nature. Bright red mucous membranes.

Other Causes of Seizures

Hypothalamic syndrome	Hypothermia or hyperthermia, polyuria, polydipsia. Occasional seizures with postseizural confusion. Electroencephalography is useful for diagnosis.
Tetanus	Muscular stiffness, hypertonus of extensor musculature, ears pulled back, nictitating membranes protruding.

*From Hoerlein, B. F.: Canine Neurology, 2nd ed. Philadelphia, W. B. Saunders Co., 1971, pp. 494–495.

TABLE 11. DRUGS, DOSAGES, ADVANTAGES AND DISADVANTAGES OF THE MOST COMMONLY USED ANTICONVULSANT DRUGS*

Drug	Indication Uses	Dose Availability	Dose Range	Advantages	Disadvantages
Diphenyl hydantoin (Dilantin)	Generalized major motor seizures, minor motor seizures and behavioral seizures	Capsules: 30 mg. 100 mg. 100 mg. with 0.25 gr. pheno- barbital	2 mg./lb./day 50 mg./lb./day	Absence of sedation Effectiveness in a high per cent of cases Low toxicity and ab- sence of many side effects noted in humans Low cost Not a controlled sub- stance (BNDD) Worldwide availability In combination with phenobarbital, is not a controlled sub- stance	Transient ataxia Rapid metabolism, difficulty in main- taining adequate blood levels; possibly is poorly absorbed in dogs Some polyphagia, polydipsia, polyuria Relatively toxic in cats; generally not desirable as an anti- convulsant in cats Does not stop initial ictal discharge

Table continues on following pages.

TABLE 11. DRUGS, DOSAGES, ADVANTAGES AND DISADVANTAGES OF THE MOST COMMONLY USED ANTICONVULSANT DRUGS* (Continued)

Drug	Indication Uses	Dose Availability	Dose Range	Advantages	Disadvantages
Phenobarbital	Generalized major motor seizures, minor motor seizures and behavioral seizures	Tablets: 0.125 gr. 0.25 gr. 0.5 gr. Liquid Injectable: 0.5 to 1 gr./ml.	0.125 gr. twice daily to 2 gr. four times daily	High efficacy Rapid action, few hours Low toxicity in animals Can be administered by several routes (intravenously, intramuscularly and orally) Generally the most effective drug in status epilepticus Low cost Worldwide availability Drug of choice in cats	Sedative effects Restricted drug Long-term prescription not honored Polyphagia, polydipsia, polyuria Reverse effects, irritability and restlessness Length of sedation precluding a neurologic examination, following intravenous, intramuscular and oral administration, is often several hours
Primidone (Mysoline), (Mylepsin)	Generalized major motor seizure, minor motor seizure	Tablets: 50 mg. scored 250 mg. scored	4 mg./lb./day 20 mg./lb./day May vary both up and down	High level of efficacy Rapid action Useful in most clinical seizure disorders	Sedation dramatic and severe in many animals; sedation may be transient as the

				Advantages	Disadvantages
				Not controlled by BNDD Widely available	patient becomes accustomed to the medication Great variability in dose tolerances Only one form available; no parenteral form Only two size tablets available (50 mg. and 250 mg.)
Diazepam (Valium)	Control of the exacerbation of seizures Control of status epilepticus Feline seizure epilepticus	Tablets: 2.5 mg. 5 mg. 10 mg. Injectable: 5 mg./ml. in 2-ml. vials	2.5 to 100 mg. intravenously or intramuscularly to effect	Effectiveness in stopping status epilepticus and other generalized seizure disorders Rapid action Safety Relative brevity of action; neurologic evaluation can be done shortly afterwards; few hours if further seizures do not occur Useful in cats, parenterally or orally Can be used as a tranquilizer	Relatively short action; often needs to be repeated several times in status epilepticus management Cannot control violent status epilepticus Relatively expensive Controlled by BNDD Seldom used for oral prevention and control Reverse effects sometimes seen, restlessness, viciousness

*From Kay, W.: Epilepsy. In Kirk, R. W. (ed.): Current Veterinary Therapy V. Philadelphia, W. B. Saunders Co., 1974.

References

Cunningham, J. G.: Canine seizure disorders. J.A.V.M.A., *158*:589–597, March 1, 1971.
Kay, W.: Epilepsy. *In* Kirk, R. W. (ed.): Current Veterinary Therapy V, Philadelphia, W. B. Saunders Co., 1974.

I–19. POISONINGS

GENERAL APPROACH TO TREATMENT (ARONSON)

With several hundred thousand potentially toxic substances on the market, it is impossible to remain knowledgeable of their toxicities. However, poison control centers located throughout the United States and Canada do maintain readily available information. *For additional information, contact the nearest Poison Control Center.*

Poison Control Centers*

The poison control centers have been organized to aid physicians, veterinarians, and others in health-related fields. Some are equipped to administer expert treatment to poisoned human patients, but all are centers of information on poisons and the treatment of poisoning.

All available information on the toxic ingredients in thousands of medicines, insecticides, pesticides, and other registered commercial products has been placed confidentially by the government in these poison control centers. As new products are marketed, information regarding the toxic ingredients is forwarded to the centers.

It has been conservatively estimated that 500,000 different household trade-name products are currently on the market, and that 1500 new items are added each month.

TELEPHONE INSTRUCTIONS

Give the following first aid instructions, as applicable, when a client calls about a poisoned animal.

---

*From Directory of Poison Control Centers, U.S. Department of Health, Education, and Welfare, Public Health Service, Division of Direct Health Service, National Clearinghouse for Poison Control Centers, Washington, D.C.

1. Induce vomiting (5 ml. of hydrogen peroxide orally or 1 teaspoonful of salt placed in the mouth) and save the vomitus. Do not induce vomiting if it appears that the animal has ingested corrosive materials, such as strong acid, alkali, or kerosene.

2. If the animal was in physical contact with toxic or corrosive material, wash its skin clear with profuse quantities of water.

3. For excitement or convulsions, try merely to protect the animal from injuring itself.

4. Bring the sample of suspected poison to the hospital with the patient.

I–19–A.   General Treatment Principles

Ideally, try to treat the specific poison when possible; however, remember that many poisons do not have specific antidotes. Immediate supportive care in poisoning cases can be life saving.

Prevent Further Absorption

Emetics

Administer intravenously apomorphine, 20 μg./lb. (0.04 mg./20 lb.).

Gastric Lavage

This is possible only on anesthetized or comatose patients.
1. Pass an endotracheal tube and inflate the cuff.
2. Pass a large size stomach tube and alternately inject and aspirate 100 to 300 ml. of tap water to rinse out the stomach contents.

Absorbents

Introduce and allow to remain in the stomach a thick slurry of activated charcoal, prepared by adding five heaping teaspoonsful of charcoal to 200 ml. of water. The universal antidote is not particularly effective.

Laxatives

Sodium sulfate, 0.3 to 0.4 mg./lb., should be given orally one hour after the charcoal slurry. Colonic irrigations with saline or mild soap solutions may be helpful.

Text continued on page 120.

TABLE 12. SPECIMENS REQUIRED FOR SPECIFIC TESTS*

Poison or Analysis Requested	Specimen Required	Amount of Specimen Desired	Comments
Ammonia†	Whole blood	5 ml.	Frozen (1-2 drops of saturated $HgCl_2$ may be used instead of freezing rumen contents)
	Stomach contents (composite)	100 gm.	
	Urine	5 ml.	
ANTU	Stomach and intestine contents	200 gm.	Can be detected only within 12-24 hours after ingestion
	Liver	200 gm.	
Arsenic	Liver	50 gm.	
	Kidney	50 gm.	
	Feed	100 gm.	
	Stomach contents	100 gm.	
	Urine	50 ml.	
Calcium	Serum	2 ml.	Serum must *not* be hemolyzed; separate clot before transit
	Feed	25 gm.	
Carbon monoxide	Whole blood	15 ml.	
Chloride	See Sodium		
Chlorinated hydrocarbon insecticides	Body fat	100 gm.	Must not be contaminated with hairs or stomach contents; preferable to use chemically clean glass jars; avoid plastic containers
	Stomach contents	100 gm.	
	Liver	50 gm.	
	Kidney	50 gm.	
	Whole blood	10 ml.	

Copper	Kidney	50 gm.	Freeze specimen promptly in air-tight container
	Liver	50 gm.	
	Whole blood	10 ml.	
	Feces	100 gm.	
Cyanide	Whole blood	10 ml.	One kidney, both in small animals
	Liver	50 gm.	
	Forage, silate	100 gm.	
	Other materials	100 gm.	
Ethylene glycol	Serum	10 ml.	
	Kidney (in formalin)	Whole organ	
	Urine	10 ml.	
Fluoroacetate	Stomach contents	All available	Frozen
	Kidney	One whole	
	Urine	50 gm.	
	Liver	50 gm.	
	Other materials	100 gm.	
Nitrates	Water	50 ml.	
	Forage, silage	100 gm.	
	Whole blood (methemoglobin)	10 ml.	
	Other materials	100 gm.	

*From Buck, William B.: Use of laboratories for the chemical analysis of tissues. *In* Kirk, R. W. (ed.): Current Veterinary Therapy V. Philadelphia, W. B. Saunders Co., 1974.

†A total of 5 ml. of nonhemolyzed serum is sufficient to conduct several clinical tests.

Table continues on following pages.

TABLE 12. SPECIMENS REQUIRED FOR SPECIFIC TESTS (*Continued*)

Poison or Analysis Requested	Specimen Required	Amount of Specimen Desired	Comments
Organophosphorous insecticides	Body fat	50 gm.	
	Stomach contents (composite)	50 gm.	
	Blood (heparinized)	10 ml.	
	Urine	50 gm.	
	Feed	100 gm.	
Oxalates	Fresh forage	6–8 plants.	Do *not* chop plants; freeze promptly
	Kidney (in formalin)	Whole organ	One kidney, both in small animals (qualitative test only)
Phenols	Stomach contents	500 gm.	Pack in air-tight container
	Other materials	200 gm.	
Phenothiazines	Feed or other materials	50 gm.	
Phosphates	Serum	5 ml.	

Thallium	Bone	25 gm.
	Other materials	100 gm.
	Urine	10 ml.
	Kidney	50 gm.
	Liver	50 gm.
Urea	Feed	100 gm.
	Other materials	500 gm.
	See also Ammonia	
Warfarin	Liver	100 gm.
	Feed	100 gm.
	Other materials	100 gm.
Zinc	Liver	50 gm.
	Kidney	50 gm.
	Other materials	100 gm.

Detoxify and Remove Absorbed Poisons

Chemical antidotes react with a specific poison to form a relatively nontoxic product that may be excreted.

1. Edathamil calcium-disodium (CaEDTA) for lead poisoning.
2. 2,3-Dimercaptopropanol (BAL) for arsenic poisoning.
3. Sodium nitrite and sodium thiosulfate for cyanide poisoning.
4. 2-Pyridine aldoxime methiodide (PAM) for organophosphate poisoning.

Improving the function of excretory organs may enhance the removal of absorbed poisons.

1. Improve ventilation (see Sections IV-18, IV-19, and IV-20), clean the skin, and administer laxatives or diuretics.
2. Diuresis with mannitol, 5 per cent in isotonic saline is particularly effective in dogs. Give mannitol, 0.5 gm./lb. intravenously over 30 to 60 minutes.
3. Peritoneal dialysis (see Section IV-16-G) may be helpful with thalium or phenobarbital poisonings.

Carry Out Supportive Therapy

This may consist of symptomatic treatments that are given to produce pharmacologic effects opposite to those of the poison and are aimed at preserving vital functions.

1. Control nervous system activity.
   a. For pain, administer analgesics (Demerol hydrochloride, 5 mg./lb.).
   b. For seizures, administer anticonvulsants or anesthetics (Pentobarbital, 12 mg./lb., or diazepam [Valium], 5 mg. intravenously).
   c. For depressed cardiovascular and respiratory centers, administer stimulants. Of questionable value, however, are intravenous injections of caffeine sodium benzoate, 50 mg., or amphetamine, 2 mg./lb.
2. Maintain respiration.
   a. Maintain airway with endotracheal tube.
   b. Use a mechanical respirator and ordinary air, unless oxygen is indicated.
3. Control body temperature.
   a. Careful use of blankets, heat lamps, and heating pads will maintain body heat; however, burns are easily produced.
   b. Alcohol rubs, cool water enemas, and fluids by intravenous injection combat hyperthermia and dehydration.
4. Maintain cardiovascular function.

a. The maintenance of ventilation, hydration, and body temperature together with frequent turning may be the most effective means of maintaining cardiovascular function. For other measures, see Sections I-8 and I-9.

I–19–B. Medicolegal Considerations

Records

Complete, dated, and signed records should include notations of history, physical findings, and laboratory or autopsy reports.

Specimens for Toxicologic Analysis

1. Wide mouth plastic bottles or plastic bags that have not been used before are convenient containers for storage of specimens. No preservatives should be added, but tissues can be frozen to prevent putrefaction.

2. Vomitus, gastric washings, or colonic lavage solutions should be saved. Blood and urine should also be retained.

3. If the patient dies, the liver, brain, kidneys, and muscle should be saved. It is desirable to weigh each organ, label, and store it (or an aliquot) in a separate container.

4. When specimens are sent for toxicologic analysis, a history and request for specific poisons should be included. Costs vary from $20 to several hundred dollars for a complete analysis.

I–19–C. Treatment of Specific Poisons

The following toxic substances are arranged alphabetically. Note, too, that the number following the name of the poison or toxic substance refers to *page number,* not to subsection heading.

Acetic acid, 124
Acetone, 123
Acetylsalicylic acid, 129
Aldrin, 132
Algae toxins, 125
Alkalies, 125
Alkaloids, 126
Alpha-napthylthiourea, 128
Amanita toxin, 126

Ammonium hydroxide, 125
Amphetamine sulfate, 126
Anesthetics, local, 127
Aniline dyes, 128
Ant pastes, 165
ANTU, 128
Arsenic, 129
Arsenic trioxide, 129
Aspergillus mycotoxins, 152

I–19–C–1. ACETONE (DIMETHYL KETONE, PROPANONE)

Source

Acetone is a potent solvent and paint remover. Inhalation of fumes or ingestion may produce toxicity.

Signs

1. Acetone or ketone odor to breath.
2. Severe vomiting and diarrhea.
3. Depressed pulse, respiration, and blood pressure.

Treatment

1. Give emetics and gastric lavage with water.
2. Support treatment with caffeine sodium benzoate, 0.05 gm.

I–19–C–2. ACIDS (ACETIC, CARBOLIC, HYDROCHLORIC, LACTIC, NITRIC, SULFURIC, TRICHLOROACETIC)

Exceptions are oxalic (see Section I-19-C-65) and tannic acids.

Source

These acids are used in cleaning and etching procedures.

Signs

Externally there is abdominal pain, vomitus that may be blood-stained, rapid breathing, and systemic acidosis.

Treatment

1. Externally:
a. Flush with copious amounts of water and apply a paste of sodium bicarbonate.
2. Internally:
a. Neutralize by administering magnesium hydroxide, egg white, or soap solution. Sodium bicarbonate may cause gastric distention. Do not use emetics if concentrated acid was ingested.
b. Administer olive oil orally.
c. Administer meperidine hydrochloride intramuscularly for pain.
d. Perform a tracheotomy if pharyngeal and laryngeal edema is severe (see Section IV-18).

I–19–C–3. ALGAE TOXINS

Source

Obtained by drinking water containing the blue-green algae (northern lakes of U.S. and southern Canada).

Signs

1. Onset rapid, death within 24 hours (often after only an hour or two).
2. Vomiting, prostration.
3. Muscular tremors, convulsions, paralysis, death.

Treatment

None.

I–19–C–4. ALKALIES (SODIUM HYDROXIDE, POTASSIUM HYDROXIDE, AMMONIUM HYDROXIDE)

Source

Alkalies are constituents in cleaning preparations, grease dissolvents, refrigerants, and dehorning and escharotic pastes.

Signs

1. External signs are pain, erythema, and maceration of the skin.

2. Internal signs are abdominal pain, nausea with blood-flecked vomitus, and systemic alkalosis.

Treatment

1. Externally:
a. Flush with copious amounts of water and apply vinegar or dilute acetic acid. Apply topical emollients.
2. Internally:
a. Neutralize with vinegar or acetic acid.
b. Do not use emetics if concentrated solutions of alkalies were ingested.
c. Give olive oil or egg white as demulcents.
d. For relief of pain administer meperidine hydrochloride intramuscularly.

I–19–C–5. ALKALOIDS (GENERAL DRUG CLASS)

Treatment

1. To inactivate the drug, administer orally 1 ml. of tincture of iodine in 120 ml. of water.
2. Use gastric lavage with potassium permanganate diluted 1:2000 in water.
3. Support treatment with heat and cardiovascular stimulants such as caffeine sodium benzoate.

I–19–C–6. AMANITA TOXIN (AMANITA PHALLOIDES)

Source

Dog eats the fungus. The toxin has a latent period of 10 to 12 hours; the course may take many days.

Signs

Sudden severe abdominal pain, vomiting and diarrhea with blood and mucus in feces.

Treatment

1. None specific—use symptomatic support.
2. Saline laxatives and enemas.
3. Atropine may be helpful.

I-19-C-7. AMPHETAMINE SULFATE (BENZEDRINE, DEXEDRINE)

Source

Amphetamine sulfate is a component in stimulant and diet pills.

Signs

In mild cases the signs are delirium, hyperpyrexia, bounding pulse, and dilated pupils. In severe cases, convulsions, circulatory collapse, coma, and death result. The LD 50 is estimated at 4 to 10 mg./lb. orally.

Treatment

1. Administer chlorpromazine, 1 mg./lb. intramuscularly.
2. Administer an intravenous injection of pentobarbital sodium until the desired level of sedation is obtained only if chlorpromazine is inadequate to control the patient.
3. Use lavage to empty stomach. Leave activated charcoal slurry in stomach. One hour later give saline laxative.
4. Administer 40 per cent oxygen (or air) with a respirator to support breathing.
5. Since amphetamines are weak bases, acidifying the urine may increase urinary excretion.
6. Keep patient under constant observation for 24 to 48 hours.
7. Cool baths or enemas may be needed to control body temperature.
8. After six hours, prognosis improves.

I-19-C-8. ANESTHETICS, LOCAL (PROCAINE, XYLOCAINE)

Source

Used as local anesthetics, but excessive amounts orally, topically on denuded skin, or by injection may cause toxicity.

Signs

The signs are excitement, delirium, tachycardia, dyspnea, convulsions, and cardiovascular collapse.

Treatment

1. Sedation. Intravenous pentobarbital is usually effective.

2. Support breathing with a respirator as needed.
3. Treat cardiovascular collapse if needed (see Section I-8).

I-19-C-9. ANILINE DYES

Source

Used as a dye ingredient in crayons, pencils, and shoe polish.

Signs

The signs are apathy, dyspnea, vomiting and convulsions, and methemoglobinemia.

Treatment

1. Emetics and gastric lavage. Give saline laxative.
2. Analeptics, e.g., Doxapram, 2.5-5.0 mg./lb., intravenously.
3. Oxygen therapy.
4. Whole blood transfusion.
5. Methylene blue solution, 1 per cent, in sodium sulfate, 1.8 per cent. Slowly administer 3 to 10 ml. intravenously.
6. Survival for 24 hours is usually followed by complete recovery.

I-19-C-10. ALPHA-NAPHTHYLTHIOUREA (ANTU)

Source

A powerful rat poison, now rarely used. Mortality high.

Signs

1. Profuse salivation.
2. Vomiting.
3. Pulmonary edema and dyspnea.
4. Muscular weakness and ataxia.

Treatment

1. Give emetics like hydrogen peroxide, 6 to 8 ml. orally every 15 minutes.

2. Give an intramuscular injection of atropine sulfate, 0.05 mg./lb. every four hours.

3. Provide oxygen therapy if needed (see Section IV-20).

4. Do not give fluids.

I-19-C-11. ARSENIC (ARSENIC TRIOXIDE, CALCIUM ARSENATE, SODIUM ARSENITE)

Source

Arsenic is used in ant poisons, herbicides, insecticides, smelters' drugs, paints, and food additives. A single toxic dose for a dog is 100 to 150 mg. of As_2O_3, and 50 to 100 mg. of sodium arsenite.

Signs

1. Vomiting, restlessness, extreme abdominal pain, and weakness.
2. Vomitus has garlic odor.
3. Dysphagia and diarrhea (often bloody).
4. Cyanosis and weak pulse.
5. Shock and collapse, coma.

Treatment

1. In early case give sodium bicarbonate or sodium sulfate orally and follow immediately with an intravenous injection of apomorphine, 20 μg./lb.

2. If absorption has occurred, inject intramuscularly BAL (2, 3-Dimercapto-1 propanol), 2 mg./lb.; repeat dose every four hours. BAL is a specific antidote for arsenic poisoning. BAL should not be used on cats.

3. For pain, administer meperidine hydrochloride.

4. Intense fluid support is mandatory (see Section IV-16).

I-19-C-12. ASPIRIN (ACETYLSALICYLIC ACID, OTHER SALICYLATES)

Source

Children's aspirin is commonly sugar- or flavor-coated; animals may readily eat them.

Signs

Weakness, vomiting, panting, seizures, petechial hemorrhage (hypoprothrombinemia), acetone odor to breath, acidosis, and collapse.

Treatment

1. Emetics to empty stomach (intravenous injection of apomorphine, 20 μg./lb., or hydrogen peroxide, 6 to 8 ml. orally).
2. Gastric lavage with potassium permanganate diluted 1:2000.
3. Support respirations, if needed.
4. Treat acidosis intravenously or orally with sodium bicarbonate.
5. Use sedatives (barbiturates) as needed.
6. Do not use derivatives of morphine.
7. Apply heat and keep patient under constant supervision for 24 hours.
8. Improve renal output by fluid therapy (see Section IV-16). Glucose may be useful.

I–19–C–13. ATROPINE SULFATE

Source

Medication incorrectly or accidentally administered.

Signs

Dry mucosa, dilated pupils, increased temperature, delirium, and collapse.

Treatment

1. Give emetics early (apomorphine, 20 μg./lb. intravenously; hydrogen peroxide, 6 to 8 ml. orally).
2. Gastric lavage with potassium permanganate diluted 1:2000.
3. Sedation with barbiturates if needed.
4. Small doses of pilocarpine are permissible if given with discretion.
5. Reduce body temperature by means of alcohol rubs. Control convulsions.
6. Survival for 24 hours usually means recovery.

I–19–C–14. BARBITURATES

Source

Accidental or incorrect administration of sedative medications.

Signs

Ataxia, followed by delirium, depression, and coma. Initial respirations are rapid but subsequently become depressed. Hypotension, shock, and death result from respiratory failure.

Treatment

1. Emetics are helpful if given early (see Section I-19-A).
2. Administer a gastric lavage (see Section I-19-A).
3. Administer oxygen, 40 per cent, or air with a positive pressure respirator.
4. Improve renal function by stimulating diuresis (see Section IV-16).
5. Support circulation with intravenous injections of ephedrine sulfate, atropine sulfate, or fluid infusions of Aramine.
6. Treat shock (see Section I-9) and cardiac arrest (see Section I-8).
7. Peritoneal dialysis may be helpful with barbiturates other than pentobarbital, which is protein-bound.
8. Analeptic drugs, if used at all, should be used with discretion. Doxapram, 2.5 to 5 mg./lb., administered intravenously, seems to be the best drug of this type. Rebound effect following analeptic drugs is often severe.

I–19–C–15. BENZENE (BENZOL, NAPHTHA, TOLUENE, TOLUOL, XYLENE, XYLOL)

Source

Benzene is used as a solvent, cleaning agent, and fuel. The fumes as well as the liquid phase are toxic. A drug form is used as an oral ascaricide.

Signs after Inhalation

1. Acute conjunctivitis, nausea, and vomiting.
2. Depression, cyanosis, and weak pulse followed by convulsions and collapse.

Treatment after Inhalation

1. Remove animal to fresh air. Give oxygen resuscitation if necessary (see Section IV-20).
2. Wash animal's eyes with copious amounts of water and apply an antibiotic-steroid ophthalmic ointment.

Signs after Ingestion

1. Nausea, vomiting, and fixed pupils.
2. Ataxia, depression, and coma.

Treatment after Ingestion

1. Gastric lavage with sodium bicarbonate solution, 5 per cent.
2. Oral administration of olive oil.
3. Oxygen therapy and treatment for pulmonary edema (see Section IV-20).
4. Subsequent treatment for anemia will be needed.

I-19-C-16. BENZENE HEXACHLORIDE (LINDANE, BHC, GAMMEXANE, CHLORDANE, TOXAPHENE, STROBANE, DIELDRIN, OLDRIN, HEPTACHLOR, ALDRIN)

Source

Benzene hydrochloride is used as an insecticide. Cats are particularly susceptible.

Signs

Restlessness, fasciculations, muscle spasms, convulsions, and fever followed by cyanosis, depression, coma, and death.

Treatment

1. If animal was topically exposed, wash it thoroughly with soap and water.

2. If animal ingested material, administer emetics (see Section I-19-A), perform gastric lavage (see Section I-19-A), and leave magnesium sulfate in the stomach.

Poisoning by Either Route

1. There are no specific antidotes.

2. Control seizures. Sedate with pentobarbital intravenously.

3. Administer intravenously calcium gluconate, 10 per cent, 3 to 10 ml.

4. Support respiration with a respirator if needed.

5. Administer Aramine or ephedrine sulfate to support circulation.

6. Reduce body temperature with cold water baths or sprays if needed.

7. Give saline laxative if ingested; wash with soap if dermal exposure.

I–19–C–17. BLEACHES (HYPOCHLORITES, CHLOROX, DAKIN'S SOLUTION, SODIUM PERBORATE)

Source

Bleaches are used as disinfectants owing to their oxidizing action.

Signs

Concentrated solutions have a caustic action (see Section I-19-C-3); mild solutions cause mild gastrointestinal symptoms. Bleaches are also irritating to the skin.

Treatment

1. Empty stomach by emetics or lavage (see Section I-19-A).

2. Administer olive oil or egg white as a demulcent.

3. Recovery is usually complete unless high concentrate solutions were ingested.

4. Sodium thiosulfate, 5 per cent solution, will decompose hypochlorite solutions.

I–19–C–18. CARBOLIC ACID

See phenol, Section I-19-C-68.

I–19–C–19. CARBON MONOXIDE

Source

Exposure of animals to exhaust fumes, as when dogs are transported in the trunks of automobiles.

Signs

History of exposure, depression, muscular twitchings, increased temperature, and dusky or cherry-red mucosa.

Treatment

1. Artificial respiration if needed, followed by positive pressure oxygen resuscitation.
2. Intravenous administration of dextrose, 50 per cent, 1 ml./lb.
3. Do not give methylene blue.
4. Do not give narcotics, sedatives, atropine, or analeptics.
5. Keep patient hospitalized for at least 48 hours.

I–19–C–20. CARBON TETRACHLORIDE

Source

Carbon tetrachloride is used in fire extinguishers, cleaning solutions and dry shampoos.

Signs

1. Nausea, delirium, and acute hepatic failure.
2. Collapse, coma, and death.

Treatment

1. Following inhalation of fumes provide animal with fresh air; use oxygen resuscitation if needed (see Section IV-20).

2. Following ingestion:

a. Induce vomiting, use gastric lavage with potassium permanganate diluted 1:2000.

b. Give magnesium sulfate orally as a laxative.

3. In poisoning by either route:

a. Administer intravenously calcium gluconate, 10 per cent, 3 to 10 ml.

b. Administer intravenously dextrose and water, 5 per cent, 20 ml./lb. Treat oliguria which develops.

c. Do not give fats, oils, or alcohol.

d. Give methionine, 2 to 4 gm. per day.

I-19-C-21.   CHENOPODIUM

Source

Used in anthelminthic preparations.

Signs

1. Nausea and vomiting.

2. Abdominal and lumbar pain (kidney damage).

3. Depression, delirium, and seizures.

4. Cheyne-Stokes respirations leading to death from respiratory paralysis.

Treatment

1. Administer emetics (see Section I-19-A) and gastric lavage with potassium permanganate, diluted 1:2000. Follow with magnesium sulfate as a saline laxative.

2. Resuscitation with oxygen if needed (see Section IV-20).

3. Intravenous administration of dextrose in water, 5 per cent, 20 ml./lb.

4. Response to treatment is poor.

I-19-C-22. CHLOROPHENOTHANE (DDT)

Source

Chlorophenothane is used in insecticidal preparations.

Signs

1. Cats show stiffness and extensor rigidity followed by tremors, pilomotor stimulation, and convulsions.
2. Dogs show primary signs of ataxia and convulsions.

Treatment

See Section I-19-C-16.

I-19-C-23. CLEANING FLUIDS AND COMPOUNDS

Benzene, Section I-19-C-15.
Carbon tetrachloride, Section I-19-C-20.
Gasoline, Section I-19-C-36.
Kerosene, Section I-19-C-43.
Oxalic acid, Section I-19-C-65.
Stoddard solvent, Section I-19-C-43.

I-19-C-24. CYANIDES

Source

Cyanides are used in herbicides: they are general protoplasmic poisons, and cause death almost instantaneously.

Signs

1. Deep coma.
2. Odor of bitter almonds.

Treatment (Usually Futile)

1. Administer oxygen therapy under positive pressure.
2. By mouth, give activated charcoal, and hydrogen peroxide, 1 part, to sodium thiosulfate, 5 per cent, 5 parts.
3. Administer intravenously sodium thiosulfate, 5 per cent, 3 to 8 ml., and alternate every 10 to 15 minutes with 3 to 8 ml. of a solution of methylene blue, 1 per cent, in sodium sulfate, 1.8 per cent.

I-19-C-25. CRAYONS

Source

Children's wax and chalk crayons are usually required by law to be harmless. Some marking crayons, however, contain aniline dyes, a toxic substance.

See aniline dyes, Section I-19-C-9.

I-19-C-26. DDT (CHLOROPHENOTHANE, DICHLORODIPHENYLTRICHLOROETHANE)

See Section I-19-C-16.

I-19-C-27. DEODORANTS OR DEODORIZERS

Source

Common cosmetic preparations contain alcohol, aluminum salts, and boric acid. Household deodorizers often contain naphthalene, formaldehyde, and essential oils.

Signs

The material is usually nontoxic unless large amounts have been ingested.

Treatment

1. Administer emetics or lavage (see Section I-19-A).
2. See naphthalene, Section I-19-C-57.

I-19-C-28. DICHLOROBENZENE

Source

The ortho isomer is used as a wood preservative, the para isomer as an insecticide.

Signs and Treatment

See Section I-19-C-59.

I-19-C-29. DIGITALIS

Source

Iatrogenic overdosing or accidental ingestion of medications.

Signs

1. Nausea, vomiting, and diarrhea.
2. Depression.
3. Slow pulse, and changes in EKG tracings (prolonged P-R interval, ectopic beats, and sinus block).

Treatment

1. Withhold the drug.
2. Administer potassium salts orally, but only until serum level reaches 5.0 m Eq./L.
3. Inject atropine sulfate, 0.05 mg./lb.
4. Provide oxygen therapy (see Section IV-20).
5. Consider use of propranolol and diphenylhydantoin for ventricular irregularities (see Section I-8).
6. Recovery likely if patient survives 24 hours.

I-19-C-30. DINITROPHENOL (DNP)

Source

Dinitrophenol is used in worming medicaments.

Signs

1. Increased body temperature.
2. Restlessness; rapid, deep breathing.
3. Convulsions and coma resulting in death from respiratory failure.

Treatment

1. If material has been ingested, administer emetics and gastric lavage (see Section I-19-A).
2. Reduce body temperature by cold sprays and enemas.
3. Administer intravenous injection of dextrose, 5 per cent, in water (20 ml./lb.).
4. Provide oxygen therapy (see Section IV-20).

I–19–C–31. ETHYLENE GLYCOL (PERMANENT ANTIFREEZE, PRESTONE, ZEREX)

Source

Ethylene glycol is used in antifreeze. Toxic effects result from the breakdown of ethylene glycol to oxalic acid, crystals of which subsequently cause renal tubular obstruction. Minimum lethal dose for the cat is 1.1 ml./lb., and for the dog 3.3 ml./lb.

Signs

1. Delirium and rapid pulse, ataxia.
2. Dyspnea, vomiting.
3. Ataxia, convulsions, and coma.
4. Anuria or oliguria, dehydration.

Treatment

1. Start treatment at once; do not wait for signs to appear.
2. Induce vomiting with apomorphine or hydrogen peroxide.
3. Lavage stomach with quantities of potassium permanganate solution diluted 1:2000.
4. Administer fluids like dextrose (5 per cent) in water to stimulate urine output, but avoid excess if oliguria is present.

   5. Ethyl alcohol is a potent competitive inhibitor of the oxidation of ethylene glycol, preventing the conversion of ethylene glycol to oxalate. Utilize a 50 per cent solution of pure ethyl alcohol and administer the solution intravenously until the animal is comatose and insensitive (test by pinching a toe). Repeat administration of the solution as needed when the dog shows positive response to stimulus. Maintain level of ethyl alcohol for three days. Control metabolic acidosis with systemically administered sodium bicarbonate.

   6. If renal failure occurs, institute peritoneal dialysis (see Section IV-20-G).

I–19–C–32. FIRE EXTINGUISHERS

   The types of extinguishers in common use and the toxic ingredients each contains are:
   1. Dry type—magnesium stearate, tricalcium phosphate.
   2. Foam type—aluminum sulfate, methyl bromide.
   3. Gas type—carbon dioxide gas.
   4. Liquid type—carbon tetrachloride, dichloromethane, chlorobromomethane, and trichlorethylene.

I–19–C–33. FLUOROACETATES

Source

   Fluoroacetates are highly toxic and cause slowly developing convulsions. They are a constituent of rodenticides and are used only by licensed exterminators. Toxic dose for a dog is 0.05 to 0.5 mg./kg.

Signs

   1. Nausea, vomiting, dyspnea, defecation, wild running and barking.
   2. Muscular twitching and tetany.
   3. Convulsions and cardiac arrhythmias.
   4. Seizures are not accentuated by external stimuli.

Treatment

   1. Treatment is usually unsuccessful unless small amounts have been ingested.

2. Give an emetic (apomorphine) if tetany or seizure has not started.

3. Anesthetize with an intravenous injection of pentobarbital and maintain for 24 hours.

4. Administer orally calcium gluconate, 10 per cent, 10 to 50 ml.

5. Administer intravenously calcium gluconate, 10 per cent, 3 to 20 ml.

6. Administer intravenously dextrose, 5 per cent, and water.

I–19–C–34. FURNITURE POLISH

Furniture polish commonly contains mineral seal oil, the toxic effects of which are similar to those of gasoline (see Section I-19-C-36) and kerosene (see Section I-19-C-43).

I–19–C–35. GARBAGE TOXINS

Source

Access to rodents or spoiled food, especially ham, chicken, milk, and some vegetables. Active agents are histamine or staphylococcus toxins or enterotoxins or *Cl. botulinum* toxin.

Signs

Staph enterotoxin: nausea, prostration, abdominal pain and diarrhea within four hours. Rarely fatal.

Staph lethal toxin: Unsteadiness, dyspnea, and violent convulsions within five to 15 minutes to 24 hours. Fatal *Cl. botulinum* toxin: motor paralysis, coma, death.

Treatment

Staph toxins:
1. Enemas and lavage.
2. Fluid support.
3. Nothing specific.

Cl. botulinum toxin: Antitoxin if early in course. Dogs are fairly resistant to botulism.

I-19-C-36. GASOLINE

Source

Inhalation, swallowing, or contact of large areas of the body with gasoline can induce toxicosis.

Contact with Skin:

By contact it removes fat and lowers resistance to infection. Absorption from large areas of skin causes systemic toxicity similar to inhalation.

Treatment

1. Wash affected area thoroughly with soap and water.
2. Give symptomatic support.

Inhalation

1. The skin is flushed, the patient ataxic and dazed.
2. Removal of the animal to fresh air at this time may effect recovery.
3. If muscular twitching develops followed by dilated pupils, delirium, and convulsions, the prognosis is poor.
4. Treatment is symptomatic—use oxygen and support circulation and renal function.

Ingestion

1. This is highly irritating and causes salivation, nausea, vomiting, and diarrhea.
2. If absorption has occurred, muscular twitching and seizures may be present.
3. Administer gastric lavage with olive oil followed by warm water. If this is done before absorption has occurred, prognosis is good. Symptomatic care to support respiration and renal function is initiated by giving fluids and antibiotics.

I–19–C–37. HEPTACHLOR

Signs and Treatment

See Section I-19-C-16.

I–19–C–38. HEXACHLOROPHENE

Source

Mainly soaps containing hexachlorophene. Also antiseptic agents, deodorants, etc.

Minimum toxic oral dosage in the dog has been reported to be 13 mg./kg.

Signs

Similar to those in phenol poisoning—nausea, vomiting, abdominal cramping, diarrhea, dehydration, and hypertension. In experiments in which hexachlorophene-containing soaps were fed to dogs, vomiting frequently occurred one to six hours after ingestion, and evidence of toxicity was not seen.

Treatment

1. A specific antidote for hexachlorophene poisoning is not known.
2. Emetics and gastric lavage can be used within the first hour following ingestion.
3. Maintain general supportive treatment, using fluids and anti-convulsants if necessary.

I–19–C–39. HEXAETHYLTETRAPHOSPHATE (HETP)

Signs and Treatment

See Section I-19-C-63.

I-19-C-40. HOMATROPINE

Source

An overdose of ophthalmic and intestinal medications may be given or ingested accidentally.

Signs and treatment are similar to those for atropine (see Section I-19-C-13) except that action is short and recovery is the rule within 12 hours after medication is stopped.

I-19-C-41. ISOPROPYL ALCOHOL (RUBBING ALCOHOL)

Source

Isopropyl alcohol is used as a solvent and in various waxes, perfumes, and cosmetics.

Signs

1. Ataxia and weakness.
2. Slow pulse and low blood pressure.
3. Acute vomiting and diarrhea.
4. Anuria and uremia.

Treatment

1. Early treatment consists of gastric lavage with tap water.
2. Stimulants such as caffeine sodium benzoate, 0.05 gm., may be administered intramuscularly, or sedation induced with pentobarbital or phenobarbital.
3. Subsequent measures may include blood transfusions, glucose injections, or treatment for uremia.

I-19-C-42. IVIES, LARGE LEAF (PHILODENDRON, DIFFENBACHIA)

Source

Animal chews on plant.

Signs

1. Irritation of mucous membranes.
2. Copious salivation; paralysis of tongue.
3. Dyspnea and dysphagia.
4. Debilitation; listlessness.

Treatment

None known other than symptomatic support.

TABLE 13. POTENTIALLY DANGEROUS ORNAMENTAL PLANTS

Common Name	Scientific Name	Toxic Constituent or Characteristic
Amaryllis	*Amaryllis* spp.	Alkaloid
Autumn crocus	*Colchicum autumnale*	Alkaloid
Avocado (some varieties)	*Persea americana*	—
Baptisia	*Baptisia* spp.	Quinolizidine alkaloids
Black-eyed Susan, goldenglow, coneflower	*Rudbeckia* spp.	—
Bleeding heart	*Dicentra spectabilis*	Isoquinoline alkaloids
Bloodroot	*Sanguinaria canadensis*	Isoquinoline alkaloids
Box (hedge)	*Buxus sempervirens*	Alkaloids
Caladium	*Caladium* spp., *Xanthosoma* spp.	Irritant, stomatitis
Candelabra cactus	*Euphorbia lactea*	Irritant sap
Castor bean	*Ricinus communis*	Phytotoxin
Cherry laurel	*Prunus laurocerasus*	HCN
Chinaberry tree	*Melia azedarach*	Resinoid
Christmas rose	*Helleborus niger*	Purgative glycoside
Crown-of-thorns	*Euphorbia millii*	Irritant sap
Daffodil, narcissus	*Narcissus* spp.	—
Daphne	*Daphne* spp.	Irritant glycoside
Dumbcane	*Dieffenbachia* spp.	Irritant, stomatitis
Euonymus	*Euonymus* spp.	Purgative principle
Flax	*Linum usitatissimum*	HCN
Foxglove	*Digitalis purpurea*	Cardioactive glycosides
Fritillaria	*Fritillaria meleagris*	Alkaloids
Glory or climbing lily	*Gloriosa superba*	Alkaloids
Goldenchain, laburnum	*Laburnum anagyroides*	Quinolizidine alkaloids
Horse chestnut	*Aesculus hippocastanum*	Glycosides
Hyacinth	*Hyacinthus orientalis*	—
Hydrangea	*Hydrangea* spp.	—
Iris	*Iris* spp.	Gastrointestinal irritant
Ivy, English	*Hedera helix*	—
Jerusalem cherry	*Solanum pseudocapsicum*	Solanaceous alkaloids
Jessamine	*Cestrum* spp.	Tropane alkaloids
Jimsonweed, thornapple	*Datura metel*	Tropane alkaloids
Lantana	*Lantana camara*	—
Larkspur, delphinium	*Delphinium* spp.	Diterpenoid alkaloids
Laurels	*Kalmia* spp.	Resinoid
Lily-of-the-valley	*Convallaria majalis*	Cardioactive glycosides

TABLE 13. POTENTIALLY DANGEROUS ORNAMENTAL PLANTS
(Continued)

Common Name	Scientific Name	Toxic Constituent or Characteristic
Lobelia, cardinal flower	*Lobelia* spp.	Alkaloids
Lupine, bluebonnet	*Lupinus* spp.	Quinolizidine alkaloids
Mistletoe	*Phoradendron flavescens*	Amines
Monkshood, aconite	*Aconitum* spp.	Diterpenoid alkaloids
Oleander	*Nerium oleander*	Cardioactive glycosides
Pencil tree	*Euphorbia tirucalli*	Irritant sap
Poinciana	*Poinciana gilliesii*	Irritant substance
Poinsettia	*Euphorbia pulcherrima*	Irritant sap
Poppy	*Papaver* spp.	Isoquinoline alkaloids
Precatory bean (seeds)	*Abrus precatorius*	Phytotoxin
Privet	*Ligustrum vulgare*	—
Rhododendron	*Rhododendron* spp.	Resinoid
Rhubarb	*Rheum rhaponticum*	Oxalates
Snowdrop	*Galanthus nivalis*	—
Snow-on-the-mountain	*Euphorbia marginata*	Irritant sap
Spurges	*Euphorbia* spp.	Irritant sap
Star-of-Bethlehem	*Ornithogalum umbellatum*	Alkaloids
Tansy	*Tanacetum vulgare*	Vesicant oil
Tobacco, flowering	*Nicotiana tabacum*	Nicotine
Virginia creeper	*Parthenocissus quinquefolia*	—
Wisteria	*Wisteria* spp.	Gastrointestinal irritant
Yew	*Taxus* spp.	Alkaloid

I–19–C–43. KEROSENE

Source

Kerosene is used as a fuel, solvent, and cleaning agent. It is also a common vehicle for insecticides and garden sprays, and is highly toxic.

Signs

1. Vomiting and diarrhea.
2. Circulatory collapse.
3. Depression and coma (sometimes convulsions).
4. Aspiration pneumonia is a common sequela.

Treatment

1. Gastric lavage, if vomiting was not profuse.
2. Sodium sulfate laxative (0.3 gm./lb.) by mouth.

3. Oxygen therapy if needed (see Section IV-20).
4. Caffeine sodium benzoate, 0.05 gm. intramuscularly, if needed.
5. Treatment for pneumonia that may follow.

I-19-C-44.   LEAD SALTS (LEAD ARSENATE)

Source

Lead salts are present in insecticides, linoleum, golf balls, paint, lead sinkers, putty, ceramics, and poorly glazed china. The toxicosis is commoner than is usually realized. Toxic dose for the dog is 10 to 25 mg./kg.

Signs

1. Vomiting, diarrhea, colic, anorexia, anemia, hemoglobinuria.
2. Neurologic signs that usually predominate are irritability, hysteria, listlessness, blindness, convulsions, paralysis, and coma.
3. Blood levels above 0.8 ppm. or urine levels above 10 ppm. are indicative of toxicosis.

Treatment

1. Lead poisoning is usually chronic in nature. If onset is recent, emetics and saline laxative may be used to prevent absorption.
2. Administer CaEDTA, 12 mg./lb. every six hours subcutaneously for five days. Commercial preparations of CaEDTA should be diluted to 10 mg./ml. to minimize pain at the injection site.
3. Barbiturate sedation may be needed to control neurologic irritability.
4. Parenteral fluids or oral alimentation are necessary measures in supportive therapy.

I-19-C-45.   LIME (CALCIUM OXIDE, UNSLAKED LIME, BURNT OR QUICKLIME)

Slaked lime is harmless, but quicklime is a potent caustic that liberates heat when exposed to moisture.

Signs and Treatment

See Section I-19-C-4.

I–19–C–46. LINDANE

Signs and Treatment

See Section I-19-C-16.

I–19–C–47. LYE

Source

Lye is a term applied to strong alkalies (sodium hydroxide, potassium hydroxide) and is found in washing powders, pipe cleaners, and paint removers.

Signs and Treatment

See Section I-19-C-4.

I–19–C–48. MALATHION

Source

Malathion is an insecticide of relatively low toxicity.

Signs and Treatment

See Section I-19-C-63.

I–19–C–49. MATCHES

Source

Safety matches (phosphorus trisulfide or sesquisulfide) are inert and relatively harmless. The phosphorus compound is on the striking surface of the box.

"Strike anywhere" matches contain potassium chlorate, antimony sulfide, and phosphorus, and are toxic.

Signs and Treatment

See Section I-19-C-69.

I-19-C-50. METALDEHYDE

Source

This toxic material is used for snail baits or in compressed tablets to fuel small heaters.

Signs

1. Lack of coordination; anxiety.
2. Muscle tremors which may be continuous.
3. Muscle spasms (like those observed in strychnine poisoning but not accentuated by auditory or tactile stimulation).

Treatment

1. General anesthesia to control spasms (Surital followed by Metofane or pentobarbital).
2. Thorough gastric lavage with tap water.
3. Administer bismuth-pectin solution orally for gastritis.
4. Administer intravenously sodium lactate, one-sixth molar, 10 ml./lb., to combat acidosis.
5. Maintain anesthesia from 12 to 24 hours (to 72 hours, if necessary).
6. Prognosis is fair.

I-19-C-51. METHOXYCHLOR

Source

Used as a relatively nontoxic chlorinated hydrocarbon insecticide.

Signs and Treatment

See Sections I-19-C-16 and I-19-C-23.

I–19–C–52. METHYL ALCOHOL (METHANOL, WOOD ALCOHOL, CARBINON, WOOD NAPHTHA, COLONIAL SPIRIT)

Source

Methyl alcohol is used as a solvent, antifreeze, and fuel, and is highly toxic if taken internally.

Signs

1. Nausea, vomiting, and gastric pain.
2. Reflex hyperexcitability with opisthotonus and convulsions.
3. Fixed pupils.
4. Acute peripheral neuritis.

Treatment

1. Emetics like apomorphine 20 μg./lb. intravenously.
2. Gastric lavage with sodium bicarbonate, 4 per cent.
3. Sodium sulfate as saline laxative, 0.3 gm./lb. orally.
4. Meperidine hydrochloride to control pain.
5. Oxygen therapy and caffeine sodium benzoate, 0.05 gm. intramuscularly.
6. Sodium bicarbonate solution, intravenously.
7. Prognosis is very poor.

I–19–C–53. METHYL BROMIDE

Source

This volatile liquid is used in fire extinguishers and as an insecticide and a refrigerant. Inhalation of fumes is toxic within four to eight hours; topical application causes primary irritation.

Signs

1. Nausea, vomiting, and gastric pain.
2. Depression and weakness.
3. Muscular twitching and temporary paralysis.
4. Temporary blindness.
5. Convulsions.
6. Pulmonary edema and circulatory collapse.

Treatment

1. Remove subject from exposure.
2. Wash skin with soap and water if topical contact was made.
3. Administer oxygen if indicated.
4. Give barbiturate sedation for seizures.
5. Use caffeine sodium benzoate or metaraminol bitartrate (Aramine) for circulatory collapse.
6. Watch for pulmonary edema and treat as needed (see Section I-20-B).

I–19–C–54. MORPHINE

Source

Intoxication is usually iatrogenically caused. The drug is especially toxic to cats in doses usually suggested for dogs (0.5 to 1.0 mg./lb.).

Signs

1. Pinpoint, nonreactive pupils.
2. Lowered body temperature and depressed respirations (collapse).
3. In cats, severe CNS stimulation and convulsions.

Treatment

1. Give atropine sulfate, 0.05 mg./lb., either intravenously or intramuscularly.
2. Nalorphine hydrochloride acts as a specific antagonist (but not in cats), and can be administered intravenously, 2 to 5 mg.
3. If required, support respiration by oxygen therapy (see Section IV-20).
4. Administer intramuscularly caffeine sodium benzoate, 0.05 gm.

I-19-C-55. MUSCARINE (MUSHROOM POISONING)

Source

Muscarine is a toxic alkaloid present in certain varieties of mushrooms. It has a latent period of one to three hours.

Signs

Rapid onset of parasympathetic stimulation:
1. Lacrimation and salivation.
2. Miosis.
3. Dyspnea and abdominal pain.
4. Vomiting and diarrhea.
5. Muscle paralysis.

Treatment

1. Induce vomiting and perform gastric lavage using potassium permanganate diluted 1:2000 (see Section I-19-A).
2. Administer atropine sulfate (0.05 mg./lb.); repeat dose hourly until effect is evident.
3. Administer saline laxative (sodium sulfate, 0.3 gm./lb.).

I-19-C-56. MYCOTOXIN OF ASPERGILLUS OR PENICILLIUM

Source

Ingestion of grain or food contaminated with mycotoxin. Need repeated exposure within 20 to 30 days.

Signs

1. Anorexia, listlessness.
2. Icterus (fatty degeneration of liver and bile duct proliferation).
3. Weakness, prostration.

Treatment

None, other than symptomatic support.

I-19-C-57. NAPHTHALENE

Source

Naphthalene is the toxic ingredient in mothballs and insect repellents.

Signs

1. Nausea and vomiting.
2. Severe depression.
3. Subsequent development of hemolytic signs.

Treatment

1. Induce vomiting (apomorphine or hydrogen peroxide).
2. Give demulcents (egg white) orally.
3. Force fluids orally or by injection to improve urine output.
4. Avoid administering fatty substances orally.
5. Blood transfusions may be needed during the hemolytic stage.

I-19-C-58. NEUROTOXIN OF DERMACENTOR VARIABILIS

Source

Tick releases neurotoxin into dermis.

Signs

1. Onset when tick is fully engorged with blood. Recovery 24 to 96 hours after tick is removed.
2. Weakness or complete flaccid paralysis.

Treatment

1. Remove tick carefully.
2. Dip dog in acaricidal solution.
3. Symptomatic nursing care.

I-19-C-59. NEUROTOXIN OF TOADS OR LIZARDS

Source

Saliva from parotid gland of *Bufo marinus* or *Bufo alvarius* is ingested. The blue tail lizard and the Gila monster are also poisonous.

Signs

1. Toxin absorbed by oral mucosa.
2. Onset within minutes; death may occur within 15 to 20 minutes.
3. Salivation, head shaking.
4. Prostration, convulsions.

Treatment

1. Atropine, 0.25 to 1.0 mg. subcutaneously.
2. Prednisolone, 0.5 to 10 mg./lb. intramuscularly.
3. Tranquilization or sedation as needed (propriopromazine or mepenidine at bedtime).

I-19-C-60. NITROBENZENE

Source

This is a common ingredient in shoe polish and dyes and is often combined with aniline dyes.

Signs

1. Vertigo and ataxia.
2. Nausea and vomiting.
3. Dyspnea and cyanosis.
4. Convulsions and coma.

Treatment

1. Administer emetics, followed by gastric lavage with sodium chloride, 0.9 per cent.

2. If required, provide oxygen therapy.

3. Administer fluids intravenously to improve urine output.

4. Give saline laxatives (sodium sulfate, 0.3 gm./lb.).

5. If patient is cyanotic, inject intravenously 3 to 10 ml. of methylene blue, 1 per cent, in sodium sulfate solution, 1.8 per cent.

I–19–C–61. OLEANDER (NERIUM OLEANDER LINNEUS)

Source

This ornamental shrub contains glycosides acting on cardiac muscle. The active principles of oleander are oleandrin, neriine, and other glycosides.

Signs

1. Autonomic and central nervous system symptoms.
2. Myocarditis.
3. Gastrointestinal tract irritation.
4. Pronounced salivation and vomiting.
5. Muscular tremors, uneasiness.
6. Frequent defecation, urination.
7. Bradycardia and/or sinus arrest.
8. Ectopic heart beats progressed to deficient grade and A-V block.

Treatment

Atropine, 0.035 to 0.07 mg./kg., and propranolol, 0.5 to 2.0 mg./kg., two to six doses of each agent over a 24-hour period.

I–19–C–62. OPIUM (LAUDANUM, PAREGORIC)

See Section I-19-C-54.

I-19-C-63. ORGANIC PHOSPHATES [TRITHION, CIODRIN, COUMAPHOS (CO-ROL), DICHLORVOS (DDVP, VAPONA), DIAZINON (ETHION), DIMETHOATE (CYGON), DIOXATHION (DELNAV), THION, FENTHION, IMIDRAN, MALATHION, PARATHION, PHOSPHAMIDON, RONNEL (ECTORAL), RUELENE, TRICHLORFON (NEGUVON, FREED, DYREX, DYLOX, DIPTEREX)]

Source

These are acetylcholinesterase inhibitors used as insecticides or systemic parasiticidal agents.

Signs

1. Signs vary depending on the drug, dose received, and individual sensitivity.
2. Salivation, muscle fasciculations, and tremors.
3. Ataxia and convulsions.
4. Vomiting and diarrhea.
5. Miosis, lacrimation, excessive respiratory secretions, broncho-constriction, dyspnea, cyanosis.

Treatment

1. Administer intravenously atropine sulfate, 0.02 mg./lb. Repeat dose at once subcutaneously. Repeat dose as needed (every one to two hours) to control excessive muscarinic activity. Large doses of atropine may be needed frequently to produce atropinization.
2. Administer 2-pyridine aldoxime methyl (2-PAM) iodide, 20 mg./lb. intravenously, over a period of more than two minutes. The dosage can be repeated in 12 hours if necessary. Administration of 2-PAM is contraindicated in carbamate (Sevin) toxicity.
3. If the medication was applied topically, wash the skin with soap and water.
4. If the medication was ingested, give saline laxative.

5. Sedation with barbiturates may be needed if the patient is excited or convulsing.

6. Support treatment with fluids and oral alimentation.

I-19-C-64. ORTHODICHLOROBENZENE

Source

This material is used as a wood preservative.

Signs and Treatment

See Section I-19-C-57.

I-19-C-65. OXALIC ACID

Source

Oxalic acid is the active agent in bleaches, cleaning agents, ink eradicators, and the leaves of rhubarb. Do not treat as a typical acid poison.

Signs

1. Erosion of mouth and esophagus.
2. Bloody vomitus and profuse diarrhea.
3. Severe dehydration.

Treatment

1. By mouth give calcium lactate chalk solution, egg white, or olive oil. *Do not give alkalies*.

2. Give apomorphine as an emetic (20 μg./lb. intravenously).

3. Repeat step number 1.

4. Control pain with meperidine hydrochloride or use morphine sulfate as emetic *and* analgesic.

5. If needed, support circulation with ephedrine sulfate or metaraminol bitartrate.

6. Be prepared to do a tracheotomy if pharynx or glottis is eroded and edematous.

I–19–C–66. PAINT REMOVERS

See:
Acetone, Section I-19-C-10.
Benzene, Section I-19-C-15.
Carbon tetrachloride, Section I-19-C-20.
Lye, Section I-19-C-47.
Methyl alcohol, Section I-19-C-52.
Turpentine, Section I-19-C-86.

I–19–C–67. PARIS GREEN

See Section I-19-C-11.

I–19–C–68. PHENOL (CARBOLIC ACID)

Source

Phenol is used for cautery or as a germicide. It may be toxic topically or by ingestion, especially to cats.

Signs

1. Odor of phenol.
2. Skin or mucous membranes become white.
3. Nausea, vomiting, and severe abdominal pain.
4. Circulatory collapse.

Treatment

1. Remove the poison:
a. Wash skin with tap water, then neutralize phenol by rinsing affected area with alcohol, 10 per cent.
b. Administer lavage, using either tap water or alcohol, 5 to 10 per cent.
2. Give olive oil by mouth.
3. Inject intravenously lactated Ringer's solution.
4. Support circulation by intramuscular injection of caffeine sodium benzoate, 0.05 gm.

I-19-C-69. PHOSPHORUS

Source

Phosphorus is an ingredient in rat or roach poisons, fireworks, imported or "strike anywhere" matches, or on the striking surface of books of safety matches.

Signs

1. Garlic odor.
2. Vomiting and diarrhea; vomitus may be luminescent.
3. Severe abdominal pain.
4. Circulatory collapse.
5. Liver damage and hemorrhage are seen three days after initial recovery.

Treatment

1. Administer an emetic followed by a gastric lavage using copper sulfate solution, 1 per cent. Follow this by lavage with potassium permanganate solution diluted 1:2000.
2. Administer mineral oil orally.
3. Administer a solution of dextrose in saline, 5 per cent, 20 ml./lb., intravenously or subcutaneously.

I-19-C-70. PINE OIL

Source

Pine oil is a complex terpene alcohol that causes hemorrhagic gastritis, central nervous system depression, and respiratory failure.

Treatment

See Section I-19-C-86.

I-19-C-71. POTASSIUM OXALATE

Source

Potassium oxalate is the active agent in many cleaning and bleaching formulas.

Signs

1. Salivation, dysphagia, and edema of the glottis.
2. Vomiting and severe abdominal pain.
3. Muscular fibrillation and circulatory collapse.
4. Uremic convulsions.

Treatment

1. Administer orally either a chalk solution or calcium lactate.
2. Administer a gastric lavage with lime water.
3. Leave magnesium sulfate in stomach.
4. Administer intravenously calcium gluconate solution 10 per cent, 3 to 10 ml.
5. Force fluid intake or injection to improve urine output and prevent oxalate crystalluria.

I-19-C-72. PYRETHRUM

Source

By itself pyrethrum is not dangerous, but it is almost always mixed with insecticides or vehicles which *are* dangerous.

I-19-C-73. QUATERNARY AMMONIUM SALTS (BENZALKONIUM CHLORIDE)

Source

Dilute solutions (0.01 to 1.0 per cent) are used as antiseptics, deodorants, and fungicides.

Signs

1. Large amounts of concentrated solutions cause pain in the mouth and stomach.
2. Restlessness, dyspnea, and cyanosis.
3. Muscle weakness and circulatory collapse.

Treatment

1. Give an emetic followed by gastric lavage with milk or soapy water.
2. Administer demulcents (milk, egg white) orally.
3. Administer pentobarbital for seizures.
4. If required, provide oxygen therapy.

I-19-C-74. RED SQUILL

Source

Red squill is used as a rodenticide.

Signs and Treatment

See Section I-19-C-29.

I-19-C-75. RESORCINOL

In its effects and reactions, resorcinol is similar to, but not as severe as, phenol (see Section I-19-C-68).

I-19-C-76. RICIN OF CASTOR BEAN

Source

Animal fertilizer that contains meat meal and castor bean meal. Toxin is absorbed and may produce immunity.

Signs

1. Nausea, violent diarrhea.
2. Dull, ataxic, tetanic spasms.
3. Pounding pulse.

Treatment

1. Specific antisera.
2. Sedative, fluids.
3. Treat shock.

I–19–C–77. ROACH PASTES

See Sections I-19-C-11 and I-19-C-84.

I–19–C–78. RODENTICIDES

See:
Arsenic, Section I-19-C-11.
Red Squill, Section I-19-C-74.
Strychnine, Section I-19-C-82.
Thallium, Section I-19-C-84.
Warfarin, Section I-19-C-87.
Zinc phosphide, Section I-19-C-88.

I–19–C–79. SHELLAC

Source

Shellac contains rosin, arsenic, and alcohol.

Treatment

See Sections I-19-C-11 and I-19-C-52.

I–19–C–80. SOAPS AND DETERGENTS

Source

White, unperfumed soaps are relatively harmless even in massive amounts. Perfumes and coloring additives may cause nausea and diarrhea. Laundry soaps contain sufficient caustic alkali to be toxic (see Section I-19-C-4). Hexachlorophene soaps like ''Dial'' are highly toxic if ingested. Detergents are divided into three classes:

Class I. Light-duty, high-sudsing formulas for dishes and delicate laundry; slightly toxic.

Class II. All-purpose high-sudsing formulas for general laundry; moderately toxic.

Class III. Automatic laundry, low-sudsing formulas for machine use; relatively high toxicity.

Treatment

Class I and II detergents:
1. Induce vomiting if it has not occurred.
2. Administer demulcents like olive oil or milk.
3. Administer intravenously calcium gluconate solution, 10 per cent, 3 to 10 ml.

Class III detergents:
1. Induce vomiting.
2. Administer gastric lavage with copious amounts of water.
3. If needed, provide oxygen therapy.
4. If required, perform a tracheotomy.
5. If needed, treat pulmonary edema.

I–19–C–81. SPIDER BITES (BLACK WIDOW OR BROWN RECLUSE SPIDERS)

Source

Spiders inhabit woodpiles, old buildings and refuse areas. Onset of signs within one hour.

Signs

1. Cutaneous edema, hyperemia and pain in local area of bite.
2. Pain in muscles, joints and abdomen.
3. Occasionally nausea, weakness, fever, hemoglobinuria.

Treatment

1. Enforce rest with sedative analgesics, such as meperidine.
2. Apply cold packs to local area.
3. Give calcium gluconate, 10 per cent (1 to 10 cc.), intravenously.

4. Give prednisone, 0.5 to 1.0 mg./lb., intramuscularly (symptomatic relief only).

5. Antihistamines have been used.

6. Recovery is usually complete in 24 hours.

I–19–C–82. STRYCHNINE

Source

Strychnine is used in rat poison and in some of the older patent medicines. Toxic dose for a dog is 0.75 mg./kg. Onset within 15 minutes to two hours after exposure.

Signs

1. Dyspnea and cyanosis. Dilated pupils. Rapid weak pulse.
2. Tonus, clonus, and opisthotonus.
3. Respiratory paralysis and death.
4. Seizures initiated by noise or touch.

Treatment

1. *If no signs of toxicity are evident,* induce evacuation of stomach contents by intravenous injection of apomorphine, $20\mu g$. Subsequently, potassium permanganate 1:4000 or tannic acid, 1 or 2 per cent, can be given orally to neutralize any residual strychnine.

2. If nervous stimulation is evident, anesthetize the patient intravenously with pentobarbital.

3. Administer gastric lavage to empty stomach.

4. Keep animal heavily sedated in a quiet dark cage for as long as 48 hours.

5. Do not use caffeine, opiates, synthetic narcotics, cathartics, or diuretics.

I–19–C–83. TAR

All derivatives of tar are toxic because of their cresol content (see Section I-19-C-68).

I-19-C-84.   THALLIUM

Source

Thallium is the active ingredient in certain rat, ant, and roach poisons, and in depilatory creams.

Signs

1. Doses of 2.5 mg./lb. may be lethal to dogs.
2. Chronic toxicity is evidenced by skin lesions, hair loss, erythema, and necrosis of the skin near the mucocutaneous junctions and in friction areas. Ten days or longer for onset.
3. More acute toxicity begins with diarrhea, salivation, and vomiting. Mucous membranes may ulcerate and dyspnea, muscle weakness, and even convulsions may occur. One to four days for onset.
4. Confirming diagnosis can be based on chemical analysis of thallium in the urine.

Treatment

1. Recently, prussian blue (potassium ferric hexacyanoferrate II) has been utilized in experimental animals and in man to treat thallium poisoning. Prussian blue is administered orally, 0.2 gm./lb./day (suggested dose) subdivided into three doses. The drug binds thallium in the intestinal tract, preventing reabsorption. Good gastrointestinal motility must be present for Prussian blue and bound thallium to be eliminated.
2. Diphenylthiocarbazone (35 mg./lb.) and diethyldithiocarbamate (15 mg./lb.) orally every eight hours, as well as potassium chloride (2 to 6 gm. daily) orally have been helpful in enhancing thallium excretion and may also be useful. Clinical experience has been disappointing, however.
3. Perform peritoneal dialysis (see Section IV-16-G).
4. Administer sodium bicarbonate orally and force patient to take fluids orally or parenterally.
5. The clinical course of the poisoning lasts from seven to 21 days and prognosis in acute cases is poor.

I–19–C–85. THIOCYANATES (SULFOCYANATES, LETHANE, THANITE)

Source

Organic (aliphatic) derivatives are used as contact insecticides with kerosene or toluene vehicles.

Treatment

For methyl, ethyl, and isopropyl thiocyanate poisoning, see Section I-19-C-24. For all other thiocyanates treat as follows:

1. Administer gastric lavage, first with copious amounts of tap water, then with mineral oil.
2. Leave some mineral oil and sodium sulfate, 0.3 gm./lb., in the stomach.
3. Use pentobarbital to combat convulsions.
4. If needed, provide oxygen therapy.

I–19–C–86. TURPENTINE

Source

Turpentine is used as a common solvent and vehicle. Toxicity due to various terpenes may be caused by inhalation, ingestion, or cutaneous absorption.

Signs

1. Characteristic odor.
2. Severe abdominal pain, vomiting, and diarrhea.
3. Hematuria, proteinuria, and violet odor to urine.
4. Coma resulting in death from respiratory failure.

Treatment

1. Give liquid petrolatum by mouth.
2. Give gastric lavage with weak sodium bicarbonate solution.
3. Administer barbiturates to curb excitement.
4. Administer a sodium sulfate laxative orally (0.3 gm./lb.).

5. Give paregoric (3 to 4 ml.) for intestinal pain.
6. Force fluids by mouth or by injection.

I-19-C-87. WARFARIN [3-(Δ-ACETONYL-BENZYL)-4-HYDROXYCOUMARIN], PINDONE

Source

Warfarin is used as a rodenticide. Toxic dose: single, 20 to 50 mg./kg. Warfarin; 75 to 100 mg. Pindone. Multiple dose, 1 to 5 mg./kg. for five to 15 days.

Signs

1. Depression, fever, multiple hemorrhages associated with increased blood clotting time.
2. Ecchymosis of skin and conjunctiva, anemia, weak rapid pulse.
3. Dyspnea and, in the terminal stage, asphyxial convulsions, paralysis.
4. Death in one to 10 days.

Treatment

1. Give fresh, whole blood transfusions.
2. Administer intravenously a stable emulsion of Vitamin K_1 in dextrose, 5 per cent. Dosage ranges from 10 mg. to 25 mg.
3. Ascorbic acid may be helpful during recovery.
4. Keep patient warm and quiet.

I-19-C-88. ZINC PHOSPHIDE

Source

Zinc phosphide is used as a rodenticide. Toxic dose is 20 to 40 mg./kg.

Signs

    1. Vomiting and diarrhea, abdominal pain.
    2. Acute dyspnea and pulmonary edema.
    3. Tonic convulsions, coma.

Treatment

    1. Give emetics and gastric lavage with potassium permanganate solution diluted 1:2000.
    2. Allow patient to rest in an oxygen chamber.
    3. Give an intravenous injection of dextrose (5 per cent) in saline unless pulmonary edema has developed (see Section I-20-B).
    4. Administer caffeine sodium benzoate (0.05 gm.) intramuscularly.
    5. No specific or effective treatment.

I–19–D. Poisonous Substances in Common Household Items*

Polishes and Waxes for Furniture and Floors

Petroleum Distillates

Kerosene
Mineral seal oil
Mineral spirits
Naphtha, high boiling
Spindle oil
Stoddard solvent
Summer black oil

Other Toxic Substances

Antimony chloride
Caustic alkali
Cellosolve
Isopropyl and butyl alcohols
Nitrobenzene
Oxalic acid
Turpentine

Paint Solvents and Related Products

*Paint Brush Cleaners
and Preservatives*

Acetone
Caustic alkalis
Cresols and higher phenols
Dipentene
Methanol

*Removers of Paint, Wax,
Lacquers, Grease Spots*

Amyl acetate
Alcohols—amyl, butyl, ethyl
Amylene dichloride
Benzene
Butyl acetate

*Adapted from *American Druggist*. From Kirk, R. W. (ed.): Current Veterinary Therapy V, Philadelphia, W. B. Saunders Co., 1974.

Naphthalene
Sodium chromate
Toluol
Turpentine

Paints, Putty, Varnishes

Arsenic
Chromium
Iron
Lead
Titanium
Zinc

Carbon tetrachloride
Caustic alkalis
Ethyl acetate
Ethylene dichloride
Kerosene
Methyl alcohol
Methylene chloride
Toluene

Cleaning, Polishing and Bleaching Agents

Dry Cleaning Fluids

Acetone
Amyl acetate
Benzene
Carbon tetrachloride
Ethylene dichloride
Kerosene
Methyl alcohol
Naphtha, heavy petroleum
Petroleum distillates
Stoddard solvent
Toluene
Trichlorethylene

Detergents for Dishware,
Glassware, Laundry

Strong Alkaline Solutions

Sodium hydroxide
Sodium metasilicate
Sodium perborate
Sodium phosphate glass
Tetrasodium phosphate

Others

Ethylene glycol
Sodium hypochlorite

Metal Cleaners and Polishes

Strong Acids & Alkalis

Ammonia water, caustic soda
Hydrochloric acid, dilute
Phosphoric acid, dilute
Soda ash
Sulfamic acid
Sulfuric acid, dilute

Others

Alkyl aryl sulfonate
Oxalic acid
Potassium chlorate
Potassium cyanide
Thiourea

Cosmetic Preparations

Skin Tonics and Lotions

Aluminum salts
Camphor or menthol
Methylated spirits
Zinc phenolsulfonate
Zinc sulfate

Sun Tan Lotions

Denatured alcohol
Methyl salicylate
Para-aminobenzoic acid esters

Hair Preparations

Brilliantines

Industrial methylated spirit
  (contains wood naphtha)
Kerosene deodorized

Permanent Wave Solutions

Sodium carbonate
Sodium sulfite
Thioglycollate salts

Neutralizers

Acetic acid
Potassium bromate
Sodium hexametaphosphate
Sodium perborate

Lacquers

Denatured alcohol
Shellac resin

Hair Dyes, Tints, Colorings

Ammonium hydroxide
Ammonium nitrate
Metallic dyes
Para-phenylenediamine
Pyrogallol
Sodium hypochlorite sol.

Shampoos

Denatured alcohol
Sodium hexametaphosphate

Hair Lotions

Beta-naphthol
Cantharidin
Denatured ethyl alcohol
Glacial acetic acid
Industrial methylated spirit
Isopropyl alcohol
Pilocarpine
Salicylic acid
Tertiary butyl alcohol

Depilatories

Calcium thioglycollate
Soluble sulfides

Nail Preparations

Organic Solvents

Alcohols—ethyl, isopropyl *n*-butyl
Esters
Ketones

Lacquers
Plasticizers, Resins

Dibutyl phthalate
Nitrocellulose
Sulfonamide resins

Cuticle Removers

Dilute caustic alkalis

Other Types of Household Products and Chemicals

Antifreeze, Carburetor Cleaners

Chlorinated benzene
Alcohols—denatured, isopropyl,
    methyl
Ethylene glycol

Deodorizing Tablets

Formaldehyde

Anti-Rust Products

Ammonium sulfide
Hydrofluoric acid
Naphtha
Oxalic acid

*Leather Preservatives, Polishes
    and Dyes*

Benzene
Methanol
Neatsfoot oil
Naphtha
Talloil

Shoe Cleaners and Polishes

Nitrobenzene
Shellac
Titanium dioxide
Turpentine

Inks

Iron gallate
Phenol
Silver nitrate
Soda ash

*Jewelry and Watch
    Cleaners and Cements*

Ammonia
Isopropyl alcohol
Nitrocellulose in ketone
Petroleum solvent

Fire Extinguishing Fluids

Carbon tetrachloride
Naphtha

Typewriter Cleaner

Cellosolve
Methanol

Laundry Blue

Prussian blue
Oxalic acid

Rug Adhesives

Latex
Sulfur zinc oxide
Synthetic rubber

Plastic Menders, Glues

Cellulose acetate
Ethylene dichloride
Formaldehyde
Nitrocellulose

Wax Crayons

Para red

Christmas Bulb Fluid

Methylene chloride

References

Additional information may be found in the following sources:

Aronson, A. L.: General approach to the treatment of poisoning. *In* Kirk, R. W. (ed.): Current Veterinary Therapy V. Philadelphia, W. B. Saunders Co., 1974.

Aronson, A. L.: Chemical poisonings in small animal practice. Vet. Clin. North Amer., Vol. 2, No. 2, May, 1972.

Flint, T., Jr.: Emergency Treatment and Management, 4th ed. Philadelphia, W. B. Saunders Co., 1970.

Radeleff, R. D.: Veterinary Toxicology. Philadelphia, Lea and Febiger, 1964.

Scott, D. W., Bolton, G. R., and Lorenz, M. D.: Hexachlorophene toxicosis in dogs. J.A.V.M.A., *162*:947–949, 1973.

Wacker, W. E., Haynes, H., Druyan, R., et al: Treatment of ethylene glycol poisoning with ethyl alcohol. J.A.M.A. *194*:1231–1233, December, 1965.

I–20. RESPIRATORY EMERGENCIES

Respiratory emergencies threaten the life of the clinical patient by producing severe hypoxia or hypercarbia. The conditions most often encountered are obstruction to airflow in the respiratory tract, lack of pulmonary expansion or collapse, interference with alveolar gaseous exchange and altered pulmonary circulation.

I–20–A. Epistaxis

Severe epistaxis may result from trauma to the nasal area, nasal tumors, coagulation disorders, or violent sneezing. Epistaxis and resultant nasal blockage may be well tolerated for a short period of time. More prolonged epistaxis can interfere with normal respiration because of the development of anemic hypoxia and the aspiration of blood into the respiratory passageways.

In the initial treatment of epistaxis, place ice packs over the nasal passages, utilize tranquilizers to sedate the animal and lower blood pressure, and place tampons soaked with 1:10,000 epinephrine in the nasal passages. Protracted epistaxis requires a more complete diagnostic workup for blood coagulation (see Section V-3-J) and radiographs of the nasal passageways.

I–20–B. Obstructions

Obstructions from tumors, trauma, deformities, infection, and foreign bodies are found in small animals. All are serious, and those that have an acute onset require immediate care.

Foreign bodies can often be removed from the nose or pharynx with an alligator forceps. General anesthesia is usually needed, particularly if the foreign object is in the trachea or larynx. In any obstructive emergency, always be prepared to pass a small endotracheal tube (see Section IV-23) or perform a tracheotomy and administer oxygen (see Sections IV-22 and IV-24-A).

Foreign objects lodged in the trachea are small and often act like a ball valve, causing episodic collapse or anoxia. In attempting to remove these objects, suspend the patient with the head down. The object may be situated just posterior to the larynx, and a sharp blow to the head or chest may dislodge it.

Deformities like prolapsed lateral ventricles; laryngeal collapse, bilateral laryngeal muscle paresis and paralysis due to recurrent nerve injury, section or degeneration; elongation of the soft palate; or stenotic nares may produce acute difficulties that can be corrected only by appropriate surgery.

Fractures of the hyoid bones, trauma to the larynx, tracheal collapse, edema, chemical burns, and tumors all produce obstruction and possible anoxia. Severe inspiratory stridor with cyanosis that becomes more severe with effort suggests laryngeal obstruction. A tracheotomy may have to be performed for temporary relief until definitive treatment can be accomplished. Tracheal collapse may present as an acute respiratory emergency in small breeds, particularly Chihuahuas, Pomeranians, miniature poodles and Yorkshire terriers. The condition is exacerbated by excitement, elevated environmental temperature and overexertion. A cool oxygen tent, humidification and tranquilization are very beneficial. Additionally, corticosteroids and aminophylline, 2 to 4 mg./lb. intravenously, should be administered.

Infections and tumors rarely cause acute obstructions. Treatment should be decided on only after a careful diagnostic appraisal.

I-20-C. Pulmonary Edema

Although pulmonary edema develops as a secondary complication usually as a sequela to left heart failure, acute smoke inhalation, or electrocution, immediate treatment to supply the oxygen requirements and support circulation (and thereby prevent more transudation) are essential emergency procedures.

1. Administer oxygen effectively in a chamber (see Section IV-20).
2. To reduce frothing, nebulize ethyl alcohol (12 per cent) into the chamber.

3. Administer morphine sulfate, 0.1 mg./lb. subcutaneously.

4. If the patient has congestive heart failure, administer digitalis glycosides and injectable mercurial diuretics (see Section I-8-C).

5. If anaphylaxis is present, inject full doses of epinephrine, antihistamines and corticosteroids.

6. If organic phosphate poisoning or brain damage has occurred with attendant bradycardia, small doses of atropine may be repeated frequently.

I–20–D. Anaphylactic Shock

1. Immediately inject epinephrine hydrochloride, 0.1 to 0.5 ml. diluted 1:1000, intravenously.

2. Give an intravenous injection of hydrocortisone sodium succinate (50 to 100 mg.) and repeat in four to six hours.

3. Systemic use of an antihistaminic drug is desirable.

4. Administer oxygen in a chamber (see Section IV-20).

I–20–E. Pneumothorax

Presence of air within the pleural cavity is called pneumothorax. It is classified as (1) open pneumothorax—an open chest wound; (2) closed pneumothorax—tears in the visceral pleura; (3) valvular pneumothorax—air entering the pleural cavity during inspiration, which leads to (4) tension pneumothorax; (5) traumatic pneumothorax—frequently associated with rib fractures and possibly hemothorax; and (6) bilateral pneumothorax—from extensive unilateral injuries to the pleura and lung.

Pneumothorax results in dyspnea, diminished breath sounds and hyperresonance to percussion. Radiographs of the chest reveal collapse of one or more lobes of the lung, free air surrounding the dorsal borders of the lung and a dorsal shift of the heart.

1. Treatment should be aimed at reestablishing negative pressure in the thorax. In mild cases, cage rest and avoidance of heavy exertion may be curative within several days.

2. Perform thoracentesis (see Section IV-7) and remove air until dyspnea is relieved. Small, visceral pleural tears often will seal following removal of air from thorax. If dyspnea returns because of a recurrent pneumothorax, the use of a chest tube and Heimlich valve may be indi-

cated so that air will be removed over a protracted period of time. Repeated episodes of pneumothorax that are uncontrollable call for an exploratory thoracotomy.

3. If dyspnea is severe and the tidal volume low, the patient may benefit from resting in an oxygen chamber for 24 to 48 hours.

4. Systemic treatment with antibiotics is indicated.

I–20–F. Rib Fractures (See also Section I–22–E).

Fractures of one or more ribs are uncommon. Fracture of a series of ribs in more than one place may destroy the normal function of the chest wall, so that there is chest wall movement in response to intrapleural pressure rather than to the muscles of respiration. This condition is known as "flail chest."

Rib fractures are characterized by localized pain, possible subcutaneous and bone crepitus and painful respiratory movements. Radiographs are helpful in confirming the diagnosis.

Most rib fractures can be treated by sedation, cage rest and occasionally bandaging the chest to provide added stabilization to the chest wall. Flail chest is a more difficult situation to treat (for a complete discussion of this topic, please refer to Ballinger).

I–20–G. Diaphragmatic Hernias

The most common type of diaphragmatic hernia in small animals is produced by rupture of the diaphragm secondary to trauma. The tear in the diaphragm may be unilateral or bilateral and may vary in shape; however, the tear often begins at one of the hiatuses. Additionally, tears may occur costally or transsternally.

The contents of the hernia may vary with the size and location of the tear and activity of the animal. Changes in the condition of an animal with a diaphragmatic hernia may occur very rapidly. Although on initial presentation an emergency situation may not be present, the degree of tissues herniated through the diaphragm may increase, producing acute respiratory distress.

The chief sign associated with diaphragmatic hernia is dyspnea, although this may be masked by shock in acute trauma cases. The degree of dyspnea depends on the extent of displacement of lung tissue by herniated visceral contents. Auscultation of the thorax reveals that normal respiratory sounds are muffled and peristaltic sounds may be heard. Frequently there is pleural effusion.

The diagnosis of diaphragmatic hernia is based upon history (especially that of trauma), clinical signs and radiographs (see Section I-20-G). Contrast radiographs made following the administration of barium may occasionally be needed to localize a portion of alimentary tract in the chest; however, the characteristic radiographic finding of an alteration in the diaphragmatic line can be visualized on plain films.

Treatment of acute diaphragmatic hernias is designed to stabilize normal patterns of respiration, control shock, and prepare the patient for surgery. Drainage of fluid from the chest and relieving an existing pneumothorax can greatly assist in establishing normal respirations. Elevation of the forequarters may also be helpful. Additionally, correction of fluid and electrolyte disturbances prior to surgery is very helpful.

I–20–H.   Feline Bronchial Asthma

1. Acute emphysema secondary to bronchial spasm and bronchiolar obstruction from mucus and cellular debris is characteristic of felines with bronchial asthma (Carpenter).

2. Place the cat in an effective oxygen chamber and administer aerosol detergents (see Section IV-20-B).

3. Administer prednisolone, 1 mg./lb. daily, intramuscularly.

4. Support treatment with systemic administration of antibiotics.

5. Do not handle, exercise, or excite patients more than is necessary.

6. Do not depress the cough reflex.

References

Additional information may be found in the following sources:

Ballinger, W. F., Rutherford, R. B., and Zuidema, G. D.: Management of Trauma, 2nd ed. Philadelphia, W. B. Saunders Co., 1973.
Flint, T., Jr.: Emergency Treatment and Management, 4th ed. Philadelphia, W. B. Saunders Co., 1970.
Harvey, C. E., and O'Brien, J. A.: Management of respiratory emergencies in small animals. Vet. Clin. North Amer., Vol. 2, No. 2, May, 1972.

I–21. SNAKE BITE TREATMENT

NONPOISONOUS SNAKE BITES

1. Identify the offending reptile, if possible.
2. Signs—the bite is usually "U"-shaped, multitoothed, and relatively painless. Adjacent reaction is negligible. Bites appear as superficial scratches and do not produce signs of a poisonous snake bite (see below).
3. Treatment:
a. Clip hair, clean wound carefully with surgical soap, and apply a sterile, dry dressing.
b. Since the mouths of snakes contain a profuse bacterial flora including Clostridia, systemically administer antibiotics (penicillin and streptomycin) and tetanus antitoxin.
c. Observe the patient closely for at least three hours after the bite was inflicted if the identity of the offending reptile is in question. Modify treatment appropriately if signs of venom toxicity appear.

POISONOUS SNAKE BITES

If possible, identify the reptile.

All venomous snakes are dangerous, but deadliness depends on the venom's toxicity, the size of the snake, the volume of venom injected, and the nature of the venom (neurotoxic, hematoxic, or both).

Coral snake venom (*Micrurus*) contains no common antigen with venom of rattlesnakes.

TABLE 14. RELATIVE TOXICITY OF VENOMS

Species of Snake	Lethal Dose (Intramuscular) Per Gram of Mouse
Naja Naja (common cobra)	0.38 μg.
Vipera Russeli (Russell's viper)	2.50 μg.
Crotalus scutulatus (Mohave rattler)	2.70 μg.
Crotalus terrificus (S. American rattler)	2.70 μg.
Crotalus adamanteus (Eastern diamondback)	11.0 μg.
Crotalus atrox (Western diamondback)	11.0 μg.
Bothrops atrox (fer-de-lance)	12.8 μg.
Agkistrodon piscivorus (cotton mouth)	18.0 μg.

Local Signs

Usually two fang marks are present. Immediate severe pain in the area causes patient to resent palpation. Edema, petechia, and ecchymosis in the area develop rapidly. Subsequently, the region becomes anesthetic and paralytic.

General Signs

Nausea, vomiting, vertigo, epistaxis hematuria, melena, and convulsions followed by coma result in death. If the animal has been untreated for more than four hours following the bite, prognosis is poor.

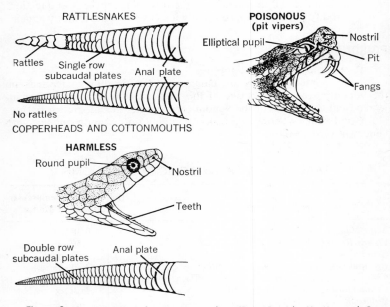

Figure 8. Characteristics of poisonous snakes. (From Parrish, H. M., and Carr, C. A.: Bites by copperheads *(ancistrodon contortrix)* in the United States. J.A.M.A., Vol. 201, No. 12, 1967, pp. 927–932.)

Treatment*

Treatment should be initiated as soon as possible after the bite was inflicted.

Containment of the Venom

Apply a flat tourniquet between the location of the bite and the heart so that venous and lymphatic circulations are impeded but arterial circulation is not. The tourniquet is properly adjusted if a finger can be inserted under it easily. It should be left intact until definitive treatment is provided, or a maximum of two hours. Keep the patient passive; do not allow it to exercise.

Removing the Venom

Leaving the tourniquet in place, excise an area of skin and superficial tissue to the level of the underlying muscle. The tissue removed should be elliptical in shape and extend 1 inch equidistant from the fang marks. All phlegmons or hemorrhagic tissue should be excised. The wound should be covered lightly with sterile gauze but left unsutured.

Neutralization of the Venom

Wyeth's polyvalent snake antivenin should be injected into the artery—radial, femoral, or carotid—that will carry it most promptly to the injured area. One vial is diluted with 100 ml. of saline with 100 mg. of hydrocortisone hemisuccinate and administered under pressure during an interval of 20 minutes. It is best to leave the tourniquet in place during the injection (except in the neck region) and perform a cutdown on the artery if necessary.

An alternate but much less effective method is the administration of one vial of antivenin intravenously, and one vial subcutaneously around the site of the bite. Antivenin is a horse serum product and because sensitivity reactions are possible, hydrocortisone is added to help prevent the reaction.

Symptomatic Therapy

Administer narcotic analgesics as needed (meperidine). Treat shock with corticosteroids and volume expanders. Anticipate clostridial

*Treatment principles generally follow those found in Knowles, R. P., and Snyder, C. C.: Bites of Poisonous Snakes. *In* Kirk, R. W. (ed.): Current Veterinary Therapy V. Philadelphia, W. B. Saunders Co., 1974.

infection, administer antibiotics systemically, and clean local wounds. Preferred antibiotics are cephaloridine (Loridine) intramuscularly every 12 hours initially, followed by doxycycline (Vibramycin) orally every 12 hours. Administer tetanus antitoxin. *Antihistamines may be synergistic with snake venom and are contraindicated, as is alcohol.* Hospitalize patient a minimum of 24 to 48 hours.

I-22. ACUTE SOFT TISSUE INJURIES

Assessment of the Injured Animal

Acute soft tissue injuries in small animals are a common occurrence. When the animal is first presented, make a quick, initial survey of the state of consciousness, respiratory function, heart action, and the presence of bleeding or shock. The comatose animal may be suffering from acute central nervous system injury, acute blood loss, or hypoxia, all of which predispose to shock. Acute respiratory distress may be caused by respiratory obstruction, blood loss, heart failure, or damage to the central nervous system.

Preliminary treatment must include measures to keep the animal alive: assure an adequate airway and assist ventilation if necessary, control hemorrhage, and replace any deficit in circulatory volume (see Section I-9).

Once initial treatment for shock has been instituted, hemorrhage controlled, and adequate respiration established, a more detailed examination of the patient may be carried out.

Initial Examination (See Section I-3)

Priority of Treatment

In animals with multiple injuries, try to recognize all the injuries at the outset and establish a priority for their treatment. Decide what supportive treatment is needed. Limit radiographic examinations to those basic procedures that will permit treatment of the acute injury.

Anesthesia in Acute Soft Tissue Injury

Carefully evaluate the patient's general condition before deciding whether to administer a general anesthetic. Establish a patent airway and stabilize the animal's cardiovascular system. If hydrothorax or pneumothorax are present, these should be treated (see Section I-20-E). If the animal's stomach is full, the animal should be intubated immediately after anesthesia is induced. Remove any blood, secretions, or vomitus from the mouth and pharynx. Oxygen may be administered to comatose animals by intubation or a nasopharyngeal tube. If the blood pressure is very low and no veins are accessible for venipuncture, perform a cutdown and insert an indwelling catheter. If gastric dilatation or retention of food or fluid is present or suspected, insert an endotracheal tube and inflate the cuff. Intubation of the trachea may be accomplished under sedation with neuroleptanalgesia if the oropharynx is anesthetized topically with lidocaine, 4 per cent. When small doses of narcotics such as Numorphan are given they should be injected intravenously, since absorption by other routes is unpredictable in shock.

Minor operations like debridement and suturing of skin lacerations may be done using an injection of a narcotic or a neuroleptanalgesic agent, provided the animal is not in shock and the respiratory system is stabilized. If general anesthesia must be used, the anesthetic selected should not jeopardize the patient. The plane of anesthesia depends on the physical state of the patient and should be as light as is consonant with the procedure being performed (Tables 130 and 131).

Care of Open Wounds

When examining the wound avoid further contamination; use rubber gloves and sterile instruments and avoid unnecessary manipulation of the wound.

Handle the animal gently to avoid further injury. Immobilize fractured limbs before the animal is moved, and if a spinal cord injury is suspected move the animal on a flat board.

Clip the area around the wound and gently clean it. Cover the wound with a sterile dressing while the hair is clipped. The wound edges should then be gently washed and cleaned with surgical soap and water. Irrigate the wound with several rinses of sterile saline.

Remove destroyed or devitalized tissue and foreign bodies. Conserve viable tissue, especially the skin. If the wound is sharply incised, the skin edges do not need to be excised. If, however, the skin edges are jagged, they should be trimmed.

Most wounds can be primarily closed. Wounds not amenable to primary closure are those seen from eight to 12 hours following injury, those that are grossly contaminated, and those involving extensive muscle damage. In cases of gross contamination, or if there is excessive dead space or extensive muscle damage, a Penrose drain should be placed in the wound. If there is not enough skin present to close the wound, skin grafts or rotation flaps may be needed.

Place a compression dressing over the soft tissue injury. This, along with a Penrose drain, serves to decrease infection, control edema and oozing, obliterate dead space, and keep the animal from mutilating the area.

If extensive soft tissue injuries involve a limb, the part should be put at rest by suitable splinting methods.

I–22–A. Prophylaxis Against Infection

Regard all open wounds resulting from traumatic incidents as contaminated by bacteria. The degree and severity of wound infection can be influenced by numerous factors, such as the amount of damaged tissue and the degree of interference with local circulation, the depth of the wound, the elapsed time between injury and treatment, the presence of alimentary or genitourinary contents in the wound, multiple injuries, and shock.

Give antibiotic therapy to all animals with severe wounds. Animals with extensive wounds can be given sulfonamides systemically or antibiotics like procaine penicillin, and streptomycin intramuscularly. Antibiotic therapy should be continued for at least four or five days after all clinical signs of infection have disappeared.

Even though animals are receiving systemically high levels of antibiotics, constant observation of the animal is necessary. Take frequent temperature readings, drain abscesses that develop, and debride necrotic tissue. If the infection does not respond to the initial antibiotic therapy, perform culture and sensitivity tests. Animals developing septicemias should have a blood culture carried out. If the organism recovered on culture is not sensitive to the antibiotic being used (penicillin in many instances) substitute an effective antibiotic (see Section V-5).

I–22–B. Muscle, Tendon, and Joint Injuries

Muscle injuries include contusions, lacerations, and ischemic necrosis. Before repairing muscle injuries, assess damage to the bones, joints, nerves, and tendons. Injured, nonviable muscle should be removed from open wounds. If possible, place sutures in lacerated muscles through the overlying fascia.

Tendons may be repaired with double armed, nonabsorbent sutures such as silk, stainless steel, or plastic. Tendons may be sutured by the technique of Mason or Bunnell. Following reapposition of the tendon, immobilize the part in a position such that the tendon is relaxed.

Open wounds of joints can be caused by traumatic lacerations or by penetration of a fractured bone. Treatment of these wounds includes aseptic cleaning and wound debridement, taking radiographs to delineate bone fractures, suturing tendons when necessary, and administering antibiotics. Under strict aseptic conditions surgically explore the joint and remove any foreign bodies, bone chips, blood clots, or devitalized tissue. Close the synovial sac with fine, absorbable suture material. If the synovial membrane is extensively damaged, closure can be performed using full thickness or split thickness skin flaps as temporary coverage. Immobilize the joint, systemically administer antibiotics, and instill crystalline penicillin G potassium into the joint cavity.

I-22-C. Wounds of the Trachea

Penetrating or perforating wounds of the trachea are usually accompanied by emphysema of the surrounding soft tissues. These wounds must be exposed, cleaned, sutured, drained, and covered with muscle and skin.

I-22-D. Penetrating and Nonpenetrating Abdominal Injuries (See Section I-5)

I-22-E. Chest

The initial management of thoracic injuries includes correction of conditions incompatible with life, such as obstruction of the respiratory passages and loss of normal negative intrapleural pressure. These conditions may be the result of the pleural space being filled with air or blood, or by impairment of the neuromuscular mechanism controlling contractions of the diaphragm, or injuries to the heart causing hemopericardium.

Initial Inspection and Examination

Examination of the animal with a chest injury should be performed carefully, gently, and rapidly so as to avoid aggravating any injuries. Do not muzzle the animal; it may interfere with his respiration. Initial inspection of the patient includes assessing the color of the mucous membranes, determining the presence of dyspnea, observing the thoracic walls during breathing, noting not only any difference between left and right sides, but also if breathing is labored during inspiration and expiration, and examining for evidence of wounds to the thoracic wall. Auscultation and percussion, and palpation of the chest may reveal the presence of fluid or air in the pleural cavity or pericardial sac, bronchial breathing over the collapsed lung tissue, the presence of soft tissue emphysema, and injuries to the ribs or soft tissue of the thorax.

Following a rapid examination of the patient, make a roentgenographic examination of the chest. Whenever possible, take both lateral and dorsoventral radiographs. Pneumothorax is best visualized with films taken at full inspiration. If fluid in the thoracic cavity is suspected, standing lateral roentgenograms are indicated.

Specific Treatment of Respiratory Injuries

Insure a clear respiratory passageway by clearing the pharynx of blood, mucus, or vomitus and pulling the tongue forward. If laryngeal obstruction is present, an endotracheal tube can possibly be inserted or a tracheostomy performed (see Sections IV-18 and IV-19).

Open or sucking wounds of the chest lead to a replacement of the normal negative intrapleural pressure by atmospheric pressure. As an emergency procedure close the wound with a sterile gauze dressing, making it impervious to air. Additional treatment of open chest wounds must be performed in the operating room under positive pressure anesthesia.

Severe pneumothorax is best treated by aspiration of air, as described in Section IV-7. If large amounts of air continue to leak into the thoracic cavity following aspiration, it is probable that a wound of the trachea or a bronchus exists and will require thoracotomy for repair. A chest tube should be utilized first with replacement therapy to try to control bleeding. If surgery is necessary, a sternal splitting incision will expose both sides of the chest. Mild cases of pneumothorax require no treatment except enforced rest and sedation.

Hemothorax demands immediate attention. Aspiration is the initial treatment of choice (see Section IV-7). Thoracentesis may have to be repeated in a few hours if blood continues to accumulate. If blood accumulates rapidly in the thorax following treatment for shock and thoracentesis, a thoracotomy may be required to locate and control the source of bleeding. However, a chest tube with a one way valve (Heimlich valve) or underwater seal will control the pneumothorax until the patient has stabilized, and may even allow the hole to seal. Occasionally a massive blood clot will form in the thorax; since it cannot be aspirated it must be removed by a thoracotomy.

Closed fractures of one to three ribs seldom produce any serious signs except pain from movement of the chest wall. Multiple rib fractures and penetration of the thoracic cavity by fractured ribs must be repaired, the pneumothorax or hemothorax corrected, and the ribs stabilized by a pressure dressing or insertion of K wires.

Cardiac tamponade may result from penetrating and perforating wounds of the heart, allowing blood to fill the pericardial sac. Characteristically, heart sounds are muffled, cardiac output and blood pressure are reduced, the veins of the neck may protrude, the heart rate is slowed, and radiographic examination reveals a large, globular heart shadow. Aspiration of the pericardial sac will bring prompt relief of signs (see Section IV-7). If the blood has clotted in the pericardial sac or if tamponade recurs rapidly, a pericardiotomy is indicated.

In every thoracic or abdominal injury, the possibility of a thoracoabdominal wound through a diaphragmatic rupture or tear should not be overlooked. The initial scout films of the thorax may reveal a diaphragmatic hernia. In some cases oral contrast media may have to be given in order to outline loops of intestine within the thorax.

Reference

Additional information may be found in the following source:

Ballinger, W. F., Rutherford, R. B., and Zuidema, G. D.: The Management of Trauma, 2nd ed. Philadelphia, W. B. Saunders Co., 1973.

I-23. VASCULAR EMERGENCIES

I-23-A. Arterial Injuries

ARTERIAL LACERATION

Laceration of an artery, if open, can result in the loss of large quantities of blood or, if closed, in the development of a hematoma.

Hemorrhage may be controlled by any one or a combination of the following methods:

1. Application of a pressure bandage.
2. Location of the bleeding vessel, clamping it with a hemostat and ligating it.
3. Application of a tourniquet to an extremity proximal to the injury. The pressure of the tourniquet must be higher than systolic blood pressure.

Once bleeding is stanched, treat the animal for shock (see Section I-9) and soft tissue injury.

INTRACRANIAL BLEEDING (See Section I-18-A)

EMBOLUS

An embolus from the heart or any other site in the body may obstruct normal arterial circulation and lead to infarction. In cats, emboli which form in the left heart frequently lodge in the terminal portion of the aorta, or in the femoral or brachial artery. When the occlusion lodges in the posterior portion of the aorta, the animal is in acute distress and suddenly becomes paralyzed in the hind legs. If complete obstruction of the aorta occurs the femoral pulse is absent and the hind feet are cool to the touch. The animal exhibits signs of shock and if renal blood flow is disturbed, death may follow quickly.

Treatment of a complete aortic embolism involves surgical removal. Recurrent formation is very common and the owner should be apprised of this probability before surgery is carried out.

Reference

Ballinger, W. F., Rutherford, R. B., and Zuidema, G. D.: The Management of Trauma, 2nd ed. Philadelphia, W. B. Saunders Co., 1973.

II

INTERPRETING SIGNS OF DISEASE

II–1. THE DIAGNOSTIC CHALLENGE

Each time the clinician faces a new patient he deals with the challenge of making a correct diagnosis. In many cases the challenge is small and the answer is provided easily. Occasionally, patients' pose questions of great complexity. This section does not pretend to give detailed diagnostic methods. Rather it has taken a group of common *signs,* which often are *presenting complaints,* and attempted to define and explain them further. Fundamental causes are outlined and conditions for differential or diagnostic consideration are discussed. These steps should give the clinician further insights into possible diagnoses, but specific details about each entity must be found by consulting other references.

II–2. ANEMIA (See Section V–3–B.)

II–3. FLUCTUATIONS IN BODY WEIGHT

WEIGHT LOSS

Physiologic Considerations

Decreased food intake results in metabolic changes within the body designed to conserve energy. These changes influence the activity, temperature, temperament and overall health of the animal. Increased environmental temperature and activity (physical and emotional) create greater energy demands which must be met by an increased caloric intake.

Diagnosis and Tests

It may be difficult to confirm an owner's complaint about an animal's weight loss especially if the diet varies, the animal was overweight to begin with, or previous weight records are unavailable. The two major considerations in weight loss are changes in appetite or food consumption, and evidence of disordered gastrointestinal function such as vomiting or diarrhea. The magnitude of the weight loss and the time during which it has taken place are important considerations. Anorexia can occur in such a wide variety of conditions that this sign in itself is not helpful in reaching a diagnosis. However, decreased absorption of food may occur in pancreatic or hepatic disease, enteritis, or malabsorption syndromes. Weight loss with gastrointestinal disorders may accompany general illness such as distemper, hepatitis, renal disease, and neoplasms of the alimentary tract. Fever, itself a sign of disease, increases the caloric requirements of the animal and may result in severe weight loss. Weight loss accompanied by polyuria suggests diabetes mellitus, diabetes insipidus, or chronic renal disease.

Weight loss without a significant change in food consumption may suggest a hypermetabolic state such as hyperthyroidism or a psychogenic state such as extreme nervousness created by a new environment or the introduction of new pets into the household.

Weight loss may frequently occur because of underfeeding. Although an animal may be receiving large quantities of food, the caloric density of the food and the total calories may not be enough to fulfill the animal's need. An animal's caloric requirements fluctuate with its activity, the environmental temperature and humidity, body temperature, environmental and emotional stress, and such specific conditions as pregnancy.

Diagnosing the cause of weight loss demands a careful investigation of the animal's diet, when and how much the animal is fed, how much it eats, its environment, and its general health. Carefully kept weight records are necessary to follow the course of a patient who is losing weight.

WEIGHT GAIN

A gain in weight reflects excessive accumulation of fat tissue or of fluid and may be either local or general.

Tests and Diagnostic Considerations

A normal caloric intake accompanied by a reduced energy expenditure may result in weight gain. Underactivity resulting from hypothyroidism, hypoestrogenism, diseases such as osteoarthritis that limit physical activity, or advancing age may produce weight gain. Older animals with a reduced basal metabolic rate and reduced physical activity tend to put on excessive weight.

Excessive caloric intake results in the deposition of fat. On occasion, compulsive eating may be caused by damage to the hypothalamus with attendant loss of control over appetite. Hypoglycemia is a potent stimulus to the ingestion of food and excessive food intake may be a compensatory mechanism to hyperinsulinism and pancreatic tumor. Most instances of weight gain due to excessive caloric intake are caused by the animal's being fed too much or having access to outside sources (such as garbage cans).

A sudden increase in weight suggests the accumulation of fluid in the body (ascites) and is commonly indicative of underlying renal, cardiac, or hepatic disease (see Section II–4).

References

Additional information may be found in the following sources:

Harrison, T. R. (ed.): Principles of Internal Medicine, 6th ed. New York, Blakiston Division, McGraw-Hill, 1970.
Kirk, R. W. (ed.): Current Veterinary Therapy V. Philadelphia, W. B. Saunders Co., 1974.

II–4. ASCITES

Ascites is the abnormal accumulation of fluid within the peritoneal cavity.

Physiologic Considerations

Ascites is the result of two or more interacting forces; namely, portal hypertension, a lowered plasma colloid osmotic pressure, hypoalbuminemia, excessive sodium retention and aldosteronemia.

Physical Signs

In most instances, the first recognizable sign of ascites is abdominal enlargement. On percussion, a fluid thrill can be felt. Movement of the animal may result in a change in position of the fluid and therefore a change in body contour. Considerable abdominal enlargement may go unnoticed for some time because of the insidious accumulation of fluid, which has not caused any discomfort to the animal. Localized pain, anorexia, depression, vomiting and either diarrhea or constipation may become evident as the fluid mass begins to interfere with normal body function. A concomitant dyspnea may exist if the fluid exerts pressure on the diaphragm and leads to pleural effusion.

Inspection of the abdomen is an important part of every examination. In generalized ascites the abdomen may be tensely distended, with tightly stretched skin, and the flanks may bulge. The venous channels on the ventral abdomen may become quite pronounced. Balottment of the abdomen will reveal a fluid thrill. A fluid wave which changes in position as the animal moves is associated with accumulation of fluid in the peritoneal cavity. Small amounts of fluid accumulation may be very difficult to detect, especially in the obese animal. A carefully performed abdominal paracentesis is indicated as part of the routine examination in every patient with ascites (see Section IV-7). Dyspnea may be present if the fluid exerts pressure on the diaphragm. Concomitant signs of heart disease (see Section III-4), liver disease (see Section V-4) and anemia (see Section V-3-B) may be present.

Diagnosis and Tests

Right-sided congestive heart failure with resultant increased venous pressure is a common cause of massive liver congestion and ascites in the dog. Both primary liver disease, such as hepatitis, lymphosarcoma, and carcinoma, and secondary liver disease, such as cirrhosis secondary to the ingestion of liver toxins, can result in ascites; disturbances in hepatic venous circulation and a lowering of the plasma albumin level contribute to its development. Part of the transudate that characterizes the ascites of liver disease leaks into the peritoneal cavity from the splanchnic capillary bed and part weeps from the liver itself.

Hypoproteinemia with total serum albumin below 1.0 gm./100 ml. may also result in ascites. Hypoproteinemia can be caused by liver disease, chronic fever, infection or parasitism, inadequate intake of protein, and nephritis or nephrosis. Obstructions to normal lymph flow or venous drainage such as can be produced by abdominal or thoracic tumors can also result in ascites.

In many instances, the cause of ascites will be apparent. The characteristics of the ascitic fluid are very helpful in reaching a diagnosis (see Section V-9). Exudates reveal that an inflammatory process such as peritonitis is responsible for the ascites. Feline infectious peritonitis frequently produces large quantities of ascitic fluid. Transudates indicate disease of the heart, liver, or other organs that interferes with normal circulatory or osmotic mechanisms in the body.

References

Additional information may be found in the following sources:

Harrison, T. R. (ed.): Principles of Internal Medicine, 6th ed. New York, Blakiston Division, McGraw-Hill, 1970.
Sodeman, W. A., and Sodeman, W. A., Jr.: Pathologic Physiology, 5th ed. Philadelphia, W. B. Saunders Co., 1974.

II–5. COMA

Coma is a state in which the patient appears to be asleep but is unable to respond to external stimuli or to inner needs. It is not an independent disease entity, but rather a symptomatic expression of disease.

Clinically, sleep and coma resemble each other, but sleep can be interrupted by adequate stimulation.

Consciousness implies the ability of an animal to be aware of its surroundings, to perceive environmental stimuli and to respond appropriately to them. *Wakefulness* implies the ability to respond immediately, fully and effectively. *Lethargy* means a state of drowsiness, inaction and indifference, in which the patient responds in an incomplete and delayed manner. A further degree of dulled indifference while still awake is *obtundation*. *Stupor* is a condition in which the patient is not wakeful. He can be aroused with vigorous stimulation; but upon cessation of the stimuli, he returns to a state of unawareness.

The rostral reticular formation is primarily responsible for maintenance of consciousness. Hemorrhages in the midbrain and pons are relatively frequent in dogs following severe head injury. These dogs usually are comatose and exhibit decerebrate rigidity (extensor hypertonus of all limbs). The pupils are often constricted but responsive to light.

Physiologic and Etiologic Considerations

Only a few mechanisms that disturb consciousness have been identified. In some disease processes there is direct interference with metabolic activities of the nerve cells in the cerebral cortex. Hypoxia, hypoglycemia, and Vitamin B complex deficiencies are well-known examples. Endogenous intoxications, such as uremia, hepatic coma and diabetic acidosis, produce coma by reducing the metabolic rate. Concussion and space-occupying lesions may interfere with consciousness by direct destruction of nervous tissue or by indirect trauma or herniation.

Causes of coma are:

1. Diseases that cause no focal neurologic signs or changes in cerebrospinal fluid, such as drug intoxications, metabolic disturbances (uremia, diabetic acidosis, hepatic coma, hypoglycemia, hypoxia, hypocalcemia and hypoadrenocortical crisis), systemic infections, shock, epilepsy, hypothermia or hyperthermia.

2. Diseases that do cause focal neurologic signs, with or without cerebrospinal fluid changes, such as brain hemorrhage, abscess, contusion, tumor, thrombosis and subdural hemorrhage.

3. Diseases that cause meningeal irritation with the presence of either blood or leukocytes in the cerebrospinal fluid, usually without focal signs, such as meningitis and subarachnoid hemorrhage.

Coma may be further categorized:

I. Primary brain disease
   A. Space-occupying lesion (neoplasm, hemorrhage, abscess)
   B. Injury (concussion, epidural or subdural hematoma, cerebral edema, brainstem contusion)
   C. Infarction (diffuse cerebral or brainstem lesion)
   D. Infection (meningitis and/or encephalitis)
   E. Degenerative disease (lipodystrophy, terminally)
   F. Hydrocephalus

II. Secondary encephalopathy
   A. Renal disease (uremia, acidosis)
   B. Liver disease (hypoglycemia, hyperammonemia)
   C. Pancreatic disease
      1. Beta cell neoplasm hypoglycemia
      2. Diabetes mellitus hyperglycemia
   D. Myocardial disease (ischemic anoxia)
   E. Pulmonary disease (anoxic anoxia, acidosis)
   F. Nutritional deficiency (thiamin)
   G. Anemia (carbon monoxide poisoning, hemorrhage)
   H. Endocrine disease (hypoadrenocorticoidism, hypothyroidism)
   I. Postictal depression
   J. Exogenous toxicity
      1. Sedative drugs, barbiturates, tranquilizers
      2. Hexachlorophene, lead
      3. Ethylene glycol, methyl alcohol.
III. Abnormal osmotic states
   A. Hyperosmolar states
      1. Hyperglycemia, diabetes mellitus
      2. Hypernatremia, diarrhea, diabetes insipidus, severe water loss
   B. Hyposmolar states, such as water intoxication (in man or iatrogenic)

Physical Signs

There is much variation in the depth of depression. The animal may appear to be asleep and yet be responsive to stimulation of some reflexes. At other times no reaction of any kind can be elicited. The history and type of onset are important in evaluating the physical signs.

Tests and Diagnostic Considerations

1. Before diagnostic procedures are instituted, a few emergency measures should be employed. Be sure the patient has a patent airway, is not in shock, and is not bleeding. Treat these problems at once before proceeding with a detailed examination. Be certain to check for head injuries or spinal trauma before moving the animal or manipulating the head or neck.

2. Determine temperature, pulse, and respiration; inspect the skin

TABLE 15. DIAGNOSIS OF GLUCOSE ABNORMALITIES

	Hypoglycemia	Hyperglycemia and Ketoacidosis
Onset	sudden	gradual
Cause	excess insulin	too little insulin
	excess exercise	infection
	delayed meal	stress
Respiration	normal	Kussmaul
Skin	pale	flushed
	cool and moist	hot and dry
Hydration	normal	dehydrated
Pulse	firm and bounding	weak and thready
Urine sugar	negative	positive
Urine ketone	negative	positive
Blood sugar	low	high
Plasma ketone	negative	positive
Response to treatment	rapid	slow
Neurologic signs	Ataxia, seizures, or depression	depression variable

for bruises, petechia, or edema; and smell the breath for the odor of uremia or poisonous chemicals.

3. Perform a neurologic examination (see Section III-8).

4. If poisoning is suspected lavage the stomach and save the contents. Collect urine for urinalysis. Check glucose, acetone, specific gravity, and albumin levels.

5. Take a radiograph of the skull or spine if indicated.

6. If indicated, collect blood or cerebrospinal fluid for analysis (see Sections IV-1 and IV-3).

References

Additional information may be found in the following sources:

Byrne, J. J. (ed.): Management of shock and unconsciousness. Surg. Clin. N. Amer. *48*:247, 1968.

Flint, T., Jr.: Emergency Treatment and Management, 4th ed. Philadelphia, W. B. Saunders Co., 1970.

Harrison, T. R. (ed.): Principles of Internal Medicine, 6th ed. New York, Blakiston Division, McGraw-Hill, 1970.

Plum, F., and Posner, J. B.: Diagnosis of Stupor and Coma. Philadelphia, F. A. Davis Co., 1972.

II-6. CONVULSION (SEIZURES)

A convulsion is a violent, involuntary contraction or series of contractions of the voluntary muscles. It is usually accompanied by disturbances of consciousness and autonomic hyperactivity. Seizures may be divided into two types: symptomatic (or secondary) and idiopathic. Idiopathic seizures are those seizures that are suspected to be of a hereditary nature and are prevalent in German Shepherds, St. Bernards, Irish Setters, Poodles and Beagles.

Obtaining a complete history is very important in making a distinction between symptomatic and idiopathic seizures. Be especially concerned about history of an aura in the preseizure state, the frequency of seizures, and any associated abnormal neurologic signs, such as circling, wandering, restlessness, visual impairment, ataxia, or personality changes. Changes in water consumption and in defecating and urinating habits are also important.

Physiologic Considerations

Seizures result from abnormal local neuronal discharges that are sporadic and sudden. They quickly spread to normal brain, brainstem, and spinal cord tissue.

Seizure foci may be produced by congenital defects, trauma, biochemical changes, neoplasia, abscesses, and changes caused by vascular and infectious disease processes. These foci may remain quiescent for long periods, but can be activated by such factors as emotional stress, fatigue, and nutritional deficiencies as well as by endocrine and electrolyte changes, blood-gas tensions, and blood glucose levels.

Physical Signs

All true epileptic seizures are preceded by an aura or sign that may be helpful in localizing the underlying disease. It may be recognized as a staring expression, licking the lips, twitching in a special muscle group, restlessness, nervousness, salivation, wandering, hiding or affection. The duration of the aura may be a few seconds to hours, and it may be hard to detect the presence of the aura. The generalized convulsion or "fit" begins with clonic twitches or tonic muscle contractions. It continues with the animal's suddenly losing consciousness and falling to the ground. There can be violent spasms of the muscles, with running motions, frothing of saliva, and clamping motions of the jaws. The eyes may roll about and there may be urinary and fecal incontinence.

The ictus (fit) can last from a few seconds to several seconds or may be continuous, developing into status epilepticus. Immediately following the seizure there is a period of confusion, disorientation, pacing, salivation, unresponsiveness to external stimuli and temporary visual impairment.

Seizures may be repeated frequently in groups of two or three or occur singly. If a series of convulsions occurs without the patient's regaining consciousness in between, the condition is called status epilepticus. It is a rare but ominous development (see Section I-18-D).

Although many seizures in dogs are classified as major (gran mal), there are seizures of a focal motor type and psychomotor type which may go largely unrecognized.

Tests and Diagnostic Considerations

Seizures in young animals commonly may be caused by developmental abnormalities, hydrocephalus (age three to nine months), idiopathic epilepsy (normal until six to 18 months), encephalitis (distemper), toxoplasmosis or lead poisoning. Seizures in young dogs characterized by hysterical behavior and running fits accompanied by gastrointestinal disturbances are very suggestive of lead poisoning. Seizures associated with cerebral neoplasms are usually progressive in frequency and occur in older patients. Seizures may develop at any age in an animal with a history of exposure to poisons or trauma or with special metabolic defects. Convulsions with characteristic signs of the underlying disease commonly accompany toxoplasmosis, tetanus, and organophosphate, chlorinated hydrocarbon, cyanide, carbon monoxide, and strychnine poisonings. Convulsions may be seen three to six months after severe head injuries, and metabolic defects like hypoglycemia and hypocalcemia manifest typical histories.

A complete neurologic examination should be performed in seizure cases (see Section III-8). Symptomatic seizures associated with underlying neurologic disease may present other neurologic deficits. Focal motor, sensory or visual deficits may indicate the presence of a space-occupying lesion.

A good general medical workup is also indicated in seizure cases. Electroencephalograms taken in centers equipped for such studies may help diagnose seizures caused by neoplasia, hydrocephalus, encephalitis or trauma. Skull radiograms, fecal examinations, special toxicology tests, ocular examination, cerebrospinal fluid tests, cultures, or blood titers may be needed in special cases. In some patients an absolute diagnosis will be impossible, but circumstantial evidence, breed, age, and history will permit a probable diagnosis.

References

Additional information may be found in the following sources:

Hoerlein, B. F.: Canine Neurology, 2nd ed. Philadelphia, W. B. Saunders Co., 1971.
Kay, W.: Epilepsy. *In* Kirk, R. W. (ed.): Current Veterinary Therapy V. Philadelphia, W. B. Saunders Co., 1974.
Redding, R. W.: The diagnosis and therapy of seizures. J.A.A.H.A., Vol. 5, No. 2, May, 1969.

II–7. SYNCOPE

Syncope (or fainting) is a transient, sudden loss of consciousness. It is much more common in man than in animals, since in man psychic, orthostatic and vasodepressor mechanisms are etiologic. The usual cause is a temporary decrease in cerebral blood flow, but brief disturbances in consciousness may also be due to changes in the chemical composition of the blood, as in hypoglycemia, anoxia, or hypocapnia caused by hyperventilation. Atrioventricular heart block, mediastinal pressure from a dilated esophagus or bloating, severe organic heart disease, and paroxysms of severe coughing may be etiologic in animals.

Syncope may be confused with asthenia, or with akinetic epileptic seizures such as petit mal attacks. A careful history with emphasis on pre- and postsyncopal manifestations is helpful in differentiation. EKG, EEG and blood glucose and calcium determinations are also useful.

Syncope	Asthenia
Sudden onset	Chronic weakness
Normal between attacks	Fatigue constant
Usually rapid recovery	Slow recovery
Loss of consciousness	Consciousness often intact

II-8. CONSTIPATION

Constipation can be defined as the infrequent or difficult evacuation of the bowel. When constipation becomes so severe that no feces can be passed, obstipation has occurred.

Physiologic Considerations

Two principle forms of constipation are recognized; one due to impaired motility of the colon, the other to rectal insensibility or a change in the natural mechanism involved in defecation. These two types may frequently be combined in the constipated animal. Diminished gastric and intestinal motility from many causes may lead to constipation.

Tests and Diagnosis

Constipation may result from a disturbance in the neural or vascular supply of the large bowel and colon, from mechanical obstruction of the small intestine, from painful anal lesions, or from fecal impaction.

Constipation may be acute or chronic. The acute form is usually associated with fecal impactions resulting from the ingestion of excessive roughage in the diet, faulty bile production, acute intestinal obstructions, or pelvic and lumbar vertebral fractures. Protrusion or herniation of an intervertebral disc with resulting paresis or paralysis can produce constipation. Male cats with urethral blockage strain excessively to urinate and may appear to be constipated.

Chronic and progressive constipation may be associated with prostatic hypertrophy, perineal hernias, developing tumors in the large bowel and anus, megacolon (as in Hirshsprung's disease), large masses of internal parasites, abscessed anal sacs, perianal fistulas, or may be a sign of age.

Diagnosis of the cause of constipation depends on history, palpation of the large intestine and colon, digital examination, barium enemas, and gastrointestinal x-rays of the upper tract.

Reference

Additional information may be found in the following source:

Sodeman, W. A., and Sodeman, W. A., Jr.: Pathologic Physiology, 5th ed. Philadelphia, W. B. Saunders Co., 1974.

II-9. COUGH

A cough is a reflex response to irritation of the respiratory mucosa. It begins with a deep inspiration and is followed by forced expiration against the closed glottis. The glottis is suddenly opened, producing an explosive outflow of air at high velocity. (Sneezing is a similar reflex with a continuously open glottis.)

Physiologic Considerations

Cough is an important clinical sign, a warning that disease is present. In general, it has a protective function, but excessive coughing may be harmful and cause bronchial trauma, or force bronchial secretions deeper into the lungs. Persistent coughing may be physically exhausting, and the repeated episodes of high intrathoracic pressure during coughing interfere with venous return to the heart and result in reduced cardiac output.

Cough may be caused by:

1. Infectious agents such as bacterial, viral, deep mycotic, or parasitic agents producing pneumonia.

2. Chemical irritants (smoke, sprays, gases) and foreign agents (dust, oil, foreign bodies) producing bronchitis or pneumonia.

3. Obstructive phenomena such as tight collars, foreign bodies, anatomic defects (trachea and epiglottis), tumors, laryngeal occlusions and fibrosis, congestion, and emphysema or edema of the lungs.

There are two general types of cough:

1. A soft, moist, or productive cough is associated with exudates or transudates. It is found in bronchiectasis, pulmonary edema, and some types of pneumonia.

2. A harsh, dry, nonproductive cough is associated with congestive heart failure, bronchitis, bronchial asthma, emphysema, pulmonary fibrosis, and some types of pneumonia.

Physical Signs

A cough is a noisy, hacking sound that (if productive) may be mistaken by owners for vomiting. The animal gasps, puts its head down, and retches, but ejects only a few milliters of mucus. This is a productive cough. It may be intermittent or progressive.

A dry cough usually is repeated rapidly as a harsh, grating, short sound. The dog often extends his head and neck while coughing. This type of cough is often aggravated by exercise or cold air. It may progress to the productive type or remain chronic, persistent, and non-productive.

Hemoptysis refers to the expectoration of blood from the respiratory passages. Some conditions that may produce hemoptysis are: penetrating injuries of the thorax and lungs, crushing injuries to the chest, damage to blood vessel walls by neoplasms, infarctions and fungal or parasitic granulomas, and chronic bronchitis.

Tests and Diagnostic Considerations

The differential diagnosis of a cough depends on many of the following factors:

1. In the history, the type of onset, duration, persistence and periodicity, exposure to other animals, and vaccination history are all important.

2. In the physical examination, determining whether the cough is productive, and ausculating the lungs carefully are useful in determining the presence of exudation, strictures, consolidation, and other changes affecting sound transmission.

3. Chest radiographs in two planes are most helpful in delineating consolidation, fluid or air, foreign bodies, and many other abnormalities.

4. Culture of bronchial washings and routine hemograms, EKG, and microfilaria examinations should be carried out. Fecal analysis should be carried out in cases of chronic cough to detect the presence of lung worms.

5. Special tests of the cardiopulmonary system (see Section III-4-A) such as special contrast radiograms, circulation time, bronchoscopy, tracheal smears, and exploratory thoracotomy may be needed in certain cases.

Reference

Additional information may be found in the following source:

Harrison, T. R. (ed.): Principles of Internal Medicine, 6th ed. New York, Blakiston Division, McGraw-Hill, 1970.

II-10. CYANOSIS

Cyanosis results in a bluish discoloration of the mucous membranes (and skin) due to excessive concentration of reduced blood hemoglobin in the capillaries. Cyanosis is most obvious in the mucous membranes and in thin, unpigmented skin with a sparse hair covering. The reduced hemoglobin concentration of the blood must exceed 5 gm./100 ml. to be recognized. In general, cyanosis is a late sign of pulmonary disease, occurring when arterial oxygen saturation is less than 80 per cent. Animals that are severely anemic will not show clinical signs of cyanosis.

Cyanosis is not synonymous with hypoxia, although it may be one of its clinical signs.

Causes

Central cyanosis results in delivery of cyanotic blood to the tissues. It may be caused by a reduced airway, depression of rate or depth of breathing, reduction of the effective size of the lungs (tidal volume), reduction in alveolar membrane permeability, and reduction of oxygen pressure of the inhaled air. Administration of oxygen may be beneficial in these cases of cyanosis. Central cyanosis can also be caused by arteriovenous shunts (blood passing through unventilated areas of the lung) or by arteriovenous blood being mixed within the heart (congenital cardiac and vascular anomalies). Oxygen therapy is rarely beneficial in these conditions.

Peripheral cyanosis results when normally oxygenated blood is delivered to the tissues but is delayed in passage through the capillaries, or when too little blood is delivered so that excess oxygen is extracted (shock, congestive heart failure, thrombosis, tourniquets, or external pressure on veins).

Cyanosis due to chemical transformation of hemoglobin and formation of methemoglobin may result from poisoning by acetanilid, cyanide, nitrate, or chlorate.

Physical Signs

The dark blue pigmentation of cyanosis is most apparent in mucous membranes or unpigmented skin. Examination must be made in daylight or under strong artificial light. Color changes in the blood can often be noted directly during surgery. Since the pigment of cyanosis is inside the vessels, finger pressure to ''blanch'' an area of mucous membrane by driving out the blood also decreases the cyanosis. Pigment in tissue outside vessels cannot be removed in this way.

Diagnostic Considerations

Further elaboration of conditions outlined under causes should include foreign bodies, laryngeal edema, pulmonary edema or exudates, tight collars, tumors or hematomas, drug depressions, air, fluid, pus or blood in the thorax, pneumonia, asthma, diaphragmatic hernia, high altitude, and other conditions listed under dyspnea (see Section II-12).

Reference

Additional information may be found in the following source:

Ganong, W. F.: Review of Medical Physiology, 6th ed. Palo Alto, California, Lange Publishing Co., 1973.

II–11. DIARRHEA

Diarrhea refers to an alteration in the normal pattern of defecation that results in the frequent passage of unformed stools. It should not be regarded as a diagnosis but only as a sign of an underlying disease process.

Physiologic Considerations

Physiologically, diarrhea may be produced by local irritation of the intestinal tract, faulty absorption of food, excessive bulk formation, or hypermotility.

Tests and Diagnostic Considerations

Etiologic factors of diarrhea can be divided into three groups:

1. Functional disorders—food or drug allergy, defective digestion, defective absorption and psychogenic aspects.

2. Generalized or metabolic disease affecting the intestines secondarily—uremia, congestive heart failure, liver cirrhosis, hypoadrenal-corticism, heavy metal poisoning.

3. Intrinsic disease of the intestine—bacterial, fungal, protozoan or metazoan parasites; nonspecific inflammatory disease.

Diarrhea may be caused by localized diseases of the intestinal tract such as bacterial (proteus, salmonella, staphylococcus) and viral infections (distemper, hepatitis) together with protozoan infections (coccidiosis, giardiasis, trichomoniasis, amebiasis) and spirochetal organisms (Borrelia and Spirillum species). Parasites such as ascarides, hookworms, strongyloides, whipworms, and tapeworms and intestinal neoplasms and obstructive lesions such as incomplete intussuception may also produce diarrhea. It may be a manifestation of a generalized systemic disease such as hepatitis, distemper, leptospirosis, uremia, or poisoning. Diarrhea can be caused by specific inflammatory diseases such as eosinophilic enteritis and granulomatous colitis. Overeating, food allergies, ingestion of spoiled foods, and sudden dietary changes may produce diarrhea. Defective pancreatic secretions, uremia, chronic liver disease, abdominal neoplasia, and nervousness may produce chronic diarrhea.

The diagnosis of the cause of diarrhea depends on careful history

TABLE 16. CLINICAL SIGNS ASSOCIATED WITH THE ORIGIN OF CHRONIC DIARRHEA*

Sign	Small Intestine	Colon
No. of stools per day	Normal or increased	Frequent
Stool quantity	Large amounts of watery or bulky	Small amounts (often)
Flatulence	Present	Infrequent
"Belch"	Present	Not present
Bloated or enlarged abdomen	Present	Absent
Tenesmus	Absent—present if secondary proctitis develops	Present (projectile diarrhea)
Gross exam of stool		
Blood	Dark black (digested)	Red (fresh)
Mucus	Absent	Present
Fat	May be present	Absent
Rectal exam	Negative	Mucus or fresh blood—foreign body (bone chips) palpated

*Courtesy of M. D. Lorenz, D.V.M.

taking and physical examination, which should include dietary history, appetite, duration of current illness, and previous illness, environmental changes, vaccination history, past treatment for diarrhea, the daily number of bowel movements, and a careful examination of the feces in which consistency, color, odor, and the presence of blood or mucus are noted. An assessment of the animal's general health should be made and the alimentary system carefully examined (see Section III-3).

Diarrhea may be acute or chronic. Acute diarrhea is manifested by the appearance of a watery, sometimes bloody stool in an animal who has previously been healthy. Diarrhea accompanied by fever, depression, anorexia, increased peristalsis, or gastric pain suggests an inflammation of the gastrointestinal tract. In dogs, the ingestion of garbage or spoiled food is a common cause of acute diarrhea.

(*Text continued on page 210.*)

TABLE 17. DETERMINATION OF DEPTH OF COLON LESIONS*

	Mucosal	Transmural
Depth of lesion	Epithelium, colon glands, lamina propria, and muscularis mucosae	Lamina propria, submucosa and lymphatics, blood vessels, muscle layers and subserosa
Lymph node involvement	None	Frequently affected
Proctoscopic appearance	Glistening surface, friable epithelium, and small ulcers with smooth edges. Colon distends evenly with air. No shortening or strictures evident.	Firm corrugated mucosal surface; deep or large rough-edged ulcers. May not distend easily with air. Strictures often present.
Barium enema	Serration and spiculation of profile. No strictures, fistulae or shortening of colon.	Strictures, fistulae, shortened colon. Decrease in lumen diameter.
Direct smear of feces	Erythrocytes and often numerous leukocytes	Erythrocytes and rarely leukocytes
Response to treatment	Usually good	Poor—a stormy course is to be expected
Diseases	Trichuris colitis, amebic colitis, allergic colitis, spastic colon syndrome	Granulomatous colitis, protothecal enterocolitis, lymphosarcoma, adenocarcinoma

*Courtesy M. D. Lorenz, D.V.M.

TABLE 18. DIFFERENTIAL DIAGNOSIS OF PANCREATIC INSUFFICIENCY AND MALABSORPTION*

Test	Normal Value	Pancreatic Insufficiency	Malabsorption Syndrome
Stool exam			
Fat droplets	2/3/LPF	Numerous of large size	Absent to fewer in number. May be smaller in size. Severe cases—numerous
Fatty acid crystals	Absent	Absent	May be present
Muscle fibers	Occasional	Numerous	Occasional
Starch granules	Absent to occasional	Numerous	Absent to occasional
Trypsin gel test	Liquefication of gelatin	Absent	Present
24-hour fat excretion	4–7 gm./24 hr.	> 7 gm.. may be as high as 20–50 gm.	> 7 gm./24 hr.
D-Xylose test	9–12 gm./5 hr. in urine	Normal	Decreased in most cases, test jejunal function in man
Glucose tolerance test	↑ blood glucose by 30–35 mg. per 100 ml. (minimum)	Normal or diabetic response	Flat curve, false normals occur
Gross fat absorption	Gross lipema 2 hr. after feeding	Absent	Absent
[131]I-Triolein	8–15% absorption (11%)	Low uptake	Low uptake
[131]I-Oleic acid	10–15% (13%) absorption	Normal uptake	Low uptake
Intestinal biopsy	Normal histology	Normal	Clubbing and flattening of villi; thickening of mucosa, dilation of lymphatics

*Courtesy M. D. Lorenz, D.V.M.

TABLE 19. ETIOLOGY OF MALABSORPTION IN MAN AND COUNTERPART REPORTED IN DOGS*

Disease in Man	Site of Lesion	Histologic Lesion	Etiology	Counterpart in Dog or Cat
Sprue, celiac disease, idiopathic steatorrhea	Jejunum	Flattening of villi, clubbing of villi	Gluten	Jejunum and ileum, etiology unknown
Tropical sprue	Jejunum	As above plus inflammatory cells in mucosa, lamina-propria, and submucosa	Dietary (B_{12} and folic acid) infectious agent	None
Whipple's disease	Jejunum and ileum	Thickening of submucosa and wall of gut; enlarged mesenteric nodes; dilated lymphatics; infiltration of wall with macrophage with PAS material	Infectious agent Allergic reaction	Colitis (hemorrhagic); ileum; etiology unknown; granulomatous colitis is similar

Regional enteritis	Terminal ileum	Inflammation of gut wall, obstruction of lymphatics	Psychological, infectious, dietary	Eosinophilic enteritis; jejunum, ileum and colon—mild inflammation (G. Sheps with psychogenic induced diarrhea)
Lymphosarcoma	Jejunum and ileum	Obstruction of lymphatics and thickening of gut wall; size of mesenteric nodes	Viral	Cat—jejunum and ileum
Lymphangectasia	Small bowel	Dilation of lymphatics (protein-losing enteropathy)	Unknown (dietary)	Ileum

*Courtesy M. D. Lorenz, D.V.M.

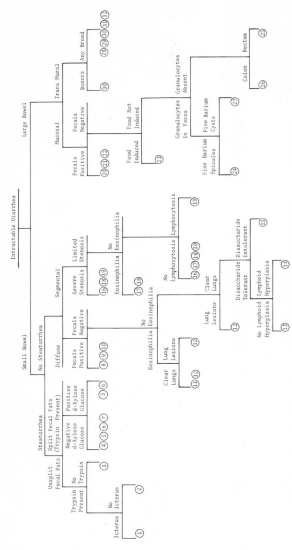

Figure 9. Flow sheet for differential diagnosis of intractable diarrhea. (From Van Kruiningen, H. J., and Hayden, D. W.: Interpreting problem diarrheas of dogs. Vet. Clin. North Amer., Vol. 2, No. 1, p. 30, January, 1972.)

1. Bile duct occlusion
2. Stagnant loop syndrome
3. Pancreatic insufficiency
4. Primary malabsorption syndrome
5. Filled villi: diseased lamina propria with secondary malabsorption
6. Intestinal lymphangiectasia with secondary malabsorption
7. Destructive mucosal lesion with secondary malabsorption
8. Endoparasitism
9. Schistosomiasis
10. Protozoa
11. Eosinophilic gastroenteritis
12. Visceral larva migrans
13. Lymphocytic—plasmacytic enteritis
14. Benign intestinal lymphoid hyperplasia
15. Disaccharide intolerance
16. Strictures
17. Segmental ulcerative ileitis
18. Regional enteritis
19. Primary intestinal lymphosarcoma
20. Trichuris typhlitis and colitis
21. Amebic colitis
22. Balantidial colitis
23. Food-induced allergic colitis
24. Mucosal colitis with crypt abscesses
25. Self-limited proctitis
26. Lymphocytic mucosal colitis
27. Colitis cystica profunda
28. Histoplasma colitis
29. Protothecal enterocolitis
30. Granulomatous colitis (boxer dogs)
31. Regional enteritis of the colon
32. Primary lymphosarcoma of the colon

Diagnostic aids may include fecal examination for parasites (see Section V-7), wet smears of the feces to look for protozoa, spirochetes and undigested food particles, fecal cultures (see Section V-8), enzyme function tests (see Section V-8), fat and glucose absorption tests (see Section V-2), radiologic examinations (see Section IV-14), hematology and blood chemistries (see Section V-3-L), liver function tests (see Section V-4), proctoscopy (see Section IV-12), and exploratory laparotomy.

References

Additional information may be found in the following sources:

Catcott, E. J. (ed.): Canine Medicine, 2nd ed. Santa Barbara, California, American Veterinary Publishing Co., 1967.
Harrison, T. R. (ed.): Principles of Internal Medicine, 6th ed. New York, Blakiston Division, McGraw-Hill, 1970.
Kirk, R. W. (ed.): Current veterinary Therapy V. Philadelphia, W. B. Saunders Co., 1974.
Van Kruiningen, H. J., and Hayden, D. W.: Interpreting problem diarrheas in dogs. Vet Clin. North Amer., Vol. 2, No. 1, pp. 29–47, 1972.

II–12. DYSPNEA (See Section III-4-A.)

Dyspnea is difficult or labored breathing.

Causes

The causes for dyspnea can be separated into two major categories: (1) stimulus for increased ventilation, which could be created by arterial hypoxemia, arterial hypercapnia, arterial acidemia, muscular exercise, fever, increased metabolic rate and heart disease; and (2) reduction of ventilatory capacity, which could be caused by low total lung volume, weakened respiratory muscles, or increased resistance to air flow.

Physical Signs

Severe signs include a rapid respiratory rate with the mouth open. The subject may salivate, its tongue thrust out, its head extended. Many subjects sit or stand but refuse to lie down. The intense effort to breathe is evidenced by "heaving activity" of the respiratory muscles. Cyanosis, pallor, or injection may be observed in the skin and mucous membranes.

Tests and Diagnostic Considerations

1. *Be certain the airway is open.* Look for tumors, foreign bodies, tight collars, laryngeal edema, stenosis, or pulmonary exudates. Hold a mirror or a wisp of cotton in front of each nostril to determine relative patency.

2. A history and physical examination will be useful in determining the most probable causes of dyspnea. It is especially helpful to determine the type of dyspnea, i.e., inspiratory, expiratory, or mixed (see Section III-9).

3. Disease of the lungs and thorax should be eliminated as causes. Usually auscultation and radiographic examinations of the chest are most helpful, but thoracentesis, percussion, palpation, and the presence or absence of pain offer additional clues to the cause. The following conditions should also be considered: pneumothorax, hydrothorax, hemothorax, pyothorax, pulmonary edema or thrombosis, pneumonia, thoracic tumors, fractured ribs, diaphragmatic hernia, pulmonary emphysema, bronchitis, and asthma. More details about these conditions can be found under examination of the respiratory system (see Section III-9).

4. Next, diseases of the heart should be investigated. Very often dyspnea, as a consequence of heart disease, is slowly progressive in its course and directly proportional to the amount of physical exertion. Ascites, hydrothorax, and hydropericardium may be obvious in advanced congestive heart failure. Circulation time, EKG, auscultation, and radiographs can be used in establishing a diagnosis (see Section III-4). In addition to congestive heart failure and the conditions producing it, one should consider the following factors in a differential diagnosis: heart base tumors (hydropericardium), chronic myocarditis or degeneration, aortic thrombosis (cats), congenital defects, and dirofilariasis.

5. Certain laboratory tests are useful in evaluating anemia, shock, acidosis, hypocalcemia, and other metabolic disorders that may produce dyspnea (see Sections V-3-B and V-3-L).

II–13. FEVER

Fever or pyrexia is an abnormally high body temperature. It is thought to be caused by the action of exogenous or endogenous pyrogens or toxins on the hypothalamus. In fever the thermoregulatory mechanisms behave as if the body thermostat were adjusted to a higher level. Temperatures above 106° F. for prolonged periods result in permanent brain damage. Temperatures above 109° F. are associated with a high mortality.

Cause

Excessive heat production by muscular activity, convulsions, excitement, and hyperthyroidism causes increased temperatures.

Impairment of heat loss by interference with transpiration from the skin (coating with oils or grease) or by interference with cooling by panting are important. Stenosis (brachycephalic breeds), paralysis, or tracheal intubation may cause the latter problem. Confinement in a hot, humid, or poorly ventilated environment may inhibit heat loss too (heat stroke).

Septicemia, infectious disease, and neoplastic degeneration are three of the common causes of fever in dogs.

Physical Signs

The obvious criterion for fever is a body temperature above 103° F. Subjects are commonly depressed, anorexic, and have a languid eye or expression. Some may act as if they are cold and shiver but usually they feel hot and seek a cool place in which to lie down. Feverish dogs may have either a wet, cool nose or a dry, warm one. Usually attendant on the fever is an increase in cardiac and respiratory rates.

Tests

In addition to the rectal temperature, a total and differential white blood count and an erythrocyte sedimentation rate are useful in initial tests. Most fevers can be explained after a careful physical examination and a complete history have been obtained. Heat, swelling, localization of pain, and disturbed locomotion as revealed by the physical examination and radiographic studies that show accumulations of pus may be diagnostic pearls.

Diagnostic Considerations

Consideration should be given to infectious diseases, chronic endocarditis and myocarditis, urinary infections, metritis, abscesses (accumulated pus under tension), subperiosteal hemorrhage (osteodystrophy), extensive tissue necrosis (emboli and infarction, neoplastic necrosis), postsurgical infection, osteomyelitis, encapsulated foreign bodies, leukemia, traumatic or neoplastic brain damage, severe dehydration, and pyrogen reactions.

Many of the forenamed entities are obscure conditions but they may be the cause of a so-called fever of unknown origin. A fever of unknown origin (F.U.O.) is defined as a temperature exceeding 103° F. of two weeks' duration and for which no established diagnosis can be made after one week of hospital investigation.

In considering causes, geographic factors are important, as diseases common in Africa, Asia or certain regions of the U.S.A. would be different from those seen in urban America. In man, infection causes 40 per cent of F.U.O.'s, neoplastic disease 20 per cent, and collagen-vascular disease 15 per cent.

Major Causes of Fever of Unknown Origin

I. Infections
  A. Systemic: Endocarditis, toxoplasmosis, disseminated mycoses, brucellosis (?), T.B. (?), psittacosis (?), meningeal infections (?), histoplasmosis
  B. Localized: liver, or abdominal organ, prostatic abscess, cholecystitis, pyelonephritis, chronic urinary infection
II. Neoplasms, especially lymphosarcoma or large masses with tissue necrosis
III. Collagen and vascular disease (in man)
  A. Rheumatoid arthritis
  B. Lupus erythematosus

Less Common Causes

I. Drug fever: tetracycline, allopurinol, sulfonamides, quinidine, iodides, diphenylhydantoin
II. Inflammatory bowel disease: granulomatous colitis, regional enteritis
III. Pulmonary emboli (or other infarcted tissues)
IV. Undiagnosed

Reference

Additional information may be found in the following source:

Jacoby, G. A., and Swartz, M. N.: Current concepts: fever of undetermined origin. New Eng. J. Med., *289*:1407–1410, 1973.

II–14.   ICTERUS (See Section V–4.)

Icterus is the abnormal accumulation of bile pigments in the blood or tissues.

Physiologic Considerations

The degree of icterus (tissue staining with bile pigments) depends on the type and level of bilirubin present in the serum, and is influenced by the type of tissue and duration of the disease. Conjugated bilirubin stains the tissues much more readily than does free bilirubin.

Physical Signs

Careful examination of the mucous membranes will reveal clinical icterus. Signs in hemolytic diseases may include weakness, increased respiratory and heart rate, anemic cardiac bruits, and petechial or ecchymotic hemorrhaging. Liver disease may produce ascites, hepatomegaly, abdominal pain, weakness, vomiting, diarrhea, and bleeding tendencies. Increased hemolysis may result in dark brown or black stools whereas simple biliary obstruction produces clay-colored stools.

Tests and Diagnostic Considerations

Icterus may result from increased production of bilirubin, impairment of the liver's capacity to take up, conjugate, transport, and excrete bilirubin, or obstruction to bile drainage. For the metabolism of bile pigments, see Section V–4.

Classification of icterus is based on the underlying alteration of pigment metabolism, namely those types in which conjugated bilirubin is found (direct reacting) in the blood and those types in which unconjugated (indirect reacting) bilirubin is found (see Section V–4).

Excess unconjugated or indirect reacting bilirubin may be produced by an increased destruction of circulating red blood cells as occurs in lymphosarcoma, sepsis, parasitism, or with the production of hemolysins. Increased destruction of sequestered red blood cells can occur in the absorption of hematomas or intraperitoneal blood, the absorption of blood in massive infarctions, following burns, in autoimmune hemolytic anemia, and in transfusion reactions.

Elevated levels of conjugated or direct reacting bilirubin can be produced by the impaired transport and excretion of bilirubin conjugates as happens in hepatitis, toxemias, cirrhosis, fatty degeneration, and dysfunction of the liver. Obstruction to biliary drainage, either extrahepatic or intrahepatic, will also cause elevated levels of conjugated bilirubin.

The type of icterus can usually be determined by a clinical examination for the presence of anemia, color of the feces and urine, bleeding tendencies, changes in liver size, and the presence of pain over the liver. A total white blood cell count, differential, hematocrit, hemoglobin, and Vandenbergh test will aid in correctly classifying the type of icterus.

For further discussion of the interpretation of icterus, see Section V-4.

References

Additional information may be found in the following sources:

Harrison, T. R. (ed.): Principles of Internal Medicine, 6th ed. New York, Blakiston Division, McGraw-Hill, 1970.
Kirk, R. W. (ed.): Current Veterinary Therapy V. Philadelphia, W. B. Saunders Co., 1974.

II–15. PAIN

Pain is a relatively localized sensation of discomfort, distress, or urgency resulting from the stimulation of specialized nerve endings. In animals, pain is not a subjective manifestation, but rather a condition that can be measured only by the observer in light of signs evidenced by the animal. Important clues in recognizing the cause of pain are to find what precipitates the pain and what relieves it. In addition, the following considerations are all very important.

Physiologic Considerations

Pain is one of the earliest signs of disease. The sensation of pain depends upon receptors located in the skin and deeper structures. Adequate stimuli for visceral pain are different from those that cause cutaneous pain. The skin is sensitive to pricking, cutting, and burning whereas visceral pain is caused by local trauma of an engorged or inflamed mucosa, distention or spasm of smooth muscle, and traction upon mesenteric attachments. Local ischemia and prolonged contraction of muscles may also be a cause of pain.

Physical Signs

Animals in pain may become listless, move constantly, continually get up and lie down, refuse to stay in one place, groan, and whimper. Some animals become phlegmatic when in pain; others have a stark or frightened expression, resent any handling or forced movement, and will "favor" the painful part (carrying an injured leg, holding the neck stiffly and moving the head as little as possible in a cervical disc protrusion, or keeping the abdominal musculature tensed when suffering from visceral pain).

Tests and Diagnostic Considerations

Pain may not be noticed until some normal physiologic act is provoked. Thus swallowing, coughing, chewing, defecating, or any bodily movement can induce pain. It should be determined if the pain is associated with a normal physiologic act or seems to be constant even in the absence of a provoking act. The mode of onset may be helpful in making a diagnosis. Sudden acute pain is usually associated with fractures, rupture or torsion of hollow visceral organs, acute inflammation, or the sudden loss of blood from an organ. Slowly developing pain is associated with osteoarthritis, slowly developing tumors, and chronic inflammation. In any given disease, as well as among different breeds of animals, there is a wide variation in tolerance and in response to pain. One should not judge the severity of a disease process by the pain response of the animal.

Palpation is an important procedure in trying to localize pain, but may be confusing, as when pain referred from a visceral injury simulates musculoskeletal injury over the lumbar area.

Pain is a way of following the course of a disease process, and its complete alleviation may not always be desirable. For example, alleviation of pain in osteochondritis dissecans would allow an animal full utilization of a diseased part that should ordinarily be kept inactive. However, pain that causes the animal to mutilate itself or to suffer great discomfort must be immediately ameliorated.

References

Additional information may be found in the following sources:

Breazile, J. E., Kitchell, R. L.: Pain perception in animals. Fed. Proc., Vol. 28, No. 4, July-August, 1969.
Harrison, T. R. (ed.): Principles of Internal Medicine, 6th ed. New York, Blakiston Division, McGraw-Hill, 1970.
Sodeman, W. A., and Sodeman, W. A., Jr.: Pathologic Physiology, 5th ed. Philadelphia, W. B. Saunders Co., 1974.

II–16. POLYDIPSIA

Polydipsia is a condition of excessive thirst, especially one that persists for long periods of time. Although these figures are unreliable, an average dog's total oral water input is approximately 23 ml./lb./day and an average cat's, 36 ml./lb./day.

Physiologic Considerations

Water intake is under the control of the thirst center in the hypothalamus. Cells in the hypothalamus called *osmoreceptors* are stimulated by an increased osmotic pressure of the body fluids to initiate thirst and drinking. Decreases in extracellular fluid volume also stimulate thirst.

Physiologic thirst may be reported by owners who substitute dry products (8 per cent water) for moist foods (70 per cent water). Since a normal animal has a fairly constant water intake, it will drink more water if less is ingested in the food. This is particularly noticeable when animals have fasted. Most dogs drink a large share of their daily water ration shortly after eating. Most cats drink very little water unless they are on a dry food diet.

Animals with excessive water loss will ingest more fluid to balance the loss. Conditions such as fever, diarrhea, vomiting, draining wounds, nervousness (diarrhea and panting), and urinary losses are of major concern. Included in the last category are osmotic diuresis (diabetes mellitus, high salt diet), lack of antidiuretic hormone (diabetes insipidus), or any renal damage that precludes water conservation.

High doses of corticosteroids, gastritis, pharyngitis, ascites, psychogenic water drinking, and toxemias like pyometra are miscellaneous causes of polydipsia.

Physical Signs

The history of polydipsia is often vague. Animals drink from ponds, streams, toilet bowls, and other sources besides their water bowls, so that the owner's description of the problem is usually incorrect. The most accurate information is obtained by confining the animal and actually measuring his water consumption for several days.

Tests and Diagnostic Considerations

Since water intake and output are closely related, several days' data on these parameters should be evaluated. Water measurements should be made with the patient in a metabolic cage, but a few days of acclimation is desirable before the test period begins (see Section II-18).

The urinary system is usually involved in serious polydipsia, and examinations should emphasize kidney function tests (see Section V-12).

II–17.   POLYPHAGIA

Polyphagia is a condition of excessive or voracious eating. (Its opposite, anorexia, is so common and found in so wide a variety of disease states that it cannot be covered in a brief outline.)

Physiologic Considerations

Hunger is controlled by the interaction of two centers in the hypothalamus. The feeding center, which stimulates appetite, is thought to be chronically active but its activity is transiently inhibited by activity of the satiety center after ingestion of food. Probably, the activity of the satiety center is directly related to its cellular utilization of glucose (and to the blood glucose level).

A cold environment and contractions of the empty stomach stimulate, a hot environment and distention of the gastrointestinal tract depress appetite. The act of chewing and swallowing has a vague satiety effect, whereas environment, habit, sight, smell, and taste all stimulate food intake. Usually these regulatory mechanisms adjust food intake so that the animal's caloric intake equals its energy needs.

Polyphagia can be ascribed to conditions preventing receipt, absorption, or utilization of nutritional elements or to factors increasing requirements or losses. In the first category are inadequate or imbalanced diet, malabsorption syndromes, chronic pancreatitis, enteritis, or colitis, diabetes mellitus, brain lesions, and anatomic abnormalities of the gastrointestinal tract.

Factors that increase losses or intake requirements are pregnancy and lactation, heavy work, extreme parasite loads, nervous diarrhea, anxiety, chronic bleeding or wound drainage, a cold environment, renal or ascitic losses of protein, and hyperthyroidism.

Physical Signs

A ravenous appetite and pica, which is eating foods unusual for the species (lettuce or fruit, for example, in carnivores), are obvious signs. These should be evaluated in conjunction with water intake and with the patient's general physical condition.

Tests and Diagnostic Considerations

1. Establish base line weights, and record weight gain or loss with dates if possible.

2. Determine the average diet and daily food intake together with housing and exercise data.

3. Perform fecal tests (see Section V-8) to determine parasite load and degree of digestion and absorption of key nutrients.

4. Evaluate patient for anemia and renal (see Section V-12) and liver function by appropriate laboratory screening tests (see Sections V-3-B, V-4, and V-12).

II–18. POLYURIA

Polyuria is the passage of a larger than normal volume of urine during a given period of time. Although these figures are unreliable, one can estimate an average dog's urine output to be 10 ml./lb./day, and an average cat's to be 20 ml./lb./day.

Physiologic Considerations

Urine volume ordinarily is influenced by the water and nutritional intake, the excretory load, and by renal and hypothalamic regulation. The kidney performs the most critical regulation of urine volume; consequently renal disease has a marked effect on urine volume.

The most spectacular urine volume changes, however, are mediated by antidiuretic hormone (ADH) secretion. This hormone increases the permeability of the collecting tubules and allows reabsorption (and conservation) of water. ADH is stored in the posterior pituitary gland and released by neural control from the hypothalamus. Osmoreceptors in the hypothalamus are stimulated by increased plasma osmotic pressures to release ADH. (It is not known if these are the same receptors that control thirst; however, much larger increases in plasma osmolarity are needed to stimulate thirst.)

Lowered extracellular fluid volume also stimulates ADH release and water retention. This stimulus overrides the osmotic mechanism. It is important as a possible cause of postsurgical water retention and hyponatremia, and as a cause of water (and salt) retention in congestive heart failure, cirrhosis of the liver, and nephrosis. Pain, trauma, emotions, and drugs such as morphine and barbiturates also cause ADH secretion. Cold and alcohol decrease ADH secretion.

Polyuria can be caused by factors increasing the water intake such as gastritis, nervousness, and psychogenic water drinking. It can also be caused by factors which inhibit the kidneys' capacity to conserve water. These factors are commoner in animals, and the excess water lost as urine often predisposes to polydipsia. Hyperadrenal corticism may present with severe polyuria. Osmotic diuretics such as urea, salt, and glucose (in diabetes mellitus) may produce polyuria. Renal damage, with or without uremia, such as chronic interstitial nephritis, glomerulonephritis, nephrosis, amyloidosis, glomerular sclerosis, poisonings, and toxemias such as pyometra, pyelonephritis, polycystic kidneys, renal cortical hypoplasia, and renal infarcts may result in polyuria. The specific renal function tests or biopsy should be employed to pinpoint the physiologic or anatomic renal abnormality (see Section V-12).

Physical Signs

The history of polyuria often begins with the owner's recognition of nocturia or "accidental" urination in the house caused by the animal's need to urinate frequently.

An appreciation of concomitant polydipsia may be an early sign of input-output abnormalities.

TABLE 20. DIFFERENTIATING COMMON CAUSES OF POLYURIA

	Chronic Renal Insufficiency	Diabetes Insipidus	Diabetes Mellitus	Excessive Water Consumption
Urine volume	Increased	Increased	Increased	Increased
Urine specific gravity	Decreased	Decreased	Variable (normal)	Decreased
Urine glucose	Negative	Negative	Positive	Negative
Blood urea nitrogen	Increased	Normal	Normal	Normal
Effect of water deprivation on specific gravity of urine	None	None	Increased	Increased
Effect of anti-diuretic hormone on specific gravity of urine following water deprivation	None	Increased	—	—

The passage of a large volume of light-colored urine of low specific gravity is often the only clinical finding. However, hematuria, dysuria, frequency, and signs of systemic disease (such as uremia, acidosis, glycosuria, emesis, lethargy, and wasting) may be evident.

Tests and Diagnostic Considerations

1. Most commonly, a distinction must be made between chronic interstitial nephritis, diabetes insipidus, diabetes mellitus, and factors causing increased water consumption.

2. Tests used to differentiate these entities are the urine or blood glucose determination (see Section V-2-E), the response of the specific gravity or osmolarity of urine to water deprivation and ADH (see Section V-2-B), BUN determination (see Section V-3-L-5), and urinalysis (see Section V-11).

3. More sophisticated tests may be needed to delineate less common urinary abnormalities accurately. These tests include renal biopsy (see Section V-12), creatinine clearance (see Section V-3-L-6), phenol-sulfonphthalein (PSP) excretion (see Section V-12), intravenous pyelogram (see Section IV-14-C), and the pneumocystogram (see Section IV-14-D).

Reference

Additional information may be found in the following source:

Osborne, C. A., Low, D. G., and Finco, D. R.: Canine and Feline Urology. Philadelphia, W. B. Saunders Co., 1972.

II–18–A. Urinary Incontinence

Urinary incontinence is the loss of voluntary control of micturition, resulting in frequent or constant passage of urine. It is a sign of bladder and/or urethral dysfunction. Owners often confuse it with dysuria (difficult or painful urination), with pollakiuria (abnormally frequent urination) or with polyuria (passage of large volumes of urine per day).

Physiologic Considerations

Normal micturition depends on normal smooth and skeletal muscles of the urinary tract and normal neural reflexes between the bladder and the spinal cord and between the spinal cord and the brain.

The external urethral sphincter is skeletal muscle; the detrusor muscle of the bladder, trigone and proximal urethra is smooth muscle.

Urine entering the bladder is accommodated by relaxation of the detrusor muscles of the bladder, due to central inhibition of parasympathetic fibers. There is little increase in intravesical pressure until a critical volume is reached. Central recognition of this increased pressure initiates an integrated contractile system which stimulates contraction of the detrusor muscle via the parasympathetic system (pelvic nerves) and relaxation of the external sphincter via the pudendal nerves. These stimuli must be maintained to assure complete evacuation of the bladder.

Urinary incontinence may be classified as neurogenic, nonneurogenic, paradoxical, and miscellaneous.

Neurogenic bladder may be caused by nerve damage, such as trauma, neoplasia or congenital anomalies of the vertebrae or the spinal cord. A paralytic bladder usually results, with overdistention and dribbling. Urine can be easily expressed by manual compression of the bladder. A "cord bladder" is caused by a lesion between the brain and the spinal reflex center of micturition. There is usually temporary bladder paralysis, but later, increased vesical pressure causes reflex but involuntary micturition.

Non-neurogenic urinary incontinence may be due to anomalies (ectopic ureter, patent urachus) or to endocrine imbalance in spayed females. Because the nerve supply is intact, there is no overdistention of the bladder, and the animal urinates normally.

Paradoxical incontinence occurs in patients with partial urethral obstructions (calculae, strictures, neoplasms). In these patients, the bladder is overdistended, there is dribbling and there is difficulty in expressing urine or in passing a catheter.

Severe diseases of the bladder itself due to neoplasia, severe cystitis or fibrosis may cause the bladder to become indistensible and insensitive to normal pressure stimuli.

Tests and Diagnostic Considerations

Careful palpation of the bladder, passage of a catheter or sound, a pneumocystogram, radiographs of the pelvis and spine, urinalysis

TABLE 21. CLASSIFICATION OF URINARY INCONTINENCE*

Type	Normal Micturition	Involuntary Dribbling	Overdistended Bladder	Contracted Bladder	Ability to Pass Catheter
Neurogenic	Absent	Present	Present	Present	Easy
Non-neurogenic	Present	Present	Absent	Absent	Easy
Paradoxical	Absent	Present	Present	Absent	Difficult
Miscellaneous	Absent	Present	Absent	Present	Variable

*From Osborne, C. A., Low, P. G., and Finco, D. R.: Canine and Feline Urology. Philadelphia, W. B. Saunders Co., 1972.

TABLE 22. DIAGNOSIS AND TREATMENT OF URINARY INCONTINENCE*

Signs	Etiology	Diagnosis	Treatment
Continuous	Ectopic ureter, hypospadias	Age of onset, physical examination, radiography	Surgery
	Overflow: Neurogenic bladder	Physical and neurologic examination, CMG and sphincter EMG	Manual expression, catheterization
Intermittent	Neurogenic	See above	Manual expression, catheterization
	Obstructive	Catheterization, radiography	Catheterization, surgery
	Loss of urethral resistance: Structural	Radiography	Surgery or artificial sphincter
	Neurogenic	Neurologic examination	
	Estrogen deficit	Radiography, CMG, EMG	Estrogen replacement
Inappropriate	Physiologic, behavioral	History, treatment	Training
	Neurogenic: Cortical Cerebellar Spinal cord	History, all tests normal History, physical and neurologic examination, CMG and EMG	Removal of cause, frequent voiding, anticholinergic medication

*From Oliver, J. E., Jr., and Bradley, W. E.: Treatment of urinary incontinence. *In* Kirk, R. W. (ed.): Current Veterinary Therapy V. Philadelphia, W. B. Saunders Co., 1974.

and cultures and possibly cystometry may be helpful in arriving at a correct evaluation of the problem.

One should always remember that patients with retention of urine are highly susceptible to urinary infection. Instrumentation should be avoided if possible, and antibacterial prophylaxis is always indicated. The bladder should be emptied with assistance as needed (at least every six hours).

Reference

Additional information may be found in the following source:

Osborne, C. A., Low, D. G., and Finco, D. R.: Canine and Feline Urology. Philadelphia, W. B. Saunders Co., 1972.

II–18–B. Hematuria–Hemoglobinuria

Hematuria is the gross or microscopic presence of erythrocytes in the urine. A few red blood cells per high power field in a specimen of urine may be normal. Large numbers indicate hemorrhage, inflammation, trauma, necrosis, ulceration or neoplasia of the urinary tract. Hematuria found uniformly throughout a urine sample suggests a lesion high in the urinary system. Blood found primarily at the beginning of micturation suggests a lesion of the genital or distal urinary tract. Hematuria most obvious at the end of micturition suggests a bladder lesion, since red blood cells tend to collect in the bottom of the bladder.

In addition to the general causes already listed, hematuria is often found with urinary calculi, iatrogenic trauma, infection (especially viral infection, in cats), renal infarcts, parasites (*Dictophyma renale, Capillaria plica*) and systemic diseases involving hemorrhagic tendencies and platelet deficiencies. These include leptospirosis, warfarin poisoning, lupus and hemophilia. Normal estrum or genital trauma may give the appearance of "urinary bleeding" at times.

Hemoglobinuria is the presence of free hemoglobin in the urine. It usually occurs as a result of high levels of plasma hemoglobin. Unlike man, dogs usually pass large quantities of hemoglobin freely into the urine. Tubular blockage usually is not a serious problem following severe hemolytic crises in dogs. Hemoglobinuria can be differentiated from hematuria by centrifuging a sample of the urine. In the former, the entire sample of urine will retain its deep red color. Intravascular hemolysis, such as is caused by autoimmune hemolytic anemia, snake venom, babesiasis, bacterial toxins, hemolytic diseases of the young and transfusion reactions will cause gross hemoglobinuria. Low specific gravity or highly alkaline urine may cause hemolysis of excess erythrocytes in the urine sediment.

Red-colored urine can be produced following medication with certain drugs (neoprontosil) or test dyes such as phenosulfonthalein (PSP).

Tests and Diagnostic Considerations

Blood or hemoglobin in the urine is a very serious sign and steps to determine the cause should be prompt and thorough. Careful palpation, endoscopic examination and radiographic evaluations are useful. Urinalysis, cultures and exfoliative cytology of urinary sediment may be diagnostic.

Reference

Additional information may be found in the following source:

Osborne, C. A., Low, D. G., and Finco, D. R.: Canine and Feline Urology. Philadelphia, W. B. Saunders Co., 1972.

II–19. VOMITING

Vomiting is a coordinated visceral and somatic muscular reflex controlled by a vomiting center in the medulla. It starts with salivation and nausea. The glottis closes, the patient holds his breath (ribs fixed), the abdominal muscles contract (to raise intra-abdominal pressure), the cardia relaxes, and the gastric contents are ejected. Dogs may initiate this reflex easily.

Projectile vomiting is the violent ejection of stomach contents without nausea or retching.

Regurgitation is the expulsion from the esophagus of undigested food. It is caused by esophageal (and sometimes gastric) action without retching and forceful contraction of abdominal muscles.

Gagging, or a "reverse sneeze," is often mistaken by owners for vomiting, since a small amount of mucus is expelled.

Physiologic Considerations

Although the central vomiting center initiates vomiting, it must first be stimulated. Even when it is drug-induced, this stimulation is not accomplished directly, but by stimulation of a medullary chemoreceptor trigger zone that forwards impulses to the vomiting center, and vomiting can occur only if the center is intact. Emetic impulses can be mediated by many sensory nerves; therefore, intense pain (especially abdominal), nervous (psychic) stimuli, disagreeable odors, tastes, and smells, sensations from the labyrinth and pharyngeal areas, toxins, drugs, and presumably metabolic retention products can all initiate vomiting.

The reasons for projectile vomiting are unknown. It is seen with increased intracranial pressure and high intestinal obstructions or foreign bodies.

Vomiting is very debilitating. When excessive, it causes severe extracellular fluid deficits, particularly of sodium, potassium and chloride ions and water. Protracted losses may cause systemic alkalosis.

Classifying the causes of vomiting is difficult, and this abbreviated list only serves to emphasize the complexity of this sign of disease.

1. Infectious disease—panleukopenia, hepatitis.

2. Acute abdomen—acute pancreatitis, peritonitis (from myriad causes), intestinal obstruction, penetrating wounds and ruptured visceral organs (see Section I-4).

3. Indigestion—chronic pancreatitis, overeating, spoiled foods, poisons, and esophageal or gastrointestinal deformities.

4. Metabolic disorders—acidosis, alkalosis, uremia and hypoadrenal corticism.

5. Drugs—digitalis, morphine, xanthines and certain antibiotics (see Section I-19).

6. Neurologic problems—motion sickness, cranial and vestibular lesions, nervousness (see Section I-18).

7. Pharyngeal or laryngeal irritations caused by enlarged tonsils or, in cats, by a piece of string with one end caught around the base of the tongue and the other end in the esophagus, stomach or small intestine.

Diseases Which Often Cause Persistent Vomiting

    I. Esophageal origin
       A. Cricopharyngeal achalasia
       B. Persistent vascular ring around esophagus (ligamentum arteriosum or left subclavian artery)
       C. Esophageal achalasia, megaesophagus, aperistalsis

D. Foreign body obstruction
E. Congenital or traumatic stenosis
F. Diverticula
G. Hiatus hernia
II. Gastric origin
  A. Pyloric stenosis
  B. Pylorospasm
  C. Achlorhydria
  D. Foreign body
  E. Tumor
  F. Ulcer
III. Intestinal origin
  A. Obstruction—foreign body, tumor, intussusception, adhesions
  B. Neoplasia—adenocarcinoma, leiomyoma, lymphosarcoma, pancreatic carcinoma

Physical Signs

Nausea in dogs and cats is evidenced by restlessness, frequent swallowing, salivation, licking the lips and a worried expression. A few spasmodic contractions of the abdomen usually precede actual vomiting. Some animals vomit quickly, without much apparent nausea. A large quantity of vomitus may be presented first, with smaller amounts at subsequent episodes. After much vomiting, reverse peristalsis will have delivered intestinal fluids into the stomach, and the vomitus may be stained with bile.

Tests and Diagnostic Considerations

1. The character of the vomitus and its relationship to the time of feeding may be important. A large quantity of partially digested vomitus suggests obstruction of the pylorus. Much blood suggests a tumor or ulcer (rare in dogs), and a few streaks of blood are not significant. A highly acid pH indicates that gastric juice is present, whereas a less acid or alkaline reaction suggests that the food may have remained in the esophagus. In general, the longer the interval between feeding and vomiting, the lower the lesion is located in the gastrointestinal tract. Vomiting immediately after swallowing usually implicates the esophagus, vomiting shortly after eating (30 to 60 minutes) implicates the stomach, and vomiting three to four hours after eating implicates the ileum.

Colonic lesions rarely cause vomiting. Vomiting unrelated to feeding may be associated with toxic, systemic, metabolic, or neurologic lesions.

2. Functional lesions tend to produce intermittent vomiting; organic lesions cause constant signs.

3. Radiograph examinations, usually with contrast media (air or barium), are often key procedures in a differential diagnosis (see Section IV-14-B).

4. Diet and eating habits are important, since changes in foods, hot or cold food, spoiled food (garbage), overeating and allergic tendencies all may produce vomiting.

5. Diarrhea as a concurrent sign implies a more generalized gastrointestinal involvement, such as infection.

6. Involvement of other systems may indicate that the vomiting is secondary to metabolic causes, infections or neurologic diseases.

7. Gastroscopic examination and exploratory surgery are often helpful in difficult cases.

References

Additional information may be found in the following sources:

Harrison, T. R. (ed.): Principles of Internal Medicine, 5th ed. New York, Blakiston Division, McGraw-Hill, 1970.

Pearson, H.: Differential diagnosis of persistent vomiting in the young dog. J. Small Animal Practice, *11*:403–415, 1960.

III

SPECIAL SYSTEMS EXAMINATION

MAKING THE DIAGNOSIS

Every new case presents a challenge for diagnosis. What is wrong with the patient? Everything is keyed to the proper and complete answer of that question. Only when the question is answered can one plan treatment properly and forecast the results with reasonable accuracy. Experienced clinicians often "eyeball" the patient, or arrive at possible diagnoses almost by intuition, but this approach to medicine is fraught with danger. Important, even vital, information is almost always missed.

One must collect and analyze clinical evidence methodically and accurately so no diagnostic possibility is overlooked. Diagnosis necessitates two basic steps: (1) collecting the facts and (2) analyzing the facts.

Collecting the Facts

Collecting the facts involves four steps:
1. Obtaining a complete clinical history.
2. Performing a thorough physical examination.
3. Utilizing ancillary methods for further evaluation (radiographs, laboratory data, endoscopy, and so forth).
4. Observing the course of the illness.

The first three points will be discussed in the following pages. However, the fourth point deserves comment here. In many cases, a diagnosis is not immediately evident, even after a careful case workup. Patients may be hospitalized "for observation," or the patient may be seen at appropriate intervals, serial tests performed and consultation with special colleagues arranged. As a disease progresses, more evidence becomes available, and eventually the diagnosis becomes a reality. There should be no stigma attached to delay in reaching a definitive diagnosis, but many veterinarians feel that there is; thus, they fail to utilize one of the most important aids to diagnosis: observing the course of the illness.

Analyzing the Facts

Analyzing the facts involves many steps. These are evaluated subconsciously by most diagnosticians, but in difficult cases it may be helpful to actually write out lists in working out the problem.

1. *Evaluate the data critically.* Are they reliable? Are abnormal results really significant?

2. *List the reliable findings chronologically* as they appear in the history and examination.

3. *List the reliable facts in order of their importance* (medically, not in the owner's opinion). Mark those facts which must be explained by your ultimate diagnosis.

4. *Select one or several central features of the problem* (e.g., diarrhea, dyspnea or weight loss).

5. *List the diseases in which these features are encountered.* (This is differential diagnosis.)

6. *Reach the diagnosis* by selecting, from the differential list of diseases, either the single disease that explains the facts, or several diseases, *each* of which best explains *some* of the facts.

7. *Review all the evidence* (positive and negative) to check on the final diagnosis again.

III-1.   THE ABBREVIATED EXAMINATION

Purpose

The abbreviated examination is required where shipment or transportation of a pet is intended, and is carried out to detect contagions or infectious disease that would preclude shipment. It is not a complete examination for all disease conditions.

History

Determine the presence of normal appetite, bowel and urine function, activity and alertness. Determine the absence of cough, seizures, recent medication, and exposure to sick animals.

Examination

Watch the animal walk. Note its attitude and deportment. Make sure that the eyes are bright, clear, and without discharge, and that the coat and skin are in a healthy condition. Take rectal temperature.

Atypical findings in any of these areas require that the animal undergo a thorough physical examination.

Vaccination

Administer vaccinations as required to meet the regulations of receiving localities (see Sections VI-6-D-1 and VI-6-D-2).

III–2. THE COMPLETE PHYSICAL EXAMINATION

The following information on the patient can be obtained by the hospital receptionist: type of animal, species, breed, age, sex (including whether or not the animal is intact), name, date of entry, and case number.

III–2–A. The Clinical History

It takes real skill to draw a true, unbiased history of their pet's illness from most owners. Some are good observers and can supply important information, whereas others either do not notice things or, what is worse, may purposely withhold information. It is important to impress the owner with the need of helping you help his pet. Talk to him with a vocabulary commensurate with his intelligence, background, and formal education. Ask neutral questions, ones that will not prejudice his answers, such as, "Tell me about your dog's water consumption." Direct or leading questions can be asked if you realize that bias may be introduced. Comments such as "Anything else?" "How do you mean?" or "Tell me about that." are helpful in inducing the owner to elaborate. Do not belittle his opinion of the illness or its cause.

If the same sequence of history taking and physical examination is followed each time, the procedure gradually requires less time and important facts will not be glossed over or omitted.

The Chief Complaint (C.C.)

This is the reason the patient is being presented. What should be recorded is a sign (diarrhea), not a diagnosis (enteritis) that may have been made by the owner or another clinician. Be sure also to record the duration of the sign, e.g., diarrhea for three months.

Present Illness (P.I.)

No exact description of the outline to follow can be given because of the variety of presenting complaints. It is important, however, to record data in chronological sequence *by date*. Record the type of onset and possible exposure to other sick animals. Find out if other persons or animals have become infected by contact with the patient.

If the P.I. has progressed in attacks separated by intervals of good health, obtain a history of a typical attack (onset, duration, signs, treatment). Both positive and negative data about disturbances to organic and systemic functions are important.

Past History (P.H.)

1. Infectious diseases: Distemper, hepatitis, leptospirosis, panleukopenia, pneumonitis.
2. Major illnesses: Dates of infections or severe illness, treatment, complications, and sequelae.
3. Allergies: Contact, atopy, and food and drug reactions.
4. Accidents.
5. Operations.
6. Pregnancies: The number of offspring whelped and weaned from each delivery.
7. Immunizations: Panleukopenia, pneumonitis, distemper, hepatitis, leptospirosis, rabies, dates of immunization and the products used.

Kennel History

The animal's kennel history may be obscure, but information about the present health of parents, siblings, and offspring may be of interest. Try to find out when and where subject was born and raised, the environments it has been exposed to during travel and with different owners, whether it is a working pet or a house pet, and the kind of shelter, care diet, grooming, and medications it routinely receives. Consider the person presenting the animal and providing the history; data obtained from very young or very old owners, or by a nonowner, may be unreliable.

Review of Systems (R.S.)

Questions are asked relating to major regions of the body in order to detect illness in areas other than those covered in the P.I., and to be certain unusual manifestations of the P.I. have not been omitted. Review the following structures and systems from front to rear:

1. Head, eyes, ears, nose: Look for signs of head tilt or shaking of the head, signs of blindness or deafness; a discharge from eyes, ears or nose; pain in the area.

2. Mouth and throat: Look for signs of abnormal salivation, dental problems, difficulty in swallowing, or change in voice.

3. Skin and coat: Look for evidence of scratching, loss of hair, seasonal incidence, progression of severity.

4. Cardiopulmonary: Look for evidence of dyspnea at rest or upon exertion, cough, wheezing, gagging, cyanosis, edema, ascites, or fainting.

5. Gastrointestinal: Determine if patient's appetite, digestion, and bowel movements are normal. Question owner about incidence of vomiting, diarrhea, type of stool, constipation, abdominal pain and food idiosyncrasies or allergies.

6. Genitourinary: Examine patient for, or ask owner about, urinary frequency, water consumption, presence of dysuria, hematuria, and incontinence, regularity of the estrous cycle, breeding dates and results. Find out if the animal has been neutered and if so, when.

7. Neurologic: Look for indications of nervousness, seizures, dispositional change, or paralysis.

8. Locomotor: Look for evidence of bone or joint swelling, joint pain, stiffness or restricted joint motion, or weakness.

9. Endocrine: Check for previous evidence of abnormal functioning of the thyroid, adrenal, gonadal, pituitary, and pancreatic glands. Determine loss of hair and appetite, and polyuria.

N.Y.S. VETERINARY COLLEGE – CORNELL UNIVERSITY
VETERINARY HOSPITALS
MEDICAL RECORDS

PHYSICAL EXAMINATION

ACC #____ PHONE____
OWNER____
STREET____
CITY____ STATE____ ZIP____
BORN____ SEX____ COLOR____
SPEC____ BREED____ ID____

REF. DVM____
CLINICIAN____
SECONDARY #____

(0000) GENERAL APPEARANCE	☐ Normal ☐ Abnormal ☐ Not Examined	(1000) INTEGU-MENTARY	☐ Normal ☐ Abnormal ☐ Not Examined
(2000) MUSCULO-SKELETAL	☐ Normal ☐ Abnormal ☐ Not Examined	(4000) CIRCULATORY	☐ Normal ☐ Abnormal ☐ Not Examined
(3000) RESPIRATORY	☐ Normal ☐ Abnormal ☐ Not Examined	(6000) DIGESTIVE	☐ Normal ☐ Abnormal ☐ Not Examined
(7000) GENITO-URINARY	☐ Normal ☐ Abnormal ☐ Not Examined	(X100) EYES	☐ Normal ☐ Abnormal ☐ Not Examined

| (X700) EARS | ☐ Normal ☐ Abnormal ☐ Not Examined | (9000) NEURAL SYSTEM | ☐ Normal ☐ Abnormal ☐ Not Examined | (5000) LYMPH NODES | ☐ Normal ☐ Abnormal ☐ Not Examined |

Wt. _____ T _____ P _____ R _____

Vac. _____

DIET _____

C. C. _____

HISTORY _____
_____
_____
_____
_____
_____
_____
_____
_____
_____
_____

ABNORMAL PHYSICAL FINDINGS _____
_____
_____
_____
_____
_____
_____
_____

HOSPITALIZATION: ☐ YES ☐ NO

ESTIMATE _____ Initial

(STUDENT) _____ (D.V.M.) _____

MEDICAL RECORD

PATIENT

Figure 10. Physical examination record.

III–2–B. *The Routine Physical Examination*

Record pertinent findings, normal and abnormal, in a systematic manner. Small patients are usually placed on a table in a well-lighted, quiet room, and the examination is carried out with care and gentleness. The owner should be present in order to calm and restrain the patient and to answer questions.

1. Vital signs: Temperature, pulse, respiration, and weight.

2. General appearance: Conformity, state of nutrition, apparent age, degree of grooming care, type of disposition, mental alertness, gross deformities, striking findings, e.g., severe dyspnea, weakness, and depression.

3. Skin: Inspect and palpate. Note the color, texture, degree of moisture or oil present, amount, texture and distribution of hair, pattern of alopecias, ease of epilation, presence of parasites, and sites of primary and secondary skin lesions.

4. Lymph nodes: Palpate all superficial nodes and the spleen. Note enlargement, consistency, mobility, and pain.

5. Eyes: Examine the conjunctiva and sclera for injection, exudation, and petechia. Elicit the pupillary reflex. Perform an ophthalmoscopic examination (cornea, iris, lens, and retina).

6. Ears: Look for discharge and perform an otoscopic examination for exudates or parasites. Note the appearance of the tympanic membranes.

7. Nose: Look for evidence of discharge and patency.

8. Mouth and throat: Smell the breath, note any discharges or excess saliva, and observe the color and appearance of mucous membranes, the pharynx, and the tonsils.

9. Neck and back: Assess the extent of rigidity or limitation of motion, deformities, and pain.

10. Thorax: Evaluate for conformity, symmetry, and free respiratory movements. Percuss and auscultate systematically from the dorsal to the ventral aspects.

11. Heart: Palpate, noting intensity of apex beat and the presence of thrills. Evaluate rate, rhythm, quality of sounds, bruits, or rubs. Record auscultated heart rate and femoral pulse rate if they are different. Carefully auscultate all four valvular areas.

12. Abdomen: Determine conformity, symmetry, masses, gases, fluids, rigidity or "splinting." Auscultate for peristalsis and palpate deeply.

13. Genitalia: In the male, palpate and inspect the testes and penis; in the female, palpate and inspect the vulva and the mammary glands.

14. Rectum: Palpate the confines of the pelvic canal; check the prostate for size, conformity, and consistency.

15. Extremities: Watch the animal walk. Inspect and palpate the legs and joints. Note the presence of pain, heat, swelling, deformities, or limitation of motion.

16. Neurologic: Watch the animal walk. From dorsal recumbency allow it to right itself and perform coordinated tasks. Palpate muscles and compare tonus and balance with opposite numbers. Check tendon reflexes and sensory responses.

ROUTINE LABORATORY PROCEDURES

Although more testing may be needed in many cases, the screening tests described here are usually done as part of a complete physical examination.

Blood (See Section V-3)

Erythrocyte sedimentation rate, packed cell volume, and occasionally a complete blood count. In older patients, a BUN is routine.

Urine (See Section V-11)

Routine urinalysis including specific gravity, pH, protein, glucose, and sediment examination.

Feces (See Section V-8)

Analyze for presence of parasites and for occasionally occult blood.

III–2–C. Summary of Routine Examination

1. Make a list of "problems."
2. List areas in which additional studies are indicated.
2. Make a plan for instituting specific procedures that will satisfactorily explain each item in the problem list.

III–3. ALIMENTARY SYSTEM

Diseases of the gastrointestinal tract are common afflictions of small animals. Careful examination with a systematic approach is necessary to evaluate the alimentary system completely. History taking is extremely important. Special attention should be paid to the following:

1. What is the duration of the clinical illness?
2. What is the dog's vaccination history?
3. Where did the dog come from and what is its travel history?
4. Is vomiting part of the syndrome, and what is its relationship to eating?
5. What is the diet? Is the appetite affected? What is the sequential relationship of the gastrointestinal abnormality to the dog's eating pattern?
6. Has the dog been examined for endoparasites?
7. Have any treatments already been instituted?
8. Has the animal had previous illness or surgery? Is the animal losing weight?

If diarrhea is present, eliciting answers to the following questions may be helpful in localizing the cause (see also Section II-11):

1. How many stools are there each day?
2. What is the quantity of each stool?
3. Is blood or mucous present in the stool?
4. Is there flatulence?
5. Does the stool smell peculiar or offensive?
6. Is tenesmus present?
7. Is the diarrhea projectile?

Before proceeding to examination of specific areas of the alimentary system, carefully observe the general physical status of the animal, noting especially any evidence of emaciation, abdominal enlargement or asymmetry, the position of the animal at rest and body carriage while moving (tucked up abdomen, stiffness and so forth).

ORAL EXAMINATION

In most animals, a routine examination of the mouth can be done without anesthesia or tranquilization. Gently retract the lips and examine the teeth and gums.

Dentition in the Dog (Habel)

Formula for deciduous dentition: $2\left(\text{Di}\,\dfrac{3}{3}\ \text{Dc}\,\dfrac{1}{1}\ \text{Dm}\,\dfrac{3}{3}\right) = 28$

Formula for permanent dentition: $2\left(\text{I}\,\dfrac{3}{3}\ \text{C}\,\dfrac{1}{1}\ \text{PM}\,\dfrac{4}{4}\ \text{M}\,\dfrac{2}{3}\right) = 42$

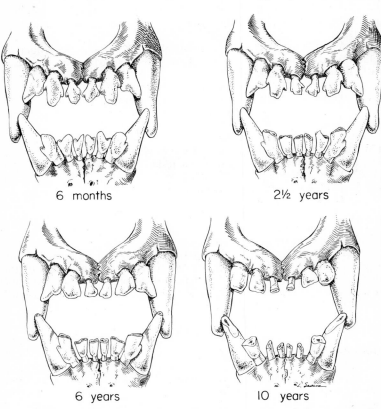

6 months   2½ years

6 years   10 years

Figure 11. Canine dentition at various ages. (From Habel, R. E.: Applied Veterinary Anatomy. Ithaca, N.Y., published by the author, 1973.)

It is possible to estimate the age of a dog up to seven to ten years by examining its teeth. It must be remembered that dogs with over- or undershot jaws or dogs who chew excessively on rocks or bones will not reflect a normal dental wear pattern.

At 5 months, permanent incisors have erupted. Third incisor is not yet in wear.

At 6 months, permanent canines have erupted.

At 1½ years, cusp has been worn off lower first incisor.

At 2½ years, cusp has been worn off lower second incisor.

At 3½ years, cusp has been worn off upper first incisor.

At 4½ years, cusp has been worn off upper second incisor.

At 5 years, cusp of lower third incisor is slightly worn; wearing surface of lower first and second incisors are rectangular. Canines are slightly worn.

At 6 years, cusp has been worn off lower third incisor. Canines are now blunt. Lower canines show impression of upper third incisor.

At 7 years, lower first incisor has been abraded to the root so that wearing surface is elliptical and the long axis is in a sagittal plane.

At 8 years, wearing surface of lower first incisor is inclined forward.

At 10 years, lower second and upper first incisors have elliptical wearing surfaces.

At 16 years, incisors are gone.

At 20 years, canines are gone.

TABLE 23. ERUPTION DATES OF DECIDUOUS AND PERMANENT TEETH (DOG)

Deciduous		Permanent	
Di1	4 to 5 weeks	I1	4 to 5 months
Di2	4 to 5 weeks	I2	4 to 5 months
Di3	5 to 6 weeks	I3	4 to 5 months
Dc	3 to 4 weeks	C	5 to 6 months
Dm2	4 to 6 weeks	PM1	4 to 5 months
Dm3	4 to 6 weeks	PM2	5 to 6 months
Dm4	6 to 8 weeks	PM3	5 to 6 months
		PM4	5 to 6 months
		M1	4 to 5 months
		M2	5 to 6 months
		M3	6 to 7 months

TABLE 24. ERUPTION DATES OF DECIDUOUS AND PERMANENT TEETH (CAT)

Deciduous		Permanent	
Di1	2 to 3 weeks	I1	3½ to 4 months
Di2	2 to 4 weeks	I2	3½ to 4 months
Di3	3 to 4 weeks	I3	4 to 4½ months
Dc	3 to 4 weeks	C	5 months
Dm2 (upper)	8 weeks	PM2 (upper)	4½ to 5 months
Dm3	4 to 5 weeks	PM3	5 to 6 months
Dm4	4 to 6 weeks	PM4	5 to 6 months
		M1	4 to 5 months

Dentition in the Cat

Formula for deciduous dentition: $2 \left(Di \frac{3}{3} \; Dc \frac{1}{1} \; Dm \frac{3}{2} \right) = 26$

Formula for permanent dentition: $2 \left(I \frac{3}{3} \; C \frac{1}{1} \; PM \frac{3}{2} \; M \frac{1}{1} \right) = 30$

Examine the teeth for caries, faulty enamel, exposure of roots, deposition of tartar, periodontitis, and loose, crooked, or sharp-edged teeth. Determine the apposition of the upper and lower jaws for prognathisn (undershot jaw) or brachygnathisn (overshot jaw).

Examine the gums for color, petechia or gross hemorrhage, hypertrophy or recession of the gums, any discharge around the base of the teeth, or any inflammation, swelling or growth.

Examine the hard palate for presence of foreign bodies, an oronasal fistula or palatoschisis.

The Tongue

Examine the tongue for the presence of any abnormal discoloration, membrane or pseudomembrane, foreign bodies, inflammation, ulcers, or growth. Note if the tongue protrudes normally and if both halves are bilaterally symmetrical. The underside of the tongue should be examined for ulcers, foreign bodies such as string wrapped around the base of the tongue (in cats), and swelling of the lingual frenulum.

Palate, Pharynx, and Buccal Mucosae

Careful examination of the palate, pharynx, and cheeks requires sedation or a short-acting anesthetic. A focal source of illumination and a tongue depressor or laryngoscope are also needed. Culturing material (see Section IV-4) and a biopsy of tissue may be done to obtain useful information.

Retropharyngeal tumors or abscesses may produce a ventral displacement of the pharynx and larynx. Careful digital exploration of the retropharyngeal area may reveal an undiagnosed mass. Fractures of the hyoid bone may occasionally occur, leading to difficulty in swallowing. Palpation of the posterior pharyngeal area may reveal crepitus and swelling. Inspiratory stridor in brachycephalic breeds of dogs is often associated with an elongated soft palate, weakened laryngeal cartilages and evagination of the laryngeal ventricles.

Tonsils

Inspect the oral mucous membranes for changes in color, hemorrhage, inflammation, abrasions, ulceration, abnormal discharges, membranes or pseudomenbranes, and abnormal growths. The tonsils should be examined for size, color, and consistency; the surrounding tissue should be examined for any abnormality. Conclusive diagnosis of the cause of tonsillar enlargement may depend on the results of a biopsy. Examine the uvula and note its length. Foreign bodies may lodge at the opening of the posterior nares and the uvula must be pulled down and forward and the posterior nares visualized. Examine the hard and soft palate with a dental mirror for the presence of tumors or foreign bodies. Fractures of the hard palate are frequently seen in cats that fall from high elevations.

Odors

Smell the breath. Mouth odors may be caused by bad teeth, ulcerations of the lip folds or the mucous membranes and tonsillitis. Uremia produces an ammoniacal odor; diabetic ketosis, a smell of acetone; and suppurative conditions of the lungs, a putrid odor.

EXAMINATION OF THE ESOPHAGUS

The esophagus starts in the posterior pharynx dorsal to the cranial portion of the trachea, and continues in a caudal direction slightly dorsal and to the left of the trachea to the thoracic inlet. Just caudal to the thoracic inlet, the esophagus becomes more ventral in position and further to the left of the trachea. At the base of the heart, the esophagus is dorsal to the bifurcation of the trachea. The esophagus then continues caudally to the diaphragm and empties in the fundus of the stomach.

Examination of the esophagus depends on the use of either a gastroscope or radiographic techniques. It is important, however, to know if the animal can swallow normally. The signs of esophageal disease are quite general and include regurgitation, abnormal or painful deglutition and weight loss associated with a caloric deficit. Regurgitation is the act of ejecting undigested food through the mouth; vomiting indicates the expulsion of gastric contents. Physical findings in esophageal disease may include distention of the cervical esophagus by food, liquid, foreign body or tumor and the possible filling of the esophagus with air when the hind legs are elevated. Dogs with regurgitation problems associated with an esophageal lesion frequently have aspiration pneumonia and pharyngitis.

Esophageal abnormalities may be produced by tumors, foreign bodies, vascular ring anomalies, inflammation, periesophageal lesion, or parasites (*Spirocerca lupi*).

III–3–A. *Examination of the Abdomen*

Observation

Stand the animal on a table, its head facing away from you. Step back and inspect the abdomen as to general contour and for swelling or retraction. Swelling can be either localized or general. The most common cause of localized swelling is a neoplasm,. General swelling can be caused by fat, fluid, flatus, or fetus.

Note whether the abdominal walls move normally during respiration. Abnormal movement may reflect pain from peritonitis. Decide if the abdominal musculature seems tense, the abdomen "tucked up." The animal will frequently stand with the hind legs drawn well forward under the body, giving an arched back appearance. When in severe abdominal pain, some animals will assume a "praying position." Look for soft tissue edema as well as abnormal venous distention of the abdominal wall, indicating circulatory interference.

Palpation

Following visual inspection, palpate the abdomen. Stand behind the animal while an assistant gently restrains the animal's head. Gain the animal's confidence by lightly moving the hands over the entire abdomen. When palpating avoid using the fingertips; use, instead, the metacarpophalangeal joints, the hand flat on the abdominal wall. Start your palpation by a very light, systematic palpation of the entire abdomen and note any localized or general rigidity or tenderness. Next, palpate the deeper structures. Palpate the liver by pressing the fingers inward and forward around the costal arches on either side. The normal dog liver is not easy to palpate. Enlargement, however, causes it to protrude beyond the costal margins and facilitates palpation. Note the amount of distention beyond the costal margins and if the edge of the liver is sharp or rounded. The spleen can be palpated in the upper left lateral region of the abdomen.

The kidneys are palpable in certain dogs. The right kidney lies ventral to the first to third lumbar vertebrae; the left kidney is ventral to the second to fourth lumbar vertebrae. In the normal cat, both the liver and kidneys can be palpated. Do not confuse the kidneys of a cat with a fetus or tumor.

The fundus of the dog's stomach is on the left side, the pylorus on the right. When moderately filled, the stomach expands to the left and the greater curvature parallels the twelfth rib. The filled stomach is distended caudoventrally so that the greater curvature lies transversely on the floor of the abdomen midway between the xiphoid cartilage and the pubis.

The duodenum passes caudad from the pylorus on the right side lateral to the ascending colon and cecum. The jejunum occupies the right ventral quadrant of the abdomen. The ileum approaches the cecum from the left and joins it at the cecocolic junction. The cecum is usually ventral to the second and third lumbar vertebrae and is in the middle of the right half of the abdomen.

The descending duodenum and the ileocecocolic junction on the right can be palpated by pressing them dorsally against the sublumbar muscles and rolling them from medial to lateral.

The descending colon can be palpated on the left and is more prominent when the dog is constipated. Intussusceptions often begin at the ileocecocolic junction. The bladder is located within the posterior portion of the abdomen and is capable of distention as far craniad as the umbilicus (Habel).

If an abnormal mass is felt while palpation is being carried out, note its position, associated pain, degree of mobility, and consistency, if possible. Upon palpation, masses like lipomas may seem to be in the abdomen when actually they are in the abdominal musculature.

Percussion

Following palpation, percuss the abdomen. The normal abdomen yields a tympanitic-like note throughout except over a solid viscus like the liver, spleen, or a full bladder. Increased accumulations of air in the stomach or abdomen will give a larger area of tympanitic sound.

Free fluid in the peritoneum (ascites) may shift as the patient is moved. When ascites is suspected, place one hand on one side of the abdomen over the lumbar area and with the other hand "flick" or tap the opposite abdominal wall. A distinct impact is felt from one hand to the other if fluid under tension is present.

Auscultation

Carry out the auscultation in a quiet room and determine if the peristaltic sounds are normal, increased, decreased, or absent.

Rectal Examination

The rectum is an elongated tube, 5 to 6 cm. in length. Its diameter varies with the breed and size of animal. The rectum traverses the pelvic canal and ends at the anal canal. Innervation to the anorectal area is supplied by the pudenal nerve (formed by S 1, 2 and 3), which also provides motor nerves to the external anal sphincter and skin of the anus and perianal region. The rectum and internal anal sphincter are supplied by nerves from the pelvic plexus.

Tenesmus and dyschezia are the primary signs in anorectal diseases. Carefully examine the external anal area and perineum for evidence of inflammation, swelling, neoplasms, and crypts at the muco-cutaneous line.

Conclude the examination of the intestinal tract by performing a rectal examination. Use a rubber glove or a finger cot lubricated with petroleum jelly. Digital examination will reveal the color and consistency of the stool in the rectum, any narrowing of the rectum, the possibility of a fractured pelvis, the size of the pelvic canal, impaction or tumors of the anal glands, and the presence of rectal polyps. In male subjects, always check the size of the prostate gland. Little discomfort should accompany this examination. Following digital examination of the rectum, direct visualization of the rectal canal can be accomplished by use of a proctoscope (see Section IV-16) or anoscope.

A careful examination of the alimentary tract and abdomen may indicate that further diagnostic work is needed. Passage of a stomach tube (see Section IV-19-B), esophagoscopy, radiography (see Section IV-18-A), test meals, proctoscopy (see Sections V-8-A and IV-16), or clinical pathologic tests may be required. Do not hesitate to perform those tests that help you to arrive at a definitive diagnosis.

References

Additional information can be found in the following sources:

Habel, R. E.: Applied Anatomy, 6th ed. Ithaca, N.Y., published by author, 1973.
Veterinary Clinics of North America, Vol. 2, No. 1, January, 1972 (gastrointestinal medicine and surgery).

III-4. CARDIOVASCULAR SYSTEM

HISTORY

Age

The age of the patient is an important clue to the diagnosis of cardiac diseases.

1. Congenital heart disease is most often diagnosed before the age of 2 years.

2. Idiopathic cardiomyopathy is generally seen between the ages of 2 and 7 years.

3. Mitral insufficiency is generally asymptomatic until 7 to 9 years of age.

4. Myocarditis and other acquired cardiac diseases generally increase in frequency with age.

Breed

There are breed predispositions toward many congenital and acquired cardiac abnormalities.

1. Congenital cardiac anomalies.
   a. Patent ductus arteriosus—Poodle, Collie, Pomeranian, German Shepherd.
   b. Pulmonic stenosis—English Bulldog, Old English Sheepdog, Fox Terrier, Chihuahua, Beagle, Schnauzer, Pointer.
   c. Aortic stenosis—German Shepherd, Boxer, Newfoundland.
   d. Tetralogy of Fallot—Keeshond, Fox Terrier.
   e. Aortic arch abnormalities—German Shepherd, Irish Setter, Weimaraner.
   f. Congenital mitral insufficiency—Great Dane.
2. Acquired cardiac abnormalities.
   a. Mitral or tricuspid insufficiency, or both—Cocker, Poodle, Schnauzer, Dachshund, Chihuahua, Pomeranian, Miniature Pinscher.
   b. Myocarditis—Boxer, St. Bernard, German Shorthair Pointer.
   c. Idiopathic cardiomyopathy—large breeds of dogs.
   d. Collapsed trachea—toy breeds.
   e. Heart base tumors—Boston Terrier, Boxer, English Bulldog.

Pertinent Questions Helpful in Obtaining Medical History

1. Any excessive weakness or tiring? An animal with clinically significant cardiac abnormality has less cardiac reserve and loses strength and stamina. The owner reports that the pet is unable to exercise as strenuously as he once could.

2. Is there coughing or dyspnea? The most frequent presenting complaint associated with heart disease is a cough, which is first noticed chiefly at night, and which is aggravated by exercise or excitement. As pulmonary congestion or edema advances, breathing may become labored. The owner notices that the pet cannot catch its breath, or that a small amount of exercise causes the pet to pant or breathe heavily for longer than would be expected.

3. How long has the problem been present? In most cases, cardiac disease is a slowly progressive problem. It usually does not begin acutely, and it may become gradually worse over a period of months or even years.

4. Is it getting worse? Cardiac disease is usually progressive, with symptoms that gradually get worse over a period of time.

5. Is the cough worse during the day or at night? The cough caused by chronic mitral valvular fibrosis is first noticed chiefly at night, because of the gravitational shift of blood from the lower portions of the

body toward the heart when the animal lies down to sleep. This shift of blood toward the heart causes an increased cardiac workload and aggravates the pulmonary congestion.

6. Does he sleep well, or is he restless at night? The gravitational shift of blood just mentioned causes the animal discomfort when the pulmonary congestion becomes aggravated. The animal feels that the room is stuffy. He may get up to move, and when he does, breathing becomes easier. Consequently, he gets up and moves often, whenever breathing becomes difficult. Recurring bouts of pulmonary edema may develop (cardiac asthma). Most of these subside within a few minutes after the animal gets up. When this becomes severe, the animal may not be able to lie down at all, and attempts to sleep standing up, or sitting down.

7. Does he expectorate material after the cough? The cardiac cough is a productive cough. The animal may expectorate a small amount of frothy white, or occasionally blood-tinged, fluid. The owner sometimes reports this as gagging or vomiting.

8. Has he had any syncopal attacks? Cardiac syncope (fainting) may occur when cardiac output falls and cerebral hypoxia occurs. This is usually caused by a severe arrhythmia. It may occur when the animal that has cardiac disease exercises too hard or becomes too excited.

9. Describe the cough. The cardiac cough is a low-pitched, resonant cough occurring in paroxysms, followed by gagging or coughing up of a white frothy phlegm which is occasionally blood-tinged.

10. If medication was given, did it help? If the dog has been treated with digitalis, diuretics, aminophylline, or low sodium diet and rest, and he responded well to this treatment, it is suggestive that his problem was cardiac oriented.

11. Are there other problems? Cardinal signs of illness should be investigated in the cardiac patient as in any other patient. These signs include anorexia, polydipsia, polyuria, vomiting, diarrhea, previous illnesses, and so on. It is well known that cardiac disease may affect the kidney and the liver, so dysfunctions of these organs must be investigated.

III–4–A. *Physical Examination*

In the evaluation of the cardiovascular competence of a patient, the clinician uses inspection, palpation, percussion and auscultation to make a tentative diagnosis. Specialized examinations are used as an aid to determine diagnosis, prognosis and treatment.

N.Y.S. VETERINARY COLLEGE — CORNELL UNIVERSITY — VETERINARY HOSPITALS

DATE_____ CARDIOVASCULAR EXAMINATION RECORD

Ward _____

Present Illness and Medications Received:

_____

ACO # _____ PHONE _____
OWNER _____
STREET _____
CITY _____ STATE _____ ZIP _____
BORN _____ SEX _____ COLOR _____
SPEC. _____ BREED _____ ID _____

REF. DVM _____
CLINICIAN _____
SECONDARY # _____

CARDIAC EXAMINATION

Inspection:
1. General Attitude ☐ Alert ☐ Depressed ☐ Prostrate
2. General Condition ☐ Normal ☐ Thin ☐ Emaciated ☐ Obese
3. Respiration ☐ Normal ☐ Dyspnea ☐ Cough
4. Mucous Membranes ☐ Normal ☐ Pale ☐ Cyanotic ☐ Jaundice ☐ Injected
5. Posture ☐ Normal ☐ Pot Bellied ☐ Abducted Elbows ☐ Head Ext.
6. Capillary Refill Time ☐ Normal ☐ Delayed

Palpation:
1. Cardiac Region:
   ☐ Normal ☐ Precordial Thrill ☐ Arrhythmia ☐ Other _____

   Point of Maximal Intensity _____

2. Abdominal Abnormalities: _____

3. Pulse:
   Venous: ☐ Jugular Pulse ☐ Venous Distention ☐ Other _____
   Arterial: ☐ Strong ☐ Weak ☐ B-B Shot ☐ Rapid ☐ Slow ☐ Arrhythmic ☐ Other _____

Auscultation:
1. *Heart Sounds:* ☐ Normal ☐ Abnormal ☐ Murmur
   Timing of Murmur: ☐ Systolic ☐ Diastolic ☐ Continuous
   Duration: ☐ Early systolic ☐ Late systolic ☐ Early diastolic ☐ Late diastolic
   Frequency: ☐ High frequency ☐ Low frequency ☐ Mixed frequency
   Loudness: ☐ Grade 1, 2(Soft) ☐ Grade 3, 4(Medium) ☐ Grade 5, 6(Loud)
   Valve Area: ☐ Pulmonic ☐ Aortic ☐ Left A-V ☐ Right A-V ☐ Radiation _____

   Other Heart Sounds _____
2. *Lung Sounds:* ☐ Normal ☐ Abnormal

   Describe _____

   _____

   _____

Signature: _____

CARDIOVASCULAR EXAMINATION RECORD

Figure 12. Cardiovascular examination record.

Inspection

In our careful inspection of the patient, there are many signs that may indicate the presence of cardiac disease.

1. Physical condition. The cardiac patient in the terminal stages is usually thin. The owner may think that the pet is fat when he really is severely ascitic.

2. Dyspnea. The dyspnea may be very subtle and easily missed, or it may be very obvious. The dyspnea may occur only during exercise.

3. Postural abnormalities. An animal with severe respiratory embarrassment may stand with the elbows abducted in an effort to expand vital capacity. Animals with pulmonary edema may sit on their haunches with forelegs and head and neck extended.

4. Abdominal distention. A distended abdomen may be caused by ascites. Palpation and percussion are helpful in making a differential diagnosis.

5. Color of mucous membranes. Some cardiac diseases, such as tetralogy of Fallot, Eisenmenger's complex and PDA with reversal of flow, may cause cyanosis of the mucous membranes. This is not a feature of chronic mitral valvular fibrosis. Capillary refill time may be checked by blanching the gums with the finger and observing how quickly the color returns when the finger is removed. Diseases that lower cardiac output may delay the capillary refill time (shock, pericardial effusion, severe mitral insufficiency and so on).

6. Venous distention. Right heart failure causes increased venous pressure. This is best judged by examining the jugular vein or the superficial mammary veins. If they are distended or engorged, right heart failure is occurring.

7. Jugular pulse. Normally a pulse in the jugular vein can only be seen as high as one-third of the way up the neck. When such a pulse is visible higher than that, it signifies slight ventricular failure, or a severe arrhythmia (atrioventricular heart block, frequent ectopic beats, ventricular tachycardia).

8. Subcutaneous edema. This is not a common feature of cardiac disease in small animals. It rarely occurs unless severe ascites is present.

9. Strength and stamina. A clinical cardiac problem may cause signs varying from lack of stamina to severe weakness, collapse and sudden death.

Palpation

Palpation provides additional clues in the examination for cardiac disease.

1. Palpation of neck area.
a. It may be possible to stimulate a cough by tracheal palpation. Palpation may reveal a collapsed trachea.
b. Masses in the area of the carotid bifurcation may cause brady-cardia via the carotid sinus reflex.

2. Thoracic palpation.
a. Palpate fractures or deformities.
b. The normal point of maximal intensity (P.M.I.) is the left inter-costal space 4 to 6 at the sternal border (mitral valve area). The P.M.I. may shift or be diminished owing to thoracic masses, diaphragmatic hernias, precordial thrills or pericardial effusions.
c. Precordial thrill is caused by loud murmurs that cause enough fremitus to be palpated (see classification of cardiac murmurs). The thrill is generally felt best over the valve that is affected.

3. Abdominal palpation.
a. Abdominal distention may be caused by masses (may be asym-metrical) that become evident on palpation. Fluid may be palpated by the hands on each side of the abdomen. One hand pushes in quickly, and a "fluid wave" may be felt against the opposite hand.
b. Try the hepatojugular reflex. Gentle compression of the abdomen increases blood flow through the liver and thus through the vena cavae. In animals with chronic hepatic congestion caused by right heart failure, pressure applied to the abdomen will cause the jugular vein to distend. This positive hepatojugular reflex confirms the presence of right heart failure.
c. In animals that have persistent aortic ring abnormalities, com-pressing the abdomen while holding the animal's nares closed will cause the dilated esophagus to bulge, usually in the left thoracic inlet.

4. Palpation of the femoral pulse requires constant practice to be-come proficient. Pulses in many instances are difficult to evaluate, but they may contribute valuable information toward making a diagnosis. Animals that have short stubby legs or that are trembling may be diffi-cult to evaluate.
a. Correlation of classic murmur with classic pulse.

(1) A jerky or "b-b shot" pulse is seen with mitral insufficiency, ventricular septal defect and patent ductus arteriosus. This is a strong pulse, easily felt, but it rises and falls rapidly.

(2) A normal pulse is seen with normal dogs, in pulmonic stenosis and in pure tricuspid insufficiency (rare). This is strong, easily felt, with an even rise and fall.

(3) A small, slow rising pulse is seen with aortic stenosis. This pulse is not strong. It rises late and falls off normally. It is difficult to evaluate.

(4) A weak, thready pulse is seen in shock, in pericardial effusion or in diminished cardiac contractility.

b. Pulse rate and rhythm.

(1) Normal pulse rate is 70 to 160 beats per minute (up to 180 in toy breeds, 220 in cats and puppies).

(2) Should be one pulse for each heart beat. A *pulse deficit* occurs when severe arrhythmias are present, such as atrial fibrillation or frequent premature contractions. A pulse deficit is present when there are more heart beats than there are femoral pulses. Generally the left hand is placed over the heart area and the right hand is placed on the femoral pulse.

(3) Sinus arrhythmia is characterized by an irregular pulse rate. It is correlated with respiration. When the animal breathes in, the pulse rate increases; when it breathes out, the rate decreases. With sinus arrhythmia, the pulse is regularly irregular (because of respiration).

(4) Other pulse irregularities that cannot be correlated with respiration indicate the need for an electrocardiogram to diagnose the arrhythmia.

Percussion

Thoracic percussion is often useful. Decreased resonance may be caused by thoracic masses, diaphragmatic hernia, cardiac enlargement, thoracic effusion or obesity. Increased resonance may be caused by emphysema or pneumothorax.

Abdominal percussion may delineate masses or determine presence of fluid.

N.Y.S. VETERINARY COLLEGE — CORNELL UNIVERSITY — VETERINARY HOSPITALS

CARDIOVASCULAR PROCEDURE SHEET

Heart Rate _____

Heart Rhythm _____

Heart Axis _____

P Wave _____

P-R Interval _____

QRS Complex _____

Q-T Interval _____

Other _____

ECG Diagnosis _____

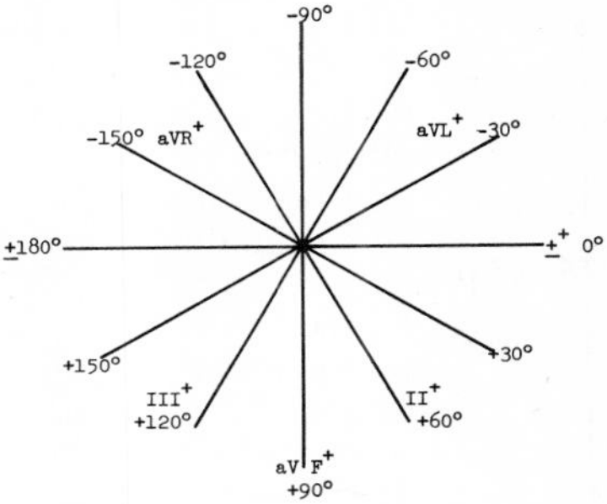

_____

_____

PHONOCARDIOGRAPHIC FINDINGS: _____

_____

_____

VECTORCARDIOGRAPHIC FINDINGS: _____

_____

_____

ROENTGENOGRAPHIC FINDINGS: _____

_____

_____

OTHER EXAM SYNOPSIS: _____

_____

_____

CARDIAC DIAGNOSIS: _____

_____

_____

RECOMMENDATIONS: _____

_____

_____

_____

Case # _____ Date _____ Owner _____ Signature _____

CARDIOVASCULAR PROCEDURE SHEET

Figure 13. Cardiovascular procedure sheet.

III–4–B. Auscultation

The last procedure during the cardiac examination is auscultation of the thorax. This should be accomplished with the dog standing up, his head facing away from the clinician. Auscultation of the heart is done in a systematic manner, by valve area (Figure 14).

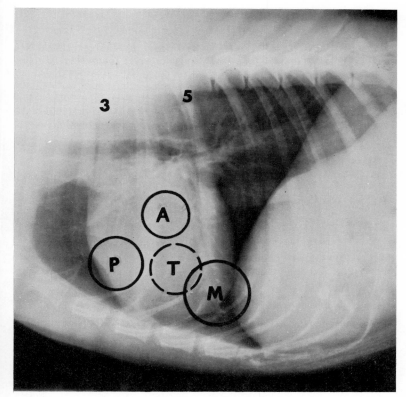

Figure 14. Left lateral radiograph of the canine thorax. Circles identify the valve areas. M, Mitral valve area; P, pulmonic valve area; A, aortic valve area; T, tricuspid valve area. Because the tricuspid valve area is located on the right side of the thorax, it is indicated by a broken circle. (From Ettinger, S. J., and Suter, P. F.: Canine Cardiology. Philadelphia, W. B. Saunders Co., 1971.)

1. Pulmonic valve area—left intercostal space 2 to 4, just above the sternal border.

2. Aortic valve area—left intercostal space 3 to 5, mid-thorax.

3. Mitral valve area—left intercostal space 4 to 6, just above the sternal border.

4. Tricuspid valve area—right intercostal space 3 to 5, mid-thorax.

NORMAL HEART SOUNDS

There are four heart sounds, designated S_1, S_2, S_3, and S_4. Normally only the first and second heart sounds are audible (S_1 and S_2). The first heart sound occurs as the ventricles begin to contract, causing closure of the left and right atrioventricular valves. The second heart sound occurs as the ventricles begin to relax, causing closure of the aortic and pulmonic valves. This is a short, high frequency "dup." The second heart sound occurs at the end of the T wave and signifies the beginning of diastole. The third heart sound is caused by the rush of blood from the atria into the ventricles during diastole. It is normally inaudible. The fourth heart sound is caused by atrial contraction, and normally it, too, is inaudible.

ADVENTITIOUS HEART SOUNDS AND MURMURS

Gallop Rhythms. Gallop rhythms are caused by the presence of either the third heart sound or the fourth. This causes three audible heart sounds and sounds like a galloping horse. In some cases both the third and the fourth sound are audible.

1. Protodiastolic gallop rhythm is the presence of S_3. This occurs *when heart failure is present,* and it is caused by the rush of blood thudding into a dilated overfilled ventricle. It is a low frequency sound best auscultated with the bell of the stethescope and is heard as a low "thud" following S_2. Loud murmurs may obliterate the second heart sound so that all that may be heard is "swoosh-thud." This sound is not spectacular and requires careful auscultation.

2. Presystolic gallop rhythm is the presence of the fourth heart sound. This also signifies *heart failure*. It is caused by the contraction of an enlarged atrium. This is also a low frequency sound and may be indistinguishable from S_3.

3. Summation gallop is the presence of both S_3 and S_4. This also signifies heart failure.

Cardiac Murmurs. The auscultation of a cardiac murmur is usually a reliable sign that there is a cardiac abnormality which might or might not be clinically significant. Characteristic defects cause characteristic murmurs. Each murmur is classified for diagnostic purposes by the following characteristics.

1. Timing. Is it systolic, diastolic, or both? In general, atrioventricular insufficiency and semilunar valve stenosis cause systolic murmurs. These comprise 95 per cent of the murmurs heard. Diastolic murmurs are often caused by atrioventricular stenosis or semilunar insufficiency. Pure diastolic murmurs are rare in small animals. In continuous murmurs, both systolic and diastolic phases are present. The classic murmur characterizing this is the patent ductus arteriosus, called the "machinery murmur."

2. Duration. Is the murmur early systolic, mid-systolic, late systolic, or holosystolic (throughout systole)? Or, when during diastole does it occur? Mitral insufficiency and ventricular septal defect have holosystolic murmurs. Aortic and pulmonic stenosis have mid-systolic murmurs. Anemic and physiologic murmurs are early systolic. Patent ductus arteriosus is holosystolic, holodiastolic.

3. Frequency (pitch). Certain murmurs may be high, low, or mixed in pitch. Low frequency is 30 to 80 c.p.s., mid frequency is 80 to 120 c.p.s. and high frequency is 120 c.p.s. and higher. Ventricular septal defect and mitral insufficiency are classic mixed frequency murmurs. Patent ductus arteriosus usually has a low rumbling quality. Pulmonic and aortic stenosis have many high frequency components. Anemic and physiologic murmurs are generally high frequency.

4. Intensity (loudness). Many systems are available for grading loudness of murmurs, and basically they are all the same.

      Soft   (Grade I) soft, barely audible.
                (Grade II) soft.
    Medium (Grade III) easily heard, but not palpable.
                (Grade IV) precordial thrill.
      Loud   (Grade V) very loud; palpable thrill present.

There is not necessarily any correlation between loudness of murmur auscultated and severity of disease. Some of the small defects create loud murmurs; very large defects may not produce any murmur.

5. Valve area. Generally, the P.M.I. will be located in the area of the valve that is affected.

6. Radiation. Certain murmurs tend to radiate their sound over the chest in characteristic directions. Mitral insufficiency murmurs tend to radiate rightward, cranial and dorsal. Aortic stenosis tends to radiate

TABLE 25. SUMMARY CHARACTERIZATION OF COMMON MURMURS

	Mitral Insufficiency	Patent Ductus Arteriosus	Aortic Stenosis
Timing	Systolic	Continuous	Systolic
Duration	Holosystolic	Holosystolic, holo-diastolic	Mid-systolic (cres-scendo-decre-scendo or dia-mond-shaped murmur)
Pitch	Mixed frequency	Mixed frequency with low frequency components	Harsh mixed frequency, with some high frequency components
Intensity	Usually moderate to loud	Usually loud	Usually loud
Valve Area	Mitral valve area	Anterior on chest in area of pulmonic and aortic valve areas; may have P.M.I. on ventral sternum cranial to left foreleg	Aortic valve area
Radiation	Rightward, cranial and dorsal	Usually to floor of sternum	Cranial and rightward; even heard over cervical vessels

rightward and cranially even up into the cervical vessels. Ventricular septal defect is heard on both sides of the chest with the P.M.I. in the mitral area on the left and at the cranial mid-thorax on the right, with the murmur being loudest on the right. The murmur of pulmonic stenosis tends not to radiate.

Miscellaneous Heart Sounds

The first or second heart sound may be split. A split first heart sound is a normal variation, heard usually in large dogs with thin chests. It is consistently related to S_1. Careful auscultation is required, for it may sound like an indistinct or sloppy S_1.

TABLE 25. SUMMARY CHARACTERIZATION OF COMMON MURMURS (*Continued*)

Pulmonic Stenosis	Ventricular Septic Defect	Anemic Murmur	Physiologic (Functional) Murmur
Systolic Mid-systolic (crescendo-decrescendo or diamond-shaped murmur	Systolic Holosystolic	Systolic Early systolic	Systolic Early systolic
High frequency	Mixed frequency	High frequency	High frequency
Usually loud	Usually loud	Usually very soft; may wax and wane	Very soft; may wax and wane; usually disappears by 8 weeks of age
Mitral area on left; anterior midthorax on right	Mitral area on left; anterior midthorax on right	Mitral area	Mitral area
Heard on both sides of chest, but P.M.I. is on right side	Heard on both sides of chest, but P.M.I. is on right side	None	None

A split second heart sound signifies pulmonary hypertension (classic disease is heartworms). It may be heard with certain arrhythmias (right and left bundle branch block, certain types of ventricular premature beats); it may occur with congenital heart disease (pulmonic or aortic stenosis, left-to-right-shunt anomalies). It is consistently associated with S_2. It may wax and wane. It is best heard at pulmonic valve area, but is difficult to auscultate, and it may seem like an indistinct or sloppy S_2.

Systolic click is of unknown significance. It seems to be a precursor of mitral insufficiency. It is heard as a high-pitched click over the mitral valve area. Sometimes it is heard closer to S_1, sometimes closer to S_2.

SPECIALIZED EXAMINATIONS

The diagnosis is generally made on the history and physical examination. Electrocardiography and radiography are useful tools that assist in determining treatment and prognosis.

III–4–C. Electrocardiography

The EKG provides us with a fast, efficient, easy way to obtain considerable data about a patient's cardiovascular status. The EKG is a clinical test and must be correlated with clinical findings.

Uses of the Electrocardiogram

1. It detects hypertrophy of any of the cardiac chambers.
2. It is useful in the diagnosis of cardiac arrhythmias.
3. It detects electrolyte imbalances.
4. It monitors response to therapy (digitalis therapy for heart failure; antiarrhythmic therapy; treatment of metabolic diseases that cause electrolyte imbalances; pericardiocentesis).
5. It is useful in the diagnosis of nonspecific diseases (myocarditis; endocarditis; metabolic diseases; neoplasia).
6. It is useful for permanent records.
7. It helps establish prognosis (estimates severity of hypertrophy and of arrhythmia; serial EKG's are helpful in determining rate of change).

Production of the EKG

1. Place animal in right lateral recumbency. Use a rubber sheet to insulate him from the table surface.
2. Tranquilization and anesthesia will not affect the EKG and may be used if necessary.
3. Limbs are held perpendicular to the body.
4. Attach leads to forelimbs on elbows and to hindlimbs on stifles. Alligator clips are not painful if bent slightly.
5. Clips are moistened with alcohol, pHisoHex or electrode jelly.
6. Standardize machine so that needle deflection of 1 mv. goes up 10 small boxes on the EKG paper (1 mv. = 1 cm.). Run the paper speed at 50 mm./sec. (Figure 16).
7. Record a few complexes of leads I, II, III, aVR, aVL, aVF. Then return to lead II and run 12 to 24 inches of paper for use as a rhythm strip.

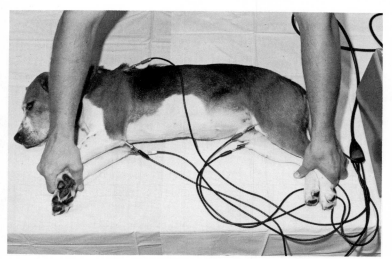

Figure 15. Dog in right lateral recumbency with EKG leads attached by alligator clips.

8. There are specialized unipolar exploring leads (V_{10}, CV_6LL, CV_6LU, CV_5RL), but these leads seldom add much information to the six basic leads. They are run by placing the exploring lead (usually marked V or C) in various locations, and recording with the V setting on the EKG machine. For CV_6LL, the electrode is placed on intercostal space 6 near the left edge of the sternum. For CV_6LU, use intercostal space 6 at the costochondral junction. For CV_5RL, use intercostal space 5 near the right edge of the sternum. For V_{10}, place the lead on the dorsal midline over the seventh thoracic vertebra.

Interpreting the Electrocardiogram

Each EKG should be read with a definite system. Begin by examining the lead II rhythm strip, and determine rate, rhythm and the measurements of the P wave, P-R interval and QRS complex. Evaluate ST segment and T wave, Q-T interval. Use all leads to determine axis and any miscellaneous criteria. Diagnosis should now be possible.

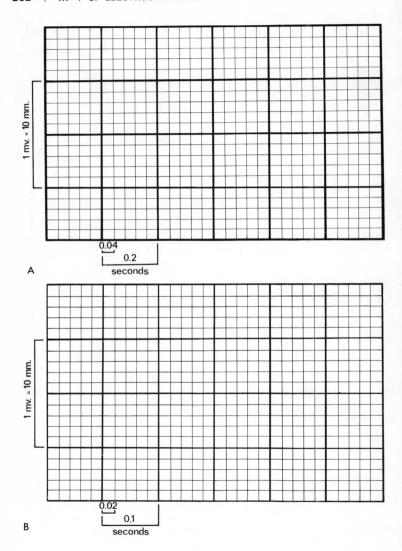

Heart Rate

Normal heart rate is 70 to 160 beats per minute, up to 180 beats in toy breeds and 220 in puppies and cats.

Determinations of Heart Rate

There are small linear marks at the top of each EKG paper. At 50 mm./sec. paper speed, the time between each mark is 1.5 seconds. By counting two of those divisions and multiplying by 20, the heart rate is calculated (Figure 17). Heart rate may also be determined by counting the number of small squares between R waves and dividing into 3000 (at 50 mm./sec. paper speed, see Figure 18).

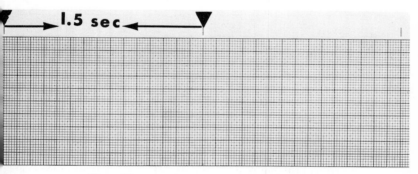

Figure 17. Normal EKG paper run at 50 mm./sec.

Figure 16. Electrocardiograph paper is divided into large squares by heavy vertical and horizontal lines at 5-mm. intervals. Within each large square are 25 1-mm.^{2} boxes. A, At the standard amplitude of 1 mv. and a paper speed of 25 mm./sec., the smallest box on the scale equals 0.1 mv. On the horizontal scale one small box equals 0.04 sec., and five boxes (the length of the large square) equal 0.2 sec. B, At the standard amplitude of 1 mv. and the faster paper speed of 50 mm./sec., the vertical axis is unchanged, each box being equal to 0.1 mv., but on the horizontal scale one small box equals 0.02 sec., and five boxes equal 0.1 sec. (From Ettinger, S. J., and Suter, P. F.: Canine Cardiology. Philadelphia, W. B. Saunders Co., 1971.)

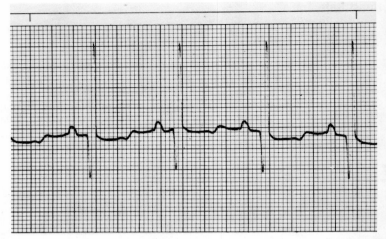

Figure 18. The distance between R waves is 20 small boxes, and 3000 ÷ 20 is 150 heart beats/min. Paper speed is 50 mm./sec.

Heart Rhythm

The normal rhythm is sinus in origin. There is a P wave for every QRS (Figure 19). The P waves are related to the QRS complexes (P-R interval is constant). Sinus arrhythmia, sinus arrest and wandering pacemaker are all normal variations of rhythm. In sinus arrhythmia, the P-P interval is irregular. The pauses are never longer than twice the usual P-P interval (Figure 20). A wandering pacemaker means that the P waves vary in height, and may even temporarily be negative (Figure 21).

Normal EKG Measurements

P Wave

Normal is 0.04 sec. by 0.4 mv. (2 boxes wide by 4 boxes tall). In P mitrale (left atrial dilatation), the P wave is wider than 0.04 seconds (Figure 22). In P pulmonale (right atrial dilatation), the P wave is taller than 0.4 mv.

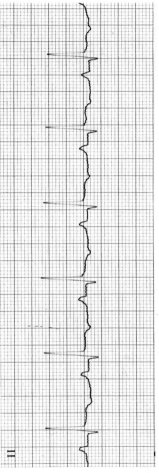

Figure 19. Normal sinus rhythm. The heart rate in this dog is 136 beats/min., and the rhythm is regular. The complexes are equidistant. (From Ettinger, S. J., and Suter, P. F.: Canine Cardiology. Philadelphia, W. B. Saunders Co., 1971.)

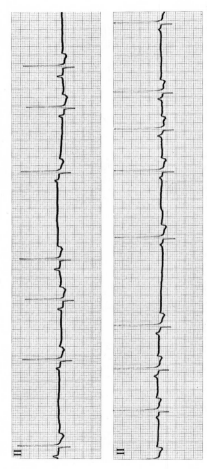

Figure 20. Sinus arrhythmia. Notice the marked fluctuation in heart rate resulting from respiratory sinus arrhythmia in recordings from two normal dogs. The rate may be described as regularly irregular. (From Ettinger, S. J., and Suter, P. F.: Canine Cardiology. Philadelphia, W. B. Saunders Co., 1971.)

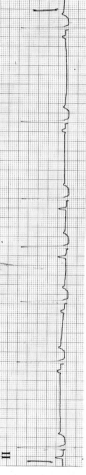

Figure 21. Wandering pacemaker. As the heart rate increases owing to decreased vagal tone, the amplitude of the P waves is increased, and the P waves originate from the sinoatrial node. As the heart rate diminishes when vagal tone increases, the form of the P waves changes, in this case becoming smaller as they arise from a pacemaker other than the sinoatrial node. The duration of the P-R interval is constant at 0.10 sec. (From Ettinger, S. J., and Suter, P. F.: Canine Cardiology. Philadelphia, W. B. Saunders Co., 1971.)

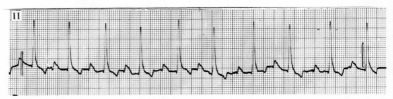

Figure 22. P mitrale. Enlarged left atria are recognized electrocardiographically by prolongation of the atrial conduction time if the P wave is greater than 0.04 sec. The P waves in this dog with chronic mitral valvular fibrosis and mitral valvular insufficiency are prolonged to 0.08 sec. Such extreme prolongation is unusual even in dogs with severe mitral valvular insufficiency. The amplitude and duration of the QRS complex are consistent with left ventricular hypertrophy. (From Ettinger, S. J., and Suter, P. F.: Canine Cardiology. Philadelphia, W. B. Saunders Co., 1971.)

P-R Interval

The P-R interval is measured from the beginning of the P wave to the beginning of the QRS complex. Normal is 0.06 to 0.13 sec. (3 to 6.5 boxes wide). In first degree heart block, the P-R interval is above 0.13 sec. (Figure 24). The P-R interval is useful in monitoring the effects of digitalis therapy.

QRS Complex

The QRS complex is measured from the beginning of the Q wave to the end of the S wave. Normal is up to 0.06 sec. by 3.0 mv. (3 boxes wide by 30 boxes tall). In older dogs of smaller breeds, normal is up to 0.05 sec. by 2.5 mv. If the QRS complex is too wide, it indicates left ventricular hypertrophy (Figure 25). If the R wave is too tall, it indicates left ventricular hypertrophy. It is measured from the baseline to the top of the R wave (Figure 26).

S-T Segment

The S-T segment is between the end of the S wave and the beginning of the T wave. Normally it lies on the baseline and then dips into the T wave. S-T slurring indicates left ventricular hypertrophy. The S wave slurs into the T wave and no S-T segment is discernible (Figure 27). The S-T segment is elevated if it lies greater than 0.1 mv. (1 box) above the baseline. This may happen with hypercalcemia or myocardial hypoxia. The S-T segment is depressed if it lies more than 0.1 mv. (1 box) below the baseline. This may be seen with myocardial hypoxia.

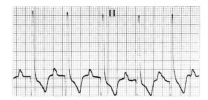

Figure 27. Left axis deviation. The mean electrical axis in the frontal plane in this dog with mitral valvular fibrosis is 35°. (From Ettinger, S. J., and Suter, P. F.: Canine Cardiology. Philadelphia, W. B. Saunders Co., 1971.)

Q-T Interval

The Q-T interval is measured from the beginning of the Q wave to the end of the T wave. Normal is 0.14 to 0.22 sec. (7 to 11 boxes wide). A lengthened Q-T interval may be seen with hypokalemia or hypocalcemia. It varies with heart rate, and it tends to be prolonged when bradycardia occurs for any reason. A decreased Q-T interval may be seen with hypercalcemia.

Axis Determination

The cardiac axis measures the direction (vector) that the cardiac ventricular impulse travels during depolarization. The QRS complex therefore is examined in leads I, II, III, aVR, aVL and aVF. These six leads determine the axis. They are arranged in a particular manner known as Bailey's Hexaxial Lead System (Figure 28). The procedure is as follows:

1. Find an isoelectric lead. This is a lead whose total number of positive (upward) and negative (downward) deflections are equal to zero (Figure 29). There won't always be a perfectly isoelectric lead. When this happens, the one that comes the closest is used.

2. Find the lead that is perpendicular to the isoelectric lead: lead I is perpendicular to aVF; lead II is perpendicular to aVL; lead III is perpendicular to aVR (Figure 28).

3. Determine if that perpendicular lead is positive or negative on the patient's EKG. If it is negative, the axis is at the negative end of that lead (each lead has a + and − pole marked in Figure 28). If it is positive it is at the end of the perpendicular lead. For example, if an aVL were isoelectric (normally it is), then lead II is its perpendicular. If lead II is + on the EKG, then the axis is +60°. If lead II were negative on the EKG, then the axis would be −120° (Figure 28).

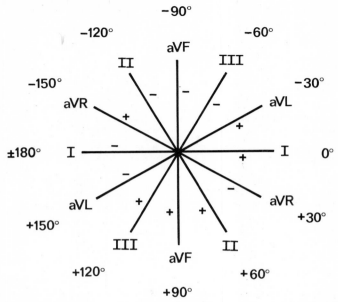

Figure 28. Bailey six-axis reference system. The lead axes are marked in 30° increments from 0° to 180° and from 0° to −180°. The six leads are marked with a + at the positive electrode and a − at the negative electrode. Notice that for leads I, II, III, and aVF the polarity and angle of the leads are positive or negative simultaneously. Leads aVR and aVL are positive at the positions of −150° and −30°, respectively, since the positive electrodes for those leads lie in the negative 0° to −180° zone. (From Ettinger, S. J., and Suter, P. F.: Canine Cardiology. Philadelphia, W. B. Saunders Co., 1971.)

Significance of Changes in Axis

Normal axis in the dog is +40° to +100°. Right axis deviation (axis is over +100) indicates right ventricular hypertrophy (Figure 30). Left axis deviation (axis is under 40°) indicates left ventricular hypertrophy (Figure 31). When there is biventricular hypertrophy, the axis usually remains normal.

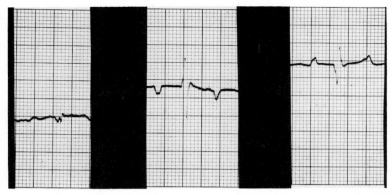

Figure 29. In each of these three leads the total positive and negative deflections equal zero. Each is considered an isoelectric lead.

Miscellaneous Criteria for Ventricular Hypertrophy

Summary of Criteria for Left Ventricular Hypertrophy

1. Left axis deviation.
2. QRS complex too wide (greater than 0.06 sec.).
3. R wave too tall (greater than 3.0 mv.).
4. S-T slurring.
5. May be associated with P mitrale, since left atrium and ventricle tend to be stressed together.

Summary of Criteria for Right Ventricular Hypertrophy

1. Right axis deviation.
2. Presence of an S wave in leads I, II and III (S_1-S_2-S_3 pattern) (Figure 32).
3. Q wave deeper than 0.5 mv. in leads II, III and aVF (Figure 33).
4. May be associated with P pulmonale, since the right atrium and ventricle tend to be stressed together.

III–4–D. Radiographic Procedures

Lateral and dorsoventral radiographs are valuable in assessing both cardiac chamber enlargement and pulmonary changes that may have occurred. This assists in determining treatment and prognosis. Heartworms is one disease that may need to be diagnosed by x-ray alone,

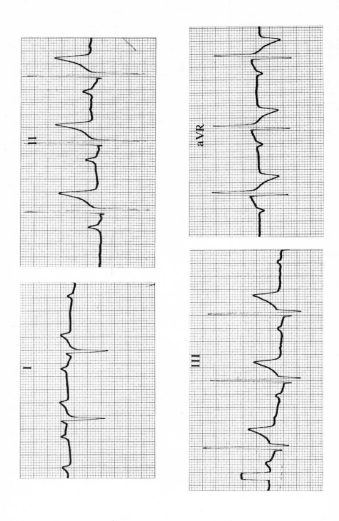

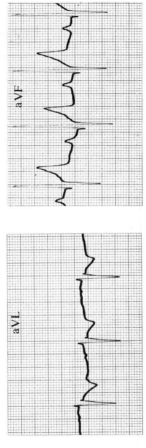

Figure 30. Notice the + 120° axis. (From Ettinger, S. J., and Suter, P. F.: Canine Cardiology. Philadelphia, W. B. Saunders Co., 1971.)

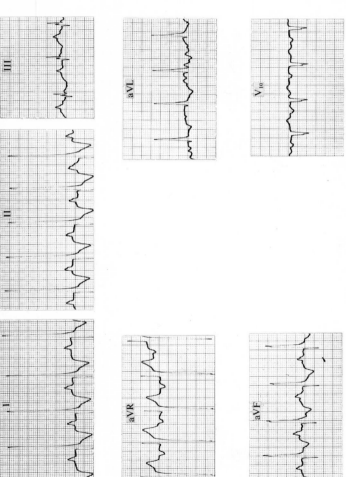

Figure 31. Left axis deviation. The mean electrical axis in the frontal plane in this dog with mitral valvular fibrosis is 35°. Notice that the R wave in lead I is tall and positive, as would be expected in left axis deviation. Also present in this tracing are P mitrale, tall and prolonged QRS complexes, and S-T repolarization changes, all of which are consistent with left atrial and left ventricular hypertrophy. (From Ettinger, S. J., and Suter, P. F.: Canine Cardiology. Philadelphia, W. B. Saunders

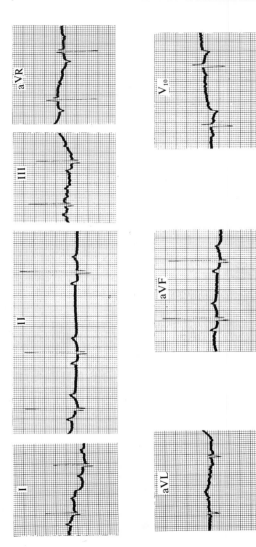

Figure 32. S_1-S_2-S_3 pattern. This tracing was made from a dog with heartworm disease. The S_1-S_2-S_3 pattern is unusual in normal dogs, and the finding can suggest right ventricular hypertrophy. Such findings warrant further study, especially in areas where heartworms are endemic. (From Ettinger, S. J., and Suter, P. F.: Canine Cardiology. Philadelphia, W. B. Saunders Co., 1971.)

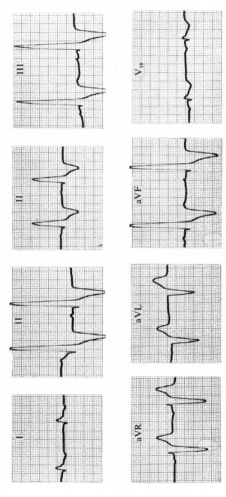

Figure 33. Electrocardiogram of dog with advanced mitral and tricuspid valvular fibrosis. The wide and notched P wave (0.05 sec.), the tall R wave (29 mm.), and wide (0.06 sec.) QRS complexes, as well as S-T repolarization changes in lead II, are consistent with left ventricular hypertrophy. The Q waves in leads II, III, and aVF are deeper than normal. (From Ettinger, S. J., and Suter, P. F.: Canine Cardiology. Philadelphia, W. B. Saunders Co., 1971.)

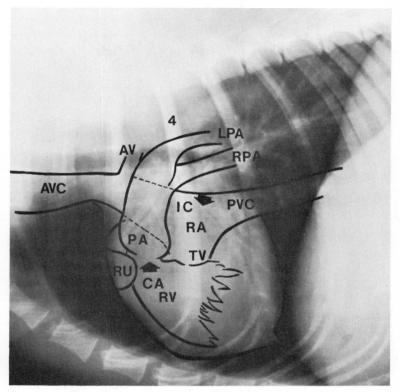

Figure 34. Left lateral radiograph of dog. Tracing delineates the structures of the right heart. The details for the tracing were obtained from angiocardiograms.

AVC—Cranial vena cava; AV—junction of the azygos vein with the AVC; RU—right auricle; RV—right ventricle; CA—conus arteriosus, or right ventricular outflow tract, extending to the tricuspid valve (arrow); PA—main pulmonary artery; LPA—left pulmonary artery; RPA—right pulmonary artery; RA—right atrium, divided dorsally by the intervenous crest, IC; arrow caudal to IC points at foramen ovale; PVC—caudal vena cava; 4—fourth rib. (From Ettinger, S. J., and Suter, P. F.: Canine Cardiology. Philadelphia, W. B. Saunders Co., 1971.)

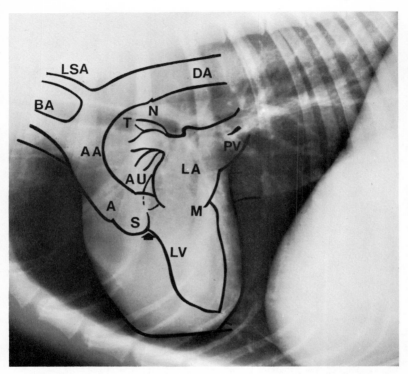

Figure 35. Lateral radiograph of dog in Figure 34. Tracing delineates the structures of the left heart. The details for the tracing were obtained from angiocardiograms.

BA—Brachiocephalic artery; LSA—left subclavian artery; AA—aortic arch; A—ascending aorta; S—sinus of Valsalva (arrow points at aortic valve); AU—small portion of the left auricle; T—tracheal bifurcation; N—notch in the descending aorta, DA, indicating the area of the ligamentum arteriosum; LV—left ventricle; M—mitral valve; LA—left atrium; PV—pulmonary veins. (From Ettinger, S. J., and Suter, P. F.: Canine Cardiology. Philadelphia, W. B. Saunders Co., 1971.)

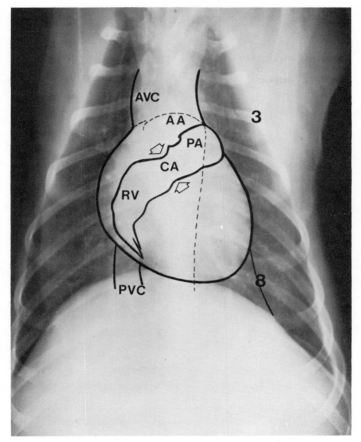

Figure 36. Dorsoventral radiograph of dog in Figure 34. Tracing delineates the right ventricle. Details for the tracing were obtained from angiocardiograms.

AVC—Cranial vena cava; AA—aortic arch; PA—main pulmonary artery, so-called pulmonary artery segment; CA—conus arteriosus, or right ventricular outflow tract; RV—right ventricle; PVC—caudal vena cava; numbers 3 and 8 indicate the respective ribs. (From Ettinger, S. J., and Suter, P. F.: Canine Cardiology. Philadelphia, W. B. Saunders Co., 1971.)

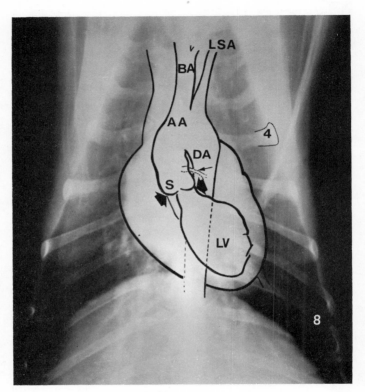

Figure 37. Dorsoventral radiograph of dog in Figure 34. Tracing delineates the structures of the left ventricle and aorta. Details for the tracing were obtained from angiocardiograms.

LSA—Left subclavian artery; BA—brachial artery; AA—aortic arch; DA—descending aorta; S—sinus of Valsalva; large arrows point at the muscular lining of the left ventricular outflow tract; small arrow indicates the origin of the left coronary artery, which is indicated by broken lines; LV—left ventricle; numbers 4 and 8 indicate the respective ribs. (From Ettinger, S. J., and Suter, P. F.: Canine Cardiology. Philadelphia, W. B. Saunders Co., 1971.)

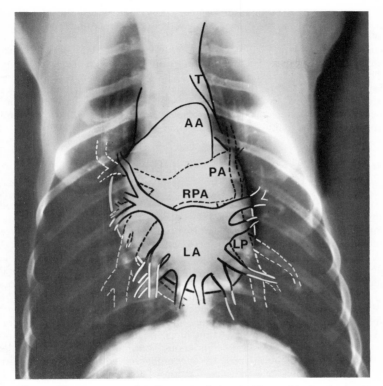

Figure 38. Dorsoventral radiograph of dog in Figure 34. Tracing outlines pulmonary arteries and the confluence of the pulmonary veins at the left atrium. Solid lines represent veins and left atrium; broken lines indicate the pulmonary arteries. Details for the tracings were obtained from angiocardiograms.

T—Thymus, seen only in growing dogs; AA—aortic arch; PA—pulmonary artery; RPA—right pulmonary artery; LP—left pulmonary artery; LA—left atrium. (From Ettinger, S. J., and Suter, P. F.: Canine Cardiology. Philadelphia, W. B. Saunders Co., 1971.)

since the blood test may be negative and the EKG may be non-contributory.

Changes in lung vasculature may be evident on radiographs. With pulmonary congestion, the pulmonary veins are engorged with blood. With pulmonary overcirculation, it is the pulmonary arteries that are engorged. Radiographically, on lateral films, the veins appear indistinct and tortuous, and are seen emanating from the area of the left atrium. The pulmonary arteries, on the other hand, appear straight and branching, like a tree. On the dorsoventral view, veins are medial and arteries are lateral. Mitral insufficiency causes pulmonary venous congestion; heartworm disease, chronic lung disease congenital left-to-right shunt anomalies cause pulmonary arterial enlargement.

III–4–E.   Cardiac Catheterization

The patient is anesthetized for this procedure, and a catheter is passed into the various cardiac chambers. Usually the catheter is passed through the jugular or the femoral vein into the right side of the heart, and through the carotid or the femoral artery into the left heart. An image intensification fluoroscopic unit helps placement of the catheters. Pressures may be taken using the catheters and a pressure transducer (Table 26). Blood samples may be withdrawn through the catheters for blood gas analysis. Angiocardiograms may be recorded by placing an injection of contrast dye into the desired area through the catheters.

Angiocardiography may be accomplished in practice by using a 2 inch, 16 gauge needle and injecting contrast media into the jugular vein. A rapid bolus of dye is used and films are taken one, two, four and five seconds after injection. This should outline the right heart. The left ventricle may be injected by accomplishing cardiac puncture with a 3 inch, 18 gauge needle. Modification of the time sequence may be necessary depending on the case. One of the more popular contrast

TABLE 26.   NORMAL CARDIAC CHAMBER PRESSURES

	PA	RV	RA	AO	LV	Wedge (LA)
Systolic	15 to 30	15 to 30	3 to 4	100 to 180	100 to 180	6 to 8
Diastolic	10	0	3 to 4	60 to 90	0	6 to 8

TABLE 27. HEART RATE AND DURATIONS OF P, P-R, QRS, and Q-T

Animal	P	P-R	QRS	Q-T	Heart Rate (Beats/Min.)	REF.
Dog						
Mean	0.07	0.12	0.06	0.21		8
Range	0.04 to 0.12	0.10 to 0.15	0.04 to 0.08	0.16 to 0.28	72 to 162	
Mean	0.06	0.106	0.045	0.187		9
Range	0.02 to 0.10	0.06 to 0.17	0.03 to 0.06	0.14 to 0.25	67 to 214	10
Cat	0.02 to 0.040	0.06 to 0.080	0.02 to 0.04	0.18 to 0.26		11
	0.038 to 0.045	0.065 to 0.090	0.035 to 0.040	0.175 to 0.325	95 to 194	

From Clark, D. R., Szabuniewicz, M., and McCrady, J. D.: Clinical use of the electrocardiogram in animals. Vet. Med., *61*:751–760, August, 1966.

TABLE 28. AMPLITUDES (MILLIVOLTS) OF THE VARIOUS ELECTROCARDIOGRAM WAVES IN DIFFERENT ANIMAL SPECIES

Lead	Animal	P	Q	R	S	T
I	DOG	0.05 to 0.40	0.00 to 1.15	0.20 to 2.22 0.00 to 0.03*	0.00 to 0.80	−0.36 to −0.63
	CAT	0.01 to 0.14	0.02 to 0.84	0.03 to 1.28 0.05 to 0.31*	0.01 to 0.42	0.01 to 0.25
II	DOG	0.03 to 0.50	0.00 to 0.89	0.30 to 3.09 0.00 to 0.19*	0.00 to 0.79	−0.27 to 0.74
	CAT	0.05 to 0.28	0.02 to 0.77	0.03 to 1.33 0.16 to 1.35*	0.03 to 0.70	0.03 to 0.35 0.07 to 0.10**
III	DOG	−0.27 to 0.39	0.00 to 0.44	0.14 to 2.43 0.00 to 0.24*	0.00 to −1.48	−0.26 to 0.81
	CAT	0.03 to 0.21	0.02 to 0.38	0.05 to 1.12 0.05 to 0.63*	0.02 to 0.65	0.02 to 0.26 0.03 to 0.14**

TABLE 28. AMPLITUDES (MILLIVOLTS) OF THE VARIOUS ELECTROCARDIOGRAM WAVES IN DIFFERENT ANIMAL SPECIES (*Continued*)

Lead	Animal	P	Q	R	S	T
aVR	DOG	−0.35 to 0.19	0.00 to 1.89	0.02 to 1.28 0.00 to 0.39*	0.00 to 2.34	−0.60 to −0.26
aVL	DOG	−0.16 to 0.24	0.00 to 1.27	0.02 to 1.79 0.00 to 0.38*	0.00 to 2.58	−0.40 to 0.36
aVF	DOG	−0.10 to 0.45	0.00 to 0.70	0.10 to −2.52 0.00 to −0.23*	0.00 to 0.67	−0.25 to 0.74
CV6LU	DOG	0.350 ± 0.114	0.570 ± 0.370	4.246 ± 1.438	0.528 ± 0.406	0.370 ± 0.554
CV6LL	DOG	0.334 ± 0.100	0.406 ± 0.276	4.766 ± 1.348	0.726 ± 0.540	0.598 ± 0.570
CV5RL	DOG	0.164 ± 0.100		2.598 ± 1.206	1.236 ± 0.766	0.724 ± 0.480

*Value for R[1] when present
**Value for Negative deflection
From Clark, D. R., Szabuniewicz, M., and McCrady, J. D.: Clinical use of the electrocardiogram in animals.
Vet. Med. *61*:861–870, September, 1966.

TABLE 29. INTRACARDIAL PHYSIOLOGIC VALUES OF DOGS

Condition	JVP	PAP	FAP	Diastolic Heart Vol. cc./kg. BW	Total Heart Weight gm./kg. BW	Blood Volume cc./kg. BW	Heart Rate (Untreated)
Normal	0–6	20–30	140–180	15–20	6–10	75–90	70–120
Mitral Insufficiency							
Mild	0 to 20	35 to 55	120–180	20 to 60	8 to 15	90 to 120	100–190
Severe			100–165				120–240
Heartworms							
Mild	0 to 25	30 to 125	120–200	20 to 60	8 to 15	90 to 125	70–120
Severe			140–200				90–190
Pulmonic Stenosis	25	115	100	36	12	122	170
Patent Ductus Arteriosus	5	60	190	—	10	—	150
	(not in congestive failure)						
Ventricular Septal Defect	20	150	150	56	15	—	140

JVP—Jugular venous pressure
PAP—Pulmonary arterial pressure, systolic
FAP—Femoral arterial pressure, systolic
BW —Body weight
Values obtained in dogs studied by the Department of Physiology, Medical College of Georgia, Augusta, Ga., under United States Public Health Service Grants HTS 5044, H 240 and AHA.
From Wallace, C. R.: Cardiac catheterization to aid in diagnosis of cardiovascular disease. Small Anim. Clin. 2:324-331, June, 1962.

medias is Hypaque (Winthrop) because of its high radiographic density and its relatively low viscosity. The dosage is 0.5 mg./lb. for 75 per cent Hypaque and 1 mg./lb. for 50 per cent Hypaque.

At the present stage of veterinary medicine, cardiac catheterization is limited clinically and is primarily a research technique. As surgical techniques are developed and refined for animals, cardiac catheterization will be a useful, informative and required piece of clinical work before open heart surgery is attempted.

Other Tests

1. *Arterial blood pressure measurements* are not routinely done on dogs. Externally, the tail or hind leg has been used, but is unreliable and requires that the animal be perfectly still. The femoral artery may be cannulated and a B-D direct blood pressure manometer used. This is usually done on an anesthetized animal or one that is in shock. When systolic pressure falls below 70 to 80 mm. Hg., the condition is critical.

2. Circulation time.

3. Laboratory work. CBC , BUN, SGPT, urinalysis and microfilaria check are advisable. Centesis fluid evaluation may be useful. The typical fluid accumulation due to congestive heart failure has the following characteristics: the transudate has a specific gravity of less than 1.018. It is usually clear, straw-colored, or slightly blood tinged. The protein content is less than 3 gm. per cent.

References

Additional information can be found in the following sources:

American Animal Hospital Association: A Manual of Clinical Cardiology, 1972.

American Animal Hospital Association: Clinical Aspects of Canine Cardiology, 1965.

Clark, D. R., Szabuniewicz, M., and McGrady, J. D.: Clinical use of the electrocardiogram in animals. Vet. Med. *61*:861–871, September, 1966.

Detweiler, D. K., and Patterson, D. F.: A phonographic record of heart sounds and murmurs of the dog. Ann. N. Y. Acad. Sci. *127*:322–340, September, 1965.

Detweiler, D. K., et al.: Diseases of the cardiovascular system. *In* Catcott, E. J. (ed.): Canine Medicine. Santa Barbara, California, American Veterinary Publications, Inc., 1968.

Ettinger, S. J., and Suter, P. F.: Canine Cardiology. Philadelphia, W. B. Saunders Co., 1971.

Kirk, R. W. (ed.): Current Veterinary Therapy V. Philadelphia, W. B. Saunders Co., 1974.

Wallace, C. R.: Cardiac catheterization to aid in diagnosis of cardiovascular disease. Small Anim. Clin. 2:324–331, June, 1962.

III-5. EYE, EAR, NOSE AND THROAT EXAMINATION

III-5-A. Examination of the Eye*

As in any type of medical examination, the detailed examination of the eyes should be preceded by a careful history. The following categories should be included in the history: 1. Chief complaint (C. C.); 2. Present illness (P. I.); 3. Review of systems (R. S.); and 4. Past history (P. H.).

EXTERNAL EXAMINATION

Inspection of the Globe and Neuromuscular Examination

A careful, systematic scheme of examination should be used when examining the eyes. A general inspection of the globe and external ocular structures should be conducted before any detailed examination of the eye is undertaken. Inspect the globe in normal daylight or room-light and observe the relationship of the globe to the orbit and the eyelids. Note if the eyes are in the same visual axis or if a tropia is present. Note any undue prominence of either or both eyes. Note the presence of any other facial lesions (e.g., facial paralysis) which may affect the symmetry of the orbit. Inspect the external ocular structures (lids, conjunctiva, cornea, sclera, and lacrimal apparatus). Note the position of the eyelids, size of the palpebral aperture, position of the membrana nictitans, the

---

*From Bistner, S. I.: Examination of the eye. Vet. Clin. North Amer. Vol. 1, No. 1, pp. 29–51, January, 1971.

presence of nystagmus, unequal pupils, blepharospasm, lagophthalmos, or ocular discharges.

The tonic eye reflexes are used in the determination of extraocular muscle function and localization of lesions in the central nervous system. The dog and cat have seven extraocular muscles: 1. M. rectus medialis; 2. M. rectus lateralis; 3. M. rectus dorsalis; 4. M. rectus ventralis; 5. M. obliquus dorsalis; 6. M. obliquus ventralis; and 7. M. retractor bulbi. Cranial nerves 3, 4, and 6 (N. oculomotorius, N. trochlearis, N. abducens) innervate the extraocular striated muscles and are examined together. Nerve 4 innervates the M. obliquus dorsalis, nerve 6 innervates the M. rectus lateralis and part of the M. retractor bulbi and nerve 3 innervates the M. rectus medialis and M. rectus ventralis, M. obliquus ventralis and M. levator palpebral superioris. Pupillary dilatation is controlled by preganglionic neurons in the first three thoracic spinal cord segments, the cranial thoracic and cervical sympathetic trunks, and by postganglionic neurons in the cranial cervical and sympathetic nerves that course through the middle ear to reach the orbit and M. dilator pupillae. Parasympathetic fibers in nerve 3 innervate the sphincter pupillae muscle.

The integrity of cranial nerve 3 may be evaluated by examining: 1. The size of the pupil; 2. The reaction of the pupil to light; 3. The presence or absence of ptosis or drooping of the upper eyelid because of paralysis of the levator palpebrae superioris muscle; and 4. The medial deviation of the eye which occurs in oculomotor nerve palsy (different than in man) possibly because the M. obliquus dorsalis muscle is stronger than the M. rectus lateralis. In oculomotor nerve palsy with a normal pupillary response, if all the extraocular muscles innervated by the 3rd nerve are affected, then an intracranial lesion should be suspected. If individual extraocular muscles are involved, then a peripheral nerve lesion may exist. If an oculomotor nerve palsy exists in association with a dilated pupil, an intraorbital and/or intracranial lesion should be suspected.

Paralysis of the trochlear nerve produces a transient strabismus resulting in a slight upward deviation of the eye (rarely seen). The affected animal may compensate for this by developing a head tilt.

Paralysis of the abducens nerve results in a medial deviation of the affected eye with inability to gaze laterally.

It is important to check tonic neck and eye reflexes when evaluating the extraocular muscles. When the nose is elevated, the forelimbs extend and the hindlimbs flex. As the nose is elevated, the eye should remain focused within the center of the palpebral fissure. Deviating the head to one side results in increased extensor tonus on that side. Normally, nystagmus should be observed on lateral deviation of the head (with the quick phase toward the side of the deviation).

Cranial nerve 2 (N. opticus) has its origin in the retina at the optic disk. In the cat, about 66 per cent of the optic nerve fibers—in the dog about 75 per cent—decussate at the optic chiasma. The optic nerve has two components; one is composed of those fibers that pass to the pupillary centers within the brainstem; the second is composed of those fibers that synapse in the thalamus, which in turn project the impulses to the visual cortex of the brain. The pupillary fibers leave the optic tract and synapse in the midbrain, where crossing occurs. Impulses reach the parasympathetic portion of the oculomotor nucleus. From here, parasympathetic preganglionic fibers exit in the third cranial nerve to synapse in the ciliary ganglion caudal to the globe. The postganglionic fibers go to the iridic sphincter and ciliary muscles. Always note and record the direct and consensual pupillary reflexes. Shine a light in the temporal portion of each eye. Note the pupillary response. Test the consensual pupillary response by shining a focal source of light in one eye and noting the effects in the opposite eye. The normal pupillary response requires that nerves 2 and 3 be intact, and involves only brainstem connections.

Assessment of Visual Function

Assessment of visual function in pet animals presents a difficult problem, and the veterinarian must depend on objective signs and reflexes to estimate vision. A common test often used to assess vision is the "menace reaction." This involves passing the hand or an object in front of the animal's eyes and noticing the presence or absence of a blink reflex. The possibility of stimulating the corneal reflex during the menace response test can be abolished by placing a clear piece of Plexiglass in front of the eye and then menacing the dog.

The response of the pupil to light also can be used to evaluate function of the visual system. Each pupil should be tested individually using a bright focal source of illumination, and the opposite eye should be covered. The consensual pupillary response also should be tested. Normal pupillary responses require only brainstem connections; therefore, cortical lesions can result in blindness with normal pupillary response to light. An obstacle course also can be very valuable in assessing visual function. Styrofoam cylinders mounted on a platform can be used to create the course. The light intensity in the examining room can be varied, and alternate patching of the eyes can be helpful in detecting lesions.

In addition to obstacle courses, the reaction to various test patterns can be used to assess visual function. A rotating optokinetic drum has, on occasion, been used to elicit a physiologic type of nystagmus in the visual animal. This form of nystagmus depends on the ability of the eyes to follow a visible pattern on a slowly rotating drum.

Examination of the Orbit

Observe the orbits for size. Look for swelling, depression, fistula, or laceration of the orbital margin. If the orbit is enlarged, note whether the swelling is hard or soft, painful or nonpainful. Retrobulbar abscesses produce exophthalmos attended by pain, immobility of the eye, chemosis, edema of the eyelids, and pain on opening the mouth. Orbital tumors may not be painful. Orbital retrobulbar hemorrhage or orbital fracture may occur following severe head trauma from automobile accidents. Enophthalmos may result from shrinkage of orbital contents (as in pthisis bulbi following ocular injury), from paralysis of the sympathetic nerve in Horner's syndrome, or from loss of retrobulbar fat in emaciation and dehydration.

Examination of the Eyelids

Note any inflammation along the margins of the eyelids and any inability to close the lids (lagophthalmos). The eyelids should touch the globe, thus preventing an accumulation of tears and debris. The cilia or eyelashes on the dog's upper eyelids are arranged in three irregular rows. The lower eyelids of dogs and both eyelids of cats are devoid of cilia. When examining the lids for the presence of entropion or ectropion, it is best not to manipulate the head, as this may distort the normal lid–globe relationship. The lids of dogs and cats have a very poorly developed tarsal plate, making manipulation relatively easy. Observe the edges of the lids for signs of entropion, ectropion, trichiasis, or distichiasis. Observe the eyelids for symblepharon or for swelling, edema, redness, or a localized inflammation, which may indicate an internal or external hordeolum. Examine the lid margins for indication of any growths.

Examination of the Eye Using Focal Illumination

In examining the anterior segment of the eye, the use of a simple optical system combining a focal source of illumination and condensing

N.Y.S. VETERINARY COLLEGE — CORNELL UNIVERSITY — VETERINARY HOSPITALS

OPHTHALMOLOGY EXAMINATION

DATE _____

History: _____

ACC# _____ PHONE _____
OWNER _____
STREET _____
CITY _____ STATE ____ ZIP _____
HOSP _____ SEX ____ COLOR _____
SPEC _____ BREED ____ ID _____

REF. DVM _____
CLINICIAN _____
SECONDARY # _____

LIDS _____

NICTITANS _____

CONJUNCTIVA _____

IRIS _____

CORNEA _____

LENS _____

OCULAR PRESSURE _____

FUNDUS EXAM _____

Summary of Findings & Diagnosis:

(Teaching   Donaldson   2X2   Pathology   Culture   Cytology   Surgery)

OPHTHALMOLOGY EXAMINATION

Figure 39. Ophthalmology examination record.

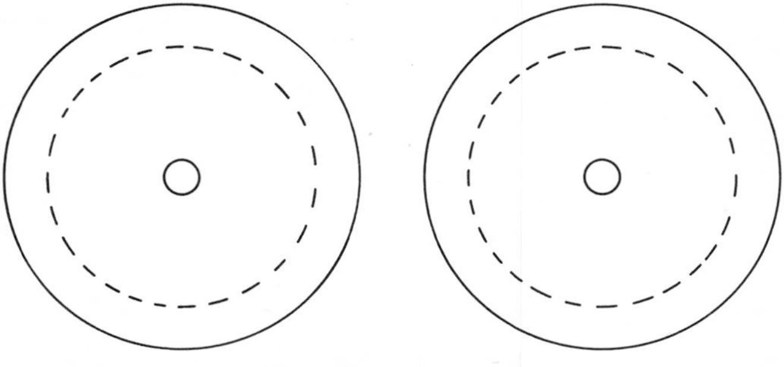

Figure 39. (Continued)

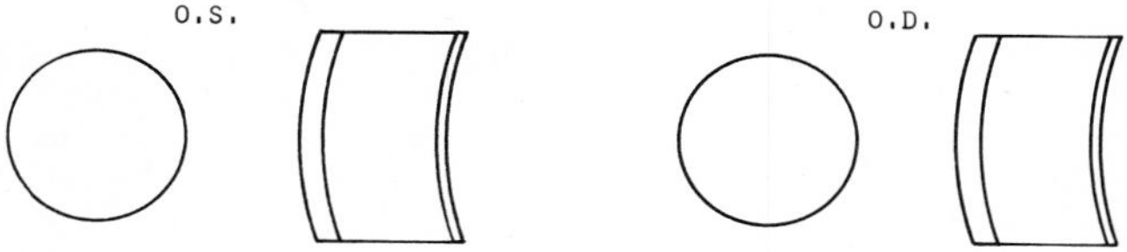

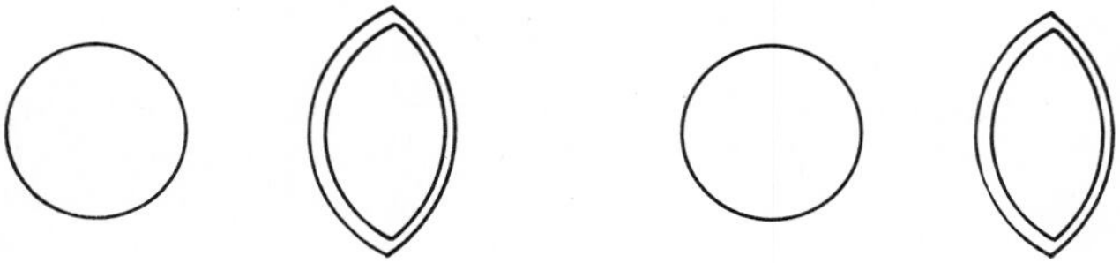

lens with an ophthalmic loupe or magnifying glass enables the observer to illuminate and examine various structures of the eye. The most highly refined source of focal illumination and magnification is the biomicroscope.

The combination of the slit lamp providing a source of focal illumination and the corneal microscope provides a method for careful and detailed examination of the eye, especially the anterior segment. The slit lamp enables the clinician accurately to locate the depth of a lesion in the cornea and lens. The major advantage of the biomicroscope is the ability to view pathologic processes in the living structure with great detail, and therefore more accurately diagnose, treat, and formulate prognosis about diseases of the eye.

In using the slit lamp for focal examination of the anterior segment of the eye there are six basic methods of illumination available: 1. Diffuse illumination; 2. Direct illumination; 3. Retroillumination; 4. Specular reflection; 5. Indirect lateral illumination; and 6. Oscillatory illumination. For clinical use in small animals, diffuse, direct and retroillumination are most valuable. Diffuse illumination permits examination of large surface areas such as the cornea, lens, and iris. In direct illumination, the focal light beam is directed obliquely into the eye and the part to be studied is illuminated. Small changes in the transparency of the optical media can be studied. In retroillumination, the focal beam of light is directed on an opaque body or reflective surface behind the tissue to be examined. The structure to be examined is then seen in the irregular reflection created by the light source.

Many types of biomicroscopes are available commercially. Most are table models and can be placed on an adjustable stand. We have found the Nikon Zoom Photo Biomicroscope on a spring-compensated Reliance table very satisfactory for examining small animals. The anterior segment of the eyes of dogs and cats can be examined using minimal restraint. The examination should not be unduly prolonged because the animal becomes restless. Magnification of 7 to 25 × usually is sufficient in small animals. The vitreous and posterior segment of the eye can be examined with the biomicroscope, provided special lenses are interposed between the eye and the instrument.

Examination of the Conjunctiva

Note whether the conjunctiva is pale, injected, pigmented, hemorrhagic, or jaundiced. The inferior or ventral conjunctiva usually is more hyperemic than the upper. Pigmentation occasionally is present, especially on the superior bulbar conjunctiva. Usually a few follicles are present on the conjunctival surface, especially that of the third eyelid.

Note if the conjunctiva is relatively smooth and dry, or excessively moist. Note any lacerations or erosions of the conjunctiva. These may be demonstrated using fluorescein. After initial inspection of the conjunctiva, additional tests may be required, such as the Schirmer tear test, culture, cytologic examination, or the use of stains.

It is important to recognize pathologic congestion of the bulbar conjunctiva. There are two forms: superficial and deep. Superficial congestion usually is characteristic of external ocular irritation from foreign bodies, bacteria, trauma, or allergic reactions. Deep congestion indicates an involvement of the cornea or the deeper structures within the eye. Normally the deeper vessels around the limbus are difficult to see, however when congested they produce a distinctive "red flush" around the eye.

When presented with a "red eye" due to conjunctival vascularization, the clinician must decide whether it is a superficial ocular condition with conjunctival congestion or a problem deeper within the eye producing ciliary congestion. Tables 30 and 31 may be helpful in differential diagnosis.

The palpebral (outer) and bulbar (inner) surfaces of the nictitating membrane should be inspected. The anterior surface of the membrane normally is smooth, and the leading edge frequently is pigmented. The bulbar surface can be examined by placing a few drops of topical anes-

TABLE 30. DIFFERENTIATION OF DEEP AND SUPERFICIAL CONGESTION

Signs	Ciliary Congestion	Conjunctival Congestion
Pain	Usually present	Usually absent
Photophobia	Usually marked	Usually absent
Location of congested area	More intense circumcorneally	More marked in fornices and tarsal conjunctiva
Course of vessels	Straight, radiating limbus	Irregular and tortuous
Mobility of vessels	Cannot be moved	Easily moved
Blanching by vasoconstriction	Not blanched	May be blanched
Discharge	Absent	May or may not be present
Pupil size	Usually contracted	Unaffected
Iris	Usually congested	Unaffected

TABLE 31. DIFFERENTIAL DIAGNOSIS OF ACUTE
CONJUNCTIVITIS, ACUTE IRITIS, AND ACUTE GLAUCOMA

	Acute Conjunctivitis	Acute Iritis	Acute Glaucoma
Onset	Gradual	Gradual	Sudden
Pain	None to mild irritation	Fairly severe	Fairly severe
Discharge	Mucopurulent or purulent	Tearing	None
Vision	Unaffected	Slightly reduced	May be markedly reduced
Conjunctiva	Superficial congestion	Deep circumcorneal and ciliary congestion	Deep conjunctival, episcleral, and ciliary congestion
Cornea	Clear	Keratic precipitates may be present	Steamy and insensitive
Iris	Unaffected	Muddy and congested; posterior synechiae may be present	Congested and displaced forward
Pupil	Normal	Contracted	Dilated
Anterior chamber	Unaffected	May contain cells, opacities and exudates	Shallow
Tenderness	Absent	Present over ciliary body	Usually absent
Tension	Unaffected	Lower than normal	Increased
Constitutional signs	Absent	Slight	Slight to moderate

thetic (proparacaine HCl) in the eye and gently using a small, atraumatic thumb forceps to evert the third eyelid. The bulbar surface usually contains a few small follicles. The following are frequently found abnormalities that may be associated with the third eyelid: eversion of the cartilage; hypertrophy; protrusion; inflammation and hypertrophy of gland of third eyelid; foreign bodies; and neoplasia.

Conjunctival Smears, Scrapings, and Cultures. Conjunctival scrapings and cytologic examination can be very helpful in establishing an etiology and outlining an effective treatment regimen in conjunctivitis. In performing conjunctival scrapings, use a platinum spatula (Kimura spatula) whose tip has previously been sterilized in the flame of an alcohol lamp. Scrape the inferior conjunctival cul-de-sac, preferably without prior topical anesthesia, since anesthetics may distort the cells. Place the material on two glass slides, and fix one in acetone-free 95 per cent methanol for 5 to 10 minutes; then stain with Giemsa stain. Heat fix the other slide and apply Gram stain.

Culturing the conjunctiva also can be a valuable aid, especially in chronic conjunctivitis. Sterile cotton applicators, fluid thioglycollate media, and blood agar media are needed to perform cultures. Evert the palpebral conjunctiva of the lower lid, and pass one side of a sterile cotton applicator, previously moistened with sterile broth or thioglycollate media, over the palpebral conjunctival surface. Streak the swab onto a sterile blood agar plate; then place it into a tube of thioglycollate broth. No topical anesthesia is used prior to culturing, since preservatives present in anesthetics can inhibit the growth of bacteria.

Examination of the Lacrimal System

Look for excessive tearing or a hypofunction of tear secretion. Note any swelling, redness, or pain in the area of the lacrimal puncta and the lacrimal sac. The nasolacrimal system can be evaluated by several basic tests. When excessive tearing exists, it must be determined if the tearing is due to: 1. Partial or complete obstruction of the excretory mechanism; 2. Increased lacrimal secretion from chronic ocular irritation, as in distichiasis or trichiasis; 3. Physiologic increase in tear production as may occur with uveitis. The first diagnostic step is the use of the primary dye test. To perform this test, place a drop of fluorescein dye from a sterile fluoro-strip into the eye. After two to five minutes, the external nares are examined with the aid of a Woods light for the presence or absence of fluorescein dye. If dye is present, one can conclude that the lacrimal excretory system is patent and functioning. If epiphora exists yet the primary dye test indicates that the lacrimal excretory system is patent, then hypersecretion of tear fluid may be implicated as the cause for the epiphora.

If no stain appears at the external nares, the primary dye test is negative, demonstrating an obstruction to normal tear flow in the excretory mechanism. Irrigation of the nasolacrimal system is then indicated. In the dog, the nasolacrimal puncta are located 1 to 3 mm. from the medial canthus on the mucocutaneous border of the upper and lower lid. In the dog, a 20- to 22-gauge nasolacrimal cannula (in the cat a 23-gauge) should be used. A 2-ml. syringe is filled with saline, and the lacrimal cannula is attached and passed into the lacrimal puncta of the upper lid. In most dogs, this can be done with the aid of topical anesthesia and local restraint. Some animals require additional sedation. The saline is injected and should exit through the lower puncta if this "arc" is patent. If the lower puncta is patent, it is held closed by digital pressure on the lower lid, and the system is again irrigated. If fluid comes out of the nose and is dye-stained, then an obstruction existed somewhere in the nasolacrimal duct and the canaliculi were patent enough to get dye part way into the excretory system. If no dye comes out the nose, a complete obstruction of the nasolacrimal system existed.

Dacryocystorhinography involves the use of radiopaque contrast material to outline the nasolacrimal system. The upper lacrimal punctum is cannulated, and the system is flushed with 0.25 to 0.5 ml. of 40 per cent Lipiodol solution. The lateral and ventrodorsal positions are used for radiography.

Several points should be made about evaluating the nasolacrimal system. First, brachycephalic breeds of dogs may on occasion have a negative primary dye test although no blockage in the nasolacrimal system exists. In flushing the nasolacrimal system of some animals, fluid may not appear at the nose, however the animal may gag and exhibit swallowing movements, indicating that the fluid has entered the mouth and the system is patent.

Basic tear secretion comes mainly from the tarsal and conjunctival glands and the accessory tarsal glands. The reflex tear secretors are the main lacrimal gland and accessory lacrimal glands. The production of normal lacrimal secretion can be tested by using the Schirmer tear test. This test is performed by placing a strip of filter paper (Whatman No. 41, 35 mm. long and 5 mm. wide, with a 5-mm. flap turned back at one end) in the inferior conjunctival cul-de-sac. The amount of wetting is measured in millimeters after a period of one minute. No topical anesthesia or drops of any kind should be used prior to conducting the test. The tear flow response in the dog as measured with the Schirmer tear test paper is a measure of corneal sensitivity and the animal's ability to produce tears. In normal dogs, wetting of the Schirmer test papers ranges from 10 to 25 mm. in one minute. Variation in the relative humidity can alter Schirmer tear test values. Values less than 10 mm. wetting in one minute when combined with the clinical signs of keratoconjunctivitis are usually indicative of keratoconjunctivitis sicca or "dry eyes." The Schirmer tear test is helpful in evaluating changes in tear secretion in animals on oral pilocarpine therapy for KCS or following surgical transposition of the parotid duct.

Examination of the Sclera

Note the color of the sclera and look for nodules, hemorrhage, lacerations, cysts, or tumors. Normal sclera is white to blue-white. The sclera may appear blue because it is abnormally thinned and the uveal tract shows through. Look for staphylomas. Look for any injection of the scleral vessels and accompanying edema. Episcleritis can produce local scleral inflammation, whereas deep-seated ocular diseases such as glaucoma and uveitis produce generalized scleral vessel injection.

Examination of the Cornea

The cornea should be smooth, moist, free of blood vessels, and transparent. Note any ulceration or opacity of the cornea. Slight opacities are termed nebulae; dense ones, leukomas. The canine cornea is oval, with a diameter of 12.5 to 17 mm. The horizontal measurement is 1 to 2 mm. greater than the vertical axis. Measurement of the corneal diameter with calipers may prove valuable when evaluating glaucoma and buphthalmia. In puppies, the cornea tends to be hazy, thus restricting ophthalmoscopic examination until four to six weeks of age. Such diseases of the cornea as corneal inflammation, pigmentation, degeneration, trauma, and neoplasia frequently may alter its transparency. To estimate the depth of a corneal lesion, observe the cornea from the side and let a focal source of light enter the cornea obliquely. Accurate assessment of the depth of corneal lesions requires the use of a biomicroscope.

Test the corneal sensitivity by touching the cornea with a wisp of dry cotton. Instill a topical anesthetic—proparacaine hydrochloride, 0.5 per cent (Ophthaine)—into the conjunctival sac of each eye. Use a small forceps to pull the third eyelid gently away from the corneal surface, and examine its inner surface for foreign bodies, hyperplastic tissue, inflammation, follicle formation, or parasites (*Thelazia*). Observe the corneal surface for the presence of foreign bodies.

External ophthalmic stains can be very helpful in diagnosing lesions of the cornea. Fluorescein does not actually stain tissues. Being somewhat acid, the normal precorneal tear film stains yellow or orange with fluorescein. The intact corneal epithelium, having a high lipid content, resists penetration of water soluble fluorescein and is not colored by it. Any break in the epithelial barrier permits rapid fluorescein penetration into the stroma, or even into the anterior chamber. When the epithelial surface has regenerated, the green color disappears, regardless of whether the underlying stroma is thickened, thinned, scarred, or irregular.

Fluorescein may be applied as a drop of 0.5 to 2 per cent solution or by placing a strip of fluorescein impregnated filter paper into the conjunctival sac until it is moistened by the tears. Excess dyes should be irrigated away with the saline solution. Fluorescein staining of the eye is transient and usually disappears in 30 to 45 minutes. Iatrogenic spread of ocular infections via fluorescein solution contaminated with *Pseudomonas* spp. is not infrequent, and for this reason individually packaged, sterilized strips are more desirable.

Unlike fluorescein, rose bengal actually stains cells and their nuclei. It selectively stains devitalized corneal and conjunctival epithelium a readily visible red. Its main use has been in identification of corneal and conjunctival lesions due to keratitis sicca.

Rose bengal is instilled as a 1 per cent aqueous solution. Application causes irritation to the cornea, and one drop of topical anesthesia prior to instillation of the dye is helpful in preventing irritation. Excess rose bengal should be removed by irrigation.

If an ulcer is present, note whether the borders are regular or irregular and whether the ulcer is superficial or deep. Ulcers that are progressive and deep present a guarded prognosis. It is advisable to culture deep ulcers and to make a scraping of their borders. The scrapings should be stained with Giemsa and the type of cells determined. If the ulcer appears to be deep, look for evidence of anterior synechia, prolapsed iris, iridocyclitis, cataract, extrusion of the lens, fistula, or hemorrhage.

Note the presence of blood vessels in the cornea. It is important to determine the depth at which vascularization is taking place, since it usually is directly related to the cause of the vascularization. Superficial vascularization commonly is associated with superficial keratitis, superficial ulcers, or pannus. Deep vascularization usually indicates a deep corneal stromal lesion, uveitis, or glaucoma.

Look for deposits on the posterior surface of the cornea (keratic precipitates). These precipitates vary in size and shape, but they usually are indicative of a disease of the uveal tract.

INTERNAL EXAMINATION

Examination of the Anterior Chamber

Examine the anterior chamber, and observe its depth; note changes in the transparency of the ocular media, such as hypopyon, hyphema, fibrin, or foreign bodies. Look for anterior synechiae.

The anterior drainage angle cannot be visualized readily in the dog without the use of a contact lens. Large tumors and some anterior synechiae can be visualized with a loupe and a focal light source.

Examination of the Iris

The color of the iris in each eye may vary. Observe the shape or size of the iris. An iris that is thickened and muddy in color indicates an infiltration of the uveal tract. Look for the presence of atrophy, tears, synechiae, persistent pupillary membranes, iridodonesis, iridodialysis, nodules, tumors, cysts, or colobomas. Examine the pupillary border of the iris for signs of atrophy or posterior synechiae to the anterior lens capsule. Complete posterior synechia results in iris bombe and secondary glaucoma.

Examine the pupil of each eye by diffuse and focal illumination. Note the pupil size and shape and its direct and consensual response to light. Note any inequalities between the two pupils. Check to see if the pupils are dilated. Find out from the owner whether the subject has had a mydriatic placed in its eye. Determine whether the pupils, when dilated, constrict when light is applied. The pupil may be dilated because of trauma, a mydriatic, fear, stimulation of the cervical sympathetic nerve, glaucoma, paralysis of the third cranial nerve, or retinal atrophy. The pupil may be contracted (miosis) because of a miotic, from synechiae, stimulation by light, in acute iritis, following the use of a narcotic, in paralysis of the sympathetic nerve, or from irritation of the third cranial nerve.

Note whether the pupil of one eye is equal in size to the pupil of the other, and whether it remains so with changes in the degree of illumination. Inequality of pupil size (anisocoria) may be physiologic or pathologic. Pathologic causes include diseases and tumors of the central nervous system.

Examination of the Lens

It is easier to examine the lens if the pupil is dilated. The lens may be examined with a focal source of illumination and a loupe, with an ophthalmoscope, or with a biomicroscope. Examine the lens for the presence of pigment, adhesions, opacities, the position of the lens (subluxation or luxation), or the absence of the lens (aphakia). Verification of the presence of the lens can be obtained by utilizing the Purkinje-Sanson's images. Hold a focal source of light in front of and just to the side of the eye. Look for the presence of three images within the eye: one is reflected from the anterior cornea and the image is erect; the second is an erect image from the anterior lens capsule; and the third is an inverted image reflected from the posterior surface of the lens if the lens is present. If the lens is opaque, the third Purkinje-Sanson's image is not seen.

The presence of the lens can also be verified by using ultraviolet illumination (Wood's light) and observing the lens fluoresce.

Ophthalmoscopy

Examination of the Retina.   Examination of the retina with an ophthalmoscope is an essential part of every complete eye examination. For adequate visualization of the fundus, dilate the iris with tropicamide solution, 1 per cent.

Examine each patient's eye grounds in a dark room. To examine the right fundus, hold the ophthalmoscope in the right hand and view the fundus with the right eye. Keep both eyes open when using the ophthalmoscope; it causes less strain to accommodation. Starting with the ophthalmoscope at 0 setting, hold the ophthalmoscope about 20 inches from the patient's eye. Observe the pupil and the tapetal reflex. Bring the ophthalmoscope to within one inch of the patient's eye and place the setting on minus 1 to 3 to view the optic disk and retina. If the disk is not immediately seen, follow the retinal vessels back to the disk. Find the setting at which the retina can be seen most clearly. Inserting more plus lenses into the ophthalmoscope focuses the lens on more anterior structures within the eye.

Direct ophthalmoscopy provides a highly magnified view of the fundus in which the image is real and upright. The magnification is 15X in an emmetropic eye, less in hyperopia, and more in myopia. The area of visualization is usually about 2 disk diameters. The extent to which the peripheral retina may be examined in dogs varies with the degree of dilatation of the pupil and the length of the muzzle. In dolicocephalic breeds, the peripheral, medial aspect of the fundus can be examined in greater detail using direct ophthalmoscopy. Indirect ophthalmoscopy permits good visualization of all areas of the fundus.

The fundus is that portion of the inner eye which includes the optic disk or papilla, the retinal vessels, tapetum lucidum, and nigrum.

Examine the optic disk and note its shape, color, and the presence of a physiologic cup. The optic disk may assume various shapes—round to triangular—and its periphery may be pigmented. The disk itself should be flat with distinct margins, and ranges from pink to gray-white. In larger dogs, the disk usually is located within the tapetum lucidum, in smaller dogs, within the non-tapetal area.

The retinal vessels can be divided into primary veins, secondary veins, and arterioles. The primary veins are the two to five largest vessels in the retina. The blood in the veins is dark red to purple. The retinal vessels should be flat as they run across the edge of the disk. Note whether the disk is depressed (cupped) or elevated as in papilledema or papillitis. If cupped, the disk may appear larger than normal, and the vessels disappear at its periphery.

The veins of the retina can be distinguished from the arteries by virtue of their larger diameters. The veins are dark red to purple in color, whereas the arteries are somewhat lighter. The cilioretinal arterioles are five to nine in number. They are bright red in color, of smaller diameter, and more tortuous than the veins, and do not anastomose within the disk. The dog does not have a central artery and vein.

The tapetum lucidum is located in the superior half of the fundus and is roughly triangular in shape. The tapetum may vary in color from blue and green to orange or yellow. The mosaic appearance is caused by the underlying pigment epithelium and choroid, which can be seen through the tapetal layer. The non-tapetal fundus (nigrum) occupies the inferior portion of the fundus and usually is brown to black in color.

The fundus of the cat differs from the dog's in that the optic disk is smaller, the tapetum lucidum occupies a much larger area, the veins and arterioles enter and leave the optic disk circumferentially, and no definite physiologic cup is visible.

The optic disk should be flat. In the dog, it normally measures about 1.5 mm. in diameter. If the disk has to be viewed by placing more convex (+) lenses in the ophthalmoscope, it probably is elevated. Papilledema is a swelling of the optic disk, is usually bilateral, and may be caused by passive congestion within the disk. The disk edges usually are blurred, the veins full and tortuous, and the arterioles smaller than normal. Papilledema need not be caused by conditions in which the intracranial pressure is elevated.

Inflammation of the optic disk is termed papillitis. It may be difficult to distinguish between papillitis and papilledema; however, in papillitis there is usually less swelling than in papilledema, often loss of vision, inflammation of surrounding retina and vitreous, and hemorrhages in the disk. Note whether the disk appears to be depressed or cupped. A small cup in the center of the disk is normal; marked depression that extends to the periphery of the disk is abnormal. Glaucoma is the most common cause of cupping of the optic disk. Both typical and atypical colombas may cause defects of the optic disk. The optic disk may appear whiter than normal in progressive retinal atrophy, optic atrophy, glaucoma, and anemia.

Observe the retina for signs of hemorrhage. Flame-shaped hemorrhages usually are situated in the superficial parts of the retina, round hemorrhages in the deeper parts. Preretinal hemorrhage usually obliterates the retinal vessels.

Pigmentation of the retina may be congenital or pathologic. Pigment usually is present in old hemorrhages, and exudates and pigment spots are present in certain types of hereditary retinal atrophy. Pigment migration may occur in retinitis and in chorioretinic scars. Depigmentation of the fundus exposes the choroid and choroidal circulation.

Many retinal detachments in animals are associated with giant retinal tears, and the retinal tissue can be seen as a wavy, white sheet in the vitreous chamber. Bullous localized detachment of the retina may be caused by exudative choroiditis or hemorrhage. Spontaneous reattachment may occur when the exudate is reabsorbed. The retina may be completely detached from the ora serrata and resemble a tent when viewed with the ophthalmoscope. In retinal detachment, the underlying tapetum, choroid, and pigment epithelium are frequently visible.

Hold the ophthalmoscope about 20 inches from the patient's eye and place the ophthalmoscope setting on 0. Direct the beam of light into the pupil. In a normal eye one should obtain a good tapetal reflex. Opacities of the cornea, hemorrhage or inflammation in the anterior chamber, or changes in the lens or vitreous may interfere with the normal tapetal reflex. Increased tapetal reflectivity is associated with some cases of progressive retinal atrophy.

Examination of the Cornea. Place the ophthalmoscope close to the eye with the +20 diopter lens before the peephole. This will enable the cornea to be visualized. Look for the presence of opacities, foreign bodies, ulcers, elevations, or vascularization.

Examination of the Anterior Chamber. By placing less + lenses in the ophthalmoscope (+8 to +20) the anterior chamber and iris can be visualized. Look for foreign bodies, hemorrhage, or exudate in the anterior chamber.

Examination of the Iris. Look for nodules or growths on the iris. Examine the iris pigmentation and look for a pupillary membrane. Assess the iris for atrophy.

Examination of the Lens. Note any opacities. Anterior opacities of the lens move down when the animal moves the eye downward and up when the eye is moved upward. Posterior opacities move in directions counter to the movement of the eye. Further estimation of the exact depth of a lens opacity requires the use of a biomicroscope. Look for dislocation of the lens or waving of the border of the iris (iridodonesis), which usually indicates lens luxation.

Examination of the Vitreous. The normal vitreous is clear and homogeneous. Examine the vitreous with lenses −1 to +8. Check for cloudiness, discoloration, or the presence of masses. Cloudiness may be due to hemorrhage, uveitis, or choroiditis. Small opacities in the vitreous may appear as "snowflakes," and move when the eye is moved. If the opacities remain stationary the condition is asteroid hyalosis. Larger masses in the vitreous may indicate retinal detachment, vitreous abscesses or tumors, or organized areas of inflammation.

Because of the constant movement of the animal's eye, scanning of the fundus by direct ophthalmoscopy is simplified; however, fixation on one portion of the fundus may be very difficult. It is important when using the direct ophthalmoscope to utilize ocular movements as an advantage and not attempt to "chase and fixate on small ocular lesions."

Recently, indirect ophthalmoscopy has been used increasingly in veterinary medicine. It has several distinct advantages. The intense illumination is of value in cases with hazy ocular media. The indirect image with less magnification allows less distortion and a much larger field of view than that obtained with direct ophthalmoscopy (35 degrees compared to 9 degrees with direct ophthalmoscopy). Indirect ophthalmoscopy permits examination at a safe distance from fractious animals. The binocular, stereoscopic indirect headsets permit the examiner to manipulate the animal's head while at the same time holding the condensing lens.

The condensing lens which supplies the greatest versatility in indirect ophthalmoscopy is the plus 20 diopter plano-convex lens with a diameter of 35 mm. The working distance of this lens is about 2 to 3 inches from the patient's eye. The convex side of the lens should be held toward the observer in order to minimize light reflections and image distortion. Right-handed examiners can hold the lens in the left hand, thus leaving the right hand free to draw pictures; or the examiner can hold the lens in the right hand and manipulate the animal's head with the left hand. Good mydriasis is essential for good indirect ophthalmoscopy. One per cent tropicamide or a combination of 2 per cent cyclogyl and 10 per cent phenylepherine have proved satisfactory as dilating agents.

When using the condensing lens in indirect ophthalmoscopy, the image that is formed is real and inverted. When first beginning to use the direct ophthalmoscope, the observer should be about 14 to 16 inches from the condensing lens. Shine the light into the eye so that the tapetal reflection is obtained. The +20 diopter condensing lens is then placed in the path of the light about 2 inches from the patient's cornea. By bringing the condensing lens away from the eye, the image will fill the condensing lens. Tilting the lens slightly will displace reflections from its surface. The light from the indirect ophthalmoscope and the condensing lens must be kept in a straight line, pivoting through the nodal point of the patient's eye. The fundus picture moves in an opposite manner to the movement of the examiner's head and indirect condensing lens. The fundus image may be lost if the lens is moved too close or too far away from the patient's eye. If diplopia occurs while using the binocular indirect ophthalmoscope, it usually can be corrected. Vertical diplopia is generally due to tilting of the ophthalmoscope. Horizontal diplopia results if the observer is too close to the patient.

SPECIALIZED DIAGNOSTIC TECHNIQUES IN OPHTHALMOLOGY

Tonometry

Glaucoma is an increase in intraocular pressure incompatible with normal ocular and visual functions. It is therefore important to be able to record changes in ocular tension in order to diagnose and treat glaucoma.

Absolute measurement of intraocular pressure involves monometry, in which a cannula is inserted into the eye and the internal pressure is recorded. Although this method is very accurate, it is of course impractical clinically. The method used clinically is tonometry, in which the tension of the outer coat of the eye is assessed by measuring the impressibility or applanability of the cornea. Because the measurements based on tonometry involve calculations which have a wide base of variations, tonometry readings are always approximations and are referred to as "ocular tension" readings, as opposed to intraocular pressure readings obtained by manometry. Ocular tension can be re-recorded in several ways.

Digital Tonometry. This method involves estimating ocular tension by judging the impressibility of the ocular coats when pressure is applied to the globe by the index fingers, which are placed on the upper eyelids of the animal. The sensation of ocular fluxation from the normal eye is learned with practice, and variations can be detected as experience is gained. This method requires much practice, is inaccurate, and usually it is impossible to detect less than 5 mm. Hg. change in intraocular tension.

Schiötz Tonometry. This tonometer has been widely used in veterinary medicine to determine ocular tension in small animals. The instrument consists of a corneal foot-plate, plunger, holding bracket, recording scale, and 5.5-, 7.5-, 10.0-, and 15.0-gm. weights. The principle of the

Schiötz tonometer is that the amount which the plunger protrudes from the footplate is related to the indentability of the cornea, which in turn is related to the intraocular pressure. The plunger is connected to a scale so that 0.05 mm. protrusion of the plunger equals one scale unit. In order to transfer the readings on the Schiötz tonometer into terms of intraocular tension, it is necessary to calibrate them against absolute readings of the intraocular pressure manometrically measured. These readings (based on measurements in humans) are available in tables which come with each tonometer.

The technique of Schiötz tonometry in dogs and cats is not very difficult. The dog is placed in the sitting or dorsal recumbent position. Topical anesthesia is instilled, and the eyelids are held open by the fingers, which are placed quite far away from the lid margins. The footplate must be placed vertically on the central aspect of the cornea. Three readings are taken in each eye and then averaged. Normal intraocular tension with the Schiötz tonometer in dogs is 15 to 25 mm. Hg.

There are many inherent defects built into the use of Schiötz tonometry in small animals: 1. The instrument itself, which must be kept clean and in good functioning order; 2. Extraocular muscle contraction and manipulation of the eyelids artificially raise intraocular tension; 3. Differences in ocular rigidity between animal eyes and those of man can greatly alter the interpretation of ocular tension; 4. Differences in curvature of the globe between man and animals can greatly affect the interpretation of readings with the Schiötz tonometer.

Applanation Tonometry. In applanation tonometry a known, very small area of the cornea is flattened by a known force. The advantage of this technique over the indentation method (Schiötz) is that the errors due to ocular rigidity and corneal curvature are greatly reduced. In dogs we have used three types of applanation tonometers. One of the oldest types was that developed by Maklakov and modified into the Tonomat tonometer. The instrument, although not expensive, requires time and skill to develop a good technique for its use. The Tonair tonometer is a hand-held applanation tonometer of constant weight that measures the intraocular tension in terms of the amount of air pressure required to flatten a small area of the cornea. The instrument is not difficult to use; however, it should always be used by the same individual so that the results obtained are repeatable. Reports indicate that when the intraocular tension is between 15 to 25 mm. of Hg. there is a linear relationship between the pressures obtained with the Schiötz tonometer and that obtained with the Tonair. The Tonair measurements were 3 to 4 mm. Hg. higher than the corresponding Schiötz measurements.

The use of the Draeger hand-held applanation tonometer in dogs and cats is still under study; however our initial investigations have shown that in the unanesthetized animal the instrument has proved difficult to use.

Gonioscopy

Glaucoma is an increase in intraocular pressure incompatible with normal ocular visual functions. Glaucoma can be caused by many different disorders—all elevating intraocular pressure. In many types of glaucoma there is an abnormality in the anterior angle of the eye (filtration angle). Gonioscopy permits one to visualize and examine the iridocorneal angle, which cannot be seen without the use of a contact lens.

It frequently is important to determine the width of the anterior angle. It may influence one's choice of treatment in glaucoma, i.e., medical vs. surgical. Examination of the angle also may influence the prognosis in glaucoma. The technique is also very valuable in examining the iris following trauma, in looking for anterior segment tumors, and in examining congenital anterior segment anomalies.

The Koeppe gonioscopic lens seems to be well suited to domestic animals. It is available in a 17-, 19- and 21-mm. size. The lens can be inserted into the eye following the application of topical anesthesia. In fractious animals a tranquilizer may be needed. The lens can be filled with 1 per cent methylcellulose or can be filled with saline. Avoid having air bubbles present, as this distorts the view. The inside of the lens is illuminated with a Barkan lamp otoscope head or binocular indirect ophthalmoscope. Magnification suitable to visualize the angle can be provided by an otoscope head, indirect ophthalmoscope, or with a Haag-Streit goniomicroscope. Photography of the angle through the gonioscopic lens can be performed using the Kowa fundus camera.

Transillumination of the Eye

If an intense light (Finoff ocular transilluminator) is placed on the sclera behind the ciliary body, the light will be transmitted to the interior of the eye and will produce a tapetal reflex in the pupil. If the light is placed over a solid mass in the eye, the light will not be scattered, and a light reflex will not be produced in the pupil. If the light is placed over a cystic area in the eye, the rays of light will not be interfered with and the light will diffuse throughout the eye. Thus, transillumination can be used to aid in differentiating solid tumor masses in the eye as opposed to cystic lesions. Transillumination also may be used to diagnose atrophy of the pigment layer of the iris. This layer normally prevents transilluminated light from going through the iris. In iris atrophy, the transilluminated light will appear in the areas of iris atrophy. To utilize the principles of transillumination, the examining room should be completely dark and the observer should be partially dark adapted.

Ocular Ultrasonography

The technique of exploring the eye with high frequency sound waves uses the principles of ultrasonography. The advantages of high frequency ultrasonographic waves (500 megacycles per second) are that they can penetrate tissues that are opaque to light, such as the sclera, edematous cornea, cataractous lens, etc., and they can delineate structures that are transparent to x-rays.

In A-mode ultrasonography, an ultrasonic probe is placed in contact with the cornea. As the sound pulse traverses the eye it is partly reflected as it passes through tissues of different acoustic density until, eventually, the transmitted energy is absorbed. The reflected sound waves are received by a microphone and converted into electrical impulses, which are then converted by an oscilloscope into light impulses. The main advantage of this technique is in the ability to analyze the contents of the posterior segment of the globe when visualization is impossible. In this way, organized vitreous hemorrhages, masses of fibrous tissue in the posterior segment, tumors, foreign bodies, or retinal detachments can be detected. The technique has proved very valuable in veterinary medicine when used in selected cases.

Angiography

Angiography of the orbit assists in the diagnosis and localization of orbital neoplasms, localized inflammations, and vascular anomalies. The infraorbital artery is cannulated at the infraorbital foramen with a 21-gauge needle. Five to 7 ml. of 50 per cent sodium diatrizoate (Hypaque) is injected, and oblique lateral and lateral positions are used.

Electroretinography

It is beyond the scope of this discussion to enter into the details of the mechanism and interpretation of electroretinography. Here we will present the basic concepts of this technique as they may be applied clinically.

The retina, like other nervous tissue, generates electrical currents. An electrical potential exists between the retina and the cornea, with the cornea being more positive. When a flash of light strikes the retina, rapid changes in retinal potentials occur and are recorded as the electroretinogram.

The electroretinogram represents the mass-response of the retina to a stimulus. The pattern of the electroretinogram can vary among different species of animals, depending on whether retinal photoreceptors are predominantly rods or cones.

Essentially, the electroretinogram in the dog consists of three major components. The a wave is a negative potential whose origin and significance is not yet completely understood. It probably originates from the photoreceptor layer. The b wave is the most important element. Its origins are probably from the Müller (glial) cells of the retina. Inactivation of the ganglion cell layer or damage to the optic nerve have no effect on the configuration of the b wave. The major component of the b wave is associated with scotopic activity, and the b wave becomes progressively larger in the dark-adapted state. The c wave may be unrelated to the actual processes of vision and appears to be associated with metabolism in the pigment epithelium.

As a clinical tool, the single flash ERG, which depends upon mass retinal response, may be of value in several ways: 1. It can be used in cases of unexplained visual loss where the fundus appears normal and where the ERG may permit differentiation between retinal disease or disease affecting the nerve fiber layer or central visual pathways; 2. When the fundus cannot be visualized because of opacification of the ocular media, the possibility of retinal degeneration can be ruled out by use of the electroretinogram.

In interpreting the significance of electroretinography as used at the present time clinically in veterinary medicine, it must be realized that the single flash ERG gives very little indication of the physiologic processes taking place in the retina. With the single flash technique testing mass retinal response, one can show whether the waves present are normal, depressed in amplitude, absent, or irregular in morphology. The investigator must be aware that selective disorders of the cone system in dogs will not be detected by the single flash ERG. To obtain information of selective damage to rods and cones, ''dynamic electroretinography'' must be applied. It is beyond the scope of this book to discuss this concept; however, it involves the use of a balanced light system and flicker fusion to obtain evidence of changes in rod and cone function.

TABLE 32. BREED PREDISPOSITION TO OCULAR ABNORMALITIES

Afghan Hound—Juvenile cataract
Basenji—Persistent pupillary membranes
Bedlington Terrier—Distichiasis, lacrimal puncta atresia, retinal dysplasia
Blood Hound—Ectropion
Boston Terrier—Hypertrophy of the nictitans gland, juvenile cataract
Boxer—Recurrent corneal erosion
Bulldog (English)—Ectropion, entropion
Chesapeake Bay Retriever—Progressive retinal atrophy, entropion
Chow Chow—Narrow palpebral fissure, entropion
Cocker Spaniel—Ectropion, hypertrophy of the nictitans gland, acute conges-
          tive primary glaucoma, juvenile cataract, progressive retinal
          atrophy
Collie—Microphthalmos, retinal detachment, progressive retinal atrophy, optic
          nerve hypoplasia, excavation of optic disk (coloboma)
English Pug—Pigmentary keratitis
English Setter—Progressive retinal atrophy
Fox Terrier, smooth—Secondary glaucoma (subluxated lens)
Fox Terrier, wire-haired—Secondary glaucoma (subluxated lens), juvenile
          cataract
German Shepherd—Pannus
Golden Retriever—Progressive retinal atrophy, entropion
Gordon Setter—Progressive retinal atrophy
Great Dane—Eversion of membrane nictitans
Irish Setter—Progressive retinal atrophy
Kerry Blue Terrier—Narrow palpebral fissure, entropion
Labrador Retriever—Progressive retinal atrophy, entropion, retinal dysplasia
Malamutes—Hemeralopia
Norwegian Elkhound—Progressive retinal atrophy
Pekingese—Distichiasis, pigmentary keratitis, corneal ulceration
Poodle—Distichiasis, lacrimal puncta and duct atresia, epiphora, microph-
          thalmos, juvenile cataract, progressive retinal atrophy
Rottweiler—Entropion
Saint Bernard—Entropion, ectropion, eversion membrane nictitans
Sealyham Terrier—Lacrimal duct atresia, secondary glaucoma (subluxated lens)
Springer Spaniel—Progressive retinal atrophy
Schnauzer, miniature—Microphthalmos, juvenile cataract
Weimaraner—Eversion membrane nictitans

III–5–B. Examination of the Ear

General Examination

Note any unusual appearance of the external ear. Compare one ear with the other. Observe the skin for signs of inflammation (swelling, redness, or desquamation of the epithelium). Movement and handling of the normal pinna should not produce pain. Look for pus or blood emanating from the external meatus.

Otoscopic Examination

An otoscope is required to examine the auditory canal. Use a clean—preferably sterile—otoscope head. Do not examine a noninfected ear with the head that was used for an infected ear, and always examine the noninfected member first.

To examine the right ear, hold the otoscope in the right hand and the pinna between the thumb and first two fingers of the left hand. Reverse the procedure for the left ear. Draw the ear flap caudally. Insert the otoscope cone carefully in a rostroventral direction but always watch the progress of the tip by looking through the otoscope. When the angle of the meatus is encountered, draw the ear laterally and turn the tip of the instrument medially to straighten the meatus. Otoscopes are usually provided with a number of specula and visualization of the ear canal is easier if the largest one that will fit the canal is used.

The ear drum is a thin membrane with a white curved bone running from the dorsal margin postventrally. The bone is the handle of the malleus (see Figure 40). The tympanic membrane consists of a small upper portion, the pars flaccida, and a large lower part, the pars tensa. The membrane separates the horizontal portion of the external auditory canal from the tympanic cavity. The posterior portion of the pars tensa is what is usually visualized to the greatest extent with the otoscope. The tense part of the tympanic membrane is dark because the dark cavity of the middle ear is seen through it. The flaccid part is opaque white with red blood vessels.

The ear drum can usually be seen in normal dogs less than one year of age. It may be difficult to visualize the eardrum in older dogs because the meatus has narrowed, because the tense part of the eardrum is obscured by the flaccid part, because the lining of the meatus obscures the eardrum or because the eardrum is ruptured. Chronic

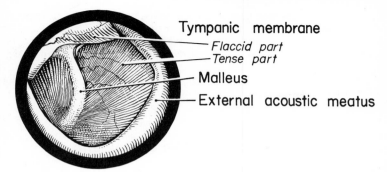

Figure 40.   Canine tympanic membrane. (From Habel, R. E.: Applied Veterinary Anatomy. Ithaca, N. Y., published by the author, 1973.)

otitis externa is a common problem in dogs, and in over 50 per cent of the chronic cases the tympanic membrane is ruptured.

Any abnormal changes in the tympanic membrane such as swelling, redness, loss of translucency, or absence of the membrane should be recorded. If the tympanic membrane has recently ruptured, a small amount of bloodstained discharge may be seen around the membrane.

Cleaning the Ear Canal

In otitis externa, the external canal is frequently blocked with cerumen, exudate, and tissue debris. In Poodles, Bedlington Terriers, and Kerry Blue Terriers, the canal contains hair that frequently obscures the view. If the canal is plugged with wax, the hair must be removed first. Instill warm olive oil or a ceruminolutic agent (Ceruminex) to soften the wax. Cotton applicators may be used to wipe the wax gently from the external meatus. If the animal resents the cleaning, administer a short-acting general anesthetic or tranquilizer. Any deep cleaning of the ear canal should be done very cautiously and gently and the patient should be adequately restrained or, preferably, anesthetized.

If the canal contains pus or other exudates, a culture should be taken to determine antibacterial sensitivity. Before the canal can be visually examined, the discharges must be removed. The recent advent of the pulsating water dental hygienic apparatus has made irrigation and careful cleansing of the ear canal a much easier process. One ounce of pHisoDerm is added to each 8 to 12 ounces of warm water. The irrigation stream is kept parallel to the external ear canal and is applied in a rotating motion. The excess water and debris can be caught in a sink or basin. The canal can then be reinspected and carefully dried with cotton.

This technique should not be used in cases of acute otitis media nor if the tympanic membrane has been ruptured.

III–5–C. Examination of the Larynx and Pharynx

General Examination

Thorough examination of the larynx and pharynx in the dog and cat requires the use of a short-acting general anesthetic. Extreme caution should be exercised when anesthetizing brachycephalic dogs who may have laryngeal problems. In these cases it may be preferable to use a tranquilizer or a combination of a narcotic and a tranquilizer.

Tonsils, Pharynx, Soft Palate, and Posterior Nares

Open the mouth with a mouth gag and gently pull the tongue forward with a tongue forceps. Examine the tonsils for size, color, and consistency. Gently wipe away any discharge in the pharynx or larynx. Observe the mucous membranes of the pharynx for color, swelling, inflammation, or follicle formation. Place the index finger on the soft palate, apply dorsal pressure and feel for abnormal swellings. This may be the site of visually concealed retropharyngeal tumors.

Inspect the posterior nares for a foreign body or tumor. Gently grasp the end of the soft palate with a tissue forceps and pull it forward. Use a dental mirror and focal illumination to view the posterior nares. Note any changes in the normally pink, moist epithelium. Insert a finger behind the soft palate and palpate the pharynx for masses or a foreign body.

Problems of the soft palate are confined largely to the brachycephalic breeds. Examine the soft palate for length. Elongation of the soft palate leads to respiratory distress, gagging, and expectoration. Look for an incomplete soft palate, a cause of chronic nasal discharge.

Larynx

The larynx can be inspected most effectively with a laryngoscope of appropriate size. Pulling the tongue too far forward will simulate collapse of the larynx. Collapse of the larynx is seen most frequently in brachycephalic dogs and is characterized by severe inspiratory distress. Examine the corniculate cartilages. Displacement ventromedially can cause collapse of the laryngeal opening. Collapse of the larynx may involve the epiglottis, the corniculate or the cuneiform process of the artenoid cartilage or any combination of defects in these structures. Severe inspiratory dyspnea accentuates the anatomical problem. Collapse of the corniculate cartilages permits them to be displaced ventromedially, causing a marked reduction in the size of the lumen of the larynx. Examine the epiglottis for length and for collapse over the laryngeal opening.

Examine the lateral ventricles of the larynx for eversion. This condition is seen in brachycephalic breeds and results from negative pressure leading to inspiratory dyspnea. Note any signs of inflammation or swelling in the laryngeal area. A more detailed examination of the trachea may be carried out with a bronchoscope (see Section IV-14-F).

III–5–D. Examination of the Nose

General Examination

Observe the muzzle and nasal area and compare both sides for any disproportion in size. Examine the external nares for changes in pigmentation or size, or abnormal discharge. If a discharge is present, note if it is bloodstained, mucopurulent or watery and whether it flows from one or both nostrils. Hold the mouth closed, place a wisp of cotton in front of each nostril, and compare the movement of the cotton on expiration. Note any deviation of the nasal septum. Stenotic nares are characterized by partial or complete occlusion of the nasal orifice and is commonly seen in brachycephalic dogs. The lateral wings of the nostril collapse upon inhalation, forcing the dog to breathe through his mouth.

Nasal Passages

Part of the nasal passages can be inspected with an otoscope and a small otoscope cone. Anesthesia or sedation is required to carry out this examination without injury to the animal. Note any signs of inflammation, ulceration, hemorrhage, or foreign bodies in the nasal passages. Hyperemia of the mucosa and pus indicate infection. A unilateral foreign body in the nasal passage frequently produces an offensive odor from the affected nasal passage. Hemorrhage from the nostrils may occur in blood dyscrasias, idiopathic thrombocytopenia, autoimmune hemolytic anemia, tumors, foreign bodies and trauma. A history of chronic partial or complete nasal obstruction and respiratory difficulty, persistent unilateral or bilateral nasal discharge, frequent episodes of sneezing and snorting could be signs of a nasal tumor. Examine the muzzle for any evidence of increase in size or pain on palpation.

Further examination of the nasal passages can be accomplished radiographically.

References

Additional information can be found in the following sources:

Habel, R. E.: Applied Anatomy, 6th ed. Ithaca, N. Y., published by the author, 1973.

Leonard, H. C.: Obstructions of the upper respiratory tract. *In* Kirk, R. W. (ed.): Current Venterinary Therapy IV, pp. 128–132. Philadelphia, W. B. Saunders Co., 1971.

Spreull, J. S. A.: Otitis media of the dog. *In* Kirk, R. W. (ed.): Current Veterinary Therapy IV. Philadelphia, W. B. Saunders Co., 1971.

III–6. GENITOURINARY SYSTEM

III–6–A. Reproductive Organs

Evaluation of the Male Breeder

History

Obtain data from owner concerning animal's age, libido, psychic problems, breeding dates, techniques and results, previous fertility studies and treatment, fertility data on related animals, treatment for disease, vaccination, and feeding and management practices.

Physical Examination

Inspect and palpate prepuce, penis, scrotum, testes, epididymis, spermatic cord, and prostate (dog). Check for the presence of pain, deformity, atrophy or fibrosis, and exudates. Collect and evaluate semen (see Section IV-8). Culture all three fractions of semen, urine, and preputial exudate.

Perform a testicular biopsy if indicated. Under general anesthesia, examine the testes, epididymis, and spermatic cord directly. Obtain a biopsy sample and place in Bouin's fluid for fixation.

Evaluation of the Female Breeder

History

Obtain data from owner concerning bitch's age, dates, action, characteristics, and duration of each period of heat, breeding dates, techniques and results, time of labor, number of offspring whelped and weaned, maternal instincts, persistence of discharge, fertility data on related animals, treatment for disease, previous medications and vaccinations administered, results of titer tests, and feeding and management practices.

Physical Examination

Inspect and palpate the breasts, vulva, and abdominal organs. Using a sterile speculum inspect the vagina and cervix. Culture and make a cytologic smear if advisable. To obtain a meaningful culture the double speculum system should be followed, and the subject should be under general anesthesia or deep sedation. In the double speculum system one sterile speculum is passed through the cleansed vulva and deeply into the vagina. A second sterile speculum is passed through the first and advanced to the cervix. The culture swab is then passed to obtain the culture specimen.

Use a sterile glove and carefully palpate the pelvic canal for size, masses, and presence of pain. It may be advisable to follow a complete heat cycle with daily vaginal cytologic studies.

Consider exploratory laparotomy to inspect the uterus, fallopian tubes, and ovaries. In addition, one should:
1. Palpate uterus and ovaries.
2. Take uterine culture and biopsy.

3. Use dilute mercurochrome solution injected into the uterus and "milked" anteriorly to determine the patency of the fallopian tubes. With patent tubes the mercurochrome can be expressed from the uterus and appears at the fimbria.

III-6-B. Urinary Organs

History

Obtain information from the owner regarding the animal's water consumption, volume of urine excreted daily, frequency of urination, incontinence, and the possibility of nocturia or dysuria. Find out if the urine is voided in a large, continuous stream or in dribbles or—as may be normal in males—is interrupted. Ascertain if clotted or frank blood is present. Ask the owner if he has noticed any abnormality in the color or odor of his pet's urine. Owners will often be ignorant of even the obvious signs in a history—a cat straining to urinate may be regarded by his owner as constipated.

Physical Examination

A physical examination involves palpating the posterior abdomen for an enlarged or painful bladder, for the absence of a palpable bladder, for evidence of general pain, abdominal fluid (urine), calculi, or tumors.

1. Examine the external urethral openings for evidence of incontinence and external irritation.

2. Elicit systemic signs of uremia (uremic breath, ulcerative stomatitis, anemia, conjunctival injection, vomiting and diarrhea, depression, or muscular twitching).

3. Pass a catheter to determine patency and to obtain urine (see Section IV-9).

Laboratory Examination

Blood

The following tests are helpful in establishing a prognosis:
BUN (See Section V-3-L-5).

Serum creatinine (see Section V-3-L-6).
PCV.
CBC (see Section V-3).
Serum chloride (see Section V-3-L-11).
Serum potassium.

Urinalysis (see Section V-11)

Specific gravity, pH, glucose, ketones, bilirubin, occult blood, proteinuria (the electrophoretic pattern may be revealing), and microscopic examination of the sediment are all vital parts of a urinalysis and deserve emphasis, as do urine cultures and antibiotic sensitivity tests (see Section V-5).

Renal Function Tests (see Section V-12)

The following tests are helpful in establishing a prognosis in cases of renal disease.

Concentration test (ADH and tubular function).
Phenolsulfonphthalein test (tubular function).
Creatinine clearance test (glomerular filtration).

Radiographs (see Section IV-14)

Flat plates, pneumocystogram.
I.V. pyelogram.

Exploratory Laparotomy

Exploratory laparotomy includes inspection, palpation, cultures, and biopsy of intra-abdominal urinary organs.

III–7. THE LOCOMOTOR SYSTEM

The locomotor system includes the muscles, bones, and joints. Diseases involving the locomotor system can be produced by alterations in muscles, bones, or joints, together with the vessels and nerves supplying these structures.

History

Obtain a complete history from the owner, examine the member that the owner believes to be abnormal, and determine the time sequence in the development of the abnormality. Traumatic injuries to bone, muscle, or tendon cause a sudden development of lameness; whereas osteoarthritis causes slowly progressive gait changes. The history may indicate that a shifting leg lameness is present. This frequently occurs in enostosis (eosinophilic panosteitis). Determine if exercise causes gait abnormality to improve or become worse.

Physical Examination

Gait

Observe the animal for any changes in gait as it is brought into the examining room. Notice which limb, if any, the animal favors. Observe whether gait change is associated with pain upon movement. As the animal walks and runs, note whether it pursues a relatively straight course or deviates from side to side.

Notice if the animal carries its head in an abnormal position as it moves. In the dog, the center of gravity never falls outside the base line. In normal stance, the dog bears 60 per cent of his weight on his front limbs. The dog is able to shift more of his weight forward by extending the head and neck and placing the forelegs farther back under the center of gravity. In severe disease of the hind legs, such as advanced hip dysplasia, 90 per cent of the weight may be carried by the forelimbs. Examine the animal's stance and gait from the lateral as well as the posterior position. Note if the forelegs assume a base-wide stance, which usually indicates rear leg lameness and pain.

Several skeletal abnormalities may be associated with characteristic changes of weight bearing and gait. In chronic medial luxation of the patellas, the femur is rotated laterally and the tibia medially; thus the animal has a "toe-in and bow-legged" (genu varum) appearance. These dogs walk with a shuffling gait because it is painful to fully extend the knee joint.

In osteochondritis dissecans of the shoulder, the stride is short and choppy because of apparent pain when the foreleg is extended.

In un-united anconeal process of the foreleg, there is pain when the elbow joint is fully extended. The animal may compensate by keeping the elbow joint in a semi-flexed position. In moving the affected leg, the animal abducts the limb.

In traumatic luxation of the elbow, the radius and ulna dislocate laterally. Tension and spasm of the brachial muscles cause the antebrachium and foot to be abducted. Flexion and extension of the joint cannot be performed.

Careful examination of the stifle joint for ligamentous injuries often requires general anesthesia. Rupture of the cranial cruciate ligament allows cranial displacement of the tibia (anterior drawer sign). Excessive outward rotation of the tibia with the limb partially flexed may indicate medial meniscal injury or rupture of the medial collateral ligaments.

Caudal cruciate rupture, which usually does not occur unless there is extensive damage to the stifle joint, permits excessive caudal tibial movement and outward rotation.

Excessive outward rotation of the tibia and abduction of the stifle joint can be produced by rupture of the medial collateral ligaments. Inward rotation of the tibia and adduction of the stifle joint can be produced by lateral cruciate rupture.

Coxofemoral luxations may assume a variety of positions. The most common is a craniodorsal luxation of the femoral head, in which the limb is rotated outward and adducted. If the femoral head is displaced caudally, the limb is rotated inward, and with dorsal luxation the limb is adducted.

Palpation and Observation

Next, examine the soft tissue and long bones of the extremities. Look for deviation from the normal shape and outline of the limb, swelling, pain and crepitation, increased heat, and sites of tenderness. The soft tissues of the digits should be examined for cuts, foreign bodies, ingrown nails, thorns, foxtails, or burns from salt. Look for indication of a penetrating soft tissue injury such as muscle swelling, pain, heat, tenderness, or a developing abscess. Check for abnormal enlargement in the diameter of long bones with attendant pain. Hypertrophic osteopulmonary arthropathy produces bone enlargement usually without pain, whereas hypertrophic osteodystrophy produces bony enlargement with pain. Palpation of the periosteum of the long bones may produce pain in eosinophilic panosteitis and osteomyelitis.

III–7–A. Inspection of the Joints

Examine the joints by inspection and palpation and determine their range of movement. Look for enlargements or irregularities of the joint. Determine if the enlarged joint is warm and tender, or firm and hard to the touch. Look for the presence of a traumatic wound in the soft tissue over the joint or a sinus tract leading from the joint. Suppurative arthritis is characterized by high fever and a pointed, hot, swollen joint with hyperemic skin overlying the joint. Palpate joint surfaces for the presence of bony growths and for grating and crepitation within the joint.

Move the joint and decide if the range of motion is normal. Limitation of movement within a joint may result from pain, muscle spasm, contractures of muscle, inflammation or thickening of the periarticular structures, effusion within the joint, bony or cartilaginous overgrowths, or bony ankylosis. Degenerative osteoarthritis is characterized by pain, joint deformity, progressive lameness, and stiffness upon rising, but symptoms become less severe with exercise. Bony proliferation and crepitation within the joint usually occurs in the hip, stifle, elbow, and spine.

An increased range of motion of a joint attended by pain and lameness is seen in dislocation of the coxofemoral and elbow joints, recurrent dislocation of the patella, and rupture of the anterior cruciate or other ligaments.

III–7–B. Muscular Diseases and Locomotor Changes

Muscular diseases can also produce locomotor changes. Myositis is characterized by severe muscular pain, swelling of the affected muscles, and difficulty in moving. Acute infection or vascular changes within the muscle may lead to necrosis with resultant fibrosis and atrophy. Eosinophilic myositis in German Shepherds severely affects the muscles of mastication and causes progressive disability. Muscular atrophy can result from disuse of the affected limb (as in fractures) or from loss of nervous innervation to the limb (as in radial paralysis), or because of primary muscle disease, resulting from vascular insults and leading to muscle necrosis and atrophy. ''Scotty cramp'' is a condition produced in Scottish and Cairn Terriers during periods of forced exercise. When forced to move, they demonstrate hypertonicity of the pelvic limb musculature that causes the hind legs to take short, jerky steps. The muscle spasm may eventually involve the forelegs and the neck muscles and the dog can no longer move. The attack usually subsides within minutes. Racing Greyhounds may suffer from acute muscle spasm of the hind legs while racing. The condition appears more frequently in poorly conditioned animals.

III–7–C. Neurologic Defects and Locomotor Changes

Neurologic defects may produce a variety of changes in gait. A cerebellar gait is characterized by a wide base stance, unsteadiness, and falling or lurching to one side or the other. Sensory ataxia is characterized by a lack of knowledge about how the limbs are positioned. Animals with this deficit will move their legs with great uncertainty, frequently cross their legs when walking, keep a wide stance, and show hypermetria. The incoordination of gait is accentuated when the animal is blindfolded. Posterior ataxia occurs, in many spinal cord diseases such as encephalomyelitis due to distemper, compressions of the spinal cord from disc protrusion or vertebral fractures, hereditary disorders such as syringomyelia and Stockard's syndrome, neoplasia of the spinal cord, or vascular and bony changes. Lesions of peripheral nerves may affect the coordinated movement of individual limbs. Injury to the brachial plexus prevents extension of the affected foreleg. Radial nerve paralysis distal to the branches of the branchial plexus that supply the triceps muscle results in a knuckling over of the dorsal portion of the foot. Femoral nerve paralysis results in inability to extend or fix the stifle joint and therefore the leg cannot support weight. Paralysis of the peroneal nerve results in a knuckling over of the affected foot so that the weight is distributed on the dorsum of the digits. Lesions of peripheral nerves are often accompanied by sensory denervation of parts of the affected limb as well as by motor paralysis (see Figures 42 and 43).

References

Additional information can be found in the following sources:

Piermattei, D. L. (ed.): Symposium on orthopedic surgery in small animals. Vet. Clin. North Amer., Vol. 1, No. 3, September, 1971.
Roy, W. G.: Examination of the canine locomotor system. Vet. Clin. North Amer., Vol. 1, No. 1, pp. 53–70, January, 1971.

III–8. THE NERVOUS SYSTEM

The nervous system is examined to ascertain the site and nature of the lesion responsible for signs of nervous disease. In examining the animal with a neurologic disorder three basic questions should be answered:

1. Where is the lesion in the nervous system?
2. What type of lesion is present?
   a. Inflammation.
   b. Degeneration.
   c. Neoplasm.
   d. Malformation.
   e. Injury.
3. What causes the lesion?

Follow an outline (Figure 41) in performing an examination of the nervous system. Examine the animal in quiet surroundings. The following equipment is helpful in performing a neurological examination: reflex hammer, 18 gauge hypodermic needle, penlight, blindfold and hemostat.

SIGNALMENT AND HISTORY

The breed, sex and age of the animal should be noted, for, considered together with the chief complaint, they may help direct the line of questioning in the historical review. Certain breeds are predisposed to specific neurologic ailments, and the age of the animal may tend to eliminate certain neurologic diseases.

The history should include a summary of all past medical and surgical illnesses and the facts surrounding the present complaint. The line of questioning will be influenced by the chief complaint.

Injury:
1. When did it occur? Was it observed?
2. Describe the animal's condition.
3. How has this changed since the accident?

Convulsions:
1. Describe completely. How do they start? How does the animal act during the convulsion? Is the animal conscious? How long does the convulsion last? How does the patient act during the recovery? Is the patient normal between convulsions? What are the intervals between convulsions? Is there a period of abnormal behavior associated with the convulsion?
2. Is there a past history of an injury?
3. When does the patient eat, and what does he eat?
4. Is there any source of intoxication, especially lead?
5. Has the patient been ill lately?
6. What is the vaccination history?

N.Y.S. VETERINARY COLLEGE — CORNELL UNIVERSITY — VETERINARY HOSPITALS

NEUROLOGIC EXAMINATION

DATE _____

History:

ACO # _____ PHONE _____
OWNER _____
STREET _____
CITY _____ STATE _____ ZIP _____
BORN _____ SEX _____ COLOR _____
SPEC _____ BREED _____ WT _____

REF. DVM _____
CLINICIAN _____
SECONDARY # _____

Gait & Posture:

Mental Status:

Cranial Nerves:

II—Menace-
    Pupillary-
    Ophthalmoscopic-

III—Pupillary   Strabismus-

V—Motor: Mand.-
    Sensory: Ophth.- Max.- Mand.-

VI—Strabismus

Muscle Tone-

Spinal Reflexes:
    1. Patellar- LH   RH
    2. Biceps- L   R
       Triceps- L   R
    3. Perineal-
    4. Flexor- LF   RF   Crossed
               LH   RH   Extensor:

    Pain Perception:

Additional Tests:

Remarks:

VII—

VIII—Cochlear-
     Vestibular—Head tilt-
     Nystagmus—Resting-
              Positional-
              Postrotatory-
              Vestibular-

IX, X—

XII—

Postural Reactions:
    1. Wheelbarrowing
    2. Hopping-   LF   RF
                 LH   RH
    3. Extensor Postural Thrust-   LH   RH
    4. Hemistands-   L   R
    5. Hemiwalks-   L   R
    6. Proprioceptive Positioning-
                            LF   RF
                            LH   RH
    7. Placing—Optic-   Tactile-
    8. Tonic Neck and Eye-

NEUROLOGIC EXAMINATION

Figure 41. Neurologic examination record.

TABLE 33. A DIAGNOSTIC PLAN FOR PATIENTS WITH EPISODIC WEAKNESS*

Disease	Diagnostic Test	Positive Result
Hypoglycemia	Fasting blood glucose	50 mg./100 ml. or less
Adrenal insufficiency	Serum electrolytes	Potassium > 5.2 mEq.
		Sodium < 135 mEq.
		Na:K ratio < 25:1
	ECG	Tall spiked T waves
		Wide QRS; absence of P waves
		Bradycardia
Hypokalemia	Electrolytes	Potassium < 2.4 mEq.
	ECG	Prolonged QT interval
Cardiac arrhythmias		
Ventricular tachycardia	ECG	Series of PVC's
Atrial fibrillation	ECG	No P waves; presence of "f" waves; rapid irregular rates
Heart block		
Third degree	ECG	P waves unassociated with QRS complexes; atrial rate normal; ventricular rate very slow
Heartworm	Modified Knott's	Microfilaria of *D. immitis*
	ECG	
	Thoracic radiograph	Right heart enlargement; enlarged pulmonary arteries; enlarged pulmonary outflow tract; right ventricular enlargement
Myasthenia gravis	Response to neostigmine testing	Improvement in weakness and greater exercise tolerance
Polymyositis	Muscle enzymes	Increase in LDH, GOT and CPK; inflammation and necrosis of muscle
	Muscle biopsy	

*From Lorenz, M. D.: Episodic weakness in the dog. *In* Kirk, R. W., (ed.): Current Veterinary Therapy V. Philadelphia, W. B. Saunders Co., 1974.

Weakness or ataxia:

1. Describe the first appearance of the signs. Was the onset sudden or gradual?

2. When did the signs begin? How have the signs changed since then? Have the signs been progressively getting worse or have they been intermittent?

3. Has the patient had periods of being normal since the first onset of the signs.

4. Have there been any convulsions or periods of abnormal behavior or other signs of disturbed cerebral function?

Puppy with neurologic signs:

1. Where the signs present at birth, or at least as soon as the pup could walk?

2. How have the signs changed since then?

Mental Status

Attempt to ascertain whether the patient is normally alert and responsive, or dull, inattentive, obtunded, even semicomatose or comatose, or hypersensitive, hysterical or convulsive.

Gait and Posture

Observe the gait for weakness or ataxia. If pelvic limb weakness prevents support, provide support by lifting by the tail and observe if any voluntary motor activity is present. If the patient is in lateral recumbency, hold the patient up in a position of support to ascertain if any strength is present or there is any abnormality of posture.

Note any abnormality of posture, such as standing with a limb resting on the dorsal surface of the paw, crossed limbs, base wide limbs, deviated vertebral column scoliosis, kyphosis, standing with the body leaning to one side or head tilting. Note any abnormal involuntary motor activity (myoclonus).

III–8–A. Cranial Nerve Examination

The 12 cranial nerves are the peripheral nerves that connect the brainstem with the head and various parts of the neck, thorax and abdomen.

TABLE 34. INHERITED METABOLIC DISORDERS OF THE
NERVOUS SYSTEM IN DOGS AND CATS*

Diseases	Breeds Affected	Lesions
Canine globoid cell leukodystrophy (Krabbe's disease)	Cairn terriers; West Highland white terriers; mixed breeds	Demyelination; globoid cells
Feline globoid cell leukodystrophy	Domestic cat	Same as canine GLD
Feline sphingomyelin lipidosis (Niemann-Pick disease)	Siamese cat	Vacuolation of neurons and macrophages in spleen, etc.
Feline metachromatic leukodystrophy	Domestic cat	Demyelination; gliosis
Feline CNS glycogenosis (Pompe's disease)	Domestic cat	Neuronal accumulation of glycogen
Canine GM_2 gangliosidosis (Tay-Sachs disease)	German short-hair pointers	Vacuolation of neurons
Feline GM_1 gangliosidosis	Siamese cats; domestic cat	Vacuolation of neurons

Terms in parentheses refer to eponyms used for analogous human disorders.
*From Baker, H. J.: Inherited metabolic disorders of the nervous system
in dogs and cats. *In* Kirk, R. W. (ed.): Current Veterinary Therapy V. Philadelphia, W. B. Saunders Co., 1974.

Cranial nerve I (olfactory) has its origin in the sensory receptors
of the nose and terminates in the pyriform lobe. The dog has a highly
developed olfactory system. Testing the integrity of the olfactory nerve
is difficult and is rarely done in dogs and cats.

Cranial nerve II (optic) has its origin in the retina at the optic disc.
In the cat, about 66 per cent of the optic nerve fibers decussate at the
optic chiasm. In the dog, this is about 75 per cent of the optic nerve. The
optic nerve has two components. One is composed of those fibers that
pass to the pupillary centers within the brainstem and the second is
composed of those fibers that synapse in the thalamus, which in turn
project the impulses to the visual cortex of the brain. The pupillary
fibers leave the optic tract and synapse in the midbrain where crossing
occurs. Impulses reach the parasympathetic portion of the oculomotor

TABLE 34. INHERITED METABOLIC DISORDERS OF THE NERVOUS SYSTEM IN DOGS AND CATS* (Continued)

Age of Onset	Signs	Biochemical Lesion
4 to 5 months	Progressive motor disability	Cerebroside accumulates; β-galactosidase deficiency
5 to 6 weeks	Same	Unknown
2 to 4 months	Same	Sphingomyelin accumulates; sphingomyelinase deficiency?
2 weeks	Same; rapidly progressing to convulsions; opisthotonus	Sulfatid accumulates; arylsulfatase deficiency?
Young adult	Unknown	Glycogen accumulates; α-glucosidase deficiency?
9 to 12 months	Ataxia; blindness; seizures	GM_2 ganglioside accumulates; hexosaminidase deficiency?
10 to 16 weeks	Tremors; incoordination; paraplegia	GM_1 ganglioside accumulates; β-galactosidase deficiency

nucleus. From here, parasympathetic preganglionic fibers exit in the third cranial nerve to synapse in the ciliary ganglion caudal to the globe. The postganglionic fibers go to the iridial sphincter and ciliary muscles.

Shine a light in the lateral (temporal) portion of each eye. Note the pupillary response. Test the consensual pupillary response by shining a focal source of light in one eye and noting the effects in the opposite eye. The normal pupillary response requires that nerves II and III be intact, and involves only brainstem connections.

The majority of fibers in the optic tract synapse in the lateral geniculate body of the thalamus. Fibers from the lateral geniculate body continue to the visual centers in the occipital lobe via the internal capsule.

Testing the animal's vision may be accomplished by:

1. Observing the animal's movements in daylight and in dim light.
2. Using a maze and alternately patching each eye.
3. Testing the menace reaction. Make a quick motion with the hand in front of the eye of the animal. Do not touch the eyelashes or create any marked air movement. A blink response indicates that cranial nerves II and VII are intact, and requires participation of the visual cortex.

Evaluation of the integrity of the optic nerve should always include an ophthalmoscopic examination of the fundus.

Cranial nerves III, IV, and VI (oculomotor, trochlear, and abducens) innervate extraocular striated muscles and are examined together. Nerve IV innervates the dorsal oblique muscle, nerve VI innervates the lateral rectus and the retractor oculi muscles, and nerve III innervates the dorsal, medial, and ventral recti, ventral oblique, and levator palpebrae muscles. Pupillary dilation is controlled by preganglionic neurons in the first three thoracic spinal cord segments, the cranial thoracic, and cervical sympathetic trunks and by postganglionic neurons in the cranial cervical ganglion and sympathetic nerves that course through the middle ear to reach the orbit and dilator pupillae muscle. Parasympathetic fibers in nerve III innervate the sphincter pupillae muscles.

The integrity of nerve III may be examined by observing:

1. The size of the pupil.

2. The reaction of the pupil to light.

3. The presence or absence of ptosis or drooping of the upper lid because of paralysis of the levator palpebrae superioris.

4. The presence or absence of strabismus with a downward and outward deviation of the eye.

Paralysis of the trochlear nerve produces a transient strabismus resulting in a slight upward deviation of the eye. (This, however, is extremely rare.)

Paralysis of the abducens nerve results in a medial deviation of the affected eye with inability to gaze laterally.

Cranial nerve V trigeminal, contains both motor and sensory fibers. The motor division innervates the muscles of mastication. Paralysis of the motor division of the fifth nerve results in the inability to chew, with a dropped jaw if bilateral paralysis is produced. Muscle atrophy accompanies the paralysis. The sensory division of the trigeminal nerve has its origin in the trigeminal ganglion and can be divided into the ophthalmic, maxillary, and mandibular branches. The function of the sensory division can be tested by pinching or pricking the skin overlying the areas innervated by these nerves.

The ophthalmic nerve supplies the skin of the upper eyelid, cornea, medial portion of forehead, and caudal portion of the nasal mucosa.

The maxillary nerve supplies the conjunctiva of the lower lid, roots of the upper cheek teeth, skin of the muzzle, hard and soft palate, and the nasal mucosa.

The mandibular nerve innervates the buccal mucosa, rostral part of the tongue, lower teeth, skin of the lateral cranium, and the base of the ear.

Cranial nerve VII (facial) is motor to all the muscles of facial expression and may be tested by the following reflexes:

1. Palpebral reflex—Touch a wisp of cotton to the cornea. If nerves V and VII are intact, the eyelids will blink rapidly.

2. Handclap reflex—Without letting the animal see you, suddenly clap the hands. If nerves VIII (cochlear branch) and VII are intact, the animal will blink its eyes.

3. Menace reflex—See discussion on the optic nerve.

Loss of facial nerve function (nerve VII) causes the muscles of the affected side of the face to sag, and the lines around the muzzle and face are lost. The eye cannot close normally and exposure keratitis develops. The ear on the affected side may droop and there is no response to stimulation of the ear. The lip and philtrum are retracted toward the intact side.

Cranial nerve VIII (vestibulo-cochlear) has two divisions, cochlear and vestibular. The cochlear nerve is concerned with balance and posture. Sound vibrations pass through the outer and middle ear and are relayed to the spiral organ (corti) in the inner ear. Deafness may indicate a lesion of the cochlear nerve, the cochlear duct, or the sound-conducting organs. Deafness can be tested by having the owner call the dog or by the handclap reflex.

The peripheral vestibular mechanism includes the labyrinthine sensory organs in the semicircular canals, the utricle and the saccule. Symptoms of disease of the vestibular system may include head tilt, rolling movements, circling, abnormal nystagmus, and an asymmetric incoordination with preservation of strength.

Nystagmus refers to the involuntary rhythmic oscillations or tremors of the eyes that occur independently of normal movements (Walsh). Nystagmus may be either pendular (the movement of the eye is at the same rate in each direction) or alternating (there is a rapid and a slow component to the eye movements). Alternating nystagmus, in which movement is chiefly in the horizontal plane, is classified according to the direction of the fast component (either right or left). The slow phase of the nystagmus is caused by labyrinthine stimulation, whereas the rapid phase is a recovery movement.

Disturbance of the vestibular portion of nerve VIII produces a marked head tilt, body tilt and concavity, and occasional falling and rolling toward the side of the lesion. A resting horizontal nystagmus directed away from the side of the lesion lasts about 72 hours, following

TABLE 35. EVALUATION OF CRANIAL NERVES*

Nerve	Diagnostic Signs of Dysfunction
I. Olfactory	Hyposmia or anosmia
II. Optic	Hesitant walking, walks into objects Anisocoria, mydriasis, miosis
III. Oculomotor	Anisocoria, mydriasis, miosis, ptosis, deviation, ventral and lateral
IV. Trochlear	Affected eye unable to move (ventrolaterally)
V. Trigeminal	Sensory—hyperesthesia on one side of face and eye Anesthesia on one side of face and eye Motor—weakness in closing mouth or unable to open mouth
VI. Abducens	Affected eye unable to move laterally. Medial strabismus may be present
VII. Facial	Asymmetry of facial expression. Eyelids and lips droop. Loss of ear motion
VIII. Acoustic	Cochlear nerve—deafness. Will not respond to sound Vestibular nerve—circling, head tilt, nystagmus, loss of balance
IX. Glossopharyngeal	Difficulty swallowing

*From Hoerlein, B. F.: Canine Neurology: Diagnosis and Treatment, 2nd ed. Philadelphia, W. B. Saunders Co., 1971.

TABLE 35. EVALUATION OF CRANIAL NERVES* *(Continued)*

Tests	Normal Response	Abnormal Response
Smell of food or volatile oil	Food—interest or attempt to eat; volatile oil—sniffing and recoiling	No reaction
Sudden object movement toward eyes	Avoidance, eye blinks	Absence of blink reflex
Point source of light in each eye	Direct and consensual pupillary constriction	Lack of pupillary responses
Ophthalmoscopic examination	Normal fundus	Retinal lesions found
Light in normal eye; light in affected eye	Direct and consensual reflex present	Direct pupillary reflex present—consensual absent. Direct pupillary reflex absent. Consensual may be present
Observation when animal follows moving object	Follows object ventrolaterally	Eye unable to follow ventrolaterally
Cold object on skin. Pinprick. Touch cornea	Slight discomfort. Eye blink both sides	Intense discomfort and recoil. May vocalize
Pinprick or cold object. Touch cornea	Slight discomfort	No response
Test muscle tension. Palpate temporalis and masseter muscles	Normal muscle tension. Normal contour to musculature	Atrophy of temporalis and masseter muscles. Trismus
Observation of eye when following moving object		Unable to follow laterally
Observation. Pinprick on side of face (trigeminal is sensory in this test)	Retraction of skin. Eye blink	No retraction, no eye blink
Sudden loud noise. EEG alerting response test	Startle reaction. Eye blink. EEG alert recordings	No response. No EEG alerting response
Observation. Caloric test?	Nystagmus	No nystagmus
Touch pharynx. Compression of throat region	Gag	No gag
	Deglutition, cough	No swallowing, no cough

Table continues on following pages.

TABLE 35. EVALUATION OF CRANIAL NERVES *(Continued)*

Nerve	Diagnostic Signs of Dysfunction
X. Vagus	Tachycardia?
XI. Spinal accessory	Few signs seen. Neck muscle weakness. Deviation of head to one side
XII. Hypoglossal	Early disease—tongue deviates toward unaffected side
	Late disease—tongue deviates toward affected side; atrophy and corrugated appearance

which a positional nystagmus can often be elicited by deviating the head laterally over the left or right shoulders. Postrotatory nystagmus is noted after an attendant holds the patient in his arms and spins rapidly for six or seven rotations. The examiner records the response. The animal's head must be held in a horizontal plane. The normal response is a horizontal nystagmus directed away from the direction of the spin, and lasts from five to 15 seconds. Rotation should be done in both directions. In deficits of the eighth cranial nerve when the animal is spun in a direction away from the lesion, the postrotatory nystagmus response is depressed. In young animals with ocular lesions the ocular nystagmus observed is characterized by equal movements in both directions (deLahunta).

Cranial nerves IX (glossopharyngeal), X (vagus), and XI (spinal accessory) are mixed motor and sensory nerves to the pharynx. They can be tested by eliciting the gag reflex and by determining the animal's ability to swallow, cough, or produce vocal sounds. In addition, the parasympathetic portion of the vagus nerve is concerned with gastrointestinal, bronchiole, and salivary secretions, slowing the heart, constricting bronchioles, increasing peristalsis, and relaxing sphincters.

Cranial nerve XII (hypoglossal) is the motor nerve to the tongue. With a unilateral lesion the tongue protrudes from the mouth toward the side of the lesion. The affected side usually atrophies.

III–8–B. *Spinal Cord and Spinal Reflexes*

In the dog there are about 36 pairs of spinal nerves. The spinal cord extends from the medulla oblongata to the junction of the sixth and seventh lumbar vertebrae, and is connected with the brain by

TABLE 35.   EVALUATION OF CRANIAL NERVES *(Continued)*

Tests	Normal Response	Abnormal Response
Pressure on eyeballs	Bradycardia (sometimes)	No bradycardia
Palpation of musculature	Muscle tone	Lack of muscle tone or atrophy
Observation. Pull tongue out	Retracts normally	Deviates

many ascending and descending tracts and with the muscles and body surface by the spinal nerves.

In testing spinal reflexes, the reflex arc is tested. The reflex arc consists of the afferent nerve, specific spinal cord segments, and the efferent nerve. In tests of limb movements, the more complete and localized the nervous dysfunction, the more peripheral the lesion usually.

Normal Spinal Reflexes

Flexor Reflex of the Forelimb (Fig. 42)

With the animal in lateral recumbency pinch a toe of the forelimb. The limb should flex, indicating intact forelimb peripheral nerves and cord segments (C6-T1). If the flexor reflex is accompanied by a crossed extensor reflex of the opposite limb, this is an indication of a lesion cranial to the reflex centers of the forelimb (C6-T1).

Flexor Reflex of the Hindlimb (Fig. 43)

With the animal in lateral recumbency, pinch a toe of the hindlimb. Flexion of the stifle and hock indicates an intact sciatic nerve and cord segments (L6-S1). Hip flexion indicates intact cord segments as far cranial as L1. If the contralateral hindlimb is extended while the opposite limb is flexed, a lesion cranial to spinal segment (L4-S2) should be suspected.

Patella Reflex

With the animal on its side, support the upper hindlimb from the medial aspect of the stifle with the stifle in moderate flexion. Strike

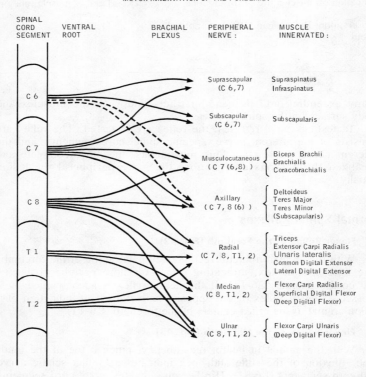

Figure 42. Motor innervation of the foreleg. (Used by permission, Alexander deLahunta.)

TABLE 36. INJURIES TO NERVES INNERVATING THE FORELIMBS*

Nerve	Sign of Paralysis
Suprascapular nerve (C6–7)	Atrophy of the supraspinatus and infraspinatus muscles
Axillary nerve (C7, 8 [6])	Weakened shoulder flexor reflex; loss of skin sensation on lateral side arm
Radial nerve (C7, 8, T1, 2)	Injury proximal to branches providing innervation to triceps muscles produces complete loss of extension of elbow. Injury distal to nerves innervating triceps muscle permits extension of elbow; knuckling of forepaw onto dorsal aspect, loss of skin sensation on dorsal and lateral parts of forearm and dorsal aspect paw
Musculocutaneous (C7 [6, 8])	Flexor reflex at elbow is weak; loss of skin sensation or medial side forearm
Median and ulnar nerves (C7, T1, 2)	Loss of active flexion of the carpus. Slight weakness of the carpus and fetlock, causing slight "sinking" of carpus and fetlock
Brachial paralysis	Extension of the shoulder with dropping of elbow and dorsal surface of carpus and digits on ground. Complete lack of any extensor activity in elbow

*See Figure 42. After Hoerlein, B. F.: Canine Neurology: Diagnosis and Treatment, 2nd ed. Philadelphia, W. B. Saunders Co., 1971.

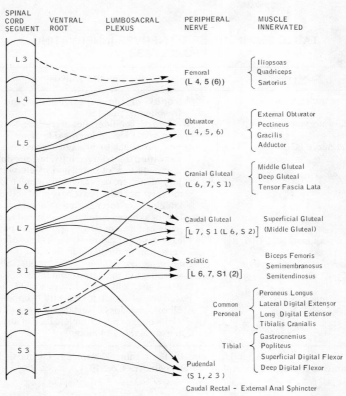

Figure 43. Motor innervation of the hindleg. (Used by permission, Alexander deLahunta.)

TABLE 37. INJURIES TO NERVES INNERVATING
THE HINDLIMBS*

Nerve	Sign of Paralysis
Obturator (L4, 5, 6)	Failure to adequately adduct the affected leg. This is especially noticeable on slippery surfaces
Femoral (L4, 5 [3])	Failure to extend or fix the stifle joint; loss of skin sensation over the medial surface of the thigh, stifle, leg and paw
Perineal nerve (terminal branch of sciatic)	Straightening of the hock and knuckling onto the dorsal surface of the fetlock and digits
Sciatic nerve (L6, 7, S1, 2)	Straightening of the entire leg, permitting weight bearing. Dorsal knuckling of the paw with excessive self-inflicted trauma. Hypesthesia of caudal and lateral aspect of leg
Pudendal (S1, 2, 3)	Related external anal sphincter and anesthesia in area of perineum, vulva, and part of scrotum

*See Figure 43. After Hoerlein, B. F.: Canine Neurology: Diagnosis and Treatment, 2nd ed. Philadelphia, W. B. Saunders Co., 1971.

the patellar ligament with a percussion hammer. Normally the stifle should extend, indicating an intact femoral nerve and cord segments L4-L6.

Perineal Reflex

Touch the skin of the perineum or the underside of the tail or anus. The external anal sphincter should contract, the vulva elevate, and the tail clamp down (except in females during heat). Normal perineal reflex indicates that sacral spinal nerves and cord segments S1-S3 are intact. Tail flexion indicates intact caudal segments.

Abnormal Spinal Reflexes

The elicitation of these reflexes indicates that the peripheral nerves and segments of the cord involved in the reflex arc are functioning but the reflex activity of the cord at this level is increased. This points to a release phenomenon caused by a lesion at a higher level (Habel).

TABLE 38. CLINICAL SIGNS AND POSSIBLE CAUSES*

Sign	Possible Causes
Nystagmus	Lesions of the semicircular canal, eighth cranial nerve, vestibular nuclei, or flocculonodular lobe of the cerebellum.
Rolling	Rolling without any sense of balance is usually caused by lesions of the semicircular canals (inner ear), eighth cranial nerve, or flocculonodular lobe. When the sense of balance is present, nystagmus is absent, and rolling is not very pronounced, rolling may be due to lesions of the basal nuclei.
Hyperalgesia	Localized hyperalgesia is usually caused by a spinal or peripheral nerve lesion. When generalized it is usually a sign of a brain (thalamus) lesion.
Hypoalgesia, analgesia	Localized hypoalgesia or analgesia is usually caused by a peripheral nerve lesion or a destructive spinal lesion.
Incoordination	Generalized incoordination is usually the result of a lesion in the cerebellum. Incoordination in one leg may be caused by injury to a peripheral nerve or the cord.
Trembling	This may be due to nervousness or a cerebellar lesion (anterior lobe).
Chorea	May be caused by a lesion in the basal nuclei. Chorea occurring during the nervous form of distemper may be caused by a lesion of the spinal cord.
Paralysis	Local unilateral paralysis is usually caused by a peripheral nerve lesion.
	Bilateral localized paralysis is usually due to spinal injuries.
	Generalized paralysis may be caused by brain lesions in the basal nuclei or reticular formation.
Extensor rigidity	Usually caused by a spinal injury, although a generalized condition may be caused by a brain injury.
Circling	If the animal has a sense of balance but continuously walks in circles, circling signifies a lesion of the basal nuclei, red nucleus, or vestibular nuclei.

TABLE 38. CLINICAL SIGNS AND POSSIBLE CAUSES* *(Continued)*

Sign	Possible Causes
Knuckling of foot	Injury to the peripheral nerve or a lesion in the motor pathways in the cord.
Blindness	A lesion in the eye, optic nerve, or cerebral cortex.
Failure of the pupils to respond to light	A lesion in the eye, optic nerve, Edinger-Westphal nucleus, pretectal nucleus, or oculomotor nerve.

*From Hoerlein, B. F.: Canine Neurology: Diagnosis and Treatment, 2nd ed. Philadelphia, W. B. Saunders Co., 1971.

1. Hyperactivity of the patellar reflex.
2. Presence of increased resistance in the limbs when they are passively manipulated in the relaxed animal.
3. Continued extension and flexion of the limb after pinching the toes once.
4. Extensor reflex of the hindlimbs. With the animal in dorsal recumbency, exerting pressure on the pads of the flexed hindlimbs results in a sudden extension of the legs. This usually indicates a lesion craniad to the reflex centers of the hindlimbs (L4-S2). The same procedure carried out on the forelimbs may indicate a lesion craniad to C6.

Testing for Pain Sensation

When spinal flexor reflexes are tested, observe whether the animal responds to pinching of its toes. Use of a hemostat on the claws provides a source of pain that is consistent in all cases and can be evaluated readily. If the peripheral nerves and ascending spinal cord tracts are intact through the brainstem to the thalamus and cerebrum, the animal will consciously react to the stimulus. If the peripheral nerves and their specific cord segments are intact, but the tracts are damaged, the flexor reflex will occur but there will be no conscious response to the pain.

III-8-C. Attitudinal and Postural Reactions

Attitudinal and postural reactions require that the peripheral nerves, local segments of the spinal cord, ascending and descending spinal cord pathways, brainstem, cerebellum, and cerebrum be intact. These reactions occur in all normal animals.

Tonic Neck and Eye Reaction

When the head and neck are extended, the forelimbs extend and the hindlimbs flex. Deviating the head to one side results in increased extensor tonus on that side. As the nose is elevated, the eyes should remain focused within the center of the palpebral fissure. Normally, nystagmus should be observed on lateral deviation of the head (quick phase toward the side of deviation).

Wheelbarrow

Lift the pelvis and hindlimbs off the ground and push the patient forward, forcing the patient to support its weight on and walk on its forelimbs. Observe the response with the head and neck in their normal position and with them extended so that vision of the path to be taken is compromised. Abnormality will be observed as an asymmetric gait with stumbling and knuckling of a paw.

Proprioception Positioning

Abduct one limb from its normal position, cross one limb in front of the other, and flex the carpus or tarsus and rest the limb on the dorsum of the paw. In each case the normal animal will immediately return the displaced limb to its normal position.

Placing Reaction

Optic. Carry the animal toward a table. On approaching the surface the animal will reach out for support. This reaction requires integrity of visual pathways in addition to the central and peripheral areas already mentioned.

Tactile. Carry the blindfolded animal toward a table. Allow the dorsum of each forepaw to strike the edge of the table. The normal animal will immediately place both forelegs on the table top to support his weight.

Extensor Postural Thrust

Hold the animal by the thorax and lower the hindlimbs toward the ground. The normal animal will extend his limbs to support his weight. If the animal is blindfolded the tactile pathways will be tested rather than the visual ones. After observing this response, back the patient up and observe for normal, symmetrical use of the limbs.

Hopping

Hold the animal with three limbs off the ground. Shift his center of gravity over the supporting limb. The normal animal will hop to keep the supporting limb under his body. Observe for asymmetry in mild deficiencies.

Hemistand and Hemiwalk

Hold up the two limbs on one side of the body, forcing the animal to support on the opposite side. Then push the patient forward and toward the opposite side and observe the normal alternate use of the limbs. Test and compare the response on each side.

Righting

Righting may be observed when the animal is released from lateral recumbency.

1. Hold the animal upside down and drop him from a height onto a padded surface. The normal animal will land on its feet.

2. Suspend the animal by his hips and pelvis and turn his body from side to side. The normal animal will hold his head in the normal position.

Righting reactions are markedly abnormal in the presence of vestibular lesions.

The above attitudinal and postural reactions are most helpful in animals with a slight alteration in their gait when it is difficult to determine whether the disturbance is neurologic or musculoskeletal in origin. Animals completely paralyzed in one or more limbs will not respond with any of these reactions in the affected limb. Animals with severe spinal cord lesions between segments T3 and L4 will be paraplegic and show no response to attitudinal reaction but will have intact spinal reflexes and an absence of pain sensation. Animals with lesion of the motor cortex or frontal lobe may show a very mild con-

TABLE 39. LEVEL OF LESION IN THE BRAIN*

I. Cerebral cortex
  A. Deficiency of placing and hopping reactions (contralateral)
  B. Alteration of mental function (recognition of owner, house training)
  C. Vision impaired
  D. Seizures
  E. Hypertonia or hypotonia in extensors (contralateral)
  F. Deficiency in voluntary movements

II. Basal nuclei
  A. Deficiency of nonvisual placing and hopping reactions
  B. Adversive turning movements
  C. Hyperkinesias (unilateral or bilateral)
  D. Hypertonia in contralateral limb

III. Diencephalon
  A. Pain, generalized or contralateral; may be intermittent
  B. Hypothalamic disorders. Changes in: eating, drinking, sleeping, or sexual behavior; cardiovascular and temperature regulation; endocrine activity
  C. Visual field defects—optic tract or chiasm

IV. Midbrain
  A. Cranial nerve III or IV
  B. Spasticity, deficiency in voluntary movement
  C. Decreased sensation (contralateral)

V. Cerebellum
  A. Ataxia—incoordination of body movements, station and gait
  B. Extensor hypertonus, acute opisthotonos
  C. Chronic muscle weakness
  D. Dysmetria—tremor with movements and other disturbances of phasic movements in chronic disorder
  E. Cerebellar nystagmus

VI. Pons
  A. Cranial nerves V, VI, VII
  B. Decreased sensation (contralateral)
  C. Deficiency of voluntary movements, spasticity (may be hypotonia if caudal pons, vestibular nucleus, or fastigial nucleus involved)

VII. Medulla Oblongata
  A. Cranial nerves VIII, IX, X, XI, XII
  B. Vestibular signs
  C. Decreased sensation
  D. Hemiparesis or tetraplegia, usually decreased tonus
  E. Cardiovascular or respiratory abnormalities, or both

*Best evidence of level of brain stem lesion is cranial nerve involvement. Cranial nerves listed with level signify possible involvement in a lesion, and not necessarily the anatomical origin of the nerve. One or more of the signs listed may not be present in a particular lesion. Losses may be total or partial. From Hoerlein, B. F.: Canine Neurology: Diagnosis and Treatment, 2nd ed. Philadelphia, W. B. Saunders Co., 1971.

tralateral hemiparesis with reflexes intact but with a deficient response to these attitudinal reactions (deLahunta).

SYNOPSIS OF NEUROLOGIC LESIONS*

Characteristics of Peripheral Nerve Lesions

1. Unilateral localized loss of sensation confined to a small area of the body.
2. Unilateral paralysis of all or part of a limb.
3. Rapid and severe muscle atrophy caused by damage to the lower motor neurons.
4. An alteration in the spinal reflex depending on the area of the body that is involved.

Characteristics of Spinal Lesions

1. Bilateral alteration in the sense of proprioception (ataxia) caudal to the lesion.
2. Paresis or paralysis that is usually bilaterally symmetrical and caudal to the spinal lesion.
3. Bilateral loss of pain perception in paralyzed animals caudal to the spinal cord lesion.

Characteristics of Brain Lesions

1. Alterations of the sensorium or behavior.
2. Generalized alterations in the motor system including inco-ordination, staggering, circling, rolling, and tumbling.
3. Presence of normal spinal reflexes and an alteration in attitudinal and postural reactions.
4. Changes in integrity of the cranial nerves.

References

Additional information can be found in the following sources:

deLahunta, A.: Small animal neurologic examination. Vet. Clin. North Amer. Vol. 1, No. 1, pp. 191–206, 1971.
Habel, R. E.: Applied Anatomy. 6th ed. Ithaca, N. Y., published by the author, 1973.

---

*After Horlein.

Hoerlein, B. F.: Canine Neurology: Diagnosis and Treatment, 2nd ed. Philadelphia, W. B. Saunders Co., 1971.

McGrath, J. T.: Neurologic Examination of the Dog, 2nd ed. Philadelphia, Lea and Febiger, 1960.

III–9. THE RESPIRATORY SYSTEM

History

Determine the presence or absence of:

Nasal Discharge. The discharge may be unilateral or bilateral.

Sneezing. Note frequency and accompanying discharge, if any.

Coughing (See Section II-9). *A true cough* (sudden forced expulsion of air through a closed glottis) is characterized by the animal's lowering its head and opening its mouth during expiration. The cough itself may be moist and productive or dry, nonproductive, and paroxysmal, and can be accentuated by collar pressure, exercise, or cold air.

Postnasal drip or *"reverse cough"* is characterized by the animal's extending its head parallel to the ground and closing its mouth during inspiration. The cough itself commonly ends with the animal's gagging, gulping, choking, or expectorating.

Dyspnea (See Section II-12). In the susceptible animal dyspnea occurs readily after exercise, abating gradually, however, as the animal takes its ease. During the distress, the subject's mouth may be open or closed. While resting, the subject commonly prefers sitting to lying down. Dyspneic animals usually exhibit an increased respiratory rate (polypnea) and depth (hyperpnea).

When considering history, specific breed predilection to some types of respiratory problems should be considered. Laryngeal problems are most often seen in brachycephalic breeds; tracheal collapse in Chihuahuas, Toy Poodles, Yorkshire Terriers and Pomeranians. Dolichocephalic breeds appear to be predisposed to nasal tumors.

III–9–A. Inspiratory Dyspnea

Breathing is through the mouth, the head and neck are extended, the ribs elevated and rolled forward, and the elbows abducted. The skin over the thoracic inlet sinks during inspiration. Inspiratory dyspnea may be caused by tumor, obstruction, or stenosis of the respiratory tract.

III–9–B. Expiratory Dyspnea

Inspiration is normal but expiration is prolonged and forced, the abdomen is actively lifted, and the anus protrudes. It may be caused by chronic emphysema, bronchitis, and pleural adhesions.

MIXED DYSPNEA

Mixed dyspnea, most commonly seen, is a combination of the inspiratory and expiratory forms and is caused by severe respiratory diseases like pneumonia, pneumothorax, and hydrothorax.

Cyanosis

The condition is most readily observed in the oral mucosa. Etiology may be respiratory or circulatory (see Section II-10).

Helpful Anatomic Landmarks

Thorax. The thorax is a laterally compressed oval, the diameter of which is greater dorsoventrally than it is either laterally or craniocaudally.

Diaphragm. The diaphragm attaches dorsocaudally at the thirteenth rib and is slanted forward to attach anteroventrally at the costal cartilage of the eighth, ninth, and tenth ribs. It bells forward as far as the sixth rib, a quarter of the way up from the sternum. In normal respiration the diaphragm moves one and one half vertebral spaces forward and back.

Lungs. Both lungs extend anterior to the first rib. The right lung consists of diaphragmatic, intermediate, cardiac, and apical lobes. A cardiac notch is situated between the cardiac and apical lobes at ribs four and five. The apical lobe ends at roughly the fourth rib; the diaphragmatic lobe begins at about the sixth rib. The intermediate lobe lies medially between the diaphragmatic lobe and the mediastinum.

Diaphragmatic, cardiac, and apical lobes comprise the left lung. A cardiac notch is absent. The apical lobe ends at about the fourth rib and the diaphragmatic lobe originates at the intercostal space between ribs five and six.

Tracheal Bifurcation. It is situated dorsal to the cranial border of the heart at the fifth rib.

Inspection

1. Note the presence, consistency, color, and quantity of any nasal discharge. The exudate may originate in the nose, chest, sinus, throat, or stomach. In the early stage of an infection the discharge is watery; in the chronic stage the discharge becomes thick, mucoid, or purulent. A rust-colored discharge indicates blood from the lung or old blood from the nose. Pulmonary hemorrhage is red and frothy; clear froth implies pulmonary edema. If hemorrhage is present look for petechiae in the skin and mucosa. Determine if both nostrils are patent. Hold a mirror in front of the nose and see if both nostrils cause fogging. In the brachycephalic breeds, examine the lateral wings of the nose for signs of collapse that might produce inspiratory difficulty. Nasal discharge may also be examined microscopically for the presence of *Lingatula serrata* or pneumonyssus mites.

2. Observe the general conformation of the thorax. Check for kyphosis, scoliosis, ricketic rosary, and fracture callus.

Chest Movements

1. Rate of respiration is normally 10 to 30 (20 at rest). Panting may go to 200 breaths per minute but tidal volume is reduced drastically to prevent hypocapnia. Cats pant as fast as 300 breaths per minute but do not compensate for carbon dioxide too effectively. An increased respiratory rate may be caused by heat, exercise, pain, anoxemia, nervous excitement, or structural changes in the lungs. A decreased respiratory rate may result from narcotic poisoning or metabolic alkalosis.

2. The rhythm of respiration may be varied voluntarily or involuntarily (as with nervous excitement). Prolonged expiration may be caused by bronchial or pulmonary disease. Note carefully the degree of effort being expended in respiration.

In Cheyne-Stokes respiration, successive respirations reach a maximum, fall off slowly to apnea, and repeat the cycle. It is a serious sign of toxemia.

3. Types of breathing include thoracic, resulting from paralysis of the diaphragm or abdominal pressure (ascites), abdominal, caused by pain in the thorax (pleuritis) and thoracoabdominal, characteristic of normal dogs and cats.

Palpation

The bones of the maxillary and frontal sinus can be palpated for any indication of fractures. The trachea can be palpated for deformities and to induce coughing. Regional lymph nodes in the neck should be palpated.

Percussion

This form of examination is of limited value in examining the respiratory tract. However, besides examining the thoracic cavity, one can percuss over the maxillary bones and sinuses and frontal sinuses, listening for changes in resonance.

Method

The middle finger, used as a pleximeter, is placed firmly on the chest and the distal phalanx is rapped abruptly with the middle finger of the right hand. Three rules must be applied in percussion:

1. In defining boundaries always move from the more to the less resonant areas.

2. The long axis of the pleximeter (finger) must be parallel to the boundary of the edge of the organ being percussed.

3. The progression of the line of percussion should be at right angles to the edge of the organ (2).

Application and interpretation of percussion is more difficult in small than in large animals. Differences in sounds are slight and it is helpful to percuss the thorax systematically by tapping the ribs while a stethoscope is held firmly against the opposite chest wall. The percussion tones are thus greatly magnified by the instrument and differences are more obvious.

Interpretation

Chest radiographs are accurate in outlining anatomic structures, but changes in resonance also offer additional helpful information.

Resonance is increased when the pleural cavity contains air and the lung is collapsed. In this case the musical "bell sound" may also be heard. A coin is held flat against the chest wall and firmly tapped by a second coin. The observer listens to the transmitted sound through a stethoscope held against the opposite thoracic wall. Resonance may also be increased by emphysema (rare).

Resonance is decreased when the lung is more solid than usual, when the pleura is thickened, when the pleural cavity contains fluid, or when an abdominal viscus is displaced into the thoracic space.

III–9–C. Auscultation

The Stethoscope

Some stethoscopes are better designed acoustically than others. The Littman is lightweight, moderately priced, well-designed, and has a reversible two-sided head. The bell transmits low-pitched sounds, e.g., heart sounds, accurately. The diaphragm, which should be infant size, transmits soft, high-pitched sound best. For best results:

Be sure the stethoscope is seated firmly in the ear.

Perform the auscultation in a room as free as possible of noise.

Hold the stethoscope firmly against the chest.

Do not breathe on the tubing.

Avoid hair friction and muscle noises. Wetting the subject's hair will help.

Listen with the animal breathing quietly, if possible.

Close the mouths of panting animals; stop the subject from shivering or trembling.

Stop cats from purring. Shake them gently or bring a dog into their view.

Concentrate on each part of the respiratory or cardiac cycle separately. Listen intently!

Character of Respiratory Sounds

Normal Breath Sounds

Normal breath sounds are of two kinds, vesicular and bronchial or tubular.

Vesicular sounds are heard as air passes through small bronchi and alveolae. The inspiratory phase is louder and twice as long in normal animals. These sounds are only heard over normal lung tissue but in dogs and cats with shallow, quiet respirations they may be inaudible.

Bronchial sounds are caused by air passing through the larger bronchi and trachea. Auscultate over the trachea of a normal dog to recognize these sounds. They are usually more pronounced on expiration, and local variations may be important signs of disease (consolidation, exudation, and effusion). The smaller the diameter of the bronchi, the softer the bronchial sounds and the higher the pitch.

Added Breath Sounds

Added breath sounds are also of two kinds, rhonchi and crepitations.

Rhonchi are prolonged noises produced by the partial obstruction of bronchi by mucosal edema or viscid secretions. In larger bronchi they are low-pitched, sonorous and almost continuous. In small bronchi they are high-pitched, sibilant or squeaky, and may be more prevalent at the end of inspiration. Rhonchi are heard in bronchitis and asthma. Coarse rhonchi may be associated with bronchiectasis.

Rhonchi or rales may be separated into dry rales, moist rales and crepitant rales. Dry rales are heard throughout both inspiration and expiration and are associated with inflammation of the mucous membranes of the bronchi and tenacious mucus occluding the bronchi. Moist rales are associated with fluid in the bronchi and produce short, discontinuous crackling sounds. Crepitant rales occur on inspiration only and are produced by the passage of air into alveoli containing fluid. They are suggestive of inflammation or pulmonary edema.

Crepitations are fine or coarse interrupted crackling noises that may be obvious during inspiration. They are caused by the opening of alveoli that are collapsed or stopped up with fluid. They are heard in early pneumonia and bronchitis. Crepitations occasionally heard in normal lungs are abolished by coughing. Crepitations can be imitated by rolling hair between the fingers in front of the ear.

Another adventitious sound in the pleural cavity is the pleuritic friction sound (rare). It is heard only when the pleura is dry and inflamed and resembles a crepitation. However, it occurs at similar times during inspiration and expiration when the roughened surfaces rub together and it is not abolished by coughing.

It is important to recognize that there are changes in breathing associated with abnormalities other than those primarily involving the respiratory system, such as heart disease, anemia, ascites, gastric dilatation, physical exertion, muscular spasms, heat and pain.

Tracheal Smears

These may be useful for preparing cultures for cell studies and for identifying parasite ova. Also carry out a fecal examination (see Section V-8).

Radiographic Study

In a radiographic study, lateral and dorsoventral views should be taken. Bronchography, using iodized oil (Dionosil) can also be utilized (see Section IV-18-G). Other specialized radiographic techniques may include pulmonary angiography, tomography and fluoroscopy.

Bronchoscopy (See Section IV-15)

Under thiamylal sodium anesthesia, the trachea and main bronchi can be visualized, or cultured. A biopsied sample can be taken.

Complete Cardiovascular Study (See Section III-4)

Thoracentesis

See Section IV-8 for technique and Section V-9 for interpretation.

Exploratory Thoracotomy

This procedure should be carried out if it is really required. However, in one step, a diagnosis can be confirmed, and in many cases—hernia, cyst, tumor, laceration of the lung, foreign body—therapy provided.

Reference

Additional information can be found in the following source:

Hunter, D. and Bowford, R. R.: Hutchison's Clinical Methods, 14th ed. Philadelphia, J. B. Lippincott Co., 1963.

IV

CLINICAL PROCEDURES

Diagnostic Procedures

IV–1. COLLECTING BLOOD

Venipuncture of the dog or cat may be accomplished by using the cephalic, jugular, femoral, or recurrent tarsal veins. In large dogs the cephalic vein is preferred. In cats and smaller dogs, the jugular vein is frequently used. A peripheral blood sample can be obtained by deep clipping of a toenail but this method is often not desirable.

It is essential to perform the venipuncture in a manner which causes as little trauma as possible so as to preserve the veins' integrity. This is vital when repeated taps must be performed. With show animals or for aesthetic reasons, it is undesirable to clip the hair over the site, but in the long-haired patients, careful clipping aids in identifying the vein. The skin should be cleansed and an effective topical antiseptic applied. The hair (if not clipped) should be parted so that the sterile needle can be placed directly on the skin.

Proper restraint of the patient is of paramount importance to successful venipuncture. Details of restraint for tapping specific veins will be discussed later. However, it is necessary for the patient to be restrained yet comfortable. The area of the vein must be held motionless, the skin stretched firmly to help anchor the vein, and the pressure applied proximal to the site of puncture to occlude blood flow.

The sterile, disposable vacutainer* system has greatly facilitated collection and processing of blood samples. In most instances, a 2 to 5 ml. blood sample is adequate for routine hematology, clinical chemistry or

---

*Becton-Dickinson Co., Rutherford, N.J.

enzyme determinations. The Vacutainer small volume tube holder with a 22 gauge by 1 inch needle is used. In small dogs and in cats, jugular vein samples are collected. For hematology, EDTA tubes are used, and for chemistry and enzyme determinations either serum or plasma obtained via a heparinized sample is used.

If the vacutainer system is not used, a dry, sterile syringe and needle are used. The syringe should be held lightly between the thumb and fingers. Some clinicians place the index finger near the tip of the syringe to help guide it. Under no circumstances, however, should the finger touch the needle.

In most cases it is best to thrust the needle through the skin just lateral to the vein. The needle is further advanced to puncture the vein from the side. Blood usually enters the syringe spontaneously, but can be encouraged to do so by applying gentle suction. Some clinicians maintain continuous suction in the syringe (after the skin and fascia have been punctured) while probing for the vein so that penetration of the vein is indicated by the appearance of blood. An inadequate flow into the syringe may be caused by too much suction, which collapses the vein, partial occlusion of the needle, circulatory failure, hematoma formation, or piercing the vein wall without entering its lumen. Occasionally the tip of the needle becomes snagged in the opposite wall of the vein. Slight retraction and rotation of the needle correct the problem. When obtaining blood the flow is often improved by alternating occlusion and release of the vein combined with slight passive motion of the leg drained by the vein.

The use of vacutainers has simplified obtaining blood samples from small animals, especially when larger-sized veins are tapped to collect blood. Do not use large volume Vacutainer containers in small veins, for the wall of the vein will collapse and samples will not be obtained.

When the needle is placed in a vein to administer fluids for long-term infusion, it must be free in the vein but firmly fixed to the leg. After venipuncture, always inject several milliliters of fluid to be certain of the needle's location. Remove the syringe and attach the previously assembled intravenous tubing. Fluid is allowed to run into the circulation (see Section IV–20).

HANDLING BLOOD SAMPLES (See Section IV-21)

Use syringe and needle or evacuated blood collection tubes (e.g., Vacutainer). All equipment must be chemically clean and *dry*.

Hemolysis is avoided by use of clean, dry equipment and also by avoiding trauma to the red cells. This is often the result of application of excessive or fluctuating suction during the aspiration procedure, excessive force in expelling blood from syringe to container, or excessive agitation of blood after collection. Whole blood should never be shipped, since trauma to red cells during shipment renders the specimen virtually useless.

Blood for Hematology

EDTA is the anticoagulant of choice for hematology. Heparin is especially to be avoided if blood films are to be made from blood mixed with anticoagulant. Heparin is acceptable for most routine procedures utilizing blood plasma. It should be remembered that the anticoagulant effect of heparin is transitory. Specimens may clot after 1 to 3 days.

Blood films should be made immediately following blood collection. Cell morphology deteriorates progressively following collection. Although blood films made immediately following addition of blood to EDTA are acceptable, a better practice is to make films from blood remaining in the blood collection needle, since this blood had not been exposed to anticoagulant. *Blood exposed to heparin should never be used for making blood films.*

Incorrect proportions of blood to anticoagulant may result in water shifts between plasma and red cells. This may alter the packed cell volume, especially when small volumes of blood are added to tubes prepared with sufficient anticoagulant for much larger volumes of blood.

Erroneous laboratory results may also be obtained when small volumes of blood are placed in a relatively large container. This is caused by evaporation of plasma water and adherance of cells to the surface of the container.

Liquid blood mixed with anticoagulant should be refrigerated after collection if there is to be a delay in making the laboratory determinations. White and red cell counts, packed cell volume, and hemoglobin can be done up to 24 hours after blood collection. Platelet counts, however, should be done within one hour after collection of blood.

Dried, unfixed blood films can be stained satisfactorily with most conventional stains 24 to 48 hours or even longer after being made. If a considerable delay before staining is unavoidable, blood films should be fixed by immersion in absolute methanol for at least 5 minutes. Such fixed films are stable indefinitely. Unfixed blood films must never be placed in a refrigerator, since condensation forming after removal from the refrigerator will ruin the film. Care should be taken to leave unfixed blood films face down on a counter top or in a closed box to avoid damage by insects. Special stains, such as peroxidase, may require fresh blood films.

TABLE 40. BLOOD SPECIMENS FOR LABORATORY TESTS

Test to be Done	Specimen Required
Blood pH, gases	Heparinized blood, preferably arterial, collected anaerobically and delivered immediately to laboratory
Blood glucose	Sodium fluoride tube must be used to prevent glycolysis. These tubes usually contain oxalate or EDTA, in addition, to prevent clotting
Electrolytes	Serum or heparinized plasma; *never use EDTA, citrate, or oxalate.* Be certain that serum or plasma is removed from cells promptly to prevent plasma or serum concentrations rising due to leakage from cells
Other chemistry	Serum is almost always appropriate and preferred. Heparinized plasma can sometimes be substituted. Occasionally EDTA plasma can be used. Check with the laboratory if other than serum or heparinized plasma is to be used
Hematology	EDTA—anticoagulant of choice Heparin—acceptable except for blood smears

Blood for Clinical Chemistry Procedures

Most clinical chemistry procedures are done on serum. This is obtained by collecting blood without any anticoagulant and allowing it to clot in a clean, dry tube. Clotting of the blood and retraction of the clot occurs best and achieves maximum yields of serum at room temperature or at body temperature. Refrigeration of the specimen impairs clot retraction. When firmly clotted, free the clot from the walls of the container by "rimming" with an applicator stick or by sharp taps on the outside of the tube. After the clot is freed, allow clot retraction to occur for approximately one hour at room temperature: then centrifuge and draw off the clear supernatant serum using a pipet and suction bulb. Serum yield is usually approximately one-third of whole blood volume.

Many clinical chemistry procedures can be done on plasma as well as serum. The advantage of using plasma is that separation of cells can be accomplished immediately without waiting for clot formation and retraction. The disadvantage of plasma is the presence of the anticoagulant, which interferes with many chemistry procedures. Plasma is often somewhat less clear than serum, which may be an additional disadvantage. Plasma and serum are virtually identical in chemical composition except that plasma has fibrinogen and the anticoagulant. For most chemical procedures in which plasma or whole blood is to be used, heparin is the anticoagulant of choice. Heparinzed blood is the only acceptable specimen for pH and blood gas studies. Although EDTA blood is acceptable for certain chemical procedures, it cannot be used for determinations of plasma electrolytes, since it both contributes electrolytes to and sequesters them from the specimen.

Serum or plasma should be separated and removed from the cells as soon as possible after blood is collected, since many constituents of plasma exist in a higher concentration in the blood cells. With time, these substances leak into the plasma and cause spurious elevations in plasma values obtained. Magnesium, potassium, phosphorus and transaminase are a few examples in which this may be a serious problem. Under no circumstances should whole blood be sent through the mail, since serum derived from such specimens is usually visibly hemolyzed and results are often inaccurate. Separate the serum and transfer to a clean, dry tube for shipment.

IV–1–A. *Venipuncture of Dogs*

To restrain a dog for a venipuncture of the cephalic vein, place him on the table in sternal recumbency. If the right vein is to be tapped the assistant stands on the left side of the dog, places his left arm under subject's chin to immobilize the head and neck, reaches across, and grasps the right foreleg just distal to the elbow joint (Fig. 44). The thumb rotates the vein laterally while the hand immobilizes the leg in slight extension. It is important to keep the dog pressed down on the table if a struggle ensues. The person making the venipuncture grasps the leg at the metacarpals and begins the skin puncture at the medial side of the vein slightly above the carpus.

For a recurrent tarsal vein tap the dog is restrained in lateral recumbency. The assistant holds the under foreleg and presses the dog's neck to the table with his forearm. The upper rear leg is held above the knee joint and in extension. The vein is not easily visualized in some animals unless the hair is clipped. It is also very mobile subcutaneously which may cause difficulty in inserting the needle.

The jugular vein in short-coated, long-necked breeds is easily visualized. Neophytes searching for the vein are often surprised at its extreme lateral location. If the dog has a heavy coat it is probably better to clip the hair. Positioning is most important to make the vein "pop out"

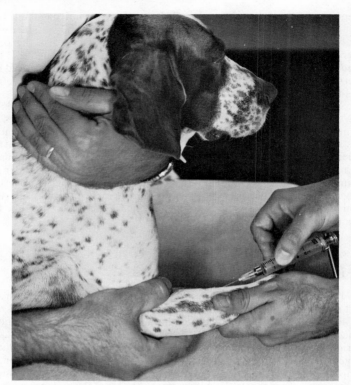

Figure 44. Cephalic venipuncture in right foreleg. A restraining arm is placed under the dog's chin, his neck and chest are held close to the assistant's body, and the cephalic vein is rolled laterally by thumb pressure. Proper restraint to prevent struggling is important.

into view, especially so for puppies and kittens less than one week old. Small breeds or puppies, feet hanging free, are held by an assistant who places his right arm under the dog's chest and holds it at his side. His right hand grasps one or both of the pup's forelegs below the elbows. The assistant's left hand is used to lift the dog's chin up and back, thus extending the neck. If the head is rotated slightly, the veins will be seen more easily. The person making the tap places his left thumb in the jugular furrow at the thoracic inlet. The right hand manipulates the syringe to

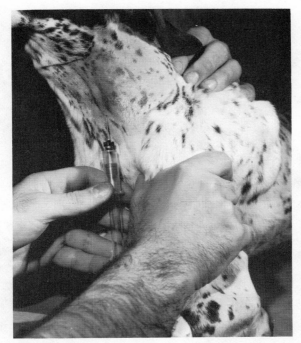

Figure 45. Jugular puncture in the dog. The hair on the neck has been clipped and the skin prepared with alcohol. The head and neck are extended and the thumb is placed in the jugular furrow to distend the vein. A Vacutainer is being used to collect blood.

make the venipuncture. Larger dogs are restrained in sternal recumbency on a table, their necks in extreme dorsal extension. (See Figure 45.)

IV–1–B. Venipuncture of Cats

Jugular puncture in the cat or kitten is accomplished in a fashion basically similar to that used for dogs. The cat bag or the wooden stocks, however, are more efficient in restraining the cat and protecting the operator. We have found that taping the front legs together and then the hind legs makes jugular punctures a much easier procedure (Fig. 46). The tape should be placed low enough on the leg to cover the claws.

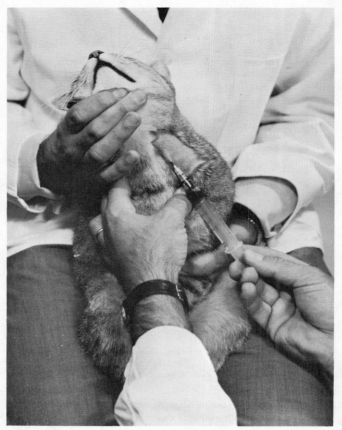

Figure 46. Jugular puncture in the cat. The legs are taped (not visible here) with the claws covered to prevent scratching. The cat is positioned comfortably on the restrainer's lap and the head and neck are extended to make the jugular vein protrude.

Puncture of the femoral vein of a cat is an effective way to obtain blood or to give medications. Because of its loose subcutaneous support, however, this vein is very mobile, and after puncture, almost always develops a hematoma. The quiet or depressed cat can be held gently on its side, the medial surface of the thigh clipped of hair and the venipuncture made with minimal restraint. The refractory animal requires more stringent measures. We prefer rolling it in a blanket and pulling out one hind leg. The medial aspect is clipped and the tap is performed as described previously.

Small amounts of blood can be collected easily from the marginal ear vein. Hair is plucked from an area of skin about half an inch in diameter at the medial dorsal edge of the ear over the vein. The skin is wiped with alcohol and pressure is applied at the base of the ear to make the vein protrude. The skin is coated with a thin film of petrolatum, which makes the blood well up in large droplets on the skin following venipuncture. The vein is incised with a lancet or number eleven Bard-Parker blade. Blood can be aspirated from the surface of the skin directly into a pipette. Hemorrhage stops quickly with gentle finger pressure. The whole procedure is quite painless and rarely upsets the patient.

IV–2. COLLECTION OF BONE MARROW
(See Section V-3-F)

This examination may prove valuable in those diseases of the blood in which examination of the peripheral blood reveals abnormal cells or cell counts. Conditions such as leukopenia, thrombocytopenia, nonregenerative anemias, agranulocytosis, pancytopenia, and leukemias may be present because of pathologic factors within the bone marrow.

Bone marrow in the young animal is very cellular and exists in the flat bones (sternum, ribs, pelvic bones, and vertebrae) and in the long bones (humerus and femur).

As the animal ages the cellular content of the marrow decreases, especially in the long bones. In older animals, bone marrow cells still exist in the flat bones; however, in conditions of stress in which new blood cells must be produced in large numbers, primitive cells in the bone marrow of the long bones again become active.

Interpretation of the bone marrow may be limited by:

1. The technique employed to obtain a bone marrow specimen. Technique is important because contamination with peripheral blood should be avoided.

2. The specialized knowledge necessary to interpret bone marrow cells.

IV-2-A. Bone Marrow Collection (Dog)

Equipment (All Equipment Should Be Sterile)

Rubber gloves.
Xylocaine, 0.5 per cent.
Skin disinfectant.
Clean glass slides.
One 20 ml. syringe.
Two 5 ml. syringes.
One 2 ml. syringe.
One scalpel.
Hemostats.
Thumb forceps.
Scissors.
Gauze.
Sponges.
Skin suture needle.
Skin suture material.
Needles, 20 and 23 gauge.
One Turkel bone marrow needle, 2 inch, 14 to 16 gauge.

Technique

In the dog, bone marrow can be obtained from the iliac crest, the sternal vertebrae or the femur. In general, bone marrow biopsy can be performed with the animal sedated or under a short-acting general anesthetic. Local anesthesia is used if the animal is only sedated.

To obtain material from the pelvis, clip an area of skin over the iliac crest and surgically prepare the site. If only tranquilization is used as restraint, infiltrate the bone marrow aspiration site with Xylocaine, 0.5 per cent, using a 23 gauge needle.

Make a small skin incision over the iliac crest and pass the Turkel bone marrow needle through the muscle over the anterior dorsal aspect of the iliac crest. By gentle pressure, along with a rotary motion, force the needle into the medullary cavity. When the needle tip penetrates the marrow cavity, remove the stylet, place a 20 ml. syringe on the needle hub, and aspirate 0.5 to 1 ml. of bone marrow material.

To perform a bone marrow aspiration from the sternum, place the animal in dorsal recumbency and clip and surgically prepare a site over the second sternebra. Infiltrate the area with local anesthetic. Using a

University of Illinois sternal needle, enter the second sternebra at a 23°
angle, stopping the needle just after penetration of the bone. Remove the
stylet and place a 20 cc. syringe on the needle and aspirate 0.2 ml. of
marrow.

Contamination of the bone marrow with peripheral blood results if
(1) the marrow is not aspirated immediately after the needle enters the
marrow cavity, or (2) too much negative pressure is placed on the syringe, thus rupturing small sinusoids in the bone marrow.

Marrow can also be obtained from the proximal end of the femur via
the trochanteric fossa.

A short-acting anesthetic (thiamylal sodium) is used. Place the animal
in lateral recumbency and clip the hair over the area of the trochanter
major and the trochanteric fossa. Surgically prepare the site.

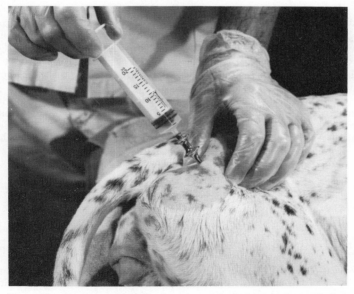

Figure 47.   Bone marrow sampling from the proximal end of the femur. The hair over
the trochanter major and the trochanteric fossa has been clipped and the site surgically
prepared. The bone marrow aspiration needle is inserted medial to the trochanter major.
By using firm pressure and an alternating rotary motion, the needle is inserted one-half
inch into the marrow cavity.

Make a small skin incision over the trochanteric fossa just medial to the summit of the trochanter major. The bone marrow aspiration needle is inserted medial to the trochanter major, using firm pressure and an alternating rotary motion. When the needle is inserted one-half inch into the femoral canal, remove the stylet from the needle and aspirate with a 12 or 20 ml. syringe (See Figure 47).

Difficulty in obtaining an adequate sample with this technique has resulted because of mixing of bone marrow with peripheral blood. This has resulted if (1) muscle hemorrhage involves the biopsy site, (2) too much negative pressure is used when aspirating marrow, or (3) too large a sample is obtained.

IV–2–B. Bone Marrow Collection (Cat)

Accessible sites for bone marrow sampling in the cat are the iliac crest and the proximal end of the femur via the trochanteric fossa. The same techniques as were previously described can be used: however, caution is advised against using vigorous restraint in a severely anemic cat. This may precipitate severe cyanosis, apnea and cardiac arrest. Adequate sedation with supplemental oxygen administration and local anesthesia usually suffices.

Smears of bone marrow should be made immediately after aspiration of material. Additionally, small pieces of marrow can be fixed in formalin for histologic preparation. Staining procedures such as new methylene blue, Wright's, or May-Grunwald Giemsa may be used. A peroxidase stain may be helpful in differentiating granulocytic elements from lymphocytes.

References

Additional information can be found in the following sources:

Melveger, B. E., Earl, F. L., and VanLoon, E. J.: Sternal bone marrow biopsy in the dog; Lab. Animal Care 19: 866-868, 1969.

Penny, R. H., and Carlisle, C. H.: The bone marrow of the dog: a comparative study of biopsy material obtained from the iliac crest, rib, and sternum. J. Small Anim. Pract. 11: 727-734, 1970.

Schalm, O. W., Jain, N. C., and Carrol, E. J.: Veterinary Hematology, 3rd ed., Philadelphia, Lea & Febiger, 1975.

IV-3. COLLECTION OF CEREBROSPINAL FLUID

In the dog, the preferred site for obtaining cerebrospinal fluid is the cerebellomedullary cistern (cisterna magna) at the atlanto-occipital articulation.

Equipment needed consists of sterile test tubes for fluid collection, an 18 to 20 gauge, 1½ to 3½ inch Pitkin spinal needle with a short bevel and stylet, a spinal fluid manometer for pressure readings, a three-way stopcock, two sterile 5 ml. syringes, and sterile sponges.

In order to perform an adequate cisternal puncture and not injure the animal, a short-acting, general anesthetic such as thiamylal sodium is required. The animal is placed in either ventral or lateral recumbency and the area of skin from the external occipital protuberance to the wings of the atlas is clipped and surgically prepared. The dog should be positioned in left lateral recumbency for right-handed individuals and in right lateral recumbency for left-handed individuals. Position the patient with the prepared area at the edge of the table. The head should be flexed ventrally and maintained at a right angle to the long axis of the neck. The flexion of the neck will serve to separate the occipital bone from the atlas.

To find the site of entrance for the needle into the cistern, an imaginary line is drawn across the neck from the prominent cranial lateral portion of the wings of the atlas. At a point where this line bisects a line drawn craniocaudally from the external occipital protuberance, the needle is passed inward at a right angle to the dorsal line of the neck (Figure 48). As the needle is advanced, the stylet is removed periodically to see whether cerebrospinal fluid appears in the hub. During this procedure the hub of the needle must be held tightly to prevent any movement of the needle. Occasionally resistance is felt just prior to when the needle passes through the dura, but this cannot be depended upon; therefore frequent removal of the stylet will avoid injury to the spinal cord. If bone is felt with the tip of the needle, the needle can be walked caudally (occipital bone) or cranially (atlas) to the atlanto-occipital space. Occasionally blood without cerebrospinal fluid is obtained. This is from puncture of a branch of the vertebral venous plexus. Obtain another clean sterile needle and repeat the procedure. This has not contaminated the cerebrospinal fluid with blood. If fresh blood appears in the cerebrospinal fluid repeat the procedure after 24 hours.

Upon entering the cisternal space and seeing fluid at the needle hub, attach the spinal fluid pressure manometer immediately and note the pressure. Next, 2 ml. of spinal fluid is removed and placed in a sterile vial. More fluid may be removed if necessary, but it should be removed slowly. Initial cerebrospinal fluid examination should include inspection for color

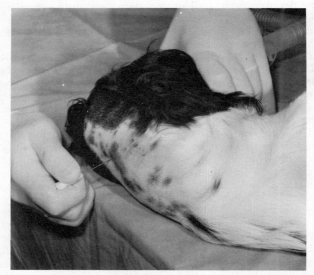

Figure 48. Collection of cerebrospinal fluid. The dog is in left lateral recumbency. The area from the external occipital protuberance to the wings of the atlas has been clipped and surgically prepared. The head is flexed ventrally. The needle is inserted at the junction of a line that bisects the cranial wings of the atlas and the external occipital protuberance.

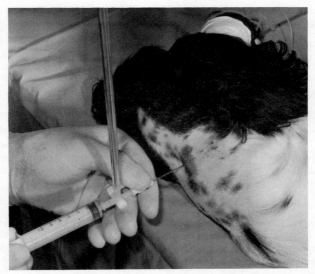

Figure 49.   Recording CSF pressure. When the cisternal space is entered and fluid is seen at the needle hub, the spinal fluid pressure manometer is attached and opening and closing CSF pressure recorded.

and turbidity, total cell count, differential, and protein determination. Further tests such as chloride content, glucose levels, differential cell count, and cultures may be indicated depending on the clinical situation.

All animals on whom a cisternal tap was performed should be closely observed for the next five to seven days for signs of adverse effects such as infection.

See Table 97, Section VI, for normal cerebrospinal fluid values.

IV–4. BACTERIAL CULTURES

Principles of Collection

Collect a representative sample and examine the material promptly.

1. Specimens should be collected from areas where organisms are most likely to be found, such as the edge of a spreading skin lesion, from incised pustules, or from contaminated cavities.

2. Specimens should be collected prior to the use of antibiotics, when possible.
3. Avoid accidental contamination of the specimen.
4. Label all specimens clearly and carefully.
5. Inoculate culture material into appropriate media *promptly*.

ROUTINE PROCEDURE FOR BACTERIOLOGIC CULTURE

Routine Smear

Prepare a smear by collecting material on a sterile cotton swab and rolling it onto a clear glass slide. Heat fix, and stain the slide with Gram stain. Fluids should be centrifuged and the sediment examined and cultured. Biopsy material may be ground in sterile sand and placed in sterile broth.

Routine Culture

Culture material on blood agar plates and in thioglycollate broth. These media serve as a basis for the isolation of most aerobic microorganisms. Selective media may be necessary for the isolation and identification of specific microorganisms.

Bacterial Cultures

Recently, multiple media plates have been developed commercially* to facilitate direct antibiotic sensitivity and tentative identification of common pathogenic bacteria.

These prepackaged, relatively inexpensive plates help the small laboratory identify pathogenic bacteria by their characteristic behavior on selective media. Some companies have different kits for different suspected infections. In general they are most useful in evaluating conjunctivitis, otitis, pyoderma, wound infections, uterine or anterior vaginal infections, fresh necropsy material and urinary infections. They are not recommended in areas having a large population of normal microbial organisms, such as the respiratory tract, throat, and vulva, nor for fecal samples or for blood cultures to determine bacteremia.

Mueller-Hinton agar is an all purpose media commonly used to evaluate antibiotic sensitivity. Table 41 gives the relative sizes of significant zones of inhibition produced with sensitive bacteria by common antibiotic discs.

---

*Bactossay Plate, Pitman-Moore Co., Washington's Crossing, N. J.; Bacti Lab Plate, Mt. View, California.

TABLE 41. THE RELATIVE SIZES OF ZONES OF INHIBITION PRODUCED WITH SENSITIVE BACTERIA BY COMMON ANTIBIOTIC DISCS WHEN USED ON MUELLER-HINTON AGAR*

Small Zone (up to 13 mm)	Medium Zone (up to 18 mm)	Large Zone (up to 25 mm)
Bacitracin (10 U)†	Lincomycin (2 mcg)	Cephalothin (30 mcg)
Colistin (10 mcg)	Sulfadimethoxine (250 mcg)	Chloramphenicol (30 mcg)
Gentamicin (10 mcg)	Methicillin (5 mcg)	Erythromycin (15 mcg)
Oxacillin (1 mcg)	Neomycin (30 mcg)	Kanamycin (30 mcg)
Polymyxin B (300 U)	Nitrofurantoin (300 mcg)	Novobiocin (30 mcg)
Vancomycin (30 mcg)	Oleandomycin (15 mcg)	Penicillin G (10 U)
	Streptomycin (10 mcg)	Tetracycline (30 mcg)
	Sulfonamides (250 mcg)	Ampicillin (10 mcg)
	Ampicillin (10 mcg) (for Gram-negative bacteria and enterococci)	(for Gram-positive organisms)

*From Bauer, H. W., et al.: Antibiotic susceptibility testing by standardized single disc method. *Amer. J. Clin. Path.* 45:493, 1966.
†Antibiotic concentration in disc.

SPECIFIC CULTURE AND SMEAR METHODS

Blood Culture

The material for culture must be collected under aseptic conditions. Clip and surgically prepare the skin over the cephalic, recurrent tarsal, or jugular vein. Use a Becton-Dickinson Vacutainer blood culture bottle, which can be used for both aerobic and anaerobic blood cultures. Add 20 ml. of blood to the culture media, following the directions carefully.

Blood cultures present many problems, and the percentage of negative results is high. A greater degree of success may be obtained if three or four carefully drawn samples are collected at intervals during one day. Relatively large amounts of blood should be collected and cultured under both aerobic and anaerobic conditions. It is especially important to secure samples prior to any antibacterial therapy, or after therapy has been withdrawn for 10 days.

Other media which may be employed as selective agents include MacConkey's agar, brain-heart infusion agar, mannitol salt agar, Streptosel agar, urea agar, blood agar, and E.-M. B. agar. Special techniques make it possible to determine total bacteria counts and whether an organism is coagulase positive or negative.

Anaerobe Culture

Because there is reason to believe that anaerobes may be present in significant numbers in positive cultures from blood, infections, wounds and urine, it may be advisable to make these special examinations. Anaerobes are in the normal flora in fecal, throat and bronchial swabs, so the anaerobic culture of these samples is rarely advisable.

Specimens for anaerobic examination should be protected from air and held at room temperature. They should be cultured as soon as possible. They should not be used with transport or enrichment media but inoculated directly from the specimen. Specimens can be held for short periods in sterile, carbon-dioxide-filled, tightly stoppered tubes or bottles. The sample should be inoculated onto prereduced anerobically sterilized media under oxygen-free gas. Streak specimens on brain-heart infusion agar in roll tubes. Incubate at 37°C and observe for 10 days before discarding as no growth.

With anaerobic organisms it is especially important to make a smear and a Gram stain and to record all morphotypes present and the relative numbers of each.

Urine Culture

Urine as it is secreted by the kidneys is sterile unless the kidney is infected. Catheterization using aseptic technique is necessary to get adequate urine samples for culture from both males and females (see Sections IV-13-A and IV-13-B). Urine to be cultured should be placed into media no later than 60 minutes after collection. Centrifuge the urine and make a Gram stain of the sediment. Spread 0.1 ml. of urine sediment on a blood agar plate or one of the multiple media plates and culture.

Puncture Fluids

Aspirate material using aseptic technique (see Sections IV-7 and IV-8). Centrifuge the aspirated material at high speed and stain a smear of the sediment with Gram stain. Culture the sediment on blood agar, in thioglycollate media, on Sabouraud's agar or on one of the multiple media plates.

Wound and Ulcers

In dealing with an abscess (except those of the eye), clip and clean the abscess site. Aspirate material from the abscess into a sterile syringe and culture in blood agar and thioglycollate or on one of the multiple media plates. In open wounds, use a sterile cotton swab and obtain fresh exudate from the deeper portion of the lesion.

Throat Cultures

It is very difficult to obtain a good representative sample from the throat without contamination from the mouth. Pass a sterile cotton swab over the tonsilar area and posterior pharyngeal walls. In some animals this may have to be done under a short-acting general anesthetic. Place swab into broth for 24 hours and subculture onto blood agar. Because of the abundant normal flora, multiple bacteria will usually grow and evaluation of pathogenicity will be difficult.

Spinal Fluid

If the spinal fluid is cloudy, make a direct smear and stain with Gram and Giemsa stains. If the fluid is fairly clear, centrifuge for ten minutes, make a smear, and stain the sediment with Gram stain. Culture the sediment on blood agar, in thioglycollate medium or on one of the multiple media plates, and on Sabouraud's agar.

Ear Cultures

Collect material on sterile cotton swabs, make a smear, and stain it with Gram stain. Place the swab into sterile broth for 24 hours, then subculture onto blood agar and thioglycollate media, or one of the multiple media plates.

Eye Cultures

Use a sterile cotton swab moistened with sterile saline or broth and pass it over the conjunctiva of the inferior fornix of each eye. Use one half of a blood agar and one half of a mannitol plate for each eye. Material should also be placed into thioglycollate medium. Alternatively, use one of the commercial multiple media plates. Make two conjunctival scrapings and stain one with Gram stain and one with Giemsa stain. Examine the slides for the presence of bacteria and for cell morphology.

References

Additional information can be found in the following sources:

Bauer, H. W., et al.: Amer, J. Clin. Path. 45:493, 1966.
Bruner, D. W. and Gillespie, J. H.: Hagan's Infectious Diseases of Domestic Animals, 6th ed. Ithaca, N. Y., Cornell University Press, 1973.
Coles, E. H.: Veterinary Clinical Pathology, 2nd ed. Philadelphia, W. B. Saunders Co., 1975.
Jawetz, E., Melnick, J. L., and Adelberg, E. A.: Review of Medical Microbiology, 10th Ed. Palo Alto, California, Lange Publishing Co., 1972.

IV-5. FUNGUS CULTURES

POSITIVE CULTURES

Obtaining positive cultures of dermatophytes involves proper selection of culture site and reduction of nonsignificant organisms. If the lesion is localized, its edge should be cleansed with alcohol, and scales, hair, and superficial keratin should be scraped onto a scalpel blade. The sample is transferred to the center of a bottle of media and implanted into the surface of the media. The bottle cap is partially closed and the culture incubated at room temperature for one to four weeks.

When the skin lesion is diffuse or not well developed in a local area, a sterile toothbrush can be rubbed vigorously over suspicious areas to collect hair, scales and skin debris. The brush can be pressed gently onto the surface of a Petri dish to transfer the sample to the media. Alternatively, the brush can be tapped into an empty sterile Petri dish to dislodge the accumulated debris. It is then collected and deposited on the surface of a bottle or Petri dish of media.

These procedures may be used to isolate dermatophytes or *Candida*. Two types of media are used. One is Sabouraud dextrose agar containing 0.5 mg. of cyclohexamide and 0.05 mg. of chloramphenicol per ml. of agar to inhibit bacterial and fungal contaminants. A new selective and differential media, Dermatophyte Test Media (DTM), contains a yellow to red pH indicator (phenol red). Dermatophytes (and *Alternaria*, a frequent contaminant) produce an alkaline reaction and a red color within several days. Most saprophytic fungal contaminants produce a yellow color. Fungal growth on this media is accelerated as compared to that on Sabouraud's media (see also Section V-6.)

Deep mycoses are so varied that generalizing about culture techniques is difficult. Growth forms in the tissues are often very different from those obtained on media, and incubation at 20°C, may produce different growth than incubation at 37°C. Usually tissue specimens or exudates from the ulcerative lesions are inoculated onto common laboratory media (nutrient agar, broth, or Sabouraud's agar). Special techniques may be needed for positive identification, and reference should be made to standard microbiology texts for specific details. Use of a state diagnostic laboratory is often very helpful in cases in which a systemic mycosis is suspected.

References

Additional information can be found in the following sources:

Carter, G. R.: Diagnostic Procedures in Veterinary Bacteriology and Mycology. Springfield, Illinois, Charles C. Thomas, Publisher, 1967.

Jawetz, E., Melnick, J. L., and Adelberg, E. A.: Review of Medical Microbiology, 10th ed. Palo Alto, California, Lange Publishing Co., 1972.

Jungerman, P. F., and Schwartzman, R. M.: Veterinary Medical Mycology, Philadelphia, Lea & Febiger, 1972.

IV–6. DERMATOLOGIC DIAGNOSTIC PROCEDURES

Skin Scrapings

This is a frequently used diagnostic procedure performed to find and identify microscopic parasites in the skin. Material required is mineral oil in a small dropper bottle, a dull scalpel blade, glass slides and a microscope.

Select undisturbed, untreated skin for a scraping site. It is best to scrape the periphery of skin lesions and avoid the excoriated or traumatized center areas. In scraping for demodectic mange, a small fold of skin should be gently pinched and the surface material collected for examinations. This procedure forces the mites out of the hair follicles and onto or near the skin surface. In scraping for sarcoptic mange, large areas should be scraped. Select sites on the elbows, hocks, and ear margins when searching for sarcoptic mange. Many or frequent scrapings may be necessary to demonstrate sarcoptic mange mites.

The accumulated material is placed on a microscope slide and mixed with a small drop of mineral oil. Examine the area with the 10× objective thoroughly and carefully.

Skin Biopsy

Histologic examination of diseased skin can serve as a means for diagnosis of cutaneous lesions. The etiological agent is often found in both acute or chronic skin infections.

Punch biopsy of the skin is a quick and accurate way to remove a small sample of diseased skin for histopathological examination. Select a site which is well developed but not traumatized or excoriated. The sample should include both normal and diseased tissue (i.e., biopsy the periphery of the lesion). The hair should be carefully clipped from the lesion. The skin should be lightly cleaned with 70 per cent alcohol. Avoid superficial trauma while cleaning the skin. Make a small subcutaneous bleb with 0.5 per cent lidocaine to deaden the area. Special equipment needed for the biopsy is a 9 mm. Keyes punch, ethyl chloride spray, and 10 per cent formalin solution. After the area has been anesthetized with lidocaine, spray the skin lightly with ethyl-chloride to freeze the skin for a clean, firm biopsy specimen. Press and rotate the Keyes punch through the skin until the subcutaneous tissue is penetrated. Remove the biopsy specimen and blot gently between two pieces of paper towel. Leave the specimen adhered to one piece of paper and drop the specimen and paper into the formalin fixative. The skin defect may be closed with one simple interrupted suture.

Skin Allergy Tests

The intradermal skin test can be employed as a means of identifying specific allergens capable of inducing immediate hypersensitivities in dogs. The test will not routinely give positive reactions for delayed hypersensitivities such as those from allergic contact dermatitis. The test also has not proved accurate for food-induced allergic dermatitis. Other diagnostic methods such as provocative exposure or patch testing must be used to identify the allergen causing food allergy or contact dermatitis.

Test antigens are purchased in concentrations of 1500 p.n.u./cc. Aqueous antigens are ordered from the manufacturer of human test antigens. The following antigen groups are suggested for routine testing:

SMALL ANIMAL DERMATOLOGY

LESIONS (circle): ☐ Photos

Macules   Papules   Pustules   Vesicles

Wheals   Nodules   Tumors   Scales

Crusts   Ulcers   Excoriations   Pruritus

Lichenification   Hyperpigmentation

Hyperkeratosis   Alopecia   Erythema

REF. DVM _____
CLINICIAN _____
SECONDARY # _____

DISTRIBUTION

CANINE

Ventral   Dorsal

FELINE

Ventral   Dorsal

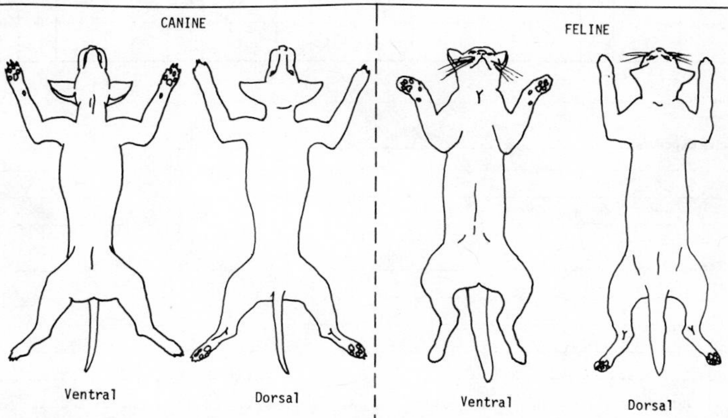

PARASITES (circle): Fleas   Lice   Ticks   Demodex   Sarcoptes   Others _____

FUNGI: Wood's Light _____   KOH _____   Culture _____

BACTERIA: Culture _____

Sensitivity _____

DIRECT SMEARS _____

BIOPSY _____

Figure 50. Dermatology examination record.

INTRADERMAL TESTS

A \\ B	1	2	3	4	5	6	7	8	9	10	11	12	13	14	15	16	17	18	19	20
5M																				
15M																				
30M																				
1h																				
2h																				
24h																				
48h																				

Interpretation _____

Provocative Exposure _____
_____
_____
_____

Special Tests _____
_____
_____
_____
_____
_____
_____
_____
_____
_____
_____
_____

Figure 51. Intradermal tests record.

Seasonal Group

1. Mixed grasses (timothy, orchard, June, red top and sweet bernal).
2. Mixed weeds (cocklebur, plantain, sorrel and elder).
3. Tall and short ragweed.
4. Mixed trees (ash, beech, birch, elm, hickory, maple, oak and poplar).
5. Fleas.

Non-seasonal Group

1. Kapok.
2. Wool.
3. Mixed feathers.
4. House dust.
5. Mixed inhalants.
6. Mixed molds.
7. Cat epithelium.

In addition, a negative diluent control and a positive histamine phosphate control are used. Seventy-two hours prior to testing, the patient should be taken off all corticosteroids, antihistamines and tranquilizers. One week may be necessary if a long-acting steroid has been given. The patient should not be tranquilized for the procedure, but can be anesthetized with short-acting barbiturates if necessary. Gently clip the hair from the lateral thorax and do not prep the skin. Make intradermal injections of 0.1 cc. of each antigen and each control. Space the injections about 4 cm. apart and mark each one with a felt pen. The reactions are recorded in terms of centimeters and are read immediately and again at intervals of 15 minutes, 30 minutes, 1 hour, 2 hours, 24 hours and 48 hours after the injection. A reaction 1 cm. larger than the negative control is proof of a positive reaction. The histamine control should be diluted 1:10 with saline before injection. This dilution will give a good 4+ reaction (2 cm. larger than negative control) in most dogs and is necessary to show that the patient is capable of responding to histamine.

A positive reaction indicates that the patient is hypersensitive to the test antigen or to a similar antigen. A negative reaction could mean any of the following: (1) the patient was not sensitive to the antigens used; (2) the antigen used was not present in sufficient quantity to give a positive reaction (combination antigens); (3) the patient is allergic but does not possess sufficient reagin antibody to give a positive skin test reaction; (4) improper technique was used; or (5) inhibitory effects of other medications interfered.

One should always remember that a negative skin test does not mean the patient is not allergic.

References

Additional information can be found in the following sources:

Baker, K. P.: Intradermal tests as an aid to the diagnosis of skin disease in dogs. J. Small Anim. Pract. *12*: 445-452, 1971.

Chamberlain, K. W.: Clinical investigations and observations on canine allergy. J. A. V. M. A., Vol. 155, No. 12, December 15, 1969.

Chamberlain, K. W. (ed.): Allergy in small animal practice. Vet. Clin. N. Amer., Vol. 4, No. 1, February, 1974.

Muller, G. H., and Kirk, R. W.: Small Animal Dermatology. Philadelphia, W. B. Saunders Co., 1969.

IV-7. ABDOMINAL PARACENTESIS

This term refers to the surgical puncture of the abdominal cavity. When abdominal fluid is to be removed, the animal should always be weighed before and after the procedure. Any subsequent gain in weight indicates a reaccumulation of abdominal fluid. The animal is placed in

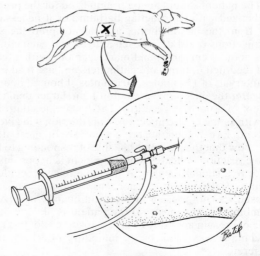

Figure 52. A three-inch square to the right of the midline between the bladder and umbilicus has been clipped and surgically prepared. Paracentesis is performed using a needle and three-way valve to facilitate fluid collection.

left lateral recumbency and restrained in this position. A 1 to 3 inch square between the bladder and the umbilicus just lateral to the midline is clipped and surgically prepared. If the bladder is distended, it should be emptied before paracentesis is performed. The paracentesis site is infiltrated with Xylocaine, 0.5 per cent, using a 22 to 24 gauge needle. Abdominal puncture can be made with a 14 to 20 gauge needle. Once the abdominal puncture has been made, the animal should be allowed to stand, as this will facilitate drainage of the fluid. Aspiration may be easier if a specially adapted needle with multiple holes drilled in the shaft is used since it is less likely to become plugged with omentum. The amount of fluid obtained should be measured and the fluid should be examined to see whether it is an exudate or transudate. Cytologic examination and culture may also be performed (see Sections IV-4 and V-13).

IV-8. THORACENTESIS AND PERICARDICENTESIS

Thoracentesis refers to the aspiration of fluid or air from the thoracic cavity. It may be performed for diagnostic or therapeutic procedures. When fluid or air is present it may be impossible to remove it all; however, as much as possible should be removed. If repeated withdrawal of air or fluid from the chest is contemplated, a chest tube is safer. The thoracic wall between the fifth to the seventh intercostal space is clipped and surgically prepared. If fluid or air is present on only one side of the thoracic cavity (a rarity in dogs and cats) only that side should be aspirated. If fluid is to be aspirated, Xylocaine, 0.5 per cent, is infiltrated into a spot low in the seventh intercostal space using a 1 inch, 22 to 24 gauge needle. An 18 to 20 gauge needle is then fitted to a two-way stopcock, which in turn is fitted to a 20 ml. sterile syringe. The needle is inserted into the thoracic cavity until the tip is just through the pleura but does not lacerate the lung. Any fluid aspirated should be saved and analyzed to determine whether it is a transudate or an exudate. Cytologic examination may be performed and cultures taken of this fluid. Thoracentesis in pneumothorax is carried out in the same manner as the aspiration of fluid; however, since air rises in the thoracic cavity, the thoracentesis puncture is made high up in the seventh intercostal space.

Pericardicentesis involves the surgical puncture of the pericardium in order to aspirate effusions. Sedate the animal with morphine or a neuroleptanalgesic agent. Surgically prepare both sides of the thorax. Place the animal in lateral recumbency with the right side down. Infiltrate the muscles of the fourth intercostal space at a level with the

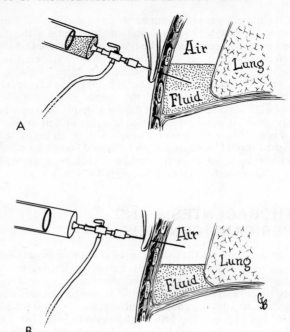

Figure 53. In thoracentesis, the needle is inserted low in the intercostal space for fluid aspiration (A) and high for aspiration of air in pneumothorax (B).

junction of the ventral and middle third of the thorax with Xylocaine, 2 per cent, using a 22 gauge needle. Use a *venocath* (16 gauge needle); place a 3-way stopcock on the syringe adapter end of the venocath. Have an assistant place a 30 cc. syringe on the 3-way stopcock and maintain negative pressure on the syringe as the chest is entered. Carefully advance the 16 gauge intercath needle into the fourth intercostal space, advancing toward the heart, while maintaining negative pressure in the syringe. When fluid enters the syringe, the pericardial sac has been entered. Thread the intercath polyethylene tubing through the 16 gauge needle so that the end of the tubing lies securely within the pericardial sac and remove the needle from the interthoracic space. Continue aspirating fluid. This technique should prevent trauma to the myocardium. The intracath tube can be heparinized and the stopcock closed and taped to the body wall, and repeated aspirations can be performed over several days if necessary. All aspirated fluid should be examined as described in Section V-9.

IV–9. BIOPSY OF THE LIVER

The diagnosis of liver disease can be made on clinical signs coupled with clinical pathological findings found when performing a "liver profile." The development of a more specific diagnosis and prognosis in liver disease may be greatly aided by information obtained in a liver biopsy. Liver biopsies are of much greater value in generalized liver disease such as cirrhosis, generalized acute hepatic necrosis or amyloidosis than in focal hepatic disease.

There are numerous procedures for obtaining liver biopsy; however, needle biopsy of the liver, when performed properly, can be very helpful. Careful physical and clinical pathologic examination should precede a liver biopsy. Abnormalities in normal hemostatic mechanisms should be detected and corrected prior to needle biopsy of the liver.

Equipment
1. Local anesthetic.
2. Franklin-modified Vim-Silverman biopsy needle.
3. Cut down tray (sterile).
4. Suitable fixative for tissue specimen.

Technique
Modified Percutaneous Liver Biopsy can generally be performed under effective sedation and local anesthesia. Prior to biopsy, the animal should be fasted, and any ascitic fluid should be removed. The animal is placed in dorsal recumbency and a local block is placed in the midline of the skin and abdomen at the caudoventral aspect of the left hepatic lobe. The incision into the peritoneal cavity should be large enough to accommodate the gloved index finger. Make a separate skin puncture site in the abdominal wall to accommodate the biopsy needle. Use the index finger to manually fix the left hepatic lobe (or other desired hepatic lobe) against the diaphragm or other adjacent structures and insert the outer cannula and stylet through the abdominal wall into the isolated hepatic lobe. Remove the stylet and rapidly insert the cutting prongs. If

properly placed, the cutting prongs should not go through the entire hepatic lobe. Advance the outer cannula over the blades of the cutting prongs, thus entrapping the hepatic tissue material within the cutting prongs. Remove the biopsy needle, using a wooden applicator stick, and very carefully place the biopsy specimen into fixative. Biopsy samples can be used to prepare slides for cytologic exam and the biopsy needle may be cultured. Close the abdominal incision in routine manner.

Blind percutaneous liver biopsy is not recommended because of the many complications that may result.

IV–10. PERCUTANEOUS RENAL BIOPSY

Renal biopsies can be valuable in confirming or eliminating a diagnosis of renal disease that is based on history, physical examination, and radiographic and laboratory data. Additionally, biopsy may be a way of arriving at a prognosis in generalized renal disease and a means of better evaluating what type of treatment should be instituted. The technique we have used for percutaneous renal biopsy in the dog is that outlined by Osborne.

Equipment

1. A Franklin modified Vim-Silverman biopsy needle (small size).
2. Sharp, pointed tissue scissors and scalpel.
3. Thumb forceps.
4. Hemostats.
5. Needle holder, skin suture, sponges.
6. Local anesthetic, surgical prep tray, small drape, formalin 10 per cent for fixation of specimen.

Technique

Many patients with generalized renal disease are critically ill and debilitated and general anesthesia is contraindicated. In these cases a neuroleptanalgesic agent may be used for sedation. If the animal is a good anesthetic risk and renal function will permit it, a general anesthetic can be used.

Surgically prepare the area over the kidney that will be biopsied. Infiltrate the skin and paralumbar muscles caudal to the last rib just below the ventral border of the lumbar muscles with a local anesthetic. Make a paralumbar incision large enough for the index finger in this site over the caudal pole of the kidney. Dissect muscle and fascia until the peritoneum is reached and enter the peritoneal cavity. With the sterile, gloved index finger examine the posterior pole and remaining portions of the kidney. Make a small stab incision in the skin just anterior to paralumbar entry into the peritoneal cavity and insert the biopsy needle into the peritoneal cavity. Guide the needle toward the posterior pole of the kidney with the index finger. Hold the kidney so that it is immobilized against the body wall and, placing the long axis of the biopsy needle away from the renal pelvis, place the needle just through the renal capsule. Replace the stylet in the needle with the cutting prongs and rapidly thrust the cutting prongs into the renal cortical tissue. Keeping the cutting prongs in their same position, move the outer cannula down over the blades, rotating the cannula. Remove the cutting prongs and outer cannula and place the biopsy specimen in fixative. Close the surgical wound, making sure that excessive hemorrhage is not present.

Reference

Osborne, C. A. (ed.): Symposium on biopsy techniques. Vet. Clin. N. Amer., Vol. 4, No. 2, May, 1974.

IV–11. PHARYNGOSTOMY

This technique allows placement of a gastroesophageal tube for repeated oral alimentation required in a wide variety of disease conditions. It obviates the necessity of repeated passage of a stomach tube and it is well tolerated by most animals.

Equipment

1. Standard surgical pack and suture material.
2. Plastic or rubber feeding tube.

Technique

A short-acting anesthetic can be utilized in those animals that are a good surgical risk. A neuroleptanalgesic agent with local anesthesia or local anesthesia alone can be used in debilitated patients. Prepare the area posterior to the angle of the mandible for surgery and hold the mouth open with a speculum. Insert the gloved index finger into the pharynx at the base of the tongue and locate the piriform fossa of the pharynx posterior to the base of the tongue and lateral to the hyoid apparatus. Replace the index finger in this location with a curved hemostat and exert outward pressure on the skin in this area. Use a small number 11 or 15 scalpel blade to incise the skin over the bulge and use the forceps to grasp the stomach tube and draw it into the incision. Place the tube in the esophagus so that the tip lies in the stomach and the proximal end is sutured into the skin of the neck, using a piece of adhesive tape as a cuff which is sutured into the skin. The tube should be capped when not being used.

The incision in the skin and entrance site of the tube should be cleansed daily with soap and water and the wound is allowed to heal by second intention when the tube is removed.

Reference

Additional material may be found in the following source:

Böhning, R. H., Jr.: et al.: Pharyngostomy for maintenance of the anorectic animal. J.A.V.M.A. *156*:611–615, 1970.

IV-12.   COLLECTION AND EVALUATION OF CANINE SEMEN

Canine semen should be collected for evaluation of a potential breeder, for investigating infertility, and for artificial insemination.

IV-12-A.   Method of Collection

Equipment

1. Sterile and warmed to body temperature (use of an incubator is acceptable):

A 3 inch glass or Teflon laboratory funnel.
Glass or Teflon test tubes.
Saline solution, 0.9 per cent.

2. Nonsterile:

Microscope slides and cover slips (warmed).
India ink (Pelican), Williams stain, buffered formalin.
Hemocytometer (counting chamber and equipment).
Microscope and light.

Collecting Semen

1. Take the male and a female (in heat if possible) to a quiet room where there will be no distractions.

2. Hold the female and allow the male to "flirt" for several minutes.

3. An assistant may be needed to hold the female and control the male by a collar and leash.

4. Grasp the male's sheath behind the os penis and apply firm, but gentle, steady pressure. Erection occurs rapidly and when pelvic motions or ejaculation begins direct the semen into the funnel. Actual contact between the penis and the funnel is undesirable. The male is usually not allowed to mount the female.

5. The ejaculate consists of three fractions:
   a. Urethral secretion—0.1 to 2 ml. within 50 seconds, pH 6.3.
   b. Sperm-containing secretion—0.5 to 3 ml. within 1 to 2 minutes, pH 6.1.
   c. Prostatic secretion—2 to 20 ml. within 30 minutes, pH 6.5.
   Total secretion—3 to 20 ml. pH 6.4.

6. Since the first and third fractions are clear, water-like material and the second fraction is thick, opaque, white material, the clinician can separate them by changing collecting tubes as each fraction is ejaculated. It is best to collect only enough prostatic fluid to rinse the sperm fraction into the test tube. Too much is detrimental to sperm longevity in storage. Settergren uses a total collection time of 5 minutes from the beginning of ejaculation. This period allows for some additional fluid collection and will also add a few more sperm to the sample.

7. The male is returned to his cage. The female is retained until the semen is examined if actual insemination is to be performed.

IV–12–B. *Evaluation of Semen*

1. Immediately after collection slowly invert the tube several times to mix the semen gently.

2. Determine motility. Place 1 drop of semen on a warmed microscope slide and mix with 1 drop of saline. Cover with a cover slip and observe under low power for general motility. There will be no "waves" but general vigorous motion should be evident. Under high power count ten different groups of ten sperm, observing the number of motile and nonmotile sperm. Total motility for a suitable sample should be 80 per cent or greater.

3. Determine the number of sperm. Although the number of sperm is determined in a hemocytometer on the basis of sperm/cu. mm., this

figure varies widely depending on the dilution by variable amounts of prostatic fluid. More important is the total number of sperm per ejaculate; it should exceed 500 million in a normal male. A minimum number of 200 million sperm per insemination is needed if average conception is to be expected.

4. Determine morphology. Place 1 drop of semen on a slide, add 1 drop of Pelican india ink, and mix carefully. The mixture is spread carefully like a blood smear and allowed to dry. The carbon particles surround the sperm and outline them so that their structure and form can be observed under high power. One hundred sperm are counted, noting normals and abnormals.

If there is any question about abnormality it would be best to evaluate 500 sperm cells. It would also be desirable to use more complex staining techniques to make more detailed examinations of the sperm. Williams stain of a semen smear is ideal for examination of the sperm heads. It is prepared as follows: make fuchsin stock of 10 gm. fuchsin and 100 cc. 96 per cent alcohol. Make phenol solution with 10 cc. liquid phenol (90 per cent) and 170 cc. distilled water. Prepare bluish eosin stock with 1 gm. blue eosin and 100 cc. 96 per cent alcohol. After filtering the fuchsin stock, take 10 cc. of it and mix with 100 cc. phenol solution. Take 100 cc. of this mixture and add 50 cc. bluish eosin solution. Leave it for 14 days and filter before using. This solution can be stored for months, but is best stored under refrigeration to prevent mold and fungal growth.

Williams Staining Method

Spread a film of fresh semen. Air dry and fix in a flame. Immerse in absolute alcohol three or four minutes. Allow to drain and dry. Immerse in one-half per cent chloramine solution until mucus is removed and the smear appears clear. Wash in distilled water and then in 96 per cent alcohol. Stain in Williams stain for 8 minutes. Wash in water and allow to dry.

The rest of the sperm cell (midpiece and tail) can best be examined by the following technique:

Dilute a drop of semen and mix with buffered formalin. Place a cover slip on the mixture and examine with a phase contrast microscope. This type of preparation is ideal for fixing and preserving semen for shipment or for later laboratory examination.

Normal canine sperm are 68 mμ long; the heads are 7 mμ long. The average percentage of abnormal sperm totals 15. Excellent samples should not exceed 20 per cent total abnormals. The differential abnormality is important, however, and the following regional abnormals

SPERM

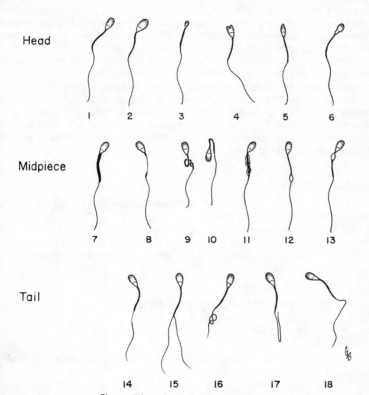

Figure 54. Chart of abnormal sperm.

Head
1. Normal
2. Giant
3. Small
4. Indented
5. Pointed
6. Pear-shaped

Midpiece
7. Thickened
8. Thinned
9. Coiled
10. Bent
11. Extraneous
12. Distal cytoplasmic droplet
13. Proximal cytoplasmic droplet

Tail
14. Thinned
15. Double
16. Coiled
17. Folded
18. Kinked

should not be exceeded in any sperm count: abnormality of the head, 10 to 12 per cent; midpiece abnormalities, 3 to 4 per cent; tail abnormalities, 3 to 4 per cent; protoplasmic droplets, 3 to 4 per cent. Abnormalities that should be counted and recorded are shown in Figure 54. It is important to note the presence and location of distal or proximal protoplasmic droplets which may indicate cell immaturity.

Damage to the cells within the testis in general are of more serious consequence and may be an indication to consider testicular biopsy for further evaluation. Damage produced after the sperm have left the testis may indicate epididymal disease or may be the result of cold, trauma or osmotic or urinary contamination. When abnormalities are found, it is always wise to obtain 2 or 3 semen samples within a few days for baseline evaluation and then repeat the studies in 4 to 6 weeks to obtain an idea of a healing or regressing trend.

Semen Production

Normal males can be used as studs according to the following schedule without reducing their sperm reserves:
1. Once every other day indefinitely.
2. Once daily for three days if two days' rest are then allowed.
3. Twice daily for one day if two days' rest are then allowed.

IV-12-C. Inseminating the Bitch

Equipment

1. Adequate semen (80 per cent motile, 80 per cent morphologically normal, at least 200 million sperm) in test tube.
2. Dry, warm, sterile 5 ml. or 10 ml. syringes; rubber adapter tubing, ¾ inch long; a 9 inch, plastic inseminating pipette; alcohol; and cotton.

Procedure

1. Determine the correct time to inseminate by test teasing with a male or by cytologic examination of vaginal smears. Breed the day after the bitch first stands staunchly to accept service and "flags" her tail, or during cytologic indications of estrum, but *before* leukocytes reappear in

the smear. *Breed at least twice at 48-hour intervals.* Repeat at these intervals as long as the bitch shows libido.

2. Clean the vulva thoroughly with alcohol swabs.

3. *Gently* aspirate semen through the inseminating pipette into the warm syringe.

4. Use no lubricants and insert the pipette through the vulva and dorsally into the vagina and forward to the cervix. With gentle manipulation the pipette may be advanced into the uterus and the semen is gently and slowly ejected. A bubble of air should be injected to push all the semen through the pipette. Deposit the semen in the anterior vagina if cervical passage is impossible.

5. The pipette is removed, and the bitch's rear quarters are elevated and held for four minutes. During this time a finger encased in a sterile glove should be inserted into the vagina and the vaginal roof "feathered" to stimulate constrictor activity. *This is important.*

6. The bitch is carefully returned to a quiet kennel.

References

Additional information may be found in the following sources:

Bartlett, D. J.: Studies on dog semen. I. Morphologic characteristics. II. Biochemical characteristics. J. Reprod. Fert. *3*:174–205, 1962.
Lagerlöf, N.: Semen examination as an aid to sexual health control in domestic animal breeding. Int. J. Fert. 9:377–382, 1974.
Settergren, I.: Personal communication, 1974.

IV–13. COLLECTION OF URINE

Urinary catheters are hollow tubes made of rubber, latex, or metal and are designed to serve four purposes:

1. To relieve urinary retention.
2. To test for residual urine.
3. To obtain urine directly from the bladder for diagnostic purposes.
4. To perform bladder lavage and instillations.

Scrupulous asepsis should be used in catheterization because one may produce a urinary tract infection through the use of unsterile equipment or faulty catheterization technique. Passing urinary catheters with a gentle technique is also important as the urethral epithelium is delicate and can be easily damaged. Catheters should be prepackaged and sterilized by ethylene oxide or autoclaving.

IV–13–A. Catheterization of the Male Dog

Equipment needed includes a sterile catheter (size 4 to 6 French and 18 inches long with one end adapted to fit a syringe); sterile lubricating jelly; pHisoHex soap or benzalkonium chloride; sterile rubber gloves or a sterile hemostat; a 20 ml. sterile syringe; an appropriate receptacle for the collection of urine; and Furacin solution in a 5 ml. syringe.

Proper catheterization of the male dog requires two people. The dog is placed in lateral recumbency on either side. The rear leg that is on top is pulled forward and then flexed (Fig. 55).

Next, the sheath of the penis is retracted and the glans penis is cleansed with a solution of pHisoHex soap, Septisol, benzalkonium chloride, or bichloride of mercury solution, diluted 1:1000. The distal 2 to 3 cm. of the appropriate size catheter is lubricated with sterile lubricating jelly. The catheter is never entirely removed from its container while it is being passed, as the container enables one to hold the catheter without contaminating it. The catheter may be passed with sterile gloved hands, or by using a sterile hemostat to grasp the catheter and pass it into the urethra.

If the catheter cannot be passed into the bladder, the tip of the catheter may be caught in a mucosal fold of the urethra or there may be a stricture or block in the urethra. In small breeds of dogs, the size of the groove in the os penis bone may limit the size of the catheter that can be passed. On occasion, a catheter of small diameter may kink and bend upon being passed into the urethra. When the catheter cannot be passed on the first try, the size of the catheter should be reevaluated and the catheter gently rotated while being passed a second time. On no occasion should the catheter be forced through the urethral orifice.

Effective catheterization is indicated by the flow of urine at the end of the catheter and a sterile 20 ml. syringe is used to aspirate the urine from the bladder. Following catheterization, 2 to 5 ml. of Furacin solution is inserted into the bladder and the catheter is removed.

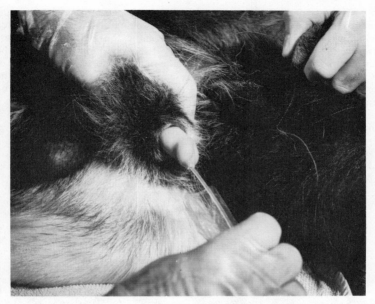

Figure 55. Male canine urethral catheter. The subject is in lateral recumbency with the upper hindleg pulled forward (to the right) and held by an assistant. The penile sheath is retracted, and the glans penis is cleaned. A sterile catheter is protected in its covering until it enters the urethra.

IV–13–B. *Catheterization of the Female Dog*

Equipment needed includes a sterile, metal or plastic female catheter; a Brinkerhoff speculum or small nasal speculum; a 20 ml. sterile syringe; Xylocaine, 0.5 per cent; sterile KY jelly; a focal source of light; appropriate receptacles for urine collection; and 5 ml. of Furacin solution. Strict asepsis should be used. The vulva is cleansed with a solution of pHisoHex, Septisol, benzalkonium chloride, or bichloride of mercury, diluted 1:1000. The instillation of Xylocaine, 0.5 per cent, into the vaginal vault helps to relieve the discomfort of catheterization. In many instances, the female dog may be catheterized in the standing position by passing the female catheter into the vaginal vault despite the fact that the urethral tubercle is not directly visualized.

In the spayed female where "blind catheterization" may be difficult, the use of a Brinkerhoff speculum or nasal speculum with a light source will help to visualize the urethral tubercle on the floor of the vagina (Figs. 56 and 57). In difficult catheterizations it may be helpful to place the animal in dorsal recumbency and pull the hind legs forward. Insertion of a speculum into the vagina almost always permits visualization of the urethral tubercle and facilitates passage of the catheter. One should be careful not to pass the catheter into the fossa of the clitoris as this is a blind passage. Following catheterization, 2 to 5 ml. of Furacin solution is injected into the bladder.

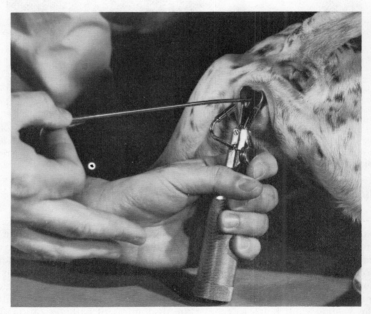

Figure 56. Female canine catheter. Subject is standing or is placed in sternal recumbency. A sterile, lighted, nasal speculum is used to visualize the urethral opening and a catheter is passed.

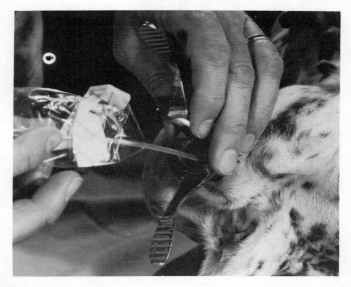

Figure 57. Female canine catheterization. The subject is in dorsal recumbency with the hindlegs pulled forward and held by an assistant. A Brinkerhoff speculum is helpful in visualizing the urethral opening. A sterile plastic catheter is being passed.

IV–13–C. Catheterization of Cats

Catheterization of the male cat without damaging the penis and urethral tissue requires the use of a short-acting anesthetic such as thiamylal sodium. Once anesthetized, the cat is placed on his back, and the hind legs are pulled forward. The penis is drawn from the sheath and gently pulled backward. A sterile, flexible plastic or polyethylene (P. E. 60 to 90) catheter is passed into the urethral orifice and gently passed into the bladder, keeping the catheter parallel to the vertebral column of the cat. The catheter should never be forced through the urethra. The presence of concretions within the urethral lumen may require the injection of 3 to 5 ml. of sterile water, saline, or dilute acetic acid to flush out the concretions so that the catheter can be passed (Fig. 58).

Catheterization of female cats can be accomplished by the use of a plastic, blunt-ended tomcat catheter. The vaginal vault is first anesthe-

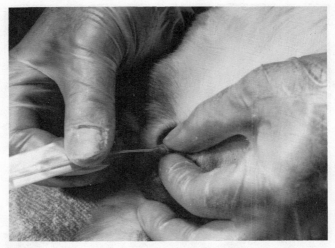

Figure 58. Catheterization of a male cat. With the cat on his back and the hindlegs pulled forward, the penis is withdrawn from its sheath and held. A sterile P.E. 90 catheter is passed into the urethra, keeping the catheter parallel to the vertebral column of the cat.

tized by instilling Xylocaine, 0.5 per cent. The lips of the vulva are cleansed with an appropriate antiseptic and are then grasped and pulled caudally. The tomcat catheter is inserted along the floor of the vagina and the tip is gently guided into the urethral orifice. The procedure is usually accomplished without difficulty.

IV–14. EXAMINATION OF THE CANINE VAGINA

Vaginal examination entails two types of procedures: collection of material from the mucosal wall for culture and exfoliative cytologic examination, and visual inspection of the vaginal mucosa.

These procedures would be useful in establishing a definitive diagnosis of a foreign body, infection, inflammation, tumor or obstruction, or endocrine abnormality.

Equipment

Short-acting anesthetic.
Clippers, surgical soap, and antiseptic solution (Zephiran).
Sterile lubricating jelly.
Sterile Welch Allyn proctoscope.
Sterile offset biopsy punch.
Sterile culture tubes, swabs, and glass slides.
Sterile female catheter.
Sterile rubber gloves.

Technique

The patient is anesthetized with a short-acting anesthetic and the perineal area is clipped, washed, and prepared as for surgery. By use of rubber gloves or sterile forceps, the lips of the vulva are parted and a sterile swab inserted deep into the vagina for culture. A second sterile swab is inserted into the vagina a distance of 1 to 2 inches via the dorsal commissure of the vulva. It is held in contact with the lateral vaginal wall and *rotated firmly* to accumulate fluid and epithelial cells. The swab is removed and *rolled smoothly* onto a chemically clean glass slide to produce a definitive smear. The smear should be fixed immediately by immersing it in 95 per cent alcohol for five minutes. It can be stored in the fixative indefinitely or stained immediately.

Staining Procedure

Wash fixative off, using tap water.
Place in Harris' hematoxylin for one-half minute.
Rinse in tap water for 5 minutes.
Put in Shorr's trichrome for 1 minute.
Put in 70 per cent alcohol for 30 seconds.
Place in 95 per cent alcohol for 30 seconds.
Place in absolute alcohol for 30 seconds.
Place in xylol for 1 minute.
Mount with cover slip, using DPX.
Hematoxylin stains the cell nuclei blue. Shorr's trichrome stains the cell cytoplasm either orange-red, if cornified, or green if noncornified. There is no cell distortion, and both nuclear morphology and the amount of cornification can be readily assessed.

There are two other staining methods, both simpler and more practical. They do not require alcohol fixation and do not produce such detailed results, but may be better for the busy clinician.

1. If vaginal fluids are abundant, they may be aspirated with an eye dropper, mixed with 0.1 per cent toluidine blue and observed as a wet mount.

2. Wright's stain can be applied to vaginal smears in a manner identical to that used for staining blood smears.

Examination

The vagina of the bitch is long and the mucosa forms longitudinal folds. The clitoris is in a well-developed fossa in the floor of the vestibule. We have found that the vagina can be completely visualized with a small sterile proctoscope. The instrument is lubricated and passed to the region of the cervix. When insufflation is performed while the vulva is compressed around the sterile proctoscope, the vagina balloons and its entire wall is envisioned completely as the instrument is withdrawn.

During the endoscopic examination, small tumors or polyps can be removed, or larger masses sampled with the biopsy punch. Ulcers or erosions can be cauterized and foreign bodies removed.

Complete vaginal examination includes careful palpation of the vaginal wall and pelvic cavity. This is accomplished by digital examination using a sterile glove.

IV–14–A. Characteristics of the Vagina During the Estrous Cycle

Anestrus

This is characterized by dryness of the mucosa and a thin vaginal wall with stratified squamous epithelial cells several layers thick but without cornification. There are noncornified epithelial cells and leukocytes in a ratio of 1 to 5 in the vaginal smear. The leukocytes are monocytes and polymorphonuclear leukocytes. The noncornified epithelial cells are 15 to 25 mμ in diameter and have round free edges, granular cytoplasm, and large nuclei with distinct chromatin granules.

Proestrus

The vaginal wall is thicker, and the mucosa shows prominent cornified squamous epithelium (20 to 30 cells thick) with rete pegging. It is impervious to leukocytes, but there is extravasation of red blood cells to the surface epithelium. Vaginal smears show predominantly erythrocytes and noncornified epithelial cells which become cornified as proestrus progresses. Leukocytes are present but decrease as estrus approaches. Debris and bacteria are abundant.

Estrus

The vagina is thick with longitudinal folds. There is abundant fluid, often blood-tinged. There is an absence of noncornified epithelial cells and leukocytes. There is a dominance of cornified epithelial cells and this seems to be related to appearance of flirting by the bitch. Leukocytes reappear at ovulation or within 36 hours afterward. Bacteria and debris are absent during estrus but they return to the smears after ovulation when leukocytes reappear.

Metestrus

Leukocytes rapidly increase in numbers; there is a decrease in cornified and an increase in noncornified epithelial cells. After five to seven days the number of leukocytes decreases to 10 to 30 per field. In nonpregnant bitches, the vaginal fluid becomes gelatinous and loses its

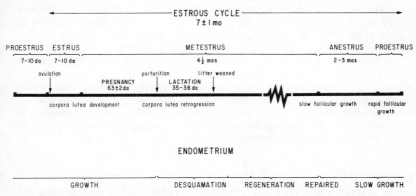

Figure 59.   Status of ovary and uterus during the estrous cycle. Data obtained from 47 beagles, one to five years of age. (From Anderson, A. C., and Simpson, M. E.: The Ovary of the Dog (Beagle). Los Altos, Calif., Geron-X, Inc., 1973.)

cornified cells by 10 to 12 days after ovulation. In pregnant bitches, the vaginal fluid remains thin and milky and a few cornified cells can be found in every smear for 15 to 20 days after ovulation.

Following parturition, much cellular debris, leukocytes, erythrocytes and a few epithelial cells will be present for several days until placental sloughing is complete. After that, the presence of masses of leukocytes (and bacteria) warns of serious metritis.

References

Additional information can be found in the following sources:

Franklund, A. L.: The collection of vaginal smears from the bitch. Vet. Record, July 24, 1971.
Gier, H. T.: Estrous cycle in the bitch; vaginal fluids. Vet. Scope, Vol. 5, No. 2, 1961 (Kalamazoo, Mich., Upjohn Co.).
Sokolowski, J. H., et al.: Canine reproduction: reproductive organs and related structures of the nonparous, parous and postpartum bitch. Amer. J. Vet. Res. *34*:1001–1013, 1973.

IV–15. LARYNGOSCOPY AND BRONCHOSCOPY

These techniques may be of value in the diagnosis of upper airway obstructions such as eversion of the lateral ventricles, collapsed arytenoid cartilages, hyperplasia of the vocal cords, the presence of nodules on the vocal cords, overly long soft palate and traumatic injuries to the neck. Lesions of the trachea and mainstem bronchi, such as collapsed trachea, mediastinal tumors, hilar lymph node enlargement, and parasitic nodules *(Filaroides osleri)* may also be diagnosed. In addition, bronchoscopy is a valuable technique that permits culturing and cytologic examination of material from bronchi involved in chronic respiratory disease. Upper airway obstruction that is not responsive to conservative therapy is an indication for more extensive diagnostic procedures, such as bronchoscopy.

Equipment

Equipment includes preanesthetic agents of choice (promazine, Innovar, Numorphan-Thorazine combination, injectable atropine, lidocaine, 2 per cent, Surital sodium), syringes, a 3 or 4 inch, 12 to 14 gauge blunt cannula, intubating laryngoscope, mouth speculum, tongue forceps, distal illuminated fiber optic bronchoscope,* portable power pack, flexible tip aspirating tube 50 cm. long, specimen collection bottles (Lukens or Morrison type, 2 cc. and 10 cc., sterilized), and a suction source.

Bronchoscopes are available in the following sizes:

3.0 mm. by 25 cm.; suitable for a 5 to 7 pound animal.

3.5 mm. by 30 cm.; suitable for a 7 to 15 pound animal.

5 mm. by 35 cm.; suitable for a 20 to 30 pound animal.

7 mm. by 35 cm.; suitable for a 30 to 50 pound animal.

8 mm. by 45 cm.; suitable for a 30 to 50 pound animal.

10 mm. by 63 cm.; suitable for an animal over 50 pounds.

Additionally, a direct vision telescope and biopsying forceps are necessary.

Preparation of the Animal

The patient should be fasted for 18 to 24 hours prior to performing a bronchoscopic examination. A suitable preanesthetic in combination with atropine should be given one half hour prior to performing bronchoscopy. If the patient is a risk for general anesthesia, local topical anesthesia of the pharynx, vocal cords, and bronchi can be instituted using lidocaine, 2 per cent, administered through a 4 inch blunt cannula, and a neuroleptanalgesic agent is utilized for general sedation. In many instances, bronchoscopy can be performed under a short-acting general anesthetic such as thiamylal sodium administered via intravenous infusion. If bronchoscopy is to be prolonged, the gas delivery tube is attached to the side arm of the bronchoscope and 4 to 6 LPM of oxygen containing 1.0 to 1.5 per cent halothane is administered.

Bronchial secretions collected by aspiration or saline lavage should be divided into two parts. One part is submitted for bacteriologic culture. The second part of the sample is transferred from the collecting tube to a centrifuge tube containing 50 per cent ethyl alcohol. The specimen is centrifuged for 30 minutes at 1500 r.p.m. and the sediment placed onto clear slides, fixed and stained for cytologic examination. Staining can be accomplished by numerous procedures, including Sano stain, Giemsa or Papanicolaou.

---

*American Cytoscope Makers, Inc., Pelham Manor, N.Y.

Reference

Additional information can be found in the following source:

Roszel, J. F., and O'Brien, J. A.: Bronchoscopy and bronchial cytology in lung diseases. Proceedings of the A. A. H. A., 1968.

IV–16. PROCTOSCOPY

Proctoscopy, the technique of examining the descending colon, rectum, and anus, is an exceedingly valuable procedure. It is helpful in the definitive diagnosis of posterior bowel lesions, such as granulomatous colitis, foreign bodies, tumors, lacerations, and other mucosal abnormalities.

Equipment

Short-acting anesthetic (thiamylal sodium).
Lubricating jelly.
A suitable proctoscope such as the Welch Allyn sigmoidoscope with distal illumination. The speculum comes in three sizes: one with a 21 mm. diameter and 25 cm. long, one with a 15 mm. diameter and 25 cm. long, and a pediatric size with a 15 mm. diameter and 14 cm. long. The complete kit usually includes all three sizes of proctoscopes together with an inflation bulb, biopsy forceps, and portable power pack. This type of set can be completely sterilized.

Technique

In order to visualize the colonic mucosa the large bowel must be empty. This can be accomplished by withholding food for 24 hours and performing a colonic irrigation two hours before examination. The material used for the enema must be nonirritating and nonoily. Mildly hypertonic saline solutions such as Fleet enemas work well if given two hours before examination so that gas and fluid can be passed completely.

If the general physical condition of the animal is poor and withholding food is not possible, then feeding a low salt diet for 12 to 18 hours preceding proctoscopy can be helpful. This diet could consist of cooked eggs, small amounts of cooked beef or chicken and small amounts of carbohydrate, such as a slice of toast or one-fourth to one-half cup of moist kibble. Maintain good hydration and eight hours before proctoscopy administer 5 to 10 ounces of magnesium citrate orally as a bulk cathartic.

The patient is given a short-acting anesthetic and placed on a tilted table in lateral recumbency with the hindquarters elevated. A digital examination of the rectum and pelvic cavity is performed to be sure that there are no strictures, polyps or other obstructions. The proctoscope is lubricated thoroughly with water-soluble jelly and passed gently through the anal sphincter. It is pressed forward slowly and carefully with a spiral motion. If any resistance is encountered the motion is stopped, the obturator removed, and the bowel inspected to determine the cause of resistance. If possible, the obturator should be replaced and forward motion continued until the instrument is passed its full length. The obturator is withdrawn and the mucosa is observed.

The major portion of the examination is conducted as the instrument is withdrawn. To view the colonic and rectal walls completely, it is necessary to move the anterior end of the proctoscope around the circumference of a small circle as it is withdrawn. Occasional insufflation with the inflating bulb is helpful in smoothing out folds of tissue. Repeated instrumentation may produce petechiae and minor hemorrhages that are not pathologic.

For examination of the terminal rectum and anus, the Hirshman anoscope provides adequate, convenient visualization.

Newer techniques for visualizing the upper and lower gastrointestinal tract are rapidly being developed and are being used in dogs. The fiber optic flexible gastroscope permits one to visualize and photograph the esophagus and stomach. One is able not only to directly visualize lesions of the upper gastrointestinal tract but also to assess motility disorders.

The development of the flexible fiber sigmoidoscope permits examination and biopsy of regions of the colon that cannot be reached by the rigid sigmoidoscope. The flexible fiber sigmoidoscope allows for injection of air and warm water into the colon. Biopsies can be taken while visualizing a lesion. We have been utilizing the American cystoscope makers' polydirectional panendoscope with excellent results.

IV–17. MEASUREMENT OF CENTRAL VENOUS PRESSURE (DOG)

Measurement of the central venous pressure in the dog is an excellent index for determining circulatory efficiency. The central venous pressure is controlled by interaction of the circulating blood volume, cardiac pumping action and alterations in the vascular bed.

Central venous pressure is not a measure of blood volume but an indication of the ability of the heart to accept and pump blood brought to it. The CVP reflects the interaction of the heart, vascular tone and circulatory blood volume. When the heart action and vascular tone remain constant, CVP reflects blood volume. When blood volume and vascular tone are constant, the CVP reflects heart action. When blood volume and heart action are constant; CVP can be used to measure vascular tone.

Additionally, the placement of a jugular catheter can be very helpful in long term fluid management and in parenteral alimentation of the critically ill patient (see Section IV-20-E).

Indications

1. Acute circulatory failure which has not responded to initial treatment.

2. Administration of large volumes of blood or fluids as may occur in acute shock.

3. As part of the monitoring procedure in poor risk surgical patients.

4. Abnormal urine production where fluids are being administered.

Equipment

One Intracath needle, 17 or 18 gauge.
One metric rule, 80 cm. long.
One three-way stopcock.
One bottle isotonic sodium chloride, 500 ml., and I.V. tubing.
One extra piece of intravenous tubing, 3 feet long.

or

A Becton-Dickinson or Batten disposable CVP set.

Procedure

In order to measure central venous pressure, a catheter must be placed in the external jugular vein so that it is in direct fluid continuity with the right atrium. Adequate measurement of the central venous pressure in the noncomatose animal requires sedation or the use of a short-acting general anesthetic.

Place the animal in lateral recumbency and clip the hair over the jugular vein. Surgically prepare the skin in the clipped area.

Make a percutaneous puncture of the jugular vein with the Intracath catheter and advance the tip to approximately the third intercostal space (tip of cather at right atrium). The catheter should be securely fastened to the neck of the patient by passing adhesive tape around the neck in incorporating the hub of the catheter needle so it comes to lie at the base of the ear. Connect a three-way stopcock to the catheter. Connect an intravenous setup of isotonic sodium chloride to one end of the stopcock and to the other end of the stopcock attach a piece of intravenous tubing which should be taped vertically to a pole or a piece of doweling (Fig. 60). The metric rule is placed so that the 0 level is aligned with the midpoint of the trachea at the thoracic inlet and the rule is taped to the vertical pole.

To fill the central venous pressure manometer, the three-way stopcock is turned so that fluid will flow from the bottle of saline into the manometer and will exceed the 15 cm. mark. Next, the stopcock is turned so that a column of fluid exists from the superior vena cava to the

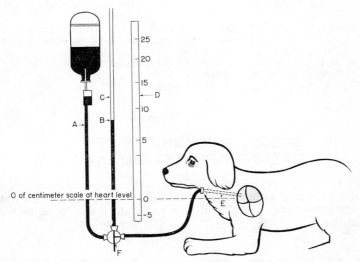

Figure 60. Central venous manometer. A, Standard intravenous infusion tube. B, Central venous pressure level. C, 30-inch intravenous extension tube. D, Centimeter scale. E, Plastic tube in great veins in thorax or right atrium via jugular vein. F, Three-way stopcock set in measuring position (open from manometer to catheter). (From Sattler, F. P.: Shock. In Kirk, R. W. (ed.): Current Veterinary Therapy III. Philadelphia, W. B. Saunders Co., 1968.)

manometer. The fluid in the manometer will fall until it reflects the level of the central venous pressure.

It is desirable to allow fluid to flow frequently through the catheter so that the catheter tip will not become plugged with a blood clot. Periodic flushing with heparinized saline will help maintain the potency of the catheter. This setup allows easy administration of fluids and medication intravenously to the patient and collection of blood if necessary.

There is no absolute value for a normal CVP. It is the trend of the CVP that should be monitored and correlated with the regimen of treatment. One must be constantly aware of the interrelationship between blood volume, cardiovascular function, and vascular tone. A range of 0 to 12 cm. H_2O is considered normal.

References

Additional information can be found in the following sources:

Jennings, P. B., Anderson, R. W., and Martin, A.: Central venous pressure monitoring: a guide to blood replacement in the dog. J. Amer. Vet. Assn. *151*:1280–1283, 15 November 1967.

Sattler, F. P.: Shock. *In* Kirk, R. W. (ed.): Current Veterinary Therapy III. Philadelphia, W. B. Saunders Co., 1968.

Whittick, W. G. : Shock. J.A.A.H.A. *8*:456–474, 1972.

IV–18. SPECIAL TECHNIQUES OF RADIOGRAPHIC EXAMINATION

In general, prolonged procedures such as intravenous urography, barium enemas, pneumocystograms, pneumoperitoneum, and myelography require the use of a short-acting general anesthetic or heavy sedation.

IV–18–A. Gastrointestinal or Small Bowel Studies

Barium swallows and esophagrams require no previous preparation of the patient except for the removal of any collars or chains around the neck. For barium swallows, the barium should be thick and pasty like marshmallow fluff. Position the patient and casette and have the x-ray technique set up. Give a tablespoonful of barium orally. Make the exposure when the patient makes his second swallow after the barium has been given.

To achieve the maximum information from a gastrointestinal study, the following preliminary steps are necessary:

1. Make sure the hair of the patient is free from exogenous dirt, paint, and foreign material. Bathe the animal if necessary.

2. Withhold food for 18 to 24 hours.

3. If the colon is filled with feces, administer a Fleet enema, which leaves no abnormal residual gas patterns in the bowel. This should be done three hours prior to the start of the gastrointestinal series.

IV–18–B. Barium Enemas

1. For the 24 hours preceding radiographs the animal should be maintained on only a liquid diet, preferably water or broth.

2. During the 18 to 24 hours before the radiographs, administer a mild high colonic enema or give a saline laxative by mouth.

3. Do not give any irritating enemas within 12 hours of the scheduled radiographic examination; however, isotonic saline solution or plain water enemas should be administered two or three times prior to the examination to make sure the bowel is clear.

4. Do not perform a proctoscopic examination on the same day as the barium enema is given.

For a barium enema, the barium should have the consistency of "top milk" (one part barium to one part water). Two to 16 ounces of barium mixture will be required, depending on the size of the dog.

The technique of performing a barium enema is as follows:

1. Insert a lubricated Bardex catheter into the rectum and inflate the cuff.

2. Put the amount of barium desired into the colon and clamp off the Bardex catheter.

3. Take lateral and ventrodorsal views.

4. Remove the catheter and allow the animal to evacuate the bowel.

5. Replace the catheter and fill the colon with air. Take lateral and ventrodorsal views.

IV-18-C.   Excretory Urography

Organic iodinated compounds in high concentrations permit visualization of the renal pelvis and ureters as the kidneys excrete the substance. Excretory urography does not reveal any quantitative information about renal function and is not a substitute for renal function tests. The degree of visualization of contrast material within the renal excretory system depends on the type of contrast material used, the injection rate, the state of hydration of the patient, renal blood flow and functional capacity of the kidneys.

Technique

1. Fast the animal for 12 to 18 hours.
2. Twelve to 18 hours prior to radiography, administer a high colonic enema or give saline laxative orally.
3. Make sure the hair is free of dirt and debris.
4. Try to limit the fluid intake for the 12 hours preceding radiography.
5. Empty the patient's bladder immediately before taking radiographs.
6. Take survey radiographs before administering contrast media.

To perform intravenous urography, sodium diatrizoate (Hypaque), 50 per cent, is administered in a dosage of 1 ml./lb. A total of 30 to 50 ml. per study can be used. If a rupture of the bladder is suspected, Hypaque should not be used, as it is irritating and may lead to peritonitis. A compression band over the abdomen, compressing the ureters, helps to retain dye in the kidneys and ureters.

Take lateral and ventrodorsal views of the abdomen following this time sequence:

1. Immediately after injection (arterial phase).
2. Two minutes after injection (venous phase).
3. Five minutes after injection (tubules, kidney pelvis, and ureters can be visualized).
4. Ten minutes after injection (the media is visible in the kidney pelvis, ureters, and bladder).
5. The urinary bladder is best visualized on 25 to 30 minute exposures.

High Dose Urography

This technique can be utilized if conventional excretory urography does not provide conclusive answers, or if the patient is uremic. High levels of the contrast agent act as an osmotic diuretic aiding in the visualization of the renal system.

1. Prepare the animal as described previously and take survey radiographs.

2. Administer 50 per cent Hypaque intravenously at a dosage of 2 to 3 cc./lb. for patients under 40 lbs. or 1.5 to 2 cc./lb. for patients over 40 lbs.

3. Take radiographs at 10, 20 and 30 minutes following injection.

IV–18–D. Pneumocystogram

1. Fast the animal for 18 to 24 hours preceding radiography.

2. Administer a high colonic enema or give saline laxative orally 12 to 18 hours prior to taking radiographs.

3. Make sure the hair is clean.

4. Take survey radiographs of the bladder and then empty the bladder of urine. Avoid the use of metal female catheters, as they may cause traumatic injury to the bladder wall.

5. Using a syringe and three-way valve, inject 50 to 150 ml. of air (depending on the size of the animal) into the bladder. Inject air until you get back pressure on the syringe barrel or leakage of air around the catheter. If air escapes during the procedure it should be replaced.

6. Take lateral and ventrodorsal views of the abdomen.

Angiography (See Section III–4–D)

IV–18–E. Myelography

Myelography is the study of the spinal cord and vertebral canal by injecting contrast media into the subarachnoid space. Ideally, the contrast material that is used should be relatively nontoxic and absorbable, should provide a good contrast and should be able to be evenly distributed throughout the subarachnoid space. Water-soluble contrast media such as methiodal sodium 40 per cent (Skiodan) provide good radiographic detail but are irritating and can be toxic. They are rapidly absorbed from the cerebrospinal fluid. The oily preparations such as Pantopaque can be used also and can give good diagnostic results, although the media may produce a chronic arachnoiditis.

Technique

1. Fast the animal for 18 to 24 hours preceding myelography.

2. Anesthetize the animal with a short-acting agent such as thiamylal sodium and maintain on gas anesthetic of choice.

3. Clip and surgically prepare the skin over the cisterna magna or in the lumbosacral area, depending on where one wishes to enter the spinal canal. For cisterna magna puncture, see Section IV-3. Lumbar puncture can be made between the fifth and sixth or between the fourth and fifth lumbar vertebrae. A short bevel spinal needle should be used.

4. Oily material (Pantopaque) and water-soluble contrast material (Skiodan sodium) are available for myelography. In performing lumbar myelograms, water-soluble Skiodan is used. Forty per cent methiodal sodium (Skiodan) is diluted with equal amounts of sterile water and Lidocaine is added to obtain a 0.1 per cent concentration. A short bevel spinal needle (20 gauge) is placed into the subarachnoid space L5-L6 and spinal fluid is aspirated. The animal should be in sternal recumbency. Then 0.3 to 0.5 ml./kg. of the Skiodan mixture is injected into the subarachnoid space. Radiographs are taken at the time of injection and over a one-minute period following injection.

In performing cervical myelograms utilizing the cisterna magna (see Section IV-3), Pantopaque is utilized. The Pantopaque should be warmed to body temperature in a water bath. The animal is placed in sternal recumbency, the muzzle deviated ventrally and the head elevated, so contrast material when injected will not flow into the lateral ventricles. A short bevel, 20 gauge, spinal needle is used and the needle opening (bevel) should be facing caudally. The needle is placed into the subarachnoid space and 5 to 6 cc. of CSF fluid is removed. The same amount of Pantopaque is then injected under pressure into the subarachnoid space. The head is maintained in an elevated position and the body slowly rotated so that the caudal end is lower than the cranial end. Radiographs are taken at the time of injection and at 10, 20 and 30 minutes following injection. Tilting the animal into an extreme position will predispose to "beading" of the Pantopaque column and poor radiographic definition.

IV–18–F. Sialography

Sialography is the radiographic examination of the salivary glands and ducts. The glands are visualized by injection of a radiopaque dye into the salivary duct. The technique can be utilized to outline (via retrograde perfusion) the parotid, zygomatic, mandibular and sublingual salivary glands. The most common indicator for sialography is the salivary mucocele. The technique is used to help locate the salivary duct tear causing the mucocele and aid in determining which gland should be removed. General anesthesia is necessary to perform sialography.

Equipment

Blunt 22, 25, and 26 gauge hypodermic needles.
Fine rat tooth forceps.
Syringes.
Mouth gag.
Sixty per cent diatrizoate sodium meglumine (Renografin-60).

The parotid duct opens into the mouth on a papilla on the labial or oral mucosa opposite the upper fourth premolar tooth. The oral mucosa just caudal to the papilla should be grasped with a fine rat tooth forceps and retracted costromedially, which will facilitate passage of a blunt 22 gauge needle. Inject 0.5 cc./10 lb. of Renografin 60 and take radiographs immediately.

The major zygomatic salivary duct opens into the mouth approximately 1 cm. caudal and slightly dorsal to the parotid duct papilla. A 25 or 26 gauge blunt needle is inserted into the duct while the mucosa around the duct opening is held with small forceps.

The mandibular ducts open into the mouth on the lateral surface of the lingual caruncles (sublingual folds). The sublingual duct enters the mouth 1 to 2 mm. caudal to the mandibular duct. The sublingual opening is smaller than the mandibular opening. It has been estimated that in one dog out of three, the two ducts (mandibular and sublingual) join before entering the mouth. In large dogs a 22 gauge blunt needle is used to cannulate the mandibular duct and in small dogs a 25 gauge needle is used. A 26 gauge blunt needle is used to cannulate the sublingual duct.

Reference

Additional information can be found in the following source:

Harvey, C. E.: Sialography in the dog. J. Amer. Radiol. Soc. *10*:18–28, 1969.

IV-18-G. Bronchography

1. Animals should be fasted for 24 hours prior to bronchography.

2. Animals should be preanesthetized with promazine, Innovar or a Numorphan-Thorazine combination and atropine. Following this, a short-acting general anesthetic (thiamylal sodium) may be given. If general anesthesia is contraindicated, lidocaine 2 per cent, may be applied topically to the pharynx, vocal cords, and bronchi.

3. Only one half of the chest is examined at a time with a 24 to 48 hour wait before the other side is examined. Aqueous Dionosil can be used, 5 to 10 ml./per side as the contrast medium. Excessive bronchial secretions must be removed by suction through a bronchoscope before the radiographic contrast material is administered (see Section IV-15).

4. Contraindications for bronchography are pneumonia and congestive heart failure.

References

Additional information can be found in the following sources:

Austin, G.: The Spinal Cord, 2nd ed. Springfield, Illinois, Charles C Thomas, 1972.

Carlson, W. D.: Veterinary Radiology, 2nd ed. Philadelphia, Lea and Febiger, 1967.

Felson, B.: Roentgen Techniques in Laboratory Animals. Philadelphia, W. B. Saunders Co., 1968.

Osborne, C. A., Low, G., and Finco, D. R.: Canine and Feline Urology. Philadelphia, W. B. Saunders Co., 1972.

Suter, P. F., et al.: Myelography in the dog: diagnosis of tumors of the spinal cord and vertebrae, Amer. J. Vet. Radiol. *12*:29–44, 1971.

Therapeutic Procedures

IV-19. ADMINISTRATION OF MEDICATIONS

IV-19-A. Oral Administration of Capsules and Tablets

Dogs

Solid medications should be given to dogs quickly and decisively so that the "pilling" is accomplished before the animal realizes what has happened. With fairly large, placid dogs the tablet is held between the tips of the second and third fingers of the right hand. The thumb of the left hand is slipped through the interdental space and presses up on the hard palate. The thumb of the right hand presses down on the space behind the mandibular incisors (Fig. 61). The pill is pushed deep into the pharynx, the hands withdrawn quickly, and the mouth is closed. Often a brusque tap under the chin startles the dog and facilitates his swallowing. When he licks his nose, you can be confident that he has swallowed.

Dogs who offer more resistance can be induced to open their mouths by compressing the upper lips against the teeth. As they open their mouths, the lips are rolled medially so that if they attempt to close, they will pinch their own lips.

Dogs that struggle and slash with their teeth are most difficult, especially if they are aggressive toward the medicator. They can often be medicated by placing the tablet over the base of the tongue with a 6 inch, curved Kelly hemostat or special pill forceps.

Cubes of canned food or dried meat can often be "pushed down" a placid but anorexic patient by using the thumb as a lever. The fingers are kept out of the mouth but the thumb is inserted behind the last molar of the open mouth and pushes the bolus down.

Cats

Two methods of pilling are useful. In both methods the cat's head is elevated and tipped back. The left hand holds the head from behind with the index finger at one commissure and the thumb at the other. The index

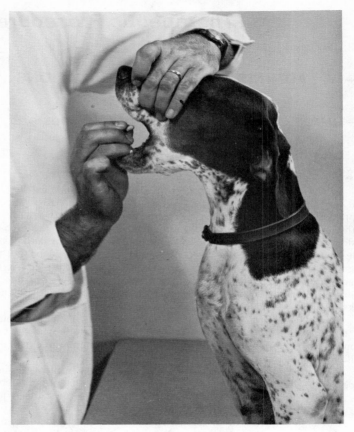

Figure 61. Administering a capsule to a dog.

finger of the right hand is used to open the mouth by pressing down on the incisor teeth. The mouth is held open by compressing inward with the fingers at the angle of the jaw. A tablet can be placed deep in the pharynx with the curved Kelly hemostat, the mouth closed quickly, and the cat tapped under the jaw to facilitate swallowing (Fig. 62). Licking of the nose signals success. The alternate method is similar except that the tablet is

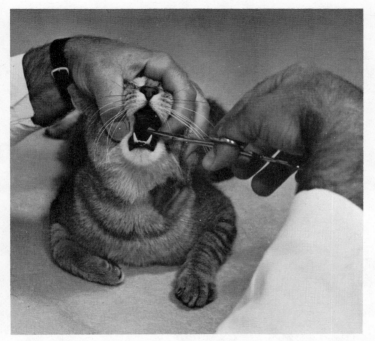

Figure 62. Administering medication to subject in pill form. A Kelly hemostat is used to place the pill deep in the mouth on the base of the tongue.

dropped deep into the mouth and the eraser-end of a pencil is used to tap the pill (or even the posterior pharynx) and stimulate the swallowing reflex.

IV–19–B. Oral Administration of Liquids

Without the Stomach Tube

Small amounts of liquid medicine can be given successfully to dogs and cats by pulling the commissure of the lip out to form a pocket (Fig. 63). The patient's head should be held level so that the medication will not ooze into the larynx. Spoons are ineffective. They measure fluids inac-

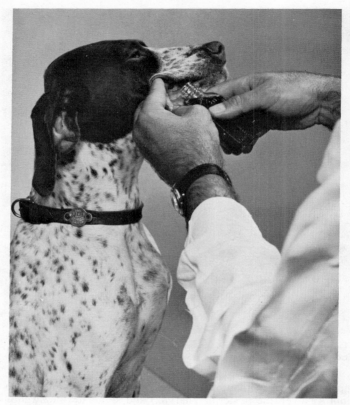

Figure 63. Administering liquid medication to a dog. The flap of the lip should be used as a funnel to direct liquids into the mouth.

curately and materials spill easily. A small prescription bottle or an old hypodermic syringe with a metal tip makes a convenient, easy to use measuring device. Often the medicine is deposited in the "cheek pouch," and it can be encouraged to flow between the teeth by using a hemostat or the metal syringe tip to push gently between the teeth. Patience and gentleness are needed for success.

With the Stomach Tube

Stomach tubes can be passed through the nostrils (nasogastric) but the small lumen limits the types of solutions that can be administered. Oragastric tubes are simpler and more practical. Little restraint is needed to pass a stomach tube in a placid or depressed dog or cat.

Gavage in puppies and kittens can be effected by passing a soft rubber urethral catheter as an orogastric tube. Size 12F is an adequate diameter to pass freely, but it is too large to enter the larynx of infant animals up to 14 days of age. The tube is marked with tape or a ballpoint pen at a point equal to the distance from the tip of the nose to the eighth rib. It is merely pushed into the pharynx and down the esophagus to the midthoracic level. A syringe can be attached to the flared end and medication injected slowly.

Larger pups and adult dogs tolerate intubation with little fuss, although they may have to be placed on a table and restrained. In some patients the finger can be used to hold the jaws slightly apart. In most, a wooden spacer-block or a partially used roll of adhesive tape should be inserted behind the canine teeth to keep the mouth open. The tube is passed through a central hole in the tape or block (Fig. 64). A 22F urinary catheter 30 inches long is an ideal tube. It is attached to a funnel, bulb, or syringe that delivers the medication. In most cases the tip of the tube should be wet, or lubricated with catheter jelly, and then gently pushed into the pharynx.

When the dog swallows, the catheter is advanced down the esophagus to the level of the eighth or ninth rib. It is advisable to measure this distance on the tube first and mark it with a ballpoint pen or with a piece of tape. It is almost impossible to pass the tube into the trachea in a conscious dog with his head held in a normal position. Always palpate the neck, however, to be certain, that the tube can be located in the esophagus!

Cats usually offer more resistance to oral intubation. They can be restrained in a bag or cat stocks, but taping the legs together seems to be more practical. With taping, the cat can be held in a vertical position by an assistant. The operator then grasps the cat's head, as for pilling, and quickly passes the prelubricated tube 6 to 10 inches down the esophagus. A 12 to 16F soft rubber catheter 16 inches long makes a suitable tube, and plastic adapter on the end for attaching a syringe makes medication easy.

For very refractory cats a block of soft wood should be used for a speculum. A vertical hole is drilled in each end of the block (wooden dowel) so that the upper and lower canine teeth can pass through. A horizontal hole in the center allows the tube to pass through. The cat is made to bite down on the block and the jaws held closed while intubation proceeds (Fig. 65).

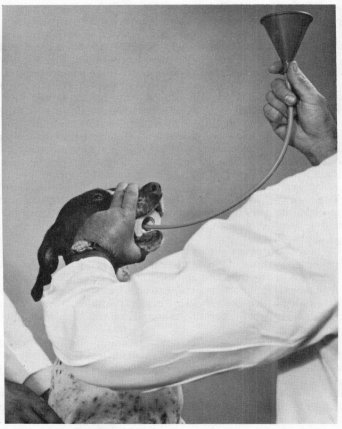

Figure 64. Administering liquid medication to a dog via a stomach tube. Note the roll of adhesive tape used as a gag.

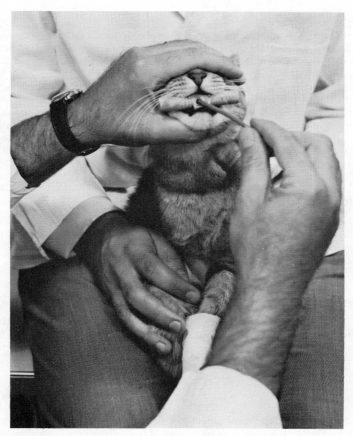

Figure 65. Administering liquid medication to a cat via a stomach tube. Note the wooden gag with a hole in the center for passage of the tube. There are vertical holes at the ends to accommodate the canine teeth.

IV–19–C. Topical Medications

Ocular

There are numerous ways of applying medication to the eyes, including drops, ointments, subconjunctival injections and subpalpebral lavage. The route and frequency of medication depends on the disease being treated.

If more than 2 drops of aqueous material is administered, the fluid will wash out of the conjunctival sac and be wasted. Most drops should be applied every two hours (or less) to maintain effect. Ointments should be applied sparingly, and their effect may last a maximum of four to six hours.

Drops should be placed on the inner canthus without touching the eye with the dropper. Ointment (⅛ inch long strip) should be placed on the lower palpebral border.

Otic

Powders and aqueous solutions are generally contraindicated in the external ear canal. Thin films of ointments or propylene glycol solutions may be effective vehicles. A few drops generally suffice, and the ear should be massaged gently after instillation.

Nasal

Isotonic aqueous drops are utilized and should be applied without touching the dropper to the nose. Oily drops are not advised because they may damage the nasal mucosa or may be inhaled and produce a lipid pneumonia.

Dermatologic

There can be several objectives that have to be met when treating dermatologic disorders: (1) eradication of causative agents; (2) alleviation of symptoms, such as reduction of inflammation; (3) cleansing and debridement; (4) protection; (5) restoration of hydration; and (6) reduction of scaling and callus. Many different forms of skin medications are available, but the vehicle in which they are applied is extremely critical.

Vehicles

1. Lotions are suspensions of powder in water or alcohol. They are used for acute, eczematous lesions. Because they are less easily absorbed than creams and ointments they need to be applied two to six times a day.

2. Pastes are mixtures of 20 to 50 per cent powder in ointment. In general, they are thick, heavy and difficult to use.

3. Creams are oil droplets dispersed in a continuous phase of water. Creams permit excellent percutaneous absorption of ingredients.

4. Ointments are water droplets dispersed in a continuous phase of oil. They are very good for dry, scaly eruptions.

5. Propyleneglycol is a stable vehicle and spreads well. It allows good percutaneous absorption of added agents.

6. Adherent dressings are bases that dry quickly and stick to the lesion.

IV–19–D. Making Injections

Preparing the Skin

Before medications are aspirated from multiple dose vials, the rubber diaphragm stopper should be carefully wiped with the same antiseptic used on the skin. This basic rule should be observed with all medication vials, even with modified live virus vaccines.

It would be admirable to prepare the skin surgically before making all needle punctures to administer medications. Since this is not practical, we should carefully part the hair and apply a good skin antiseptic such as Zephiran in 70 per cent alcohol. The needle should be placed directly on the prepared area and thrust through the skin.

Subcutaneous Injections

The dog and cat have loose alveolar tissue and can easily accommodate large volumes of material in this subcutaneous space. Infection may be introduced inadvertently or vessels may rupture, causing hematomas. Because these accidents are more difficult to handle there, and because the skin of the dorsal neck is very thick, this region should be avoided for injections. The dorsal back from the shoulders to the rump makes an ideal site for subcutaneous injection. A fold of skin in this region is picked up, prepared with antiseptic, and pinched. It is pinched a second time and the injection made simultaneously. Gentle massage of the area after the injection is completed facilitates spreading and absorption of the medication. Only isotonic, buffered, or nonirritating materials should be given subcutaneously (Fig. 66).

Intramuscular Injections

Because the tightly packed muscular tissue cannot accommodate large volumes of injectibles without trauma, medications given by this route should be small in volume. They are often depot materials that are poorly soluble and some may be mildly irritating. Intramuscular injections should never be given in the neck because of the fibrous sheaths there and the complications that may occur. We also feel that injections in the hamstring muscles may cause severe pain, lameness, and occasionally

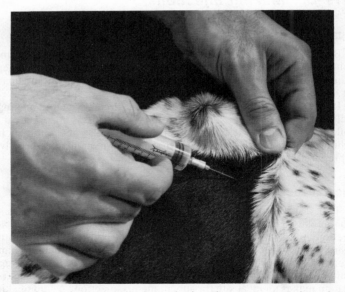

Figure 66. Subcutaneous injection in the dog. The injection site is cleaned with an alcohol swab. The fold of skin is picked up and the needle inserted under the skin.

peroneal paralysis due to local nerve involvement. Unless the animal is extremely thin, we advise giving injections into the lumbodorsal muscles on either side of the dorsal processes of the vertebral column.

After proper preparation of the skin the needle is inserted through the skin at a slight angle (if the animal is thin), or at a perpendicular angle (if it is obese). When any medication is injected by a route other than the intravenous one, it is *imperative* to retract the plunger of the syringe before injecting to be certain that a vein was not entered by mistake. This is especially crucial in oil suspension, microcrystalline suspension or potent dose medications (Fig. 67).

Intravenous Injections (See Sections IV–1 and IV–20–E)

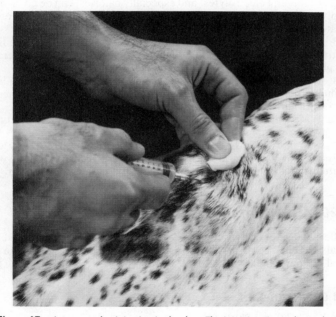

Figure 67.   Intramuscular injection in the dog. The injection site is cleaned with an alcohol swab. This injection is being made into the lumbosacral muscles.

IV-20. SIMPLIFIED FLUID THERAPY

Proper administration of fluids can be a difficult and challenging experience for the veterinarian. Proper management of fluid therapy depends upon understanding the abnormal physiology present as well as the advantages and disadvantages of the various forms of fluid therapy. Assessment of each animal's needs—his lacks and excesses—and of his renal and cardiovascular function must be made.

This section covers the basic principles of fluid therapy.

General Principles

1. Although administration of salt, dextrose, and water may ameliorate temporary emergencies, the addition of other electrolytes in balanced or especially tailored formulas is better definitive therapy.

2. Fluids and electrolytes, and especially calories, can be given more cheaply and effectively by mouth than by injection (unless contraindicated).

3. If renal function is adequate the body will adjust its needs by selectively retaining or excreting water and electrolytes. However, we must give enough. If dosage volume is a question, give more.

4. If renal function is inadequate the patient is in a critical condition and should be referred to a center with adequate laboratory and therapy facilities for intensive treatment.

5. Water and some electrolytes are in a state of constant flux between the body fluid compartments.

6. Use fluids in proper relation to the total medical problem.

7. Do not use laboratory tests routinely. Select a few that, when repeated frequently, will indicate *trends* in the patient's condition.

IV-20-A. Normal Values in Fluid Therapy

Percentage of body weight as water in the total body for the average animal is 60 per cent; for the fat animal, 50 per cent; and for the thin animal, 70 per cent.

Fluid Compartments

Total water, 60 per cent:
Intracellular water, 40 per cent.
Extracellular water, 20 per cent.

Interstitial water, 15 per cent.
Intravascular water, 5 per cent.

Rules Pertaining to Blood

1. Canine total blood volume is approximately 40 ml./lb.
2. Most dogs can donate 10 ml. blood/lb. every three weeks.
3. Total blood volume is 7 per cent of body weight.
4. Plasma volume is 4 per cent of body weight (dogs, 23 ml./lb.; cats, 21 ml./lb.).
5. Erythrocyte volume is 3 per cent of body weight.

Normal Blood Plasma Electrolytes

Cations and anions always balance, and the total approximates 155 mEq./liter (Tables 42 & 43).

TABLE 42.   NORMAL WATER TURNOVER DATA

	Dog (ml./lb.)	Cat (ml./lb.)
Total water turnover/24 hours	30	42
Input		
Oral (food and drink)	23	36
Metabolic (released from carbohydrates and fat)	7	6
Output		
Urine	10	20
Other (sweat, feces, insensible, incorporated into new protoplasm)	20	22

TABLE 43.   BLOOD PLASMA ELECTROLYTES*

Cations (mEq./liter)		Anions (mEq./liter)	
Na	143.0	HCO_3	20.5
K	4.4	Cl	106.0
Ca	5.3	HPO_4	1.6
Mg	1.8	SO_4	2.0
		Protein	14.5
		Organic acids	10.0

*Approximately 155 mEq./liter.

Major extracellular ions are Na, Cl, and HCO_3. Major intracellular ions are K, PO_4, and proteins.

IV–20–B. Types of Fluid and Electrolyte Imbalance

Water and electrolytes are lost in various proportions. There are four major types of imbalance; the fiirst two are more commonly encountered than the other two.

Water Loss

In water loss or desiccation, more water than sodium is lost. It is caused by decreased water intake or increased loss by transpiration in fevers or heatstroke. There is thirst. Urine contains large amounts of sodium and chloride ions and has a high specific gravity. There is no severe increase in shock tendency.

Sodium Loss

In sodium loss, more sodium than water is lost. It is caused by osmotic loss through vomiting, diarrhea, wound drainage, polyuria, sequestration of fluid in tissues, and diabetes. There is little thirst. Urine specific gravity is normal but has a low sodium and chloride content. Vascular volume is low and there is *great danger of shock*.

Water excess

Water excess is usually caused by treatment error, such as giving plain water for sodium loss problems. It is a rare problem.

Sodium excess

Sodium excess is associated with various states of edema. Usually it is a chronic problem refractory to treatment. It is not usually considered a problem of fluid therapy.

IV–20–C. Planning Fluid Therapy

General Considerations

1. Keep patient in water and electrolyte balance and modify treatment as the clinical course varies.

2. Recognition of trends and patterns of shifts is more important than observation of one abnormal laboratory test.

TABLE 44. NORMAL VALUES FOR LABORATORY TESTS COMMONLY USED TO EVALUATE DEHYDRATED DOGS

Test	Normal Value
Packed cell volume or hemoglobin*	37 to 55 per cent
	12 to 18 gm./100 ml.
Plasma protein*	5.3 to 7.5 gm./100 ml.
Blood urea nitrogen	10 to 20 mg./100 ml.
Plasma or serum osmolality	280 to 305 mOsm./L.
Plasma or serum sodium	140 to 155 mEq./L.
Plasma or serum potassium	3.7 to 5.8 mEq./L.
Plasma or serum chloride	100 to 155 mEq./L.
Plasma HCO_3	16 to 24 mEq./L.
Blood pH	7.30 to 7.45
Blood pCO_2	29-42 mm. Hg

*Most important in objectively evaluating fluid problems. The PCV and plasma protein values are usually considered together so that anemia (if present) will be evident as fluids are replaced.

3. With rare exceptions potassium is of much less importance in fluid problems of dogs than of man.

4. Caloric balance is difficult to obtain by any route other than oral, and is of small importance during short, acute illness since it can be corrected during convalescence.

5. Determine whether a fluid imbalance exists by history of losses, body weight loss, plasma protein, and packed cell volume.

Specific Considerations

1. Determine the volume deficit (4-6-8 rule).
   a. The loss of 4 per cent of the body weight in fluid is indicated only by a history of fluid loss. Thus, a 25 lb. dog with 4 per cent loss would have a volume deficit of 0.04 times 25, or 1 lb., or 500 ml.
   b. The loss of 5 per cent of body weight is the level at which clinical signs of dehydration are first observed. The skin lacks pliability; the mouth is dry.
   c. The loss of 6 per cent represents moderate and obvious fluid deficits. It is indicated by "tacky" skin, dry red mucosa, concentrated urine of decreased volume, etc.

TABLE 45. COMPOSITION OF SOLUTIONS*

	Glucose (gm./L.)	NaCl	Na Lactate	KCl	CaCl₂	MgCl₂	NH₄Cl
				(mEq./L.)			
5% D/W	50						
10% D/W	100						
20% D/W	200						
5% D/S	50	145					
2.5% dextrose in half-isotonic saline	25	73					
0.85% saline (isotonic saline; N/S)		145					
0.9% saline		154					
3% saline		513					
5% saline		856					
1/6 molar sodium lactate (1.9%)			167				
1/6 molar ammonium chloride (0.9%)							167
2% ammonium chloride							374
Ringer's solution		147		4	5		
Hypotonic Ringer's solution (modified)		103		5	5	3	
Lactate-Ringer's solution		103	27	4	4		

*From Rosenfeld, M. (ed.): Manual of Medical Therapeutics, 20th ed. Boston, Little, Brown and Co., 1971.

    d. The loss of 8 per cent represents severe fluid losses. The pulse may be weak, there is oliguria, and the animal is depressed.

    e. Loss of 10 to 12 per cent or even higher is extremely serious and may be life threatening. The general signs are those of shock.

  2. Determine the osmolar deficit.

The object is to determine whether the patient has lost more water than electrolytes (type one dehydration) or more electrolytes than water (type two). The clinical signs and history will give helpful clues, but determining the plasma sodium level can be useful. If the sodium is *less* than approximately 143 mEq./L., the plasma is hypotonic and the fluid losses were hypertonic (contained much electrolyte in proportion to water). If the sodium is more than approximately 143 mEq./L., the plasma is hypertonic and losses have been hypotonic. Replacement is made accordingly.

If the patient is not acidotic, the sodium level can be estimated by

TABLE 46. COMPOSITION OF ADDITIVES TO SOLUTIONS*

	Volume (ml.) in Ampule	mEq. in Ampule (Not Concentration)
7.5% sodium bicarbonate	50	45
28.0% sodium lactate	40	100
7.5% potassium chloride	20	20
14.9% potassium chloride	20	40
10.0% calcium chloride	10	14
10.0% calcium gluconate	10	4
25.0% magnesium sulfate	2	4
26.8% ammonium chloride	20	100
		Gm in Ampule
25.0% mannitol	50	12.5
50.0% glucose	50	25

*From Rosenfeld, M. (ed.): Manual of Medical Therapeutics. 20th ed. Boston, Little, Brown and Co., 1971.

adding the factor of 17 to HCO_3 and chloride levels. For example, 17 plus 20 plus 106 equals 143 (normal).

3. Determine special ion involvement.

Potassium and calcium are the clinically significant ions in this category. Very small changes may produce profound effects. Their levels are usually estimated by EKG changes or by serum levels obtained by laboratory tests. Calcium deficits cause tetany. Potassium levels are of extreme concern, especially in addisonian crisis, acidosis problems (diabetes, uremia) and when digitalis or diuretic therapy has been prolonged. However, potassium changes in dogs do not follow the data reported for man.

4. Determine the acid-base status.

The preservation of normal hydrogen ion concentration is of vital importance to normal enzyme activity, cardiac and skeletal muscle contraction and nerve conduction. Conclusions regarding clinical acid-base status are not precise, but probably are best drawn from measurements of extracellular fluids, especially arterial blood. History, clinical signs and even measurement of urine pH may be helpful.

The four states of altered acid-base physiology are metabolic acidosis, respiratory acidosis, metabolic alkalosis and respiratory alkalosis. Each of these changes induces a compensatory response in the body to minimize the changes in pH.

Metabolic acidosis is by far the most common in veterinary medicine.

TABLE 47. CONVERSION OF MILLIGRAMS PER CENT TO MILLIEQUIVALENTS*

		To Convert mg.% to Milliequivalents per Liter Multiply by:	or Divide by:	To Convert Milliequivalents per Liter to mg.% Multiply by:	or Divide by:
Sodium	Na⁺	0.435	2.30	2.30	0.435
Potassium	K⁺	0.256	3.91	3.91	0.256
Magnesium	Mg⁺⁺	0.820	1.22	1.22	0.820
Calcium	Ca⁺⁺	0.500	2.00	2.00	0.500
Chloride	Cl⁻	0.282	3.55	3.55	0.282
Bicarbonate	HCO₃⁻	0.164	6.10	6.10	0.164

*From Fluid and Electrolytes, Abbott Laboratories, North Chicago, Ill., p. 71.

It is seen in acute and chronic renal failure, diabetic ketoacidosis, acidosis of shock, ingestion of toxic acids and severe diarrheas.

Metabolic alkalosis is extremely rare in small animals but is to be expected in severe and persistent vomiting. It has rarely been documented.

Respiratory acidosis should be expected with acute or chronic lung disorders in which there is inadequate blood-gas exchange. Respiratory depression is frequently caused by anesthesia or depressant drugs. Neuromuscular disorders interfering with respiration might also be causative.

TABLE 48. FORMULAS, ATOMIC AND EQUIVALENT WEIGHTS*

Substance	Formula	Atomic or Formula Weight	Equivalent Weight
Sodium	Na⁺	23	23
Potassium	K⁺	39	39
Magnesium	Mg⁺⁺	24.3	12.2
Calcium	Ca⁺⁺	40	20
Chloride	Cl⁻	35.5	35.5
Sodium Chloride	NaCl	58.5	58.5
Phosphate	HPO₄⁻⁻	96	48
Sulfate	SO₄⁻⁻	96	48

*From Fluid and Electrolytes, Abbott Laboratories, North Chicago, Ill., p. 71.

TABLE 49. TESTS TO ASSESS SEVERITY OF DEHYDRATION

Test	Result	Interpretation
URINE		
Volume	Lower than normal.	Intake low or extrarenal loss of water is increased.
Chloride	Present.	Water depletion with little salt depletion.
	Absent or very low.	Salt depletion.
Albumin	Present with oliguria.	Dehydration.
	Present after fluid replacement.	Renal disease.
BLOOD		
Hemoglobin content and hematocrit	Raised.	Dehydration; degree helps assessment of case.
Plasma protein	Low after treatment.	1. Sodium retention and over-expansion of extracellular fluid phase.
		2. True anemia as complicating feature.
Blood urea nitrogen	Raised slightly.	Dehydration.
	High and persistent.	Renal disease.
Total carbon dioxide; chloride	Low CO_2 with normal or raised chloride.	Acidosis.
	High CO_2 with normal or low chloride.	Alkalosis.
	Low chloride level.	Suggests chloride or sodium chloride depletion.
Plasma sodium	Low.	Sodium deficit.
	High.	1. Loss of water in excess of base.
		2. After relief of dehydration: suggests excessive sodium administration.
Plasma potassium	Low.	Potassium deficit: may be due to giving sodium without potassium in replacement.
	High.	Severe dehydration despite absolute potassium deficit.
		May follow too rapid administration of potassium by infusion.
Plasma calcium	Low.	Hypocalcemia may occur after relief of acidosis, especially if animal is undernourished.

Respiratory alkalosis is common in man when he hyperventilates. In the dog, the panting mechanism reduces the tidal volume, even in heat stroke, so this state is rare.

History or diagnosis of a disease with acid-base abnormal tendencies should be considered. Metabolic acidosis is characterized by deep, sighing (Kussmaul) respirations. Initially the depth of respiration is increased and then the rate. Hyperventilation is usually greater with moderate acidosis. The patient is listless, anorexic and vomiting. As the pH falls, lethargy deepens to stupor, cardiac output falls and there is peripheral vasodilation. In man, alkalosis is associated with paresthesia, tetany, and epilepsy.

The body attempts to compensate for acid-base abnormalities by protein buffers and by carbon dioxide–bicarbonate buffer system. The latter can be modulated by the lungs and kidneys, and it can be measured easily by laboratory tests. The normal ratio of HCO_3: H_2CO_3 is 20:1, but variation of either part of the fraction can change the pH.

Implementing the Plan

1. Supply fluids to replace deficits from previous losses and to improve renal function. (Hydrate the patient!)

Use the 4-6-8 per cent rule times body weight to give volume needed.

Use the history and sodium data to estimate osmolar needs. For hypotonic needs, use water orally, or water and dextrose 5 per cent, or dextrose 2.5 per cent in half-strength lactated Ringer's solution, as these provide "free water." For isotonic needs, use lactated Ringer's solution, or 0.9 per cent saline in $\frac{1}{6}$ M sodium lactate at a ratio of 3:1. For hypertonic needs, use dextrose 5 or 10 per cent in saline, or in lactated Ringer's solution, or use 3 per cent sodium chloride solution, which is very hypertonic. Hypertonic solutions should be administered slowly to prevent circulatory overload.

TABLE 50. ACID-BASE PARAMETERS IN ACUTE UNCOMPENSATED DISTURBANCES

Disturbance	pH	pCO_2	CO_2 Combining Power	HCO_3^-	$\dfrac{HCO_3}{H_2CO_3}$
Metabolic acidosis	↓	—	↓	↓	<20
Respiratory acidosis	↓	↑	—	—	<20
Metabolic alkalosis	↑	—	↑	↑	>20
Respiratory	↑	↓	↓	↓	>20

2. Supply fluids to meet daily normal maintenance needs (for urine, feces, insensible losses). The volume should be 25 ml./lb./day, supplied as water orally, or as dextrose or invert sugar in water for injection.

Other daily requirements to meet include: sodium, 0.5 mEq./lb.; potassium, 1 mEq./lb.; protein, 2 to 4 gm./lb.; and calories, 20 to 50/lb. Protein will be used for energy unless adequate calories are provided from other sources. Replacing calories by injection is difficult. Probably it is best accomplished orally by gavage unless the need is likely to be short-term. Fat emulsions by injection are impractical for dogs and dangerous for cats. Invert sugar and fructose are retained better than dextrose, which is readily lost in the urine. Administration of 20 per cent or higher concentrations of dextrose intravenously result in a net water loss unless the rate is *very* slow.

3. Supply fluids to meet the special losses that occur during the course of treatment (vomiting, diarrhea, wound drainage). Replace these losses by selecting fluids that match the volume and composition of those lost (Table 51). Replace blood loss with fresh blood and wound drainage with plasma or lactated Ringer's solution. Give plain water for insensible losses of fevers.

In diarrhea, large amounts of Na^+, K^+, Mg^{++} and Ca^{++} and water are needed. A vomiting dog requires replacement of large amounts of Cl^-, Na^+, and K^+ and water. In vomiting, potassium is lost in gastric fluid and in the urine (Finco).

4. Supply fluids to assist in the therapy of acid-base disorders. Since most acid-base disturbances are secondary to pathologic processes, the initial therapy should be aimed at proper diagnosis and management of the primary disease. It is best not to use alkali unless the acidosis is severe and the primary disease is unresponsive. Sodium bicarbonate is the drug of choice. Sudden increases in bicarbonate can drive large amounts of potassium into the cells and can cause serious cardiac arrhythmias—especially in patients on digoxin.

Many of the standard injectable solutions (0.9 per cent NaCl, lactated Ringer's solution, Ringer's solution) have a pH below 7.0 and an addition of 5 to 10 mEq./L. of bicarbonate makes an excellent buffer that can be used routinely. When moderate to severe acidosis is present, larger amounts are indicated, and Table 52 gives useful guidelines. In all cases and regardless of the route employed, bicarbonate deficit should be corrected over a period of 24 hours. The following formula is useful in treatment of acidosis: Total HCO_3^- deficit (in mEq./L.) = body weight (in kg.) times 0.6 times $\left[20 \text{ (normal } HCO_3^-)\right]$ minus patient's HCO_3^- (in mEq./L.).

TABLE 51. COMPOSITION OF GASTROINTESTINAL SECRETIONS IN THE DOG*

	Volume ml./hr.	pH	H^+ free	Na^+ (mEq./L.)	K^+ (mEq./L.)	Cl^- (mEq./L.)	HCO_3 (mEq./L.)
Gastric	–	–	150	46 to 79	10 to 22	98 to 143	–
Jejunum	5 to 88	6.3 to 7.28	–	126 to 152	4 to 10	141 to 153	5 to 30
Ileum	11 to 42	7.61 to	–	146 to 156	5 to	68 to 88	70 to 97
Colon	1 to 10	7.94 to 8.03	–	136 to 153	6 to 9	60 to 88	86 to 93

*From Troutt, H. F.: Fluid and electrolyte therapy in diarrhea. J.A.A.H.A., Vol. 8, May, 1972, pp. 214–223.

TABLE 52. ESTIMATION OF BICARBONATE DEFICIT IN PATIENTS WITH METABOLIC ACIDOSIS*

Severity of Signs	Estimated HCO_3^- Deficit (mEq./L.)	HCO_3^- Needed to Correct (mEq./kg.)
Mild	5	3
Moderate	10	6
Severe	15	9

*Four grains sodium bicarbonate = 0.25 gm = 3.0 mEq HCO_3^-. From Finco, D. R.: General guidelines for fluid therapy. J.A.A.H.A. Vol. 8, May, 1972, pp. 166–177.

IV–20–D. Routes and Rates of Administration

Intravenous

Any solution for injection can be given by this route, but it is the only route for hypotonic or hypertonic solutions.

The rate depends on the patient but usual routines call for 4 to 5 ml./minute. Rates up to 30 to 40 ml./minute may be indicated in some patients for short periods of time.

Use special care in determining rate and volume administered to old patients with cardiopulmonary disease.

Subcutaneous and Intraperitoneal

These are "pool" routes by use of which a depot of fluid is accumulated for absorption later. Fluids used should approach isotonicity and should contain at least half (80 mEq./liter) the normal sodium level of plasma.

Large volumes can be given rapidly (100 to 200 ml. subcutaneously over a local area; 100 to several thousand milliliters intraperitoneally.)

Intramuscular

The intramuscular route is useful for administering small volumes, e.g., medications.

Frequency

Continuous infusion intravenously is necessary initially, or if peripheral circulation is poor. It may be given intermittently too.

Intermittent infusions into a "pool" should be repeated as the "pool" is absorbed. Usually every 12 hours is adequate.

IV–20–E.   Technique of Administration

Assembling Equipment

1. Use unopened, sterile equipment, pyrogen-free.
2. Provide air vent and attach recipient set with bubble trap and drip chamber.
3. Set up bottle and fill tubing to needle adapter. Be sure bubble trap is half full of fluid.

Venipuncture for Intravenous Route

1. Fill a 5 ml. syringe with saline and attach a 1 inch, 20 gauge needle, clean skin, and enter selected vein.
2. Insert needle into vein and advance to the hub. Inject solution and make sure it flows freely. Detach syringe.
3. Attach infusion tubing and allow free flow for one minute.
4. Adjust rate of flow with attached clamp.
5. Tape needle hub, tubing adapter, and looped tubing to patient's leg securely.

Use of Intravenous Catheters in Animals

The percutaneous placement of catheters into large veins such as the jugular has made the administration of fluids to animals a more feasible procedure. Additionally, the use of catheters in the jugular vein allows easy recording of central venous pressure.

Types of Intravenous Catheters Available

There are three basic types of catheters: (1) those that introduce the catheter through a needle (Fig. 68); (2) those that introduce the catheter over a needle; and (3) a combination of types (1) and (2).

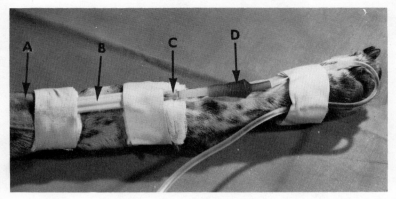

Figure 68. A Bardic* intravenous catheter has been placed in the cephalic vein of a dog. A, cephalic vein; B, needle guard; C, end of catheter; D, intravenous infusion apparatus.

We usually prefer to use a catheter that is inserted through the needle. Careful preparation of the skin site is done to avoid contamination, and if possible a percutaneous placement is made. A cut down procedure is used only when a vein of adequate size cannot be located. Catheter contamination is reduced by using a closed system. Care should be taken to avoid excess traumatic injury to vessel walls, as this predisposes to phlebitis and thromboembolism. A soft, pliable catheter reduces these risks.

Equipment

Bardic inside needle catheter* with stylet (available in various sizes. Both 18 gauge and 14 gauge are used commonly; larger sizes are best).

Technique

The catheter can be placed into the jugular, cephalic or recurrent tarsal vein (Fig. 69). Prepare the skin site by clipping the hair and clean

---

*Manufactured by Bard Hospital Division of C. R. Bard, Inc., Murray Hill, N. J., 07974.

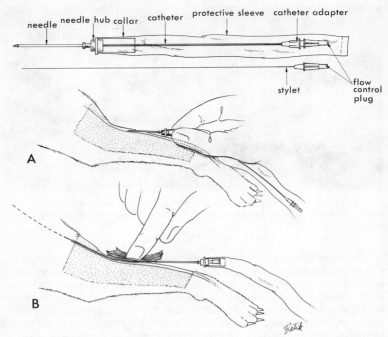

Figure 69. *A,* Percutaneous needle puncture of cephalic vein. The catheter is advanced through the needle into the vein. *B,* After placing the catheter in the vein, the needle is withdrawn, pressure applied over the venipuncture site, the catheter taped in place, and the needle guard placed around the needle.

thoroughly with antiseptic solution. Open the sterile package and remove the needle guard, which should be retained for later use. Distend the vein by appropriately positioning the animal and make a percutaneous needle puncture into the vein. Blood should enter the catheter. Place thumb in back of flow control plug and push catheter gently into the vein. Do not attempt to pull the catheter back out through the needle; the sharp edge may cut the catheter. If venipuncture is not successful, remove the needle and catheter together.

Once the catheter has been placed into the vein, remove the needle from the vein. Apply pressure over the venipuncture site for 30 seconds with a gauze sponge. Cover the venipuncture site with Neomycin-polymixin B ointment and sterile gauze sponge and tape in place. Discard collar and protective sleeve from needle hub and seat intravenous fluid adapter into needle hub. Remove stylet from catheter.

Place needle within the needle guard. Tape needle guard to skin and connect intravenous infusion set to the adapter. Check for leakage or infiltration and be sure the intravenous solution is running freely.

It is necessary to completely cover the catheter apparatus and needle holder with bandage and tape, as illustrated in Figure 70.

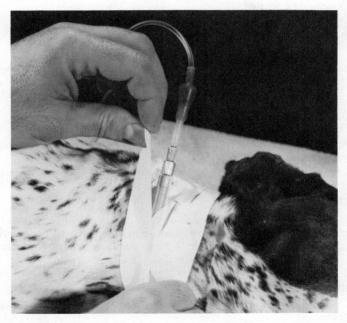

Figure 70. Placement of a Bardic intravenous catheter in the jugular vein. The needle guard and catheter are taped into place on the neck to facilitate continuous intravenous medication. When the catheter is affixed in such a manner, it is difficult for the dog to remove it.

References

Additional information can be found in the following sources:

Bland, J. H.: Clinical Metabolism of Body Water and Electrolytes. Philadelphia, W. B. Saunders Co., 1963

Finco, D. R. (ed.): Special Issue Fluid Therapy. J.A.A.H.A., Vol. 8, No. 3, May, 1972.

Goldberger, E.: Primer of Water, Electrolyte and Acid-Base Syndromes, 3rd ed. Philadelphia, Lea and Febiger, 1965.

Levin, M. L.: Disorders of acid-base relationships. Rational Drug Therapy, Vol. 6, No. 5, May, 1972. W. B. Saunders Co., Philadelphia.

Statland, H.: Fluid and Electrolytes in Practice, 3rd ed. Philadelphia, J. B. Lippincott Co., 1963.

Subcutaneous Injection

1. Use a 3 inch, 15 or 16 gauge needle attached to tubing.
2. Clean skin and push needle to entire depth under the skin in region of the shoulder, back, or loin.
3. Pull folds of skin up to the needle hub to allow needle to penetrate fully.
4. As fluid fills subcutaneous space allow skin folds to retract and gradually withdraw needle.
5. *Do not* "fan" needle under skin to spread fluid; however, needle may be redirected in a straight line in another direction.
6. Use multiple sites as needed to give additional volumes.

Intraperitoneal Injection

1. Thoroughly clip and clean skin over abdominal injection site (just lateral to the linea alba and midway between umbilicus and pelvic brim).
2. Insert a 2 or 3 inch, 16 or 18 gauge needle into peritoneal cavity.
3. Fill cavity until abdomen is distended or lesser dosage is given.

General Considerations

Solution bottles can be changed easily or Y-tube infusion sets used with impunity except in intravenous infusions. In the latter case extreme care must be used to avoid air embolism during bottle changes. Do not permit an unattended bottle to become empty.

With hypertonic or hypotonic solutions care must be exercised to avoid subcutaneous infiltration. Constant supervision is needed during intravenous infusions.

IV–20–F.   Solutions Needed

1. Use commercial solutions.
2. Use simple solutions unless you have a good laboratory and the interest to follow cases closely.

Necessary Basic Solutions

1. Dextran (plasma substitute), 500 ml.; dextran, 6 per cent, in dextrose, 5 per cent in water; or dextran, 6 per cent, in sodium chloride, 0.9 per cent.
2. ACD solution in blood collecting vacuum bottle, or CPD blood collection and administration packs (see Section IV-21).

Electrolyte Solutions (500 and 1000 ml.)

3. Dextrose, 5 per cent in water.
4. Sodium chloride, 0.9 per cent.
5. Sodium lactate, one sixth molar.
6. Lactated Ringer's solution.

Optional Helpful Solutions

1. Invert sugar, 10 per cent (5 per cent dextrose, 5 per cent fructose), in water.
2. Dextrose, 50 per cent in water.
3. Sodium chloride, 3 per cent.
4. Gastric replacement solution.
5. Duodenal replacement solution.
6. Calcium gluconate, 10 per cent in water.
7. Dextrose, 5 per cent, in sodium chloride, 0.9 per cent.
8. Amino acid solution, 5 per cent.
9. Intestinal replacement and general electrolyte solution.

IV–20–G.   Peritoneal Dialysis

The peritoneum is a semipermeable membrane with a large surface area. The rate at which substances of low molecular weight can diffuse across this membrane is related to the concentration of the substance. By varying the concentration of substances in a dialysate solution one can increase the diffusion of substances across the peritoneal membrane.

Commercially available dialysate solutions may contain 1.5 per cent, 4.25 per cent or 7 per cent glucose. Diffusion rates of solutes across the peritoneal membrane are also affected by the temperature of the dialysate solution and the length of time the dialysate remains in the abdomen. Increasing the temperature of the dialysate solution to 37°C increases the clearance rate of low molecular weight substances across the peritoneal membrane.

Peritoneal dialysis is the process of filling the peritoneal cavity with a balanced electrolyte solution and removing it two hours later. It is useful in removing urea, phenobarbital, thallium and various other toxic products from the body. The procedure must be performed under sterile conditions. The abdomen should be clipped and prepared as for surgery. Cover the area with a small surgical drape.

Empty the bladder if it is filled. Infiltrate the skin and abdominal musculature just lateral to the midline and a few centimeters posterior to the umbilicus. Commercial peritoneal dialysis sets are available* or a needle can be used. For repeated dialysis, we prefer the use of a catheter. When placed, the catheter is sutured to the skin.

Inject enough warm dialysate fluid to distend the abdomen mildly (200 to 2000 ml.). Lactated Ringer's solution with glucose added (to 2 per cent) is a satisfactory lavage fluid, but Peridial, 1.5 per cent, and Inpersol, 1.5 per cent, are balanced more correctly. There is an ever-present danger of peritonitis resulting from peritoneal dialysis. Although the prophylactic incorporation of antibiotics in the dialysate solution has not been proven to prevent peritonitis, we add crystalline penicillin and streptomycin to the lavage solution.

After one hour the abdomen is drained of solution. The dialysate is removed by siphoning it back into the original sterile container. During the first dialysing period, some fluid will be absorbed and the entire volume that was placed in the peritoneal cavity will not be collected. In severe renal failure cases, peritoneal dialysis may have to be repeated 3 to 5 times a day.

Complications of peritoneal dialysis include blockage of the catheter, causing problems with recovery of dialysate solution, and peritonitis, but this risk is lessened by using good sterile technique and a closed drainage system. Maintain the dialysis set for as short a period of time as is possible.

---

*Stylocath, Abbott Labs; Diacath, Travenol Labs Inc.

Replacement therapy with proteins may be necessary in severely debilitated patients who are losing excessive amounts of protein in the dialysate fluid.

Reference

Additional material can be found in the following source:

Osborne, C. A., and Low, D. G.: The application of principles of fluid and electrolyte therapy to patients with renal failure. J.A.A.H.A. 8:181–199, May, 1972.

IV–21. BLOOD TRANSFUSIONS

IV–21–A. Cats

Blood transfusions for cats are usually administered for medical reasons and repeated small doses of fresh whole blood are desirable. Although work is fragmentary, it appears that blood groups in cats are not important and typing or cross matching is not necessary. Never use interspecies transfusions!

Equipment

Thiamylal sodium.
Two siliconized syringes, 20 ml.
One siliconized needle, 2 inch, 18 gauge.
One scalp vein infusion set.
Adhesive tape, 1 inch wide.
Blanket.
Clear plastic bag.
Oxygen tank, flow meter, and rubber tubing.
If desired, an ACD blood collection bottle, 150 ml. or CPD plastic bag (Fenwal Blood Pak).

Technique

Donor cats can be anesthetized by barbiturates and destroyed by complete exsanguination by a left ventricular puncture with a two inch, 18 gauge needle. In such cases about 150 ml. of blood can be harvested and stored in ACD or CPD solution. In many instances a donor cat is kept in the hospital for repeated collections. These animals are lightly anesthetized with barbiturate, the left thorax prepared as for surgery, and ventricular puncture accomplished by inserting a 2 inch, 18 to 20 gauge needle through the left third or fourth intercostal space. The needle is attached to a 20 ml. siliconized glass syringe and blood is aspirated to fill the syringe. Two syringes are filled in this manner. If silicon is not available to treat the needles and syringes, heparin solution will suffice to prevent clotting.

Donor cats should be healthy, vigorous, and free of blood disorders. In these animals a 40 ml. donation can be repeated safely every three weeks.

Administering Blood

Cats needing blood are usually extremely depressed, toxic, or anoxic and require blood to correct anemias or for other medical reasons. Struggling or violent exertion may cause these patients to collapse and die. Therefore extreme gentleness and care are mandatory in handling and restraint. It is strongly advised that the patient be cradled gently on a towel or blanket and the head placed in a clear plastic bag into which oxygen is being infused at 4 to 6 L./minute.

Blood can be administered intravenously by way of the jugular, cephalic, or femoral veins, using a 22 to 24 gauge scalp vein infusion set. Intramedullary infusion is possible through the femur by way of the intratrochanteric fossa. However, this may be impractical and present dangers of intramedullary infection. Intraperitoneal infusion can be used safely with good utilization of erythrocytes. About 45 per cent of the infused red blood cells are in the circulation within 24 hours, and 65 per cent within 48 hours.

The average 4 or 5 pound cat can accept 30 to 40 ml. of blood injected intravenously over a period of 30 minutes. Small, repeated injections are safer and more desirable than a large, single injection. Single intraperitoneal injections (40 ml.) are safe and convenient.

IV–21–B. Dogs

Blood transfusions usually are given to dogs for severe blood loss and other acute conditions, but may be given for medical reasons too. Of the several canine blood types, only the A group is important antigenically. Donor blood should be A negative (universal donor) if possible.

Equipment

Thiamylal sodium.
Blood donor kit preferably a CPD containing blood pak (Fenwal)*.
Blood recipient kit containing a 5 ml. syringe with saline and an intravenous catheter.
Sterile intravenous cutdown kit containing a scalpel, thumb forceps, needle holder, sharp-pointed scissors, two pairs of mosquito forceps, curved needle, plain catgut, fine silk, and sponges.

Collecting Blood

The donor is anesthetized with thiamylal sodium. Blood may be drawn from the jugular vein of dogs, obtained via left ventricular puncture, using a 3 inch, 18 gauge needle. This is inserted through the fifth intercostal space and an area 4 inches in diameter around this site should be prepared as for surgery. If repeated collections are to be made from a single donor, we have routinely utilized the jugular vein. Blood is allowed to flow through the CPD solution while the bag is gently agitated. When the bag is filled, the tubing should be removed without allowing air to enter.

Oxygenated blood so collected can be stored under refrigeration at 4°C. In general, we do not utilize stored whole blood if it is over 3 weeks old. Plasma can be harvested from blood and frozen for later use. It is safe to collect 10 ml./lb. of donor body weight per collection, and this may be repeated every three weeks. The donor dog should be healthy, parasite free, vaccinated for the usual diseases and legally owned by the veterinarian. A mature, thin, 50 pound animal makes an ideal donor.

---

*Fenwal is a division of Baxter-Travenol Laboratories.

Administering Blood

In dogs, blood is invariably given intravenously. The cephalic vein is used commonly, but the jugular vein is routinely utilized when an intravenous catheter is placed in the animal. The recipient set should be filled so that blood in the drip chamber covers the filter. Blood can be administered at variable rates but the routine figure of 4 to 5 ml./minute is often used. Volume is given as needed, with a suggested dose of 10 ml./lb./day for medical cases. Surgical emergencies and shock may require several times this volume within a short period (see Section IV-17).

If the blood type of the patient is unknown and A negative blood is not available, any dog blood can be given to patients in acute need if they have not had previous transfusions. However, if mismatched blood is given, the patient will become sensitized to it and after nine days destruction of the donated erythrocytes will begin. In addition, any subsequent mismatched transfusion may cause an immediate reaction (usually mild) and rapid destruction of the donated cells.

Adverse reactions during transfusion appear as dyspnea, shivering, vomiting, or urticaria. If any of these appear the transfusion should be discontinued immediately.

Blood typing is important when brood bitches are to be transfused or when repeated transfusions are anticipated. Cross matching is important when the patient has experienced previous transfusions (see Section V-3-D).

Reference

Additional information can be found in the following source:

Eisenbrandt, D. L., and Smith, J. E.: Evaluation of preservatives and containers for storage of canine blood. J.A.V.M.A. *163*:988–990, October, 1973.

IV–22. TRACHEOTOMY

Indications

1. To relieve upper respiratory tract obstructions.
2. To facilitate removal of respiratory secretions.
3. To decrease the dead air space.

4. To provide a route for inhalant anesthesia when oral or facial surgery is complex.

5. To reduce resistance to respiration.

6. To reduce the risk of closed glottis pressure (cough) following pulmonary or cranial surgery.

7. To facilitate artificial respiration.

Technique

In an emergency situation with asphyxiation imminent, any cutting instrument will suffice. Moistening the hair over the ventral neck facilitates midline incision over the trachea. The first few tracheal rings (2-3, 3-4) are incised to allow placement of any firm tube (ballpoint pen barrel); or the knife blade may be rotated 90° to maintain the tracheal opening.

In less demanding circumstances, aseptic surgical technique should be followed. A midline skin incision is made just caudal to the larynx to permit incision and retraction of the paired sternohyoideus muscles, exposing the trachea. The trachea may then be elevated and immobilized by passing quarter-inch umbilical tapes around it as traction sutures. The first few tracheal rings may be incised or partially resected to allow placement of the tracheotomy tube.

Tracheotomy Tubes

Many of the shortcomings of the old curved metal tracheotomy tubes are overcome by the utilization of the newer plastic tubes. These are often far better tolerated by the patient, as they are lighter weight, more flexible, less irritating, and contoured better for the canine or feline trachea. Crusting of secretions has been less of a problem with the PVC tubes.

The uncuffed Morrant-Baker and cuffed Bassett tubes are available in a wide variety of sizes for the dog (42-21 FG), with and without adapters for connection to respirators or anesthesia machines. The infant tracheotomy tubes (Great Ormond St. Hospital pattern) have proven ideal for small dogs and cats.

Postoperative Care

1. Postoperative care is more important than the surgery.

2. Humidify the inspired air.

3. Use systemic antibiotics prophylactically (penicillin-streptomycin).

4. Cleanse the wound and the tracheal tube daily, or more often if needed. By using the traction sutures the tube can be easily removed and replaced.

5. Frequent aspiration of respiratory secretions should be performed. A soft urethral catheter (12 F) is attached to the T-tube and to a vacuum pump so that suction can be applied or released at will. This tube is passed through the wound to the large bronchi.

6. Tracheotomy wounds heal within seven to 10 days following removal of the tube.

IV–23. ENDOTRACHEAL INTUBATION

General Considerations

The two most commonly used types of endotracheal tubes in veterinary medicine are the Magill and the Murphy. The tubes are usually constructed of rubber or plastic and their appropriate size can be classified by several different scales of measurement. In selecting an endotracheal tube of appropriate size, consider the size of the animal and select the tube with the largest diameter that can be introduced without force (Table 53).

TABLE 53. RECOMMENDED SIZES FOR ENDOTRACHEAL TUBES

	Body Weight (lb.)	Magill Size	French Size	Internal Diameter (mm.)
Dogs	5	2	22	6.0
	10	4 to 5	26 to 28	8.0
	15	6 to 7	28 to 30	9.0
	20	8	32	10.0
	25	9 to 10	34 to 36	11.0 to 12.0
	30	9 to 10	34 to 36	11.0 to 12.0
	35	10 to 11	36 to 38	11.0 to 12.0
	40	11 to 12	38 to 44	12.0
	45	11 to 12	38 to 44	
Cats	2.5	00	13	4.0
	4.5	0	16	5.0
	9.0	1	20	5.0

Equipment

Materials needed include an appropriate size endotracheal tube, a laryngoscope, a mouth gag, Pontocaine cream or Cetacaine spray, gauze pads and 1-inch gauze.

Tubes should be cleansed with soap and water, both inside and outside scrubbed and thoroughly rinsed. The dry tubes may be sterilized by steam heat, liquid chemicals, or ethylene oxide gas. We prefer gas sterilization. Tubes are stored in a dry clean area.

Always check the cuff of a cuffed tube to see that there are no leaks and that it is working properly. Prior to intubation, the selected endotracheal tube should be lubricated with an anesthetic cream, such as Pontocaine. Intubation is carried out under a short-acting anesthetic or while the animal is under the influence of an analgesic-tranquilizer combination. Intubation in the dog and cat may cause an increase in sympathetic activity or vagal stimulation, resulting in cardiac arrhythmias. Various preanesthetic agents and the release of catecholamines during excitement may enhance these arrhythmias. The administration of atropine as a pre-anesthetic will serve as a vagolytic agent and will greatly minimize the hazard of arrhythmias from intubation.

Technique

Direct visualization of the larynx is the best method for intubating dogs and cats. The animal may be placed in lateral, sternal or dorsal recumbency, according to preference. Intubation of cats is more easily accomplished if they are in dorsal recumbency. Hold the laryngoscope in the left hand and open the mouth with the right hand. In large dogs or animals under light anesthesia the use of a mouth gag can be very helpful. Pull the tongue forward with the right hand, being careful not to lacerate the ventral aspect of the tongue on the lower incisor teeth. In large dogs, it may be helpful to hold the tongue between the small and ring fingers to prevent it from moving excessively. Place the tip of the laryngoscope blade at the base of the tongue at the glossoepigliotic fold. Elevate the laryngoscope blade, which will lift the epiglotitis and expose the glottis. Holding the endotracheal tube in the right hand, insert the endotracheal tube. A piece of aluminum wire temporarily placed inside a very flexible plastic tube will provide enough rigidity to make intubation simpler. Place the tube through the vocal folds, using a slight rotating motion rather than trying to push the tube through. Never try to force too large a tube into position. If partial closure of the glottis or laryngeal spasm occurs during attempted intubation, deepen the level of anesthesia or apply a local

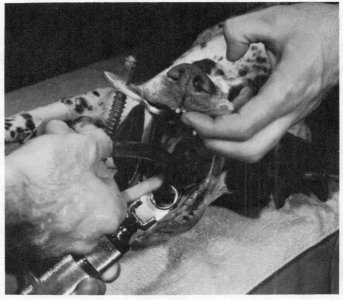

Figure 71. Endotracheal intubation in the dog. The larynx is visualized, utilizing a laryngoscope. The tongue is pulled forward, and the tip of the laryngoscope blade is placed at the base of the tongue at the glossoepiglottic fold.

anesthetic spray such as Cetacaine to the larynx.

The cuff of a cuffed endotracheal tube should be at a level just beyond the larynx. Overinflation of the cuff may lead to pressure necrosis of tracheal epithelium.

IV–24. OXYGEN THERAPY

TISSUE OXYGENATION

The basic indication for oxygen therapy is inadequate tissue oxygenation (hypoxia).

1. The partial pressure of oxygen (Po_2) is a convenient figure to use in following oxygen utilization. Inspired air has a Po_2 of 150 mm. Hg. As it is mixed with air in the alveolus the Po_2 drops to 100 mm. Hg. Arterial blood saturated with oxygen has a Po_2 of 95 mm. Hg and when tissues have been supplied, the Po_2 of venous blood is about 40 mm. Hg. Oxygen tissue levels normally approximate 35 mm. Hg.

2. Oxygen is transported in the blood in combination with hemoglobin and in physical solution in the plasma. If an adequate amount of hemoglobin is normally saturated with oxygen while breathing room air, breathing high concentrations of oxygen will increase that carried by hemoglobin only slightly. However, significant increases in dissolved plasma oxygen will be obtained. On the other hand, if inadequate hemoglobin saturation is obtained by breathing normal air, breathing high concentrations of oxygen may markedly raise hemoglobin saturation and improve tissue oxygen tensions. The additional oxygen in physical solution would be helpful, too.

SIGNS OF HYPOXIA

1. Measurement of arterial blood gases and pH is the only reliable means of measuring hypoxia. Peripheral vascular collapse (shock) and reduced oxygen carrying capacity (anemia) are serious indications of severe complications.

2. The clinical signs of hyperpnea, dyspnea, tachycardia, and cyanosis may be dominant features in some patients but they are nonspecific and unreliable.

TYPES OF HYPOXIA

Hypoxic Hypoxia

Alterations of respiratory function may lead to a lowered Po_2 of arterial blood, which in turn may be caused by:

1. *Alveolar hypoventilation*, which is the result of depressed respirations or resistance to chest movements. Hypercapnia is present.

2. *An arteriovenous shunt* within the heart or lungs due to congenital defect or to perfusion of a section of lung that is not ventilated (consolidated or atelectatic segment). If the rest of the lung is hyperventilated, hypercapnia will not develop.

3. *A diffusion defect* in which the alveolar membrane is altered by fibrosis, emphysema, or thromboembolic disease. Hypercapnia usually is not present since carbon dioxide can diffuse 20 times as fast as oxygen.

4. *Uneven blood flow and ventilation* throughout the lung may be caused by many pulmonary diseases, and is probably the most common cause of hypoxia. Hypercapnia may or may not be present.

Anemic Hypoxia

Reduced oxygen-carrying capacity of the blood may be due to low or abnormal hemoglobin.

Circulatory Hypoxia

Inadequate perfusion of tissues may be due to shock, low cardiac output, or vascular obstruction.

Histotoxic Hypoxia

Toxic tissue cells may be unable to utilize oxygen.

IV–24–A. Indications for Oxygen Therapy

1. In veterinary medicine oxygen is indicated in acute cases of respiratory insufficiency (hypoxic hypoxia) leading to a low arterial oxygen tension. It is rarely indicated for any chronic condition because of economic and practical considerations.

2. Altered ventilation-perfusion relationships are often indications for oxygen therapy. However, measures designed to treat infection, reduce airway obstruction, or improve the mechanics of breathing may reduce the need for oxygen.

3. Circulatory failures such as shock and reduced cardiac output cause hypoxia due to poor perfusion. Giving oxygen is an ancillary treatment, subordinate to the measures directed at the primary cause. However, oxygen therapy may be the critical factor in raising oxygen tissue levels above hypoxic levels.

4. In anemic hypoxia, blood transfusions are needed, and oxygen therapy is only helpful if the hemoglobin is abnormal (carboxyhemoglobin).

5. Histotoxic hypoxia is unlikely to be benefited by oxygen therapy, but it should be administered.

6. When possible, arterial blood gas analysis should be used to assess the need for oxygen therapy. Analysis should include oxygen tension, carbon dioxide tension, and arterial blood pH.

ADMINISTERING OXYGEN

1. The goal of oxygen therapy is to increase the oxygen carried in the blood by raising the arterial oxygen tension to normal in hypoxic hypoxia, and by increasing the arterial oxygen tension above normal in circulatory and anemic hypoxia.

2. Requirements of an oxygen tent environment:
    a. Usually 30 to 40 per cent oxygen is more than adequate to treat cases of hypoxia correctable by oxygen therapy. (Higher concentrations may be needed for severe circulatory failure.) Initially, high flow rates of 10 L./min. are required to wash out residual nitrogen in the cage. Maintenance flow of 5 L./min. is usually sufficient.
    b. Adequate humidification (often 4 to 60 per cent) is absolutely essential.
    c. Maintenance of carbon dioxide at less than 1.5 per cent is necessary. Oxygen tents equipped with CO_2 absorbers can maintain CO_2 levels at 0.7 per cent.
    d. Control of environmental temperature at 65 to 70°F. is necessary in almost all cases.

3. Methods of oxygen administration include face mask, tracheal catheter, nasal catheter, oxygen tent, endotracheal tube and IPPB respirator. Obviously, endotracheal intubation and IPPB can be used only in the anesthetized or comatose animal. Tight-fitting masks are usually resented by the animal, and his struggles cause further hypoxia.

Supplemental oxygen may be administered via a catheter placed either through the cricothyroid ligament or between the tracheal rings. Either of these techniques overcomes the total lack of patient cooperation so common with nasal catheters. It has proven especially useful for the administration of supplemental oxygen to dogs too large for the oxygen cages. A large, sterile, pliable male urinary catheter is utilized. Humidified oxygen at a flow rate of 5 to 8 liters per minute should achieve an oxygen concentration of 30 to 50 per cent.

4. Oxygen tent equipment to provide these conditions is rarely found in veterinary hospitals. The best equipment includes a mechanical, thermostatically controlled compressor cooling unit, a circulatory fan, nebulizers or humidifiers to moisten the air, and a CO_2 absorber. The OTC-2 intensive care oxygen therapy unit manufactured by Kirschner Scientific fulfills these requirements; other professionally designed tents meet some of the requirements. The ice-chest oxygen diffusion tents are *very poor* for long-term maintenance therapy in hypoxemic animals. Small incubator isolettes have been used with good success in cats and puppies.

TABLE 54. APPROXIMATE REMAINING HOURS OF SERVICE IN STANDARD 244 CUBIC FEET CYLINDERS OF U.S.P. OXYGEN

Full Cylinder		Contents at Diminishing Gauge Pressure		
Rate of flow in liters per min.	244 cu. ft. 2,200 lbs. 6,900 liters	183 cu. ft. 1,650 lbs. 5,175 liters	122 cu. ft. 1,100 lbs. 3,450 liters	61 cu. ft. 550 lbs. 1,725 liters
4	28¾ hours	21½ hours	14¼ hours	7½ hours
6	19 hours	14¼ hours	9½ hours	4¾ hours
8	14¼ hours	10¼ hours	7¼ hours	3½ hours
10	11½ hours	8½ hours	5¾ hours	2¾ hours
12	9½ hours	7¼ hours	4¾ hours	2¼ hours
14	8 hours	6 hours	4 hours	2 hours
16	7 hours	5¼ hours	3½ hours	1¾ hours

Examples—Full cylinder, at 2,200 lbs. pressure, flowing at a rate of 4 liters should last 28¾ hours. A cylinder with 1,100 lbs. pressure flowing at a rate of 6 liters per minute should last 9½ hours. (Courtesy of Ohio Chemical & Surgical Equipment Company, Madison, Wisconsin.)

5. The patient should be maintained in the tent continuously, not on an intermittent basis. Animals with chronic respiratory disease or hypoxemia from other causes have become adjusted to a high CO_2 level for producing their "hypoxic drive" and resultant respiratory rate. Administration of high levels of O_2 may depress the "hypoxic drive," resulting in a lowered respiratory rate of apnea and increased hypoxia. Therefore, animals with chronic hypoxia should be observed closely for respiratory depression when oxygen therapy is administered.

OXYGEN TOXICITY

Toxicity problems are not encountered with short-term, low concentration therapy. Convulsions, and atelectasis from nitrogen washout of obstructed areas of lung may be found as special complications of prolonged high concentration therapy.

IV–24–B. Nebulization Therapy

Large water particles (10 to 60 μ) in the high velocity air flow of the nose and throat settle on the mucosa of the larynx, nose, and throat. Particles smaller than 10μ (2 to 10 μ) are deposited in the bronchi but only the smallest reach the bronchioles. Ultrasonic aerosol generators are the most effective machines for nebulization.

Dense mist from an unheated jet-nebulizer contains only slightly more water than is needed to humidify air whose temperature is increased from 22 to 37°C. The evaporation of the aerosol solution can be prevented by stabilization, i.e., by heating it to 53°C or by reducing the vapor pressure by adding 10 per cent propylene glycol. Since distilled water and hypertonic solutions are irritating to the mucosa, only isotonic or half strength isotonic saline should be used.

Although continuous, low level humidification of the oxygen tent atmosphere is necessary, periodic medication by aerosol spray is permissible. High levels of water can be introduced several times daily for 10 to 15 minutes per treatment, or drugs can be added to the solution during these times. Many drugs have been used, but only isoproterenol, epinephrine, and phenylephrine have caused bronchodilatation and decreased airway resistance.

It is important to differentiate obstruction of the bronchi due to pulmonary edema from that due to bronchial secretions. In both cases the patient cannot ventilate because of fluids or semifluid liquids in the bronchi. In pulmonary edema the fluid turns to a frothy, bubbly material that produces a "rattling" in the throat. Patients suffering from pulmonary edema should be treated with antifoaming substances such as 12 per cent alcohol in water, given by nebulization. If used to treat tenacious exudates these agents increase viscosity and thus the obstruction.

Thick, inflammatory exudates, on the other hand, need to be thinned by detergent materials (such as Tergemist or Mucomyst) that liquefy bronchial secretions. However, these agents increase frothing, and, indirectly, anoxia if used in pulmonary edema.

1. In pulmonary edema, use antifoaming agents (12 per cent alcohol).
2. In bronchial exudates (thick), use detergents (liquefying agents).

References

Additional material can be found in the following sources:

Gillespie, J. R., and Martin, D. B.: Long-term oxygen cage therapy for hypoxemic dogs. J. A.V.M.A. *156*:717–725, 1970.

Goodger, W. J.: Administration of supplemental oxygen to the critically ill patient. J. A.A.H.A., *8*:434–443, 1972.

Whyte-Hedley, J., and Winter, P. M.: Oxygen therapy. Clin. Pharmacol. Therapeut. *8*:696–737, 1967.

IV-25. RADIATION THERAPY

PRELIMINARY CONSIDERATIONS

1. Radiation therapy is highly dangerous to the patient and operator unless the proper equipment is used and used correctly.

2. A correct diagnosis (including histopathologic diagnosis) should be obtained before radiation therapy is attempted.

3. Lesions should be treated with other methods first if feasible.

4. When radiation is indicated, a complete course should be planned carefully, with consideration given to the balance of risks against possible benefits.

5. Consider combination therapy; preoperative or postoperative (or both) depending upon surgical success.

Guidelines for Use

The following are *guidelines only* to the general indications and dosages for ionizing radiation. Treat cases individually.

Beta Ray Therapy

Beta rays are very "soft" and are applied by strontium-90 applicator (AEC license required).

1. Corneal vascularization—from 2500 to 3000 reps/dose repeated every fourth day. Total dose: 10,000-12,000 reps.

2. Rodent ulcer (cat labial granuloma)—from 5000 to 10,000 reps/dose repeated once. Total dose: 10,000-20,000 reps. Most lesions are too deep for beta rays.

Low Voltage Therapy

Low voltage x-ray therapy (superficial effects) is applied by a calibrated x-ray therapy machine delivering 80 to 120 K; half value layers (HVL) = 1 to 4 mm. aluminum.

1. Rodent ulcer—treat with 500 R/dose, which may be repeated once in three days. Total dose: 500–1000 R. May be repeated in four weeks if not healed.

2. Pyoderma, chronic dermatitis, otitis externa—treat with 500 R/dose repeated twice at three-day intervals. Total dose: 1000–1500 R. If lesion does not heal repeat therapy in six weeks. Results are best in acute inflammation.

Moderate Voltage X-ray Therapy (Intermediate Depth Effect)

Applied by calibrated x-ray therapy machine delivering from 120 to 200 kV, HVL = 4 mm. Al and 1 mm. Cu.

See dosage schedules for deeper therapy and general suggestions for specific lesions.

High Voltage X-ray Therapy (Deep Effect)

Applied by calibrated x-ray therapy machine delivering 200 to 400 kV, HVL = 1.8 to 3.0 mm. Cu.

Dosage schedules are as follows:

1. Treat as small an area as possible to minimize damage to normal tissue. Multiple part exposure of the lesion also helps spare normal tissue.

2. In general, with small lesions the patient can receive larger amounts of radiation per dose than with large lesions.

3. The amount of filtration used depends on the depth and tissue type of the lesion.

4. General doses:
   a. For benign lesions give a total of 500 to 1500 R in one to three doses depending on the size of the lesion.
   b. For malignant lesion give a total of 2000 to 4000 R in four to eight doses of 400 to 500 R administered every third day. This schedule varies depending on the tissue and the size and type of lesion. Weekly treatment is also possible.

GENERAL SUGGESTIONS FOR SPECIFIC LESIONS

1. *Tumors that are not responsive to radiation*: Neurofibroma—total dose (T/D), none recommended.

2. *Tumors that are resistant to radiation but may receive palliation therapy*:
   a. Carcinoma of nasal passages—T/D 3000 to 3500 R.
   b. Carcinoma of tonsils—T/D 3000 to 4000 R and nodes.
   c. Fibrosarcoma—T/D 3000 to 4000 R (may not respond).
   d. Malignant melanoma—T/D 3000 to 4000 R (may not respond).
   e. Neoplasms of skull—T/D 3500 to 4000 R with high kV and heavy filtration.

3. *Tumors that are sensitive to radiation*:
   a. Adenoma and adenocarcinoma of sweat gland—T/D 3000 to 4000 R and regional lymph nodes.

    b. Adenoma and adenocarcinoma of sebaceous gland—T/D 3000 to 4000 R. These above two lesions may show poor response.

    c. Basal cell carcinoma—T/D 3000 to 4000 R.

    d. Lymphoma and lymphosarcoma—T/D 2500 R to all affected nodes if total body irradiation is not excessive.

    e. Mastocytoma—T/D 2000 to 3000 R.

    f. Perianal gland tumors:
        (1) Benign—T/D 1000 to 2000 R.
        (2) Adenocarcinoma—T/D 3000 to 4000 R.

    g. Recurring benign tumors—T/D 1000 to 2000 R.—if surgical excision is not feasible.

    h. Salivary carcinoma—T/D 3000 to 4000 R.

    i. Squamous cell carcinoma—T/D 3000 to 4000 R (not all respond).

    j. Transmissible venereal tumor—T/D 1000 to 2000 R (treatment of choice).

Note: High doses (especially tumoricidal) of radiation produce several local changes including hair loss, poliosis, erythema, ulceration, and necrosis. Many of these are irreversible.

USE OF RADIOISOTOPES

    Radioisotope therapy for malignant tumors has many advantages but requires A.E.C. trained and licensed personnel, thus limiting its use to large centers.

    Cobalt-60, gold-198, and iodine-131 are three radioisotopes that should be effectively used in veterinary medicine.

    Radon seeds may be used. Be careful of excessive exposure doses to operator; use removable or afterloading procedures.

References

Additional information can be found in the following sources:

Banks, W. C., Roberts, R., Morris, E., and Hussey, D. H.: Radiotherapy techniques in veterinary medicine. J.A.V.M.A. *160*:446–450, 1972.

Gillette, E. L.: Veterinary radiotherapy. J.A.V.M.A. *157*:1707–1712, 1970.

Roenigk, W.: Radiation therapy. In Kirk, R. W.: Current Veterinary Therapy V, Philadelphia, W. B. Saunders Co., 1974.

IV–26. PHYSIOTHERAPY

Most of the physiotherapeutic principles outlined have a stimulating effect and their action is directed toward the musculoskeletal system or the skin.

HEAT

Effects

1. Hyperemia and dilation of cutaneous vessels.
2. Increase in pulse, blood pressure, and pulmonary ventilation.
3. Increased metabolite transfer across capillary membranes.
4. General muscle relaxation.
5. Sedative and analgesic effect.
6. Improved extensibility of connective tissue.

Contraindication

1. In the presence of trauma, swelling, and edema, circulation may be impeded and the application of heat may cause necrosis. Cold is of more benefit in early acute stages of inflammation and edema.

Moist Heat

1. Local application of hot wet packs or local immersion with the water temperature about 120°F. This is especially effective if one alternates four minutes in a hot bath and one minute in a cold bath. Repeat the cycle four or five times with the entire process repeated two or three times daily.
2. Whirlpool baths combine gentle massage with entire body immersion. Temperatures of 105 to 110°F. with low suds detergents or antiseptics added to the bath should be used. Water turbines circulate water vigorously for 15 minutes while the patient is controlled in the tub. This keeps the skin and wounds clean of exudates and excretions, is stimulating and is indicated for arthritis, myositis, fractures, and for contractures during healing, paraplegia and skin infections.

Dry Heat

1. Infrared radiation applied by lamps penetrates to superficial tissues only. Most lamps are placed 2 feet from the surface and treatment is applied for 15 to 20 minutes three or four times daily. Keep a hand in the

field to monitor the degree of heat being applied. *It is easy to burn unconscious patients*, especially if the area exposed to heat is moist.

2. Diathermy is not commonly used by veterinarians. *It is contraindicated in tissues that have metal implants*. Deeply penetrating heat is produced by high frequency electromagnetic waves passing through tissues. After the acute response to trauma subsides, this form of heat may be applied daily to sprains, strains, contusions, and other soft tissue injuries.

COLD

Ice packs or immersion in cold water can be helpful for early treatment of soft tissue injury to prevent edema and swelling. It can also be used effectively when alternated with heat as already described. Although frequently repeated treatments with cold during the first 24 to 48 hours are indicated, overtreatment should be avoided (maceration and frostbite may result).

MASSAGE

Gentle massage in the direction of venous flow may be useful to reduce edema and swelling and to promote muscle tone. When combined with passive exercise (flexing and extending joints) it may be useful to prevent contractures and hasten rehabilitation following fractures and luxations. Long, frequent sessions of massage and exercise are necessary.

ELECTRICAL STIMULATION

Low frequency alternating current (faradism) may be used to stimulate muscles. It is useful in nerve-damaged areas to exercise muscles and improve their tone but it has no effect on nerve regeneration.

ULTRASOUND

1. Ultrasonic energy is produced by transforming electrical energy to mechanical energy and a high frequency vibration results.

2. Biologic effects of the ultrasound vibration can be lethal or can destroy tissues when high levels are used.

3. Therapy is applied by moving the applicator head over the area to be treated. A coupling medium of mineral oil can be used to insure contact

between the applicator and the skin. It is best to shave the skin before treatment to enhance this contact.

With shock-proof machines it may be possible to submerge the applicator and the part to be treated in a tank of water to achieve proper coupling. Proper restraint of the patient is often difficult in these cases, however.

4. Dosage varies with each case. Most ultrasound generators have an output of 700,000 to 1,000,000 cps at intensities of 0.1 to 1.0 watt/sq. cm. It is best to use the lowest intensity possible. The maximal dosage should be 1 watt/sq. cm. for five minutes of application to the affected tissues. This can be repeated daily for five days, then every other day for five days. It should not be repeated again for at least one month.

5. Indications:
   a. *Not* for use in acute injuries, inflammations, or infections.
   b. Cervical intervertebral disc disease—0.3 watt/sq. cm. for three minutes daily for five days, then every other day for five treatments.
   c. Arthritis, bursitis, myositis—0.2 watt/sq. cm. for three minutes for joints of the lower extremities. Repeat twice weekly.

References

Additional information can be found in the following sources:

Leonard, E. P.: Physiotherapy in small animals: *In* Kirk, R. W. (ed.): Current Veterinary Therapy III. Philadelphia, W. B. Saunders Co., 1968.

Schirmer, R. G.: Ultrasound therapy. *In* Kirk, R. W. (ed.): Current Veterinary Therapy III. Philadelphia, W. B. Saunders Co., 1968.

V

INTERPRETATION OF LABORATORY TESTS

This section discusses the interpretation of results of laboratory tests that vary from normal. It provides information about the possible causes of these variations, and so touches on points of differential diagnosis. However, the discussion is *not* a complete evaluation of the differential merit of each test.

Information here is not intended to give specific directions for performing laboratory tests. For this, the reader should consult standard texts on clinical pathology.

V–1. CEREBROSPINAL FLUID

Analysis of cerebrospinal fluid is a valuable aid in establishing a diagnosis in neurologic disease. Changes in cerebrospinal fluid depend mainly on the location and extent of the lesion.

Cerebrospinal fluid (CSF) in the dog and cat is collected by puncture of the cisterna magna (see Section IV-3). Once the needle has entered the subarachnoid space, a pressure recording manometer should be attached immediately and the opening and closing pressures recorded. Once the pressure has been recorded, remove 2 cc. of CSF for further examination. Normal cerebellomedullary fluid pressure does not exceed 150 mm.

GROSS APPEARANCE

Color

Normal cerebrospinal fluid is clear and colorless. A pinkish or reddish color usually indicates hemorrhage, which may be caused by the spinal tap itself or may be due to central nervous system disease. A yellow or xanthochromic color of the spinal fluid is found in icterus, old hemorrhage, neoplasms, toxoplasmosis, and acute inflammation. In some cases of old hemorrhage, centrifuging the cerebrospinal fluid will reveal the supernatant to be yellow and the sediment to be red or brown. In other cases a clot forms so that there are few loose cells. A gray or green color may indicate suppuration.

Turbidity

A cloudy cerebrospinal fluid usually indicates the presence of a high cell count (pleocytosis). Neutrophils are found in bacterial meningitis, bacterial encephalitis, abscess and hemorrhage. Increased numbers of mononuclear cells are found in the CSF in viral encephalitis, fungal infections, postvaccinal reactions, uremia, and chronic and toxic conditions.

Cytologic examination should be done within 30 minutes after obtaining the sample; otherwise cell disintegration will take place.

Coagulation

Normal cerebrospinal fluid does not coagulate. Increased fibrinogen, found in inflammation such as acute suppurative meningitis, produces coagulation.

PROTEIN

The main protein in normal cerebrospinal fluid is albumin. Increases in the total protein in disease usually reflect increases in the globulin levels. If blood is present within the CSF, the globulin levels will also be high. Protein examination may be qualitative or quantitative. The Pandy test used for qualitative determination of proteins measures only globulins. Quantitative protein determinations are more critical measuring lower levels of protein, including both albumins and globulins. Small amounts of proteins, mainly albumins, are present in the CSF fluid (up to

15 to 25 mg./100 ml.). CSF protein levels above 25 to 30 mg./100 ml. are considered abnormal.

BACTERIOLOGIC EXAMINATION

If the cerebrospinal fluid is turbid, it should be cultured and a Gram or new methylene blue (NMB) stain made. Gram and new methylene blue will also show cryptococci. NMB will also show the capsule. Culture the cerebrospinal fluid on blood agar, in thioglycollate medium, or in Sabouraud's medium, depending upon findings in the direct smear. If the fluid is not turbid, centrifuge it before staining and culturing the sediment. India ink can be used to see the capsule of the cryptococcal organisms in a smear.

References

Additional information can be found in the following sources:

Averill, D. R., Jr.: Examination of the cerebrospinal fluid. *In* Kirk, R. W. (ed.): Current Veterinary Therapy V. Philadelphia, W. B. Saunders Co., 1974.
Kay, W. J., Israel, E., and Prata, R. G.: Cerebrospinal fluid. Veterinary Clin. North Amer. *4*:419–435, 1974.

V–2.   ENDOCRINE FUNCTION

Disturbances in the secretion of some hormones may be recognized clinically if careful attention is given to the history and physical examination. Particular attention should be paid to the rate of growth and physical development; subsequent changes in body weight and conformation and distribution of body fat; sexual development and reproductive performance; changes in physical activity and stamina; the condition of the skin and hair; and the occurrence of polyphagia, polydipsia, or polyuria.

V–2–A.   Adrenal Cortex

Cortisol, corticosterone, and aldosterone, the principal hormones secreted by the adrenal cortex, regulate carbohydrate and electrolyte metabolism. Cortisol is the main glucocorticoid produced by the adrenal cortex and its rate of secretion is controlled primarily by adrenocorticotropin (ACTH) from the adenohypophysis. Aldosterone is the main mineralocorticoid and corticosterone has both mineralo- and glucocorticoid functions.

The Effect of Mineralocorticoids

The mineralocorticoids increase reabsorption of sodium and chloride, increase the excretion of potassium, and allow an exchange of intracellular potassium with extracellular sodium.

The Effect of Glucocorticoids (Cortisol)

1. Protein catabolism is increased, resulting in increased breakdown of muscle protein, interference with the normal production of bone matrix, and increased gluconeogenesis from amino acids.

2. Antibody formation initially increases but is later decreased because of the lysis of lymphocytes and lymph nodes.

3. Blood sugar levels are increased (in some species, but *not* significantly in the dog) because of gluconeogenesis and the metabolism of hepatic fat deposits.

4. Glomerular filtration is increased and an "anti-ADH" effect results in diuresis.

5. Electrolyte effects are evidenced by retention of small amounts of sodium and excretion of potassium.

6. Arteriolar tone and blood pressure are maintained.

Inflammatory reactions are reduced because of a decrease in fibroplasia and a decrease in the production of histamine and histamine-like substances (serotonin).

In the dog only a small proportion of the urinary catabolites of cortisol have a dihydroxy-ketolic side chain and can be measured by the Porter-Silber procedure for 17-hydroxycorticosteroids (17-OHCS). Measurement of urinary 17-ketogenic steroids (17-KGS) permits quantitation of both these and the greater proportion of cortisol metabolites that have a trihydroxy side chain and is therefore preferred in the dog (Siegel).

EVALUATION OF ADRENOCORTICAL FUNCTION

Clinical Syndromes

1. Hyperadrenocorticism is characterized by bilateral, symmetrical, nonpruritic alopecia and polydipsia, polyuria, a pendulous abdomen,

abdominal muscle weakness, a soft and thin skin, and osteoporosis. Polydipsia and polyuria are the earliest signs seen.

2. Hypoadrenocorticoidism is characterized by weakness, weight loss, hypotension, dehydration, gastrointestinal upsets, and the development of a "shock-like" condition.

Laboratory Tests

The total leukocyte, differential, hematocrit, and total eosinophil count should be evaluated. Serum sodium, potassium, chloride, urea, and protein determinations may be valuable too.

In hyperadrenocorticism there is a lymphopenia, eosinopenia, and slight hyperglycemia. Electrolyte disturbances are not common but may include hypokalemia. Liver function may be altered, resulting in fatty livers and hypercholestrolemia, increased serum alkaline phosphatase, and increased serum glutamic-pyruvic transaminase.

In hypoadrenocorticism there is a relative lymphocytosis and an elevated hematocrit; eosinophilia is not a consistent finding. Hyponatremia, hypochloremia, hyperkalemia, and elevated blood urea levels may also be found.

The Electrocardiogram

1. In hyperadrenocorticism with hypokalemia, the Q-T interval is prolonged and U waves may be seen.

2. In hypoadrenocorticism with hyperkalemia (serum potassium between 6 and 7 mEq./liter) the T waves may become increased in amplitude, spike, and narrow based. Serum potassium levels of 7 and 8 mEq./liter produce a depression of the P wave. Serum potassium levels above 8 mEq./liter produce bradycardia (50 to 70 beats/minute), absence of P waves, and a widened QRS wave.

Analysis of Adrenocortical Hormones

Plasma Cortisol Determinations

Plasma cortisol levels can be valuable diagnostic aids in hyperadrenocorticism. Both fluorometric and competitive protein binding techniques are available for assaying plasma cortisols. Normal values vary for each technique. There is good evidence that a diurnal or circadian rhythm in plasma cortisol levels exists in dogs. Tests are taken both before injection and two hours after intramuscular injection of 40 units ACTH gel. Most adrenal cortical tumors are unresponsive to ACTH, and little difference is found between control and post-ACTH values.

Plasma cortisol values for the fluorometric technique are: normal dog (control), 2 to 15 μg./100 ml.; after ACTH stimulation, 3.0 to 14.9 μg./100 ml. Hyperadrenocorticism control, 7.3 to 52.4 μg./100 ml.; after ACTH, 28.4 to 92 μg./100 ml.

Plasma cortisol values for the CPB (competitive protein binding) technique are: normal dog (control), 0.2 to 2.5 μg./100 ml.; after ACTH, 0.3 to 7.3 μg./100 ml. Hyperadrenocorticism control, 1.9 to 4.8 μg./100 ml.; post-ACTH, 17.5 to 30 μg./100 ml.

Dogs with adrenal insufficiency have low normal control values and show little or no response to ACTH stimulation.

17-Ketogenic Steroid Determinations

This test measures the metabolic by-products of glucocorticoids that are excreted in the urine. Twenty-four hour urine collections are necessary. Control urinary excretion in the normal dog is 2.1 to 7.0 mg./24 hrs. After 20 units of ACTH gel is given intramuscularly, a normal response is an increase of 0.1 to 4 mg./day above the control level. Control urinary excretion in the dog with hyperadrenocorticism may be normal or elevated. After ACTH stimulation, a value at least double the control is found.

Adrenocortical tumors have been found to produce constant levels of steroids that are not increased after administering ACTH.

Dexamethasone Suppression Test

Obtain resting or control plasma cortisol value at 9 A.M. Give 0.1 mg./kg. Dexamethasone orally at 9 P.M. At 9 A.M. the following day, obtain a second plasma cortisol sample. Normal dogs show the following values after suppression: fluorometric, 1.5 to 6.5 μg./100 ml.; CPB, up to 1.2 μg./100 ml. Hyperadrenal dogs give these values following suppression: fluorometric, > 5 μg./100 ml.; CPB, > 1.5 μg./100 ml.

Most normal dogs depress to 50 per cent or greater from the resting level.

EVALUATION OF THE PITUITARY-ADRENAL AXIS

The differentiation between primary and secondary hyperadrenocorticism can be accomplished by measuring residual pituitary ACTH reserve (Fig. 72). This is done by administering Metyrapone, which inhibits β, hydroxylation by the adrenal gland, and thus decreases the

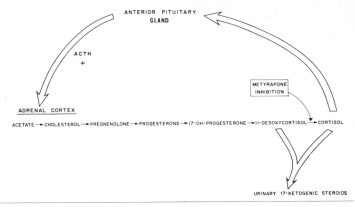

Figure 72. Evaluation of residual adrenocorticotropin (ACTH) reserve in the pituitary gland. (From Siegel, E. T.: Assessment of the pituitary-adrenal gland function in the dog. Amer. J. Vet. Res. 29: 173–179, January, 1968,)

synthesis of cortisol. Metyrapone is administered in a single oral dose of 100 mg./kg. after at least one 24 hour control collection of urine, and collections are then made for two succeeding 24 hour periods.

In the presence of a normal pituitary-adrenal gland axis, the decrease in blood cortisol levels produced by Metyrapone causes an increased secretion of ACTH. The increased ACTH production stimulates normal adrenal glands to produce elevated levels of the precursors of cortisol, which can be measured as urinary 17-ketogenic steroids. A negative or decreased response to Metyrapone can be seen in hypopituitarism, in a defect in the negative feedback mechanism, with autonomous adrenocortical tumors, or with autonomous ACTH pituitary-secreting tumors (unresponsive). An increased response to Metyrapone can be seen in primary adrenal hyperplasia, responsive pituitary tumors, and functional hyperpituitarism (Siegel).

V–2–B. The Posterior Pituitary

Antidiuretic hormone or vasopressin and the oxytocic hormone involved in parturition are both produced in the hypothalamus and released from the pars nervosa of the pituitary.

The Effect of Antidiuretic Hormone

Antidiuretic hormone release is controlled by changes in the extracellular fluid osmotic pressure, by direct nervous stimulation of the hypothalamus, and by changes in the extracellular fluid volume.

ADH increases renal tubular reabsorption of solute free water and can also raise blood pressure by constricting arteries and capillaries.

DIABETES INSIPIDUS

Diabetes insipidus is a syndrome of excessive excretion of water due to insufficient production or release of antidiuretic hormone. There are two prerequisites to a diagnosis of diabetes insipidus:

1. Persistent diuresis in the presence of stimuli that normally provoke the secretion of ADH.

2. Antidiuresis in response to administered ADH.

The release of ADH and its effect upon the urine should be measured in terms of the urine and plasma osmolality rather than in specific gravity. (Osmolality is a measurement of the number of particles in a given weight of fluid and is proportional to the osmotic pressure of that fluid. Osmolality is measured by freezing point depression in an osmometer.)

Tests for Diabetes Insipidus

Withhold food and fluids from the patient for eight hours and measure the osmolality of plasma and of urine *formed at that time*. If the urine osmolality is greater than that of the plasma at the end of this period, diabetes insipidus is eliminated as a diagnosis. The patient must be kept under very close observation during this period, as animals with diabetes insipidus or chronic interstitial nephritis may become dehydrated and decompensated rapidly. If urine osmolality is not distinctly greater than that of plasma at the end of eight hours, deprivation of food and water may be continued for an additional four hours and the measurements repeated. Animals that are debilitated or in whom it is suspected that water deprivation will precipitate a uremic crisis should not be subjected to water deprivation. The aqueous vasopressin test (although not as accurate as water deprivation and more sophisticated tests) should be used.

If there is no response to fluid restriction, the response to vasopressin should be measured.

Vasopressin Response Tests
Aqueous Vasopressin Test.

1. Inject subcutaneously one-fourth unit of aqueous vasopressin per kilogram of body weight, up to a maximum of 5 units.

2. Withhold fluids and food during test period (2 hours).

3. Empty the bladder immediately and collect all urine at 30, 60, 90, and 120 minute intervals after the administration of ADH.

Although precise responses for dogs to this test have not been established, a urine specific gravity value of 1.020 to 1.025 or higher represents a normal response.

Intravenous Vasopressin Test

1. Withhold food for 12 hours but permit water free choice.

2. Administer water load of 15 ml./lb. by stomach tube. Diuresis should occur within one hour.

3. Empty bladder one hour after water load and obtain plasma and urine sample after another 10 minutes.

4. Dilute 10 units of aqueous vasopressin (Pitressin-Vasopressin injection, Parke, Davis & Co.) in 500 ml. of sterile isotonic saline. This provides a solution containing 20 milliunits/ml. The dilute solution should be prepared immediately before use.

5. Administer 2 milliunits of vasopressin/lb. intravenously (0.1 ml. of the dilute solution/pound).

6. Empty bladder 30 minutes after injection of vasopressin and obtain urine sample and plasma sample after another ten minutes.

A rise in urine osmolality to a level above plasma osmolality demonstrates normal renal tubular responsiveness to ADH.

Infusion of Hypertonic Saline

Infusion of hypertonic saline may also be used to determine whether antidiuretic hormone can be released, but is rarely required and should be employed with some caution.

1. Withhold food for 12 hours (however, water may be given free choice).

2. Administer 15 ml. of water/pound by stomach tube.

3. One hour later, urine and plasma samples are collected and the osmolality checked. An indwelling catheter is left in the bladder.

4. Five milliliters per pound of 5 per cent saline is administered intravenously over a period of 30 minutes *under close observation*. (This infusion occasionally produces mild to moderately severe seizures and should be discontinued immediately if they occur.)

5. At the 15 and 30 minute marks after the infusion, urine and plasma

samples are collected and their osmolality checked. The hypertonic saline will cause a rise in plasma osmolality and urine osmolality must be increased to above that of the corresponding plasma sample to demonstrate antidiuretic hormone secretion (Bullock).

Differential Diagnosis of Diabetes Insipidus

Chronic interstitial nephritis and psychogenic polydipsia may simulate diabetes insipidus. In chronic interstitial nephritis there is adequate antidiuretic hormone secretion but the damaged renal tissue cannot concentrate the urine normally and there is no response to endogenous antidiuretic hormone or exogenous vasopressin. In psychogenic polydipsia, the capacity for producing antidiuretic hormone is intact but the constant intake of water suppresses the release of antidiuretic hormone. In this case, water deprivation results in a rise of urine osmolality, demonstrating adequate endogenous antidiuretic hormone as well as functioning kidneys. (See Section II-18.)

V-2-C. The Thyroid Gland

Thyroid hormone affects the rate of metabolism, growth, and development. Thyroxine and triiodothyronine are iodinated amino acids and their synthesis and secretion are principally under the control of thyroid stimulating hormone. Thyroxine is transported in the blood of the dog by at least four serum proteins. A normally functioning thyroid gland requires both adequate endogenous thyroid stimulating hormone secretion and normal glandular function to produce adequate amounts of thyroxine. Minute amounts of thyroxine are produced independently of thyroid stimulating hormone production, however.

Normal level of blood thyroxine in the dog is about 2.00 to 4.00 μg./100 ml. of serum and in the cat it is about 1.5 to 3.5 μg./100 ml. PBI levels would then be about 2.00 μg./100 ml. for the dog and around 1.60 μg./100 ml. for the cat.

EVALUATING THYROID FUNCTION

Clinical Signs of Hypothyroidism

Hypothyroidism is characterized by lethargy and easy fatigability, intolerance to cold, changes in skin and hair coat, abnormal estrous cycle, infertility, decreased libido, constipation or mild diarrhea, bradycardia, gain in weight and occasionally, mild—usually subclinical—anemia.

Laboratory Tests

1. The thyroid gland's ability to trap iodide can be evaluated by its ability to take up radioiodine (^{131}I). This procedure is limited to institutions that are equipped to perform this work. Thyroid uptake of radio-iodine in most adult dogs reaches a maximum of from 10 to 30 per cent of the dose by 72 hours (exception is the Basenji, which peaks at 24 hours). Diminished uptake of ^{131}I may be caused by primary hypothyroidism, as in atrophy of the thyroid, or by a deficiency of thyroid stimulating hormone. Recent exposure to high levels of iodine in the diet or in medications also depresses radioactive iodine uptake in the diet and hence invalidates the test.

2. Thyroid function also can be evaluated by measuring the protein-bound iodine in the blood, although this is not specific for thyroidal hormone in the dog. The high levels of inorganic iodide in the blood *of dogs* must be removed before the final protein-bound iodine assays are made.

Contamination by iodine-containing drugs and diagnostic agents must be avoided. Tincture of iodine (residues may persist for four to six weeks), disophenol (DNP residues may persist for nine to 12 months), and radiographic contrast media such as Hypaque, Diodrast, Telepaque, and thyroxine may erroneously elevate the protein-bound iodine. Mercurial diuretics interfere with the laboratory procedure, and propylthiouracil will depress protein-bound iodine levels.

Normal protein-bound iodine values in dogs range from 1.2 to 3.6 μg. per cent with a mean of 2.4 μg. per cent. The total serum iodine should be measured together with the protein-bound iodine.

Normal total serum iodine in the dog ranges from 5 to 20 μg. per cent with a mean of 10 μg. per cent. If the total serum iodine exceeds 20 μg. per cent, the protein-bound iodine value may be spuriously elevated because of an abnormally high inorganic iodide content and should not be considered valid.

In hypothyroid dogs the protein-bound iodine ranges from 0 to 2.0 μg. per cent and the total serum iodine from about 0.5 to 7.5 μg per cent. It must be emphasized that the error or variability in protein-bound iodine measurements in the dog is probably of the order of 0.5 μg. per cent even with laboratories having considerable experience and adequate quality controls. Thus, a protein-bound iodine reported to be 1.6 μg. per cent may actually be from 1.1 to 2.1 μg. per cent. This probably accounts for some of the overlap in values between euthyroid and hypothyroid dogs (i.e., values between 1.2 and 2.0 μg. per cent) and although it would appear to limit greatly the value of this measurement in diagnosis, in fact it seldom does.

3. The response to exogenous thyroid stimulating hormone injection is of some value in differentiating primary hypothyroidism from hypothyroidism secondary to hypopituitarism, and is particularly useful in the interpretation of initial protein-bound iodine values in the range of 1.2 to 2.0 μg. per cent (the range of overlap between hypothyroid and euthyroid dogs). Elevation of the protein-bound iodine (or the uptake of radioiodine) following thyroid stimulating hormone administration may be used to measure the response.

A control serum sample should be collected. Then 5 to 10 units of thyroid stimulating hormone is given intramuscularly. A second serum sample should be obtained 12 hours following the injection of thyroid stimulating hormone. With protein-bound iodine determinations following thyroid stimulating hormone administration, it has been found that euthyroid adult dogs have an average increase of 3.0 μg. per cent and animals with primary hypothyroidism rarely have an increase above 0.5 μg. per cent. Dogs with hypothyroidism secondary to hypopituitarism may need a series of injections of TSH for a three day period before a response is seen. If no response is seen after three days, primary hypothyroidism may exist.

It must be emphasized that the data on protein-bound iodine determinations quoted here pertain to tests run by two laboratories.* Results from other laboratories have *not* been consistent with those obtained from these two (Belshaw).

4. The determination of serum cholesterol values is not a specific test for hypothyroidism (see Section V-4). Although hypercholesterolemia has been found in one-half to two-thirds of the dogs with hypothyroidism, a normal serum cholesterol does not rule out the possibility of hypothyroidism. Serum cholesterol determinations should be coupled with other thyroid function tests.

In Vitro ^{131}I-Triiodothyronine Uptake (T-3)

The resin sponge uptake of triiodothyronine ([125]I T-3) from serum is an indirect indicator of thyroid function. The test indicates the saturation of thyroid-binding globulin. It has been used as a screening test in thyroid dysfunction in dogs; however, it is not extremely sensitive to small changes in thyroid function and it gives false results when there are

---

*Boston Medical Laboratory, Bay Street Road, Boston, Mass., 02115, and Leonard's Medical Laboratory, 4568 Mayfield Road, Cleveland, Ill., 44121.

abnormal levels of serum proteins or when the A-G ratio is changed. Unsaturation of thyroid binding globulin in hypothyroidism allows less ^{131}I T-3 to enter red cells in vitro. Current techniques using resin T-3 uptake have different values; however, reported values for T-3 in the dog are 42 to 60 per cent and 61 to 76 per cent in the cat.

T-4 Test

This test determines the total circulating serum thyroxine level, which is the best indicator of functional status of the thyroid. It is superior to the T-3 test, since it is not affected by the protein level of the patients. Thyroxine levels in the serum may be determined by two methods: column chromatography (T-4 column) and competitive protein binding (T-4 CPB). Normal values for the dog by T-4 column are 0.9 to 2.3 μg./100 ml. and by T-4 CPB are 2.0 to 6.0 μg./100 ml. The anthelmintic DNP will falsely elevate the T-4 column values. The only drug known to interfere with the T-4 CPB test is the anticonvulsant diphenylhydantoin. The T-4 tests (specifically competitive protein binding) are more accurate indicators of thyroid function because contaminating non-organic iodine does not influence the test. Normal values for the dog are 2.0 to 6.0 μg. thyroxine/100 ml. serum (slightly less in older dogs) and 1.50 to 3.50 μg. thyroxine/100 ml. in the cat. If laboratory results are reported in micrograms of thyroxine iodine, then these values must be multiplied by 1.53 to find the normal range.

T-4 determinations made by competitive protein binding technique are coupled with response to TSH administration to assess thyroid function. At least a two-fold increase above normal T-4 levels is expected 12 hours following TSH administration in the normal dog.

Thyroid Gland Biopsy

This procedure is very helpful in confirming the diagnosis of hypothyroidism and in distinguishing primary from secondary hypothyroidism. Since most cases of hypothyroidism in dogs are due to primary atrophy of the thyroid or destructive thyroiditis, biopsy of the thyroid is nearly equal in diagnostic value to measurement of PBI or radioiodine uptake. Furthermore, it often provides confirmatory evidence in cases in which the results of other tests are equivocal or are invalidated by iodine contamination.

V–2–D.   The Parathyroid Glands

The production of parathormone by the parathyroid glands varies inversely with the plasma level of ionized calcium. Parathormone increases calcium and phosphorus reabsorption from bones, increases calcium reabsorption and phosphate excretion in renal tubules, and increases absorption of calcium from the gastrointestinal tract. Parathyroid function can be assessed indirectly by radiographs of the long bones, the skull, and the teeth. In hyperparathyroidism, radiographs reveal generalized osteodystrophia fibrosa with bone cysts, loss of the lamina dura from around the teeth, and possible pathologic fractures. The measurement of serum calcium (see Section V-3-L-9), serum phosphorus (see Section V-3-L-12), and serum alkaline phosphatase (see Section V-3-L-17) is helpful in evaluating parathyroid function.

V–2–E.   The Islets of Langerhans

The islets of Langerhans secrete two hormones that have important functions in intermediary metabolism. Glucagon is a polypeptide hormone that elevates blood glucose by stimulating hepatic glycogenolysis. It may help maintain blood glucose levels during starvation.

Insulin is a protein hormone that lowers blood glucose levels and facilitates the entry of blood glucose into muscle and many other tissues. Changes in blood glucose levels produce reciprocal changes in the levels of these two hormones. Many other hormones are important in regulating carbohydrate metabolism.

GLUCOSE TOLERANCE TEST EVALUATING GLUCOSE METABOLISM

The glucose tolerance test is indicated to help confirm a diagnosis of diabetes mellitus when other tests are equivocal. Either the oral or the intravenous test may be used.

The oral glucose tolerance test in the dog is started by obtaining a base-line, fasting blood sugar. Next, 1.0 g. of glucose/lb. of body weight is administered in a solution through a stomach tube. Blood samples are taken at 30, 60, 120, 180, and 240 minutes. In nondiabetic animals who have been on a high carbohydrate intake for three days prior to testing, the fasting blood sugar is less than 110 mg./100 ml. It does not rise above 160 mg./100 ml. at the end of the first hour and returns to normal by the end of the second hour. In diabetic animals, the base-line, fasting blood sugar is usually over 150 mg./100 ml., rises markedly during the test, and does not return to pretest levels within two hours.

The intravenous glucose tolerance test is conducted in much the same way as the oral glucose tolerance test, but a smaller dose, 0.25 g. of glucose/lb. of body weight in a 50 per cent sterile solution, is injected intravenously over a period of five minutes. A base-line fasting blood sugar should be determined and blood samples are then taken at 15, 30, 60, 90, 120, 180, and 240 minutes following administration. In the intravenous glucose tolerance test, there is no absorptive phase and glucose levels will normally return to the base-line earlier (by one hour) than in the oral glucose tolerance test. The two hour limit applies, however, in diagnosing diabetes mellitus.

PROVOCATIVE TESTS FOR INSULIN RELEASE

Several diagnostic tests have been utilized to document the diagnosis of hypoglycemia secondary to functional beta cell tumors in dogs. The tolbutamide tolerance test and the glucagon tolerance test have proved useful.

Tolbutamide Tolerance Test

Tolbutamide directly stimulates the release of insulin from the pancreatic beta cells and is valuable in the differential diagnosis of hypoglycemia caused by a pancreatic islet cell tumor. After an overnight fast, a control blood glucose is taken. Then 1 gm. of tolbutamide/65 lb. is given intravenously in 20 cc. of saline. Blood samples for glucose are collected at 10-minute intervals for the first 30 minutes and then every half hour for 3 hours. Dogs with insulin producing neoplasms have 70 per cent or more decrease in the blood glucose level and will sustain this level for 3 hours or more. The test involves considerable risk to the patient because severe and sustained hypoglycemia is produced. Close observation of the patient is mandatory in order to prevent severe seizures or coma from developing.

Glucagon Tolerance Test

The hormone glucagon raises the blood sugar by stimulating glycogenolysis of liver glycogen. The elevation of blood glucose thus stimulates the release of insulin from pancreatic beta cells. Glucagon also has a secondary effect to directly stimulate the release of insulin from pancreatic beta cells. These two effects of glucagon are utilized in the glucagon tolerance test for functional beta cell tumors in dogs. A fasting blood sample is taken and then 0.03 mg./kg. glucagon is given intravenously. Blood samples for glucose are taken at five minutes, then 15, 30, 45, 60, 90, 120, and 180 minutes. In the normal dog, a rise in blood glucose occurs initially and returns to the control level in two to three hours. In dogs with functional beta cell tumors, an initial rise in the blood glucose occurs in five to 15 minutes. By 60 minutes, the blood glucose usually falls to levels below the control sample. On occasion, severe hypoglycemia may develop and intravenous glucose can be given to prevent seizures from occurring. This test has been used in a limited number of cases, but it appears to be a safer procedure than the tolbutamide tolerance test.

References

Additional information can be found in the following sources:

Campbell, J. R., and Watts, C.: Assessment of adrenal function in dogs. Brit. Vet. J. *129*:134-144, 1973.

Gorman, C. K.: Hypoglycemia: A brief review. Med. Clin. N. Amer. July, 1971.

Halliwell, R. E. W., et al.: The value of plasma corticosteroid assays in the diagnosis of Cushing's disease in the dog. J. Small Anim. Pract. *12*:453–462, 1971.

Hoge, W. R., Lund, J. E., and Blakemore, J. C.: Response to thyrotropin as a diagnostic aid for canine hypothyroidism. JAAHA *10*:167–170, 1974.

Kallfelz, F. A.: Comparison of the ^{125}T-3 and ^{125}T-4 tests in the diagnosis of thyroid gland function in the dog. JAVMA *154*:22–25, 1969.

Kallfelz, F. A.: Determination of total serum thyroxine in the dog by competitive protein binding of labelled thyroxine. Amer. J. Vet. Res. *30*:929–932, 1969.

Kaneko, J. J., and Cornelius, C. E.: Clinical Biochemistry of Domestic Animals, 2nd ed. New York, Academic Press, Inc., 1971.

Kirk, R. W. (ed.): Current Veterinary Therapy V. Philadelphia, W. B. Saunders Co., 1974.

Krook, L.: Metabolic bone diseases. *In* Kirk, R. W. (ed.): Current Veterinary Therapy V. Philadelphia, W. B. Saunders Co., 1974.

Osborne, C. A., Low, D. G., and Finco, D. R.: Canine and Feline Urology. Philadelphia, W. B. Saunders Co., 1972.

Siegel, E. T.: Assessment of the pituitary-adrenal gland function in the dog. Amer. J. Vet. Res. *29*:173–179, 1968.

Siegel, E. T., et al.: Cushing's syndrome in the dog. JAVMA *157*:2081–2090, 1970.

V–3. HEMATOLOGY: INTERPRETATION OF LABORATORY FINDINGS

Hematology is the branch of medicine that deals with the relationship of changes in the hemogram to underlying primary or secondary disease states and includes the study of morphology of the blood and blood-forming tissues.

Hematologic studies in veterinary medicine have five major functions:

1. To confirm the diagnosis of the presence or absence of a blood abnormality.

2. To determine the extent of the disease process.

3. To find out why there is a blood abnormality.

4. To serve as a guide in the prognosis of clinical cases.

5. To serve as a guide during therapy in the treatment of clinical disorders.

This section on hematology covers the interpretation of results obtained from hematologic examination. It includes evaluation of the erythron, evaluation of the leukogram, leukemias, sedimentation rate, coagulation disorders, blood parasites, and blood chemistry.

V–3–A. Evaluation of the Erythron

The erythron refers to the circulating erythrocytes in the blood, their precursors, and all the elements of the body concerned with their production. Abnormalities in the erythron may manifest themselves as anemia, polycythemia, hemodilution, or hemoconcentration (Fig. 73).

TESTS

There are several basic tests that enable one to evaluate the state of the erythron.

The Hematocrit (Packed Cell Volume)

This test measures the relative red blood cell mass. It is a most accurate test (error of 1 to 2 per cent). The use of the microhematocrit enables one to use a small amount of blood and conduct the test rapidly.

Following high-speed centrifugation, the blood in the hematocrit tube will be divided into three layers: the bottom or packed erythrocyte layer,

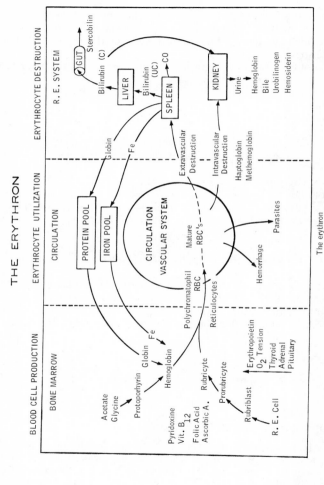

Figure 73. The erythron. (Used by permission of Dr. John Switzer.)

the middle or buffy coat containing leukocytes and thrombocytes, and the upper plasma layer.

The hemoglobin concentration can be predicted from the packed cell volume (PCV) in all conditions except iron deficiency anemia and during the remission phase of acute blood loss and hemolytic anemia. The value of the hemoglobin is approximately equal to one third the packed cell volume. The approximate total erythrocyte count (normocytic, normo- chromic erythrocytes) can be estimated by dividing the packed cell vol- ume by 1/6.

Approximate leukocyte counts can be made by measuring the buffy coat (useful only in the Wintrobe hematocrit tube). The first millimeter of the buffy coat is equal to approximately 10,000 leukocytes and each additional 0.1 mm. equals 2000 leukocytes/cu. mm. (This is only a means of obtaining a rough estimation of the total leukocyte count.)

Always examine the color of the plasma layer in the hematocrit tube: a yellow plasma may indicate icterus, a pale to colorless plasma may indicate bone marrow depression, a cloudy plasma may indicate lipemia, and a red-tinged plasma is indicative of hemolysis. The PCV varies with the age of the animal, the breed, the state of nutrition, the environment, the degree of activity, and the state of hydration. Care should be taken to avoid anticoagulant excess (EDTA), as this can result in a reduction of the PCV by as much as 25 per cent.

Hemoglobin

This test measures the oxygen carrying ability of the erythrocytes. Although many different ways of measuring the hemoglobin content are available, no one is absolutely accurate.

Erythrocyte Counts

This determination is the most inaccurate of the tests used to evaluate the erythron (the error may be as high as 20 to 40 per cent). Red blood cell numbers vary with the age of the animal and, in general, total RBC count is utilized only in obtaining red blood cell indices.

Red Blood Cell Indices

These values are based on knowing the PCV, total red blood cell count and hemoglobin. Since both the total red blood cell count and hemoglobin suffer from inaccuracies, the blood cell indices may also reflect these inaccuracies. Basically, these indices determine whether the erythrocyte population is made up of small cells, large cells or cells with adequate or inadequate amounts of hemoglobin. The average volume of erythrocytes is called the mean corpuscular volume. The average weight of hemoglobin in the average cell is called the mean corpuscular hemoglobin. The mean corpuscular hemoglobin concentration is the percentage concentration of hemoglobin in the red cell mass. The same basic information obtained in the red blood cell indices may also be obtained subjectively by careful examination of the blood smear.

$$\text{Mean corpuscular volume} = \frac{\text{PCV in ml. per 1000 ml.}}{\text{red cell count, millions per cu. mm.}}$$

$$\text{Mean corpuscular hemoglobin} = \frac{\text{hemoglobin in gm. per 1000 ml.}}{\text{red cell count, millions per cu. mm.}}$$

$$\text{Mean corpuscular hemoglobin concentration} = \frac{\text{hemoglobin in gm. per 100 ml. times 100}}{\text{PCV in ml. per 100 ml.}}$$

Blood Smears and Erythrocyte Morphology

Thin blood smears utilizing a good staining technique are needed to evaluate the morphology of red blood cells. Examine the smear and evaluate the size, shape, and color of the erythrocytes and the presence of any intra- or extracellular parasites.

Anisocytosis refers to an abnormal variation in the size of the red blood cells, owing to the presence of both mature and immature red blood cells in the circulation. It may be slight, moderate, or marked.

Poikilocytosis refers to any unusual shape of the red blood cells. This usually occurs in chronic anemia in which the red blood cells are not stable and undergo fragmentation and indicates premature destruction of erythrocytes or defective erythrocyte formation.

Polychromatophilia refers to the bluish tinge of young red blood cells.

Howell-Jolly bodies are remnants of nuclear material found in young red blood cells.

Normoblasts are immature red blood cells, both orthochromophilic and polychromatophilic, that contain hemoglobin, are nucleated and are capable of carrying oxygen. They indicate that immature red blood cells are in demand. Since nucleated red blood cells are ordinarily counted as leukocytes in the process of counting white blood cells, the white blood cell count should be corrected for circulating normoblasts.

Leptocytes are thin erythrocytes whose surface area has been increased without an increase in cell volume, giving the cell distinctive morphologic characteristics. The cells are usually seen in chronic disease leading to anemia. "Target cells" are a form of leptocyte seen most frequently in the dog.

Hypochromasia refers to a decrease of hemoglobin in erythrocytes. In Wright's or Giemsa stained smears, the cells appear abnormally pale.

Punctate basophilia or stippling of the erythrocytes may be due to degenerative changes in the cytoplasm involving RNA in the young cells. Stippling may also occur in lead poisoning.

Spherocytes are red blood cells of decreased diameter in relationship to their volume. They appear hyperchromatic, and lack central pallor. They are seen in autoimmune hemolytic anemia.

Reticulocytes are immature, nonnucleated erythrocytes that still retain basophilic staining material (RNA). These cells can only be identified by supravital staining methods, such as with new methylene blue stain. The degree of reticulocyte count indicates increased erythrogenesis. The cat has a delayed maturation time for reticulocytes. Peak levels of reticulocytes are reached after 11 days (following blood loss of 50 per cent). The normal reticulocyte count in the cat ranges from 1.4 to 10.8 per cent, with a mean of 4.6 per cent.

Erythrocyte refractile bodies (ERB) are round or angular refractile bodies seen in the erythrocytes of sick cats when the blood smears are stained with new methylene blue. The refractile bodies are 1 to 3 μ in diameter and are located at the periphery of the cell. They probably are the same as Heinz bodies and reflect denatured hemoglobin. The red cells exhibiting ERB bodies may have shortened life spans.

The life span of red blood cells for the dog is approximately 120 days, and for the cat approximately 75 days. The stimulus for increased red blood cell production is persistent anoxia at the level of the renal cortex resulting in the elaboration of the hormone erythropoietin by the kidney.

V–3–B. Anemias

Anemia is a condition in which there is a diminution in the numbers of erythrocytes or a deficiency in hemoglobin or both. It is a clinical sign of disease, not a diagnosis. The significant clinical signs associated with anemia are pallor, weakness, collapse and shortness of breath, tachycar-

TABLE 55. PRELIMINARY CLASSIFICATION OF ANEMIA*

Preliminary Classification of Anemia

Responsive

Reticulocytosis
Polychromasia
Nucleated red blood cells
Marrow — erythroid hyperplasia

Blood Loss

Platelets Normal	Platelets Decreased
Trauma	I.T.P.
G.I. bleeding	Amegakaryocytic
Hemophilia	Thrombotic t.p.
Hypofibrin	Thrombopathic
Fibrinolysins	(von Willebrand's)
G.I. parasites: hookworms	

No Blood Loss

Hemolytic
Decreased RBC life span
± Icteric

Coombs Negative		Coombs Positive
Blood parasites	No blood parasites	Increased saline fragility
Babesia	Symptomatic hemolytic anemia	Spherocytosis
Hemobartonella	Bacterial disease	
Anaplasmosis	Leptospirosis	Autoimmune hemolytic anemia
Malaria	Septicemia	Lupus erythematosus
	Subacute bacterial endocarditis	
	Viral disease	
	Equine infectious anemia	
	Hypersplenism	
	Neonatal ischemolytic anemia	
	Porphyria	
	Postpartum hemoglobinuria	
	Lead poisoning	

Nonresponsive or Inadequate Response

Erythroid Precursors Decreased or Absent

Aplastic
Hypoplastic
Myelofibrosis
Myelophthesic
  Leukemia
  Myeloma
  Reticulosarcoma
  Metastatic carcinoma

Erythroid Precursors Present

Megaloblastic
  Vit. B_{12}, folic acid
Megaloblastoid
  Vit. B_6 — sideroblastic
  Vit. E — nuclear abnormalities
Normoblastic
  Iron deficiency
  Chronic disease
    Chronic interstitial nephritis
    Liver disease
    Pancreas
    Tumors
    Abscesses
    Distemper
  Hormonal
    Thyroid
    Adrenal
    Pituitary
Refractory
  Ineffective erythropoiesis
Malabsorption
  Sprue
Erythroleukemia (di Guglielmo's)

*Used by permission of Dr. John Switzer.

dia, systolic bruits, and malaise. Anemia, a sign of disease, should not be treated without first trying to understand and eliminate the cause of the anemia.

Anemias may be classified in two basic ways: either by morphology or by etiology.

ETIOLOGIC CLASSIFICATION

Anemias can be subdivided into two categories on the basis of (1) excessive loss of erythrocytes due to hemorrhage or hemolysis, and (2) inadequate production of erythrocytes.

Blood Loss Anemias

The anemia of acute blood loss occurs when 25 to 40 per cent of the circulating blood volume is lost over a relatively short period of time. Blood loss anemia may result from overt hemorrhage following trauma or surgery, clotting defects or rupture of highly vascular malignant tumors such as hemangioendotheliomas. Chronic loss of blood from parasitism may also result in blood loss anemia. Acute uncomplicated blood loss anemia exhibits a marked regenerative response and the anemia is characteristically normochromic-normocytic. Chronic blood loss anemia associated with parasitisms, gastrointestinal bleeding, or genitourinary tract bleeding may result in a hypochromic, microcytic anemia.

The response of the dog to acute external blood loss is predictable. By the third day following blood loss, reticulocytes in increased numbers are present in the peripheral blood. Peak reticulocyte response occurs between the fifth and sixth day. Normoblasts, Howell-Jolly bodies and anisocytosis are also markedly evident at the time of peak reticulocyte response. Packed cell volume increases from the fourth day to the twenty-first day, after which it is normal. Cats do not respond as rapidly to blood loss, and the peripheral blood smears do not reflect marked polychromasia and anisocytosis.

Internal blood loss into body cavities results in marked absorption by the lymphatics so that two-thirds of the lost blood may be absorbed in 24 hours and the balance completely absorbed after 48 to 72 hours.

Hemolysis

Hemolytic anemias are characterized by an increased level of serum bilirubin, especially unconjugated bilirubin; hemoglobinuria; and an elevated icterus index.

Hemolytic anemias can be caused by parasites such as Babesia and Hemobartonella (see Section V-3-K); chemical agents such as copper, lead, and phenothiazines (see Section 1-19); infections with hemolytic agents such as *Leptospira icterohemorrhagica;* and autoimmune hemolytic anemia or isoimmunization such as neonatal isoerythrolysis.

Hemolytic anemias can be peracute, acute or chronic. In the peracute cases, all signs of regeneration are absent and jaundice and hemoglobinuria may rapidly develop. The spleen may be congested and markedly enlarged.

Acute hemolytic anemia may develop over a period of one week and regenerative signs are usually prominent; jaundice is usually present. A

TABLE 56. HEMOLYTIC ANEMIA*

Type	Red blood cell parasites	Bacterial and viral diseases	Autoimmune hemolytic anemia	Abnormal red blood cell metabolism	Symptomatic Idiopathic hemolytic
Marrow	Erythroid hyperplasia	Erythroid hyperplasia	Erythroid hyperplasia There may be depression	Erythroid hyperplasia	Erythroid hyperplasia
Peripheral blood reticulocytosis nucleated red blood cells polychromasia	Demonstration of parasites Animal inoculation	Morphology: normal siderocytes (EIA)	Spherocytes Poikilocytes Red blood cell fragments	Normochromic Normocytic	Normocytic Normochromic
White blood count	Moderate neutrophilia Atypical lymphocytes	Neutrophilia with left shift Viral – leukopenia, lymphocytosis	Moderate neutrophilia	Normal	Normal to elevated
Platelets	Normal	Normal	Normal to decreased with ITP	Normal	Normal
Saline fragility	Normal to slight increase	Normal to extreme fragility Autohemolysis marked	Increased fragility with characteristic curve	Normal Autohemolysis corrected with glucose or ATP	Usually normal
Coombs test	Negative	Negative	Positive	Negative	Negative

*Used by permission of Dr. John Switzer.

neutrophilic leukocytosis is present, indicating a generalized bone marrow response. In cases of autoimmune hemolytic anemia, rouleaux formation and spherocytosis may be present.

Chronic hemolytic anemia is usually associated with marked intracellular damage and damaged cells are removed by the spleen. Hemolysis is usually not evident when examining the plasma; however, the presence of icterus is common.

Congenital hemolytic anemia has been described in the Basenji dog. It is usually recognized in the first year of life. In this particular anemia, there is intense regeneration, characterized by marked reticulocytosis, anisocytosis and polychromasia. The MCV is elevated (80 to 110 μ^3) and MCHC is low. This form of congenital hemolytic anemia is associated with an impairment of red cell glycolysis because of abnormal pyruvate kinase. Inadequate production of ATP leads to loss of normal membrane integrity and increased osmotic fragility.

It has been demonstrated that methylene blue, present in some urinary antiseptics, can produce Heinz body hemolytic anemia in cats four to 10 days after the substance is given to the cat. The methylene blue acts on reduced glutathione to cause oxidative denaturation of the globin portion of the hemoglobin molecule.

Depression Anemia

Bone marrow depression anemias are those anemias in which erythrocytes are produced at a decreased rate, or are improperly formed within the bone marrow. The anemia may be hypoplastic if there is partial or incomplete production of erythrocytes, or aplastic if there is no development of new erythrocytes.

Bone marrow depression anemias can be caused by:

1. Adverse physical agents such as excessive irradiation.

2. Chemical agents such as arsenicals, estrogens, hydrocarbons, and antibiotics such as chloramphenicol and streptomycin.

3. Metabolic inhibition of bone marrow such as occurs with any chronic infection, chronic interstitial nephritis, chronic liver disease, and endocrine diseases (hypothyroidism and hypopituitarism).

4. Myelophthisic tumors such as lymphosarcoma.

DIAGNOSIS OF ANEMIAS

There are several major questions that should be answered in order to begin to classify anemia as to etiology:

1. *Does a true anemia exist?* This can be determined by evaluating the hemoglobin and PCV together with the presenting clinical signs.

2. *Is the anemia hemolytic or nonhemolytic?* This can be answered by examining the urine for excessive bilirubin or hemoglobinuria, presence of free hemoglobin in the plasma, the presence of icterus, increased urobilinogen in the urine and feces, and signs of increased bone marrow activity.

3. *Is the anemia responsive (are the bone marrow and other hematopoietic centers responding to the stress) or unresponsive?* A response to an anemia is indicated by increased leukocytes and a shift to the left, increased reticulocytes, nucleated erythrocytes present in the peripheral circulation, polychromatophilia, Howell-Jolly bodies, and increased platelet count.

The signs of a nonresponsive anemia are a pale or colorless plasma, decreased leukocytes, absence of reticulocytes, no nucleated erythrocytes, and normal erythrocyte indices.

Exceptions to normal erythropoietic indices would be iron and vitamin B_6 (microcytic hypochromic), or folic acid and vitamin B_{12} (macrocytic hypochromic) deficiencies.

Of primary importance in evaluating nonresponsive anemias is the bone marrow examination. The myeloid-erythroid ratio determines whether or not erythrocytic precursors are present. Examination for abnormally shaped erythroid precursors or for the presence of leukemic or tumor cells has diagnostic importance in refractory anemias.

V-3-C. Polycythemia

Polycythemia refers to an increase in the erythrocyte count, hemoglobin concentration or packed cell volume. Absolute polycythemia is an excess of erythrocytes in the circulation accompanied by an increase in total blood volume. "Relative polycythemia" refers to an increase in red blood cells associated with a decrease in the volume of plasma associated with water deprivation, vomiting, diarrhea, fever, general malnutrition or acute shock. The distinction between absolute polycythemia and "relative polycythemia" can be made by examining the hemogram.

Absolute polycythemia can be associated with physiologic changes. Physiologic polycythemia can occur when red blood reserves in the spleen are suddenly released into the peripheral circulation. This usually occurs when epinephrine is released secondary to shock, excitement or fright. Pathologic polycythemia is associated with defective oxygen saturation of the blood, which may occur at high altitudes, and with impaired pulmonary ventilation or poor circulation, such as occurs in patients with heart failure, either acquired or congenital. Congenital heart defects result in much more severe polycythemia.

Polycythemia rubra vera is a rare disease with an insidious course and of unknown etiology. There is unrestricted proliferation of red blood cells.

V–3–D. Blood Groups and Cross Matching

There are at least 8 different blood factors known in the dog (A_1, A_2, B, C, D, E, F and G). Of these, only the A factor is highly antigenic and seems to be of clinical significance in blood transfusions. Although the exact inheritance of blood groups in dogs is not known, factors A, B, C and D appear to be dominant. Thirty-seven per cent of dogs are A negative and 63 per cent of dogs are A positive. Transfusion of A positive blood into A negative dogs may lead to the development of anti A antibodies, which are potential hemolysins in both in vivo and in vitro conditons. On the first random transfusion, approximately 25 per cent of these transfusions have the potentiality for the production of anti-A antibodies. If an A negative recipient that has been previously immunized receives A positive blood, a transfusion reaction occurs within one hour and is characterized by hemoglobinemia, hemoglobinuria, thrombocytopenia, leukopenia, fever, emesis, incontinence, urticaria, and weakness.

With a second transfusion, about 15 per cent of recipients receiving blood from randomly selected donors will receive incompatible blood. The main danger is in administering A positive blood for a second and third time to an A negative recipient. An A negative bitch sensitized to A positive blood through transfusions and mated to an A positive sire may also produce puppies with neonatal isoerythrolysis after suckling.

All blood donors should be A negative dogs to prevent transfusion reactions due to the A factor. The identification of blood groups in dogs is, at present, being done by only a few people interested in this field. Typing sera for dog blood is not commercially available. Cross matching blood, however, is a technique applicable to clinical practice and it is important to cross match blood when transfusions are to be given to a patient who has had previous transfusions.

The test of the recipient's serum with the donor's red cells is known as a major crossmatch, and when the donor's plasma and recipient's red cells are used it is call minor crossmatch. Under most circumstances, a major crossmatch is performed. Fresh blood of the donor and recipient should be used in cross matching. Two drops of a 4 per cent suspension of the donor's red cells suspended in donor's serum are mixed with 2 drops of recipient's serum in a 7 × 60 mm. test tube and the tube is incubated at room temperature for 15 minutes. After centrifuging the tube for one minute at 1000 RPM, the contents are examined for hemolysis and agglutination. A control should be set up using the donor's serum and red blood cells in the same tube.

The presence of significant hemolysis or agglutination in the crossmatched tube indicates incompatibility of blood donor and recipient.

V-3-E. Coombs' Test (Antiglobulin Test)

Patients who develop autoimmune hemolytic anemia form abnormal globulins that are adsorbed to their erythrocytes or circulate in their serum. If normal canine serum, plasma, or plasma globulin is injected into rabbit, antibodies are produced by the rabbit against the canine protein and these circulate in the rabbit's serum. The rabbit serum so produced is called antiglobulin serum or Coombs' serum. This serum will react with canine erythrocytes and cause agglutination only if those cells have been coated with abnormal canine globulin.

The direct antiglobulin (Coombs' test) is carried out by mixing anti-canine globulin serum with washed erythrocytes from a patient suspected of having autoimmune hemolytic anemia. Agglutination confirms the presence of antibody on the erythrocytes.

ERYTHROCYTE OSMOTIC SALINE FRAGILITY TEST

The increased susceptibility of erythrocytes to lysis in hypotonic saline is associated with spherocytosis. The presence of spherocytes associated with autoimmune hemolytic anemia is of sufficient magnitude to produce gross changes in the saline fragility curve.

V-3-F. Interpretation of Bone Marrow

Bone marrow is the site of production of erythrocytes, granulocytes, and thrombocytes. For methods by which bone marrow can be obtained from the dog and cat see Section IV. Once the bone marrow material is obtained, a differential count of 500 nucleated cells should be made. The myeloid to erythroid (M:E) ratio should be determined by dividing the number of nucleated red cells into the sum of all cells belonging to the granulocytic series. When the total leukocyte count is within the normal range for the species the myeloid to erythroid ratio can be used to indicate depression or acceleration of erythrogenesis. When the M:E ratio is less than 1.0 there is intensification of erthyrogenesis whereas an M:E ratio that is greater than 2.5 usually indicates depression of erythrogenesis. For example, a high M:E ratio of 4.0:1.0 with a normal blood leukocyte count would indicate depressed erythropoiesis; a low M:E ratio of 0.5:1.0 with a normal or increased blood leukocyte count would mean increased erythropoiesis. Differential count of bone marrow cells can demonstrate the overproduction of one cell type that may be associated with a maturation arrest or hypoplasia of a cell series. Normal M:E ratios in the dog are 0.75 to 2.5 with a mean of 1.20:1.0. The normal M:E ratio in the cat is 0.60 to 3.90 with a mean of 1.6:1.0 (Schalm).

V–3–G. The Leukogram

Leukocytes include all the leukocytes and their precursors, i.e., the granulocytes, including neutrophils, eosinophils, and basophils, all of which are formed in the bone marrow; the lymphocytes produced in the lymph nodes, spleen, and other lymphocytic foci in the body; and the monocytes produced in the reticuloendothelial system.

Leukocytic changes in the peripheral blood can be associated with: (a) diseases that affect the bloodforming organs such as the bone marrow, lymphoid tissue, spleen, and reticuloendothelial system; and (b) diseases that affect other body tissues in such a way as to mobilize leukocytes to the area of injury or disease. In order to obtain the maximum information from leukocyte examinations, the total leukocyte count should be correlated with the differential count.

Total Leukocyte Count

1. *Leukopenia* refers to a reduction below normal in the total leukocyte count. Leukopenia can be produced by the reduction in number of a specific cell type, e.g., neutropenia, lymphopenia, or by a reduction in all cell types.

Leukopenia can be found in overwhelming infections, virus diseases, adverse drug reactions, aplastic or hypoplastic anemias, myelophthisic tumors, excessive exposure to ionizing radiation and in treatment with antimetabolites.

2. *Leukocytosis* is an increase of the total number of leukocytes. Usually only one cell type is elevated in number, usually the neutrophil. The degree of increase in the total leukocyte count is dependent on the cause of the leukocytosis, the degree of severity of an infection and the virulence of the invading organism, (overwhelming infections may not permit the body to respond with a leukocytosis), the degree of localization of the inflammatory process, and the effect of treatment.

Differential Leukocyte Count

General principles in the interpretation of the differential leukocyte count are as follows.

1. The leukocytic response to stress or to the administration of corticosteroids is characterized by a leukocytosis, neutrophilia, eosinopenia, and lymphopenia. A one- to five-fold increase in neutrophils can be seen. Neutrophils do not move out of the blood as rapidly as they normally do, and therefore more mature forms are found in the blood. A two- to three-fold increase in monocytes is usually seen.

2. Neutrophilia with a slight left shift and with the persistence of eosinophils suggests a mild infection.

3. A neutrophilia with a left shift indicates the presence of a severe disease process. However, it indicates a good response by the host.

4. A left shift without a leukocytosis is called a "degenerative shift" and is an unfavorable sign. The appearance of toxic neutrophils can also be associated with a "degenerative shift." The neutrophils are said to be toxic because of delayed maturation of their cytoplasm resulting in an incomplete utilization of RNA. These cells are diffusely basophilic and their cytoplasm has a foamy appearance.

5. Lymphocytes are immunologic cells that are subject to change with stress and immunologic abnormalities. A young dog has a higher percentage of lymphocytes than an older dog. Lymphocyte numbers falling below 1000/cu. mm. are representative of absolute lymphopenia.

6. A decreasing total leukocyte count with a decrease in neutrophils and a return of lymphocytes and eosinophils in normal numbers is a sign of convalescence from disease.

7. Monocytes originate from bone marrow cells resembling lymphocytes. The blood monocyte in body tissues will transform into a macrophage. Marked monocytosis can be associated with the destruction of cellular elements in the blood.

8. Eosinophilia may be a response to the release of abnormal quantities of histamine somewhere in the body. Injury to tissues from many

causes results in the disintegration of basophils and mast cells with the release of histamine. An increase in eosinophils in chronic disease may indicate that histamine is being produced in greater quantities than can be neutralized.

9. A marked, absolute, prolonged reduction in lymphocytes indicates the prolongation of a chronic stress condition and justifies a guarded to poor prognosis.

10. Viruses can markedly affect leukocyte values in the early stages of a disease process. Virus replication takes place in young, actively growing cells, such as lymphocytes, and interferes with normal replication, resulting in leukopenia.

Differential leukocyte counts should be analyzed by using absolute values rather than percentages.

V–3–H. Sedimentation Rate

If blood containing anticoagulant is allowed to stand in an upright tube, the erythrocytes will gradually settle to the bottom. The rate at which the settling takes place is an index of the reaction of the body to disease or injury. To interpret the sedimentation rate one must compare the obtained value with the value expected for the packed cell volume of the animal. The corrected value is expressed as "minus" when the sedimentation rate is less than expected and "plus" when it is more than expected.

There are a number of factors all of which can influence the sedimentation rate:

1. Alterations in the composition of the plasma may occur in inflammatory, neoplastic, and metabolic diseases. Increased levels of globulin and fibrinogen may produce clumping or aggregation of erythrocytes, followed by rapid settling of these cells.

2. Alterations in the numbers of erythrocytes present in the circulation can affect the sedimentation rate. Negative sedimentation values are often related to the presence of young erythrocytes in large numbers in anemia in remission. These young blood cells do not form rouleaux and they stay dispersed in the plasma. Young cells also have a lower specific gravity than mature red blood cells, which does not permit them to settle as rapidly. A reddish tinge in the lower portion of the plasma fraction of the sedimentation tube indicates the presence of young erythrocytes (diphasic reaction).

3. The size of the erythrocytes can influence the sedimentation reac-

tion. The presence of macrocytes and spherocytes increases the sedimentation rate whereas microcytes, leptocytes, and poikilocytes retard the sedimentation rate.

4. The type of anticoagulant used, the age of the blood sample (samples more than two hours old have decreased sedimentation rates), the diameter of the sedimentation tube, and the position of the tube—all will influence the sedimentation rate.

The sedimentation rate is a nonspecific test. It is a valuable procedure in determining the presence of some diseases and in following the course of a disease. A normal sedimentation rate, however, does not rule out the presence of disease.

Increased sedimentation rates can be found in:

1. Infectious diseases such as leptospirosis and canine distemper.

2. Some neoplastic diseases.

3. Systemic infections such as bacterial endocarditis, and in localized infections, like pneumonia, myocarditis, and pleuritis.

4. Parasitism such as infestation with heart worms.

5. Secondary skin disorders in which there is alteration in plasma proteins.

6. Pregnancy.

7. Radiation injury.

8. Metabolic abnormalities such as hypercholesterolemia.

References

Additional material can be found in the following sources:

Cramer, D. V., and Lewis, R. M.: Reticulocyte response in the cat. JAVMA *160*:61–67, 1972.

Penny, R. H. C., Carlisle, C. H., and Davidson, H. A.: The blood and bone marrow picture of the cat. Brit. Vet. J. *126*:459–464, 1970.

Penny, R. H. C., et al.: Some observations on the effect of the concentration of EDTA on packed cell volume of domesticated animals. Brit. Vet. J. *126*: 383–389, 1970.

Schalm, O. W.: Leukopenia and resurgence of granulopoieses in the cat. Fel. Pract., pp. 35–39, Jan.-Feb., 1973.

Schalm, O. W.: Interpretations in feline bone marrow cytology. JAVMA *161*: 1418–1425, 1972.

Schalm, O. W., Jain, N. C., and Carroll, E. J.: Veterinary Hematology, 3rd ed. Philadelphia, Lea & Febiger, 1975.

Schechter, R. D., Schalm, O. W., and Kaneko, J. J.: Heinz body hemolytic anemia associated with the use of urinary antiseptics containing methylene blue in the cat. JAVMA *162*:37–44, 1973.

Searcy, G. P., Miller, D. R., and Tasker, J. B.: Congenital hemolytic anemia in the Basenji dog due to erythrocyte pyruvate kinase deficiency. Canad. J. Comp. Med. *35*:67–70, 1971.

Sodikoff, C. H.: Heinz body anemia in a cat induced by methylene blue. Fel. Pract. *3*:38–42, 1973.

V–3–I. Hematopoietic Neoplasms

This group of blood disorders is characterized by malignant neoplasia of the hematopoietic tissues, which may include bone marrow, lymphoid tissue, the reticuloendothelial system, and the plasma cell system. The disease can be classified according to the predominant cell type; however, the parent neoplastic tissues may all be of one stem cell type.

1. Lymphosarcoma refers to a neoplastic proliferation of abnormal lymphocytes or their precursors in lymph nodes or other lymphatic tissue, resulting in enlarged lymphatic tissue and infiltration of various tissues by neoplastic cells.

2. Reticulum cell sarcoma is a neoplastic proliferation of reticulum cells of lymph nodes or other reticuloendothelial areas, resulting in tumor formation and infiltration of various tissues.

3. Myelosarcoma is a neoplastic proliferation of granulocytic leukocytes or erythrocytes originating in bone marrow or extramedullary areas of hematopoiesis (e.g., spleen, liver, lymph nodes) resulting in tumor formation.

4. Myelogenous tumor refers to the presence of primary neoplastic cells within the bone marrow.

5. Erythemic myelosis, erythroleukemia and reticuloendotheliosis refer to hematopoietic tumors of erythroid precursors.

Feline Lymphosarcoma

Lymphosarcoma is the most common type of hematopoietic neoplasm in the cat. Feline lymphosarcoma comprises 90 per cent of all feline hematopoietic neoplasms. The disease often affects cats younger than one year of age, but there appear to be two age peaks of occurrence: two years of age and 10 years. Four forms of the disease occur: (1) alimentary, involving mainly the mesenteric lymph nodes and the gastrointestinal tract; (2) multicentric, in which the tumor is generalized and spread throughout lymphatic tissue; (3) anterior mediastinal or thymic; and (4) unclassified, which includes the eyes, the skin and other organs not already referred to.

Diagnosis of lymphosarcoma in the cat depends upon what primary tissues are affected. In the gastrointestinal form, vomiting, diarrhea, constipation and anorexia are the signs most often seen. In the multicentric form, icterus and uremia are often present when there is extensive infiltration of the liver and kidneys. The anterior mediastinal form may be characterized by difficulty in swallowing, dyspnea, coughing and vomiting after eating. Often there are nonspecific signs such as lethargy, anemia, loss of weight, anorexia and dehydration.

Enlargement of peripheral lymph nodes is not commonly found in lymphosarcoma of the cat; however, all lymph nodes should be carefully examined. In addition, the liver, spleen, mesenteric lymph nodes and kidneys should be carefully palpated for any indication of enlargement. Aspiration of fluid (thoracentesis or paracentesis) may be helpful when exfoliative cytology is performed.

Examination of peripheral blood smears in cats with lymphosarcoma reveals that a pronounced normocytic normochromic anemia is present in 50 per cent of the cases. There is an absolute leukocytosis in 30 per cent of the cases, an absolute leukocytopenia in 10 per cent of cases, and an absolute lymphocytopenia in 40 per cent of cases. Leukemia is present in 10 to 30 per cent of the cases, depending on in what stage of the disease the blood samples are examined (Hardy).

Ancillary examinations that may be very helpful in confirming a diagnosis of lymphosarcoma are radiographs of the thorax and abdomen, thoracentesis and paracentesis coupled with exfoliative cytology, IVP examination, pneumoperitoneogram and biopsy of any suspicious tissue.

Large amounts of evidence collected over the past five years have shown that feline lymphosarcoma is associated with an oncogenic C-type RNA virus morphologically identical to those associated with avian and murine leukemias. Data obtained by numerous investigators support evidence for the horizontal infectious spread of FELV in cats.

FELV is capable of growing in canine tissue culture cells and in human tissue culture cells. However, FELV antigen has never been found in any human tumors thus far examined. The cat, a known harborer of an oncogenic virus, is always in very close contact with man. For this reason the public health significance of FELV is being carefully investigated. At this time there is no definitive proof that vertical transmission of FELV may occur between the cat and man; however, it is strongly recommended that cats afflicted with lymphosarcoma be euthanized and not held for treatment.

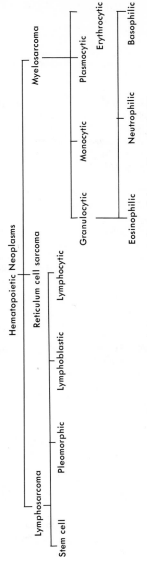

Figure 74. Classification of hematopoietic neoplasms of the cat. (From Hardy, W. D., Jr.: Newer knowledge of solid tumors and leukemias of the dog and cat. 40th Ann. Proc. A.A.H.A., San Antonio, Texas, 1973, p. 632.)

Canine Lymphosarcoma

The most common type of lymphosarcoma in the dog appears to be lymphoblastic and prolymphocytic lymphosarcoma of the disseminated type. The affected animal is usually between 5 and 10 years old. Peripheral lymphadenopathy is a common presenting sign and the disease may start with localized lymph node enlargement around the head. The signs associated with lymphosarcoma are often related to sites of involvement. Vomiting, diarrhea, weight loss, coughing, dyspnea, ascites, icterus, anemia and fever are often seen. In suspected cases of canine lymphosarcoma, all peripheral lymph nodes should be examined, the spleen and liver should be carefully palpated, and the tonsils should be visually examined.

Examination of peripheral blood smears of dogs with lymphosarcoma reveal primitive or atypical cells in more than 60 per cent of the cases. Additional examinations that may be very helpful are exfoliative cytology in lymph nodes or fluid aspirates, lymph node biopsy, bone marrow examination, radiology and exploratory surgery.

As yet, no virus has been associated with canine lymphosarcoma, although lymphosarcoma can be induced in one-day-old puppies who are inoculated with FELV.

References

Additional material may be found in the following sources:

Hardy, W. D., Jr.: Feline lymphosarcoma: a model of viral carcinogenesis and significance related to human neoplasia. *In* Animal Models for Biomedical Research IV, National Academy of Sciences, 1971.

Hardy, W. D., Jr., et al.: Feline leukemia virus: occurrence of viral antigen in the tissue of cats with lymphosarcoma and other diseases. Science, *166*:1019–1021, Nov., 1969.

Nielsen, S. W.: Spontaneous hematopoietic neoplasms of the domestic cat. National Cancer Institute Monograph, *32*:73–93, August, 1969.

Schalm, O. W., Jain, N. C., and Carroll, E. J.: Veterinary Hematology, 3rd ed. Philadelphia, Lea & Febiger, 1975.

V–3–J.   Bleeding and Blood Coagulation

The physiologic control of hemorrhage is based on an intact system of blood vessels, platelets, and the normal coagulation of blood.

Normal hemostasis of small vessels requires the presence of:

1. Normal vascular factors.

2. Platelet factors.
3. Normal plasma coagulation system.
4. Normal fibrinolysis.

Bleeding and altered mechanisms of blood coagulation may have varied manifestations, including petechial hemorrhages, epistaxis, melena, hematuria, bleeding into body cavities and joints and into the spinal cord. The clinician must determine whether the bleeding has a local cause or is the manifestation of a disease producing alteration in bleeding or clotting mechanisms. It is important to establish the site and duration of the bleeding, its history (including any previous episodes of bleeding), and whether any disease is present.

VASCULAR DEFECTS

Vasoconstriction of an injured vessel is an important factor in hemostasis. Small vessels may be abnormally fragile or fail to constrict properly, i.e., telangiectasia, thus resulting in increased and prolonged bleeding upon injury. Adhesion of platelets to collagen fibers in the damaged vessel wall along with the release of thromboplastins initiates the hemostatic mechanism.

PLATELET FACTORS

Platelets are essential for normal blood coagulation. When vasoconstriction occurs in an injured vessel, the blood flow is retarded and platelets attach to the injured endothelium, disintegrate and undergo viscous metamorphosis releasing serotonins, histamines and ADP. ADP induces platelet aggregation at the bleeding site.

Evaluation of blood platelets is based on a total thrombocyte count, a clot retraction test, and a bleeding time (Table 60). *Thrombocytopenia* results in a delayed clot retraction time and an increased bleeding time, although clotting time remains normal.

Causes of Thrombocytopenia

A decrease in the number of circulating platelets (thrombocytopenia) can result in increased bleeding time and prolonged clot retraction time. The existence of abnormal or nonfunctional platelets (thrombasthenia, thrombocytopathia) may be manifested by one or a combination of the following abnormalities: abnormal prothrombin consumption test, pro-

Text continues on page 503.

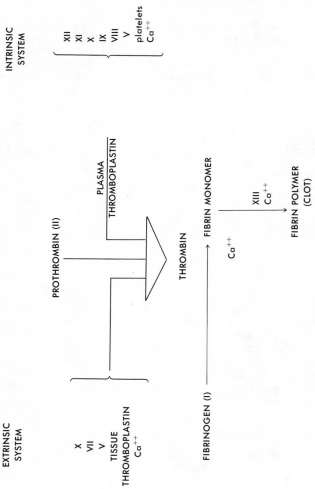

Figure 75. Factors involved in blood coagulation. (From Dodds, W. J., and Kaneko, J. J.: Hemostasis and blood coagulation. In Kaneko, J. J., and Cornelius, C. E. (eds.): Clinical Biochemistry of Domestic Animals, 2nd ed., Vol. II. New York, Academic Press, 1971.)

TABLE 57. BLOOD CLOTTING FACTORS AND SYNONYMS*

International Classification†	Synonyms
Factor I	Fibrinogen
Factor II	Prothrombin
Factor III	Tissue thromboplastin
Factor IV	Calcium
Factor V	Proaccelerin labile factor, accelerator globulin (AcG)
Factor VII	Proconvertin serum prothrombin conversion accelerator (SPCA), stable factor, autoprothrombin I
Factor VIII	Antihemophilic factor (AHF) antihemophilic globulin (AHG), platelet cofactor I, plasma thromboplastic factor A
Factor IX	Christmas factor Plasma thromboplastin component (PTC), platelet cofactor II, autoprothrombin II, plasma thromboplastic factor B
Factor X	Stuart factor Stuart-Prower factor
Factor XI	Plasma thromboplastin antecedent (PTA)
Factor XII	Hageman factor
Factor XIII	Fibrin stabilizing factor (FSF) fibrinase, Laki-Lorand factor

*From Dodds, W. J., and Kaneko, J. J.: Hemostasis and blood coagulation. *In* Kaneko, J. J., and Cornelius, C. E. (eds.): Clinical Biochemistry of Domestic Animals, 2nd ed., Vol. II. New York, Academic Press, 1971.

†As recommended by the International Committee for the nomenclature of Blood Clotting Factors (1962). The most commonly used synonym for each factor is listed first.

TABLE 58. TREATMENT OF KNOWN CONGENITAL COAGULATION DISORDERS IN DOGS*

Bleeding Disorder	Treatment†
Factor VII deficiency	Mild condition; no treatment required
Factor VIII deficiency (hemophilia A)	Fresh-frozen dog plasma, or cryoprecipitates, or special Factor VIII concentrates
Factor IX deficiency (hemophilia B)	Fresh-frozen dog plasma, or supernatant from cryoprecipitates, or special Factor IX concentrates
Factor XI deficiency	Fresh-frozen dog plasma, or supernatant from cryoprecipitates
von Willebrand's disease	Fresh-frozen dog plasma, or cryoprecipitates or supernatant from cryoprecipitates
Hypofibrinogenemia	Fresh-frozen dog plasma, or cryoprecipitates, or fibrinogen concentrates
Thrombocytopathy; thrombasthenia; thrombocytopenia	Fresh platelet-rich plasma two or three times daily until bleeding stops

*From Dodds, W. J., and Kaneko, J. J.: Hemostasis and blood coagulation. *In* Kaneko, J. J., and Cornelius, C. E. (eds.): Clinical Biochemistry of Domestic Animals, 2nd ed. Vol. II. New York, Academic Press, 1971.

†For severe hemorrhagic episodes, fresh-frozen plasma is given, 6 to 10 ml./kg. of body weight every six to eight hours until bleeding stops, followed by plasma twice a day for the next three to five days.

TABLE 59. INHERITANCE OF HEREDITARY COAGULATION DEFECTS IN ANIMALS*

Bleeding Disorder	Inheritance Pattern
Factor VII deficiency	Autosomal, incompletely dominant
Factor VIII deficiency (hemophilia A)	X-linked, recessive
Factor IX deficiency (hemophilia B)	X-linked, recessive
Factor XI deficiency	Autosomal
von Willebrand's disease	Autosomal
Hypofibrinogenemia	Autosomal
Thrombocytopathy; thrombasthenia	Autosomal, incompletely dominant

*From Dodds, W. J., and Kaneko, J. J.: Hemostasis and Blood Coagulation. *In* Kaneko, J. J., and Cornelius, C. E. (eds.): Clinical Biochemistry of Domestic Animals, 2nd ed. Vol. II. New York, Academic Press, 1971.

longed bleeding times, abnormal siliconized tube clotting time, defective clot retraction, bizarre platelet morphology.

Primary (Etiology Unknown)

1. Idiopathic thrombocytopenia purpura.
2. Autoimmune hemolytic anemia.
3. Amegakaryocytic thrombocytopenia.

Secondary

1. *Aplastic anemia.*
2. *Destruction of thrombocytes in peripheral blood due to:*
   a. Incompatible blood transfusions.
   b. Hypersplenism.
   c. Sensitivity or allergy to various drugs and chemicals.
   d. Extensive burns.
   e. Massive transfusions of citrated stored blood.
   f. Excessive platelet consumption in pulmonary thrombosis.
3. *Myelophthisic.*
   a. Leukemia.
   b. Bone marrow tumors.
4. *Abnormal platelet function, i.e., thrombocytopathic thrombocytopenia resembling von Willebrand's disease in man. This is a familial disorder in Samoyed dogs.*

TABLE 60. DIFFERENTIAL DIAGNOSIS OF BLEEDING DISORDERS*

Test	Hypopro-thrombinemia	Thrombo-cytopenia	Hemophilia	Traumatic Hemorrhage	Increased Capillary Fragility	Autoimmune Hemolytic Anemia	Normal Value for Dog
Coagulation time	Increased	Usually normal	Increased	Normal	Normal	Normal	3-8 min.
Bleeding time	Increased	Increased	Normal	Normal	Prolonged	Normal	Less than 3 min.
Thrombocyte count	Normal	Decreased	Normal	Normal	Normal	May be decreased	$2\text{-}9 \times 10^5$/ cu. mm.
Prothrombin time	Increased	Normal	Usually normal	Normal	Normal	Normal	6-10 sec.
Coombs' test	Negative	Negative or positive	Negative	Normal	Negative	Positive	
Partial thromboplastin time	Abnormal	Abnormal	Abnormal				14-22 sec.
Serum prothrombin consumption	Abnormal	Abnormal	Abnormal				18-30 sec.

*Another important disorder which can be associated with hemorrhagic tendencies is disseminated intravascular coagulation.

DISSEMINATED (DIFFUSE) INTRAVASCULAR COAGULATION

Disseminated intravascular coagulation is a disorder associated with generalized activation of the clotting mechanism resulting from the release of coagulation-initiating activity from damaged tissues, cells or vasculature. The release of tissue thromboplastin (from a wide variety of causes) can induce activation of extrinsic clotting mechanisms. Platelet aggregation and metamorphosis that also is involved with various types of tissue damage can induce the activation of intrinsic clotting mechanisms. Additionally, plasmin can be activated by tissue damage. Plasmin is the proteolytic enzyme responsible for fibrin and fibrinogen breakdown to degradation products which can have anticoagulant effects on thrombin activity. When these clotting abnormalities become generalized and severe, the available stores of labile coagulation factors and platelets can be severely depleted, leading to widespread bleeding and diathesis.

Disseminated intravascular coagulation can be associated with trauma, poisonings, hemolytic uremic syndromes, acute necrosis of tumors involving liver and pancreas, bacterial endotoxemia and septicemia, hemorrhagic shock, snake and spider bites, hemangiosarcoma and immune vasculitis.

The symptoms of DIC are a combination of simultaneous thrombotic and hemorrhagic events. The initiating process is thrombosis, with thrombotic infarctions occurring in numerous areas in the body. Labora-

TABLE 61. LABORATORY FINDINGS IN ACUTE DIC AND FIBRINOLYSIS*

Test	Acute DIC	Fibrinolysis
Platelet Count	Decreased	Normal
Clot Retraction	Defective	Normal
Prothrombin Time	Prolonged	Prolonged
P.T.T.	Prolonged	Slightly prolonged
Fibrinogen	Low	Slight decrease
Ethanol Gelation	Positive	Negative
Protamine Sulfate	Positive (high titre)	Negative or low titre
Fibrinogen split products	Positive	Positive
Fibrin split products	Positive	Negative
Thrombin Time	Prolonged	Prolonged

*From Hurvitz, A. I., Wilkins, R. J., and Kane, L.: Laboratory Newsletter, Animal Medical Center. No. 23, April, 1974.

tory findings with DIC include prolonged bleeding, prothrombin and partial thromboplastin time, low fibrinogen levels and poor clot retraction.

In the initial treatment of severe DIC, intravenous clotting must first be arrested by heparin anticoagulant therapy, even if the patient already exhibits a hemorrhagic diathesis. Once an antithrombotic state is achieved, attention can then be turned to replacing "consumed" clotting factors. Fresh, frozen whole plasma transfusion is the most effective replacement therapy for soluble clotting factors. If significant blood loss has occurred, fresh whole blood or packed cell transfusions are required in addition to plasma. While treating DIC, it is important that the precipitating cause of the problem also be managed.

The fibrinolytic syndrome results from primary activation of plasmin leading to induction of fibrinolysis. The condition may occur following massive physical injury, hemorrhagic shock, burns, transfusion reactions and surgery. Tissues with a high content of plasmin activators include lungs, kidneys, uterus, and prostate. Findings in acute, early fibrinolytic states include delayed blood clotting, accelerated clot lysis, hypofibrinogenemia and normal platelet count. In the latter stages of fibrinolysis, nonspecific proteolytic effects of plasmin can produce severe depletion of clotting factors. Fibrinolytic syndrome is treated by the use of aminocaproic acid (Amicar), which blocks the activation of plasminogen.

PLASMA COAGULATION

The coagulation of blood can be divided into three stages:

Stage I—In this stage plasma proteins interact with the phospholipid components of the platelets to produce plasma thromboplastin. Stage I can be tested by measuring the partial thromboplastin time (PTT), whole blood clotting time, and prothrombin consumption time.

Thromboplastin deficiency (stage I defect) can occur in:

1. Deficiency of factor VIII, hemophilia A. This has been reported in German Shepherds, Irish Setters, Collies, Labrador Retrievers, Beagles, Greyhounds, Shetland Sheepdogs, Weimaraners, and Chihuahuas. The defect is produced by a sex-linked recessive gene and is almost always found in males.

2. Another type of hereditary defect in which there is a factor VIII deficiency is known as von Willebrand's disease. This entity has been described in Labrador Retrievers and a family of German Shepherds. In the German Shepherds the disease was inherited as an autosomal dominant trait with variable penetrance. Patients with von Willebrand's disease have prolonged bleeding time and reduced platelet adhesiveness.

Affected animals can be transfused with either normal or factor VIII deficient plasma and will begin to synthesize their own factor VIII.

3. Deficiency of factor IX (Christmas factor or hemophilia B) has occurred in the dog and has been reported in black and tan Coonhounds, Cairn Terriers and St. Bernards. Primary bleeding times are usually normal; however, secondary bleeding times are prolonged because of an unstable platelet plug. It is inherited as a sex-linked trait.

4. Deficiency of factor VII has also occurred in the dog. Congenital deficiencies of factor VII have been reported in Beagles, although bleeding tendencies are very mild. It appears to be inherited as an autosomal characteristic with heterozygotes having 50 per cent factor VII deficiency. There is a prolonged prothrombin time and prolonged serum prothrombin consumption time.

5. Factor X deficiency has been found in the Cocker Spaniel.

Stage II—This stage is characterized by the thromboplastic conversion of prothrombin to thrombin. Stage II can be evaluated by testing the Quick prothrombin time. It can also be tested by one-stage prothrombin time (measures prothrombin and Factors V, VII and IX) and by Russell viper venom time (measures prothrombin, factors and platelet aggregation and clot retraction (Dodds and Kaneko). The stage II defect results in prolonged prothrombin, bleeding, and coagulation times. Prothrombin deficiency can be due to:

1. Liver disease caused by hepatitis, hepatic toxins, or obstructive jaundice. In infectious canine hepatitis, stage II defects usually begin on the third day of fever and persist during the febrile period.

2. Vitamin K deficiency or the inability to utilize vitamin K in the formation of prothrombin (as occurs in severe hepatocellular damage, with bile deficiency or obstructive jaundice). Extensive treatment with oral antibiotics may interfere with the bacterial synthesis of vitamin K in the intestinal tract.

3. In poisonings with drugs such as warfarin.

Stage III—This stage involves the conversion of fibrinogen to fibrin. Defects in this stage have not been found to be important in veterinary medicine at this time although increased fibrinolysins occur postsurgically and decreased fibrinogen levels are associated with liver disease.

Collection and Handling of Blood Samples To Be Used in Evaluation of Coagulation Abnormalities

1. Take all blood samples with plastic or silicone coated glass syringes by *careful* venipuncture.

2. Trisodium citrate or sodium oxalate is the anticoagulant of choice for coagulation and platelet work (e.g., 1 part 3.8 per cent trisodium citrate plus 9 parts whole blood).

3. All samples must be kept in plastic or silicone coated glass test tubes.

4. Plasma samples should be prepared from fresh blood and tested immediately or frozen for testing later. Samples should be assayed in duplicate, and kept at refrigerator temperature when tested.

5. Platelet tests must be done on fresh samples within two hours of collection. Polycarbonate is an ideal plastic surface for platelet preparation. Samples should be kept at room temperature because platelet shape is altered by heat or cold.

6. Normal control samples from the *same* species must always be measured with all test samples to check reagents (Dodds and Kaneko).

References

Additional information may be found in the following sources:

Dodds, W. J.: Canine von Willebrand's disease. J. Lab. Clin. Med. *76*:713-721, 1970.

Dodds, W. J., and Kaneko, J. J.: Hemostasis and blood coagulation. *In* Clinical Biochemistry of Domestic Animals, 2nd ed., Vol. II, pp. 179–204. New York, Academic Press, 1971.

Hurvitz, A. I., Wilkins, R. J., and Kane, L.: Laboratory Newsletter, No. 23, Animal Medical Center, April, 1974.

Marder, V. J.: Pathophysiology and therapy of disseminated intravascular coagulation. *In* Rational Drug Therapy, Vol. 5, No. 12. Philadelphia, W. B. Saunders Co., December, 1971.

Rowsell, H. C.: The hemostatic mechanism of mammals and birds in health and disease. Advan. Vet. Sci. *12*:337–410, 1968.

V-3-K. Blood Parasites (D. W. Scott, D.V.M.)

HEMOBARTONELLA FELIS (FELINE INFECTIOUS ANEMIA)

H. felis is the rickettsial agent causing a disease in cats which may be characterized by fever, anorexia, lethargy, emaciation, splenomegaly, macrocytic normochromic anemia *without* hemoglobinuria, and occasionally icterus. Cats may carry *Hemobartonella felis* and be perfectly normal; however, during periods of stress, overt clinical infection may develop. The parasite is seen as coccoid, rodlike or ring-like bodies on the red blood cells in smears stained with Wright's, Giemsa, new methylene blue or acridine orange. The numbers of parasites present in the peripheral blood at any one time can vary greatly; therefore, repeated smears may be needed (three to five consecutive days). In cases of severe infection with *H. felis* and a resultant very low packed cell volume (below 20), a whole blood transfusion can be administered (see Section IV-21). Treatment of *H. felis* is controversial. Thiacetarsamide sodium (caparsolate) may be the most effective treatment, although it is approved only for use in dogs. Caparsolate is administered intravenously, giving 0.5 cc./10 lb. the first day, skipping treatment the next day, and repeating the dosage the third day. During the course of this treatment the affected animal is hospitalized. Treatment of *H. felis* infection with tetracycline hydrochloride orally, 10 mg./lb. three times a day for 21 days or chloramphenicol orally, 10 mg./lb. three times a day for 10 to 14 days has achieved variable success.

HEMOBARTONELLA CANIS

H. canis is the rickettsial agent causing a disease in dogs which may be characterized by fever, anorexia, weakness, splenomegaly, macrocytic normochromic anemia, and (rarely) icterus. The infection is usually latent and may be activated by stress or splenectomy. The parasite is seen as coccoid or chainlike forms on the red blood cells in smears stained with Wright's, Giemsa, new methylene blue or acridine orange. The numbers of parasites present in the peripheral blood at any one time can vary greatly; therefore, repeated smears may be needed (three to five consecutive days). Treatment consists of tetracycline hydrochloride orally, 10 mg./lb. three times a day for 21 days, or oxyphenarsine hydrochloride (Mapharsen) intravenously, 2 mg./lb. in an 0.4 per cent solution.

BABESIA CANIS

B. canis is the protozoan agent causing a disease in dogs which may be characterized by recurrent fever, anorexia, lethargy, splenomegaly, macrocytic normochromic anemia, hemoglobinuria, and variable icterus. The parasite is seen as multiple, basophilic, pear-shaped bodies within the red blood cells in smears stained with Wright's, Giemsa, or new methylene blue. The numbers of parasites present in the peripheral blood at any one time can vary greatly; therefore, repeated smears may be needed (three to five consecutive days). The brown dog tick, *Rhipicephalus sanguineus,* is the principal vector in the United States. Treatment consists of quinuronium sulfate (Acaprin) subcutaneously, 0.25 mg./kg.; phenamidine subcutaneously, 0.25 cc./10 lb. in a 3 per cent solution (may be repeated in 24 hours); trypan blue intravenously, 1 cc./10 lb. in a 1 per cent solution; or diminazene aceturate (Berenil) intramuscularly, 11 mg./kg. in a 1 per cent solution (two doses, five days apart).

BABESIA GIBSONI

B. gibsoni is the protozoan agent causing a disease in dogs which may be characterized by recurrent fever, anorexia, lethargy, splenomegaly, macrocytic normochromic anemia, hemoglobinuria, and (very rarely) icterus. The parasite is seen as multiple, basophilic, annular or oval bodies within the red blood cells in smears stained with Wright's, Giemsa or new methylene blue. The numbers of parasites present in the peripheral blood at any one time can vary greatly; therefore, repeated smears may be needed (three to five consecutive days). Treatment consists of diminazene aceturate (Berenil) intramuscularly, 11 mg./kg. in a 1 per cent solution (two doses, five days apart) or metronidazole (Flagyl) orally, 250 mg./day for 10 days.

BABESIA FELIS (BILIARY FEVER OR MALIGNANT JAUNDICE)

B. felis is the protozoan agent causing a disease in cats which may be characterized by fever, anorexia, lethargy, macrocytic normochromic anemia, and icterus. The parasite is seen as multiple, basophilic, oval or round bodies within the red blood cells in smears stained with Wright's, Giemsa or new methylene blue. The numbers of parasites present in the peripheral blood at any one time can vary greatly; therefore, repeated smears may be needed (three to five consecutive days). Treatment consists of tetracycline hydrochloride orally, 10 mg./lb. three times a day, along with trypan blue intravenously, 1 cc./10 lb. in a 1 per cent solution for two days, or quinuronium sulfate (Acaprin) subcutaneously, 0.25 mg./kg.

EHRLICHIA CANIS (CANINE EHRLICHIOSIS)

E. canis is the rickettsial agent causing a disease in dogs which may be characterized by cyclic fever, lethargy, hyperkeratosis, mucopurulent oculonasorrhea, neurological signs, and normocytic normochromic anemia. The parasite is seen as basophilic, raspberry-shaped bodies within the lymphocytes, monocytes, and (rarely) other leukocytes in smears stained with Wright's or Giemsa. Treatment consists of tetracycline hydrochloride orally, 25 mg./lb. three times a day for seven to 14 days.

EHRLICHIA CANIS (TROPICAL CANINE PANCYTOPENIA)

E. canis is the rickettsial agent causing a disease in dogs which may be characterized by fever, anorexia, weakness, weight loss, epistaxis, edema of limbs and scrotum, petechiae and ecchymoses of skin and mucous membranes, peripheral lymphadenopathy, and pancytopenia. The parasite is seen as basophilic, raspberry-shaped bodies within the lymphocytes and monocytes in smears stained with Wright's or Giemsa. Treatment consists of tetracycline hydrochloride orally, 10 mg./lb. three times a day for 14 days.

HEPATOZOON CANIS

H. canis is the protozoan agent causing a disease in cats and dogs which may be characterized by cyclic fever, emaciation, anemia, and hepatosplenomegaly. The parasite is seen as basophilic, elongate, rectangular bodies with dark, red-purple nuclei and pink cytoplasmic granules within the leukocytes in smears stained with Wright's. There is no effective treatment.

V–3–L. *Blood Chemistry*

The measurement of various constituents of the blood can be an invaluable aid in confirming a diagnosis and in determining the prognosis and course of a clinical disease. There are a number of facts that should be remembered when the use of blood chemistry tests is contemplated.

1. Blood chemistry tests are only important when combined with an adequate history and physical examination.

2. Blood chemistry tests should not be used indiscriminately. Selected tests should be used to evaluate a differential diagnosis or confirm a diagnosis.

3. The clinician must realize the limitations of the test being used and must be able to interpret the results of the test.

When performing blood chemistry determinations try to:

1. Eliminate the environmental influences whenever possible, e.g., fast the animal and limit exercise.

2. Carefully obtain samples (see Section IV-1).

3. Analyze samples quickly and store them in a suitable manner.

4. If you do not perform the tests yourself, be familiar with what type of samples the laboratory needs to complete the tests.

V–3–L–1. SERUM PROTEINS

Fibrinogen, albumin and globulins constitute the major proteins of the blood plasma. In determining serum proteins, serum or plasma must be free of hemolysis. Fibrinogen is removed in coagulation; therefore fibrinogen determinations cannot be done on serum.

In general, plasma proteins are low in young animals (usually less than 5.0 gm./100 ml. of plasma). Older animals may have total plasma proteins in the range of 7.0 to 8.0 gm. per cent.

Gamma globulins are formed by the reticuloendothelial cells of the body whereas albumin, fibrinogen, prothrombin, and alpha and beta globulins are formed in the liver. (See Section IV for information on globulins and A/G ratio.)

Determination of plasma protein levels may be important when:

1. One wishes to assess the nutritive state of the animal.

2. One is trying to evaluate kidney and liver function.

3. One wants to assess the role of the reticuloendothelial system in a clinical situation.

4. One wants to determine fluid balance in states of shock, dehydration, and hemorrhage.

The albumin fraction exerts the greatest effect on the total volume of plasma protein. Decreases in albumin levels usually result in lowered total plasma volume. A decrease in total serum albumin may be the result of a lowered protein intake, deficient synthesis of albumin by the liver associated with chronic hepatic disease (see Section V-4), excessive protein breakdown that may occur with prolonged fever, diabetes mellitus, post-surgical conditions and trauma, and excessive loss of protein that may occur with acute nephritis, nephrosis, burns, parasitism, ascites, and hemorrhage.

The concentration of proteins in the blood determines the colloidal osmotic pressure of the plasma. Lipemic plasma, cloudy plasma, or hemolysis will affect the total serum protein determinations. The concentration of protein in the plasma can be influenced by the nutritional state of the animal, hepatic function (see Section V–4), renal function, blood loss, dehydration, various diseases, and metabolic abnormalities. Various individual fractions of the plasma proteins may be helpful in diagnosing certain diseases. These plasma protein fractions may be separated by plasma electrophoresis.

Hypoproteinemia may be due to poor diet; inability to absorb nutrients properly; excessive loss of body protein through draining wounds, burns, or blood loss; increased protein need as in recovery from surgery or pregnancy; metabolic destructions such as liver disease; and severe parasitism.

Hyperproteinemia can occur in dehydration, shock, and administration of quantities of concentrated amino acids; in certain neoplasms; and in some infections.

Plasma fibrinogen levels have been used in the interpretation of the response and severity of certain diseases in small animals. The normal range of fibrinogen is 200 to 400 mg./100 ml. of plasma. The total plasma protein:fibrinogen ratio is variable, depending on the age of the animal. In general, a PP:F ratio of less than 15:1.0 would indicate an increase in fibrinogen over plasma protein. A ratio below 10:1.0 indicates a marked increase in fibrinogen.

V–3–L–2. SERUM AMYLASE

In normal animals a small amount of serum amylase from the pancreas and salivary glands is present in the blood. Inflammation of the pancreas may release abnormal amounts of this enzyme into the blood. It should be remembered that conditions such as renal insufficiency, corticosteroid elevations, and factors that increase the production of pituitary and adrenal glands could also elevate serum amylase levels. It has been demonstrated that in pancreatitis in the dog, the changes in serum amylase and lipase activity often parallel each other, and elevations of both enzymes occur early in the disease. Serum amylase levels are easier to determine than lipase levels and can be done in the hospital.

V–3–L–3. PLASMA BICARBONATE

The bicarbonate-carbonic acid buffer is one of the most important buffer systems in maintaining the normal pH of the body fluids. Normally these constituents are present in a ratio of one part of carbonic acid to 20 parts of bicarbonate.

Serum bicarbonate is elevated in metabolic alkalosis such as occurs with prolonged vomiting, or in respiratory acidosis due to hypoventilation. Serum bicarbonate is reduced in metabolic acidosis in such conditions as diabetic ketosis, persistent diarrhea, renal insufficiency, shock, or respiratory alkalosis due to hyperventilation.

V–3–L–4. CARBON DIOXIDE

Serum contains HCO_3^-, physically dissolved CO_2 (proportional to the pCO_2) and H_2CO_3. At normal blood pH, the ratio of HCO_3^- to dissolved CO_2 and H_2CO_3 is 20:1. In reliably assessing acid-base status, measurement of arterial blood pH or pCO_2 and total CO_2 is desirable. Knowing the value of any two of these three parameters, a nomogram can be used to calculate the other.

Practical office evaluation of acid-base abnormalities often depends on the availability of CO_2 determinations interpreted along with clinical findings. When one measures the CO_2 content of blood allowed to be exposed to the air, the total CO_2 that is measured is almost exclusively bicarbonate. The development of rapid, inexpensive office screening procedures for CO_2 determination makes this test quite practical. A low CO_2 level may indicate either a metabolic acidosis or respiratory alkalosis and a high CO_2 level may indicate metabolic alkalosis or respiratory acidosis.

V–3–L–5. SERUM BILIRUBIN (see Section V-4)

V–3–L–6. BLOOD UREA NITROGEN (BUN)

Ammonium oxalate or "double oxalate" cannot be used as an anticoagulant if this test is to be performed, because the ammonia will be measured as urea.

Urea, an end product of protein metabolism, is excreted by the kidneys. Some 40 per cent or more of this urea is reabsorbed by the kidney tubules. Thus, blood urea levels are one indication of kidney function and can serve as a rough index of glomerular filtration rate. The BUN varies directly with protein intake and inversely with the rate of excretion of urea.

Blood urea nitrogen may be elevated in renal insufficiency (acute or chronic); increased nitrogen metabolism associated with diminished renal blood flow or impaired renal function, as may occur in dehydration and shock; adrenal insufficiency and congestive heart failure; and postrenal obstruction preventing normal urination as may occur with urethral calculi.

Repeated blood urea nitrogen tests are usually indicated to follow the progress of the patient. An elevation of blood urea nitrogen will not become evident until 70 to 75 per cent or more of the nephrons of both kidneys become nonfunctional.

V-3-L-7. CREATININE

Creatinine is derived from creatine and phosphocreatine during muscle metabolism and is excreted by way of the glomerulus of the kidney. Blood creatinine levels are not affected by dietary protein, protein catabolism, age, sex, or exercise. Any abnormality which decreases the glomerular filtration rate will cause an increase in the serum concentration of creatinine. Creatinine is eliminated more readily than urea, and therefore an increase in blood creatinine usually is seen later in the course of kidney disease. Concentrations of creatinine above 2.0 mg./100 ml. indicate a reduced GFR. Serial determinations of creatinine should be used when determining the prognosis in renal disease. The significance of an elevated creatinine can be determined only after analyzing other renal function tests. A persistently high creatinine despite appropriate therapy justifies a guarded prognosis.

V-3-L-8. URIC ACID (See Section V-4)

V-3-L-9. BLOOD CALCIUM

Calcium is necessary for normal muscle contraction, normal transmission of nerve impulses, normal blood coagulation, normal neuromuscular excitability, and cell membrane permeability. The main store of body calcium is in the bones. Serum calcium exists in two forms: one form is inactive and is combined with a serum protein fraction (mainly albumin), and the second form is active and not combined with a protein.

There are a number of clinical situations in which serum calcium levels should be determined including bone disorders, convulsions, parathyroid abnormalities, renal insufficiency, and malabsorption syndromes.

There are a number of factors that can alter the ionized (active) serum calcium levels:

1. Alkalosis lowers ionized calcium levels whereas acidosis may increase ionized calcium levels.

2. Vitamin D levels influence serum calcium levels. Deficiencies of

vitamin D may lead to low blood calcium levels. Large excesses of vitamin D cause high levels of serum calcium and may result in dystrophic calcification.

3. The parathyroid glands, by producing parathormone, can greatly influence the serum calcium levels. Parathormone controls calcium mobilization from the bones and also the renal excretion of phosphorus, thus controlling the calcium to phosphorus ratio.

4. The calcium to phosphorus ratio in the diet can also affect the serum calcium levels.

Increased serum calcium levels are seen in primary hyperparathyroidism. Primary hyperparathyroidism is very rare and is usually caused by a functioning adenoma of the parathyroid gland. It has been reported in dogs.

Secondary hyperparathyroidism may result from an improper calcium or phosphorus ratio in the diet or from renal insufficiency. The normal calcium to phosphorus ratio in the diet is 1.2:1. Excessively high phosphorus ratios, as seen in cats on all red meat diets, lead to hyperparathyroidism and mobilization of calcium from the bones. Secondary hyperparathyroidism in renal insufficiency is associated with a retention of phosphorus leading to hyperphosphatemia and hypocalcemia, which stimulates the production of parathormone. It is important to remember that in secondary hyperparathyroidism the serum calcium levels may be normal, decreased, or elevated depending on the stage of the disease.

Thus, repeated serum calcium, phosphorus, and alkaline phosphatase determinations are needed to assess the condition of an animal with secondary hyperparathyroidism.

Excesses of vitamin D can cause high blood calcium levels with the production of metastatic calcification.

Decreased levels of blood calcium can be seen in hypoparathyroidism, azotemia, hypoalbuminemia, starvation, eclampsia, rickets, vitamin D deficiency, and malabsorption syndromes. Excessive dietary calcium produces hypercalcitonism, either by increasing plasma calcium with direct stimulation of the thyroid C cells, or indirectly, via stimulation of gastrin produced by the G cells, mainly in the distal pylorus of the stomach. The ultimate results of excessive dietary calcium in balanced proportion to phosphorus are hypocalcemia, hypophosphatemia and hypophosphatasemia.

V–3–L–10. BLOOD CHOLESTEROL (See Section V-4)

V-3-L-11. CREATINE PHOSPHOKINASE (CPK)

The enzyme CPK splits creatine phosphate in the presence of ADP to yield creatine and ATP. Skeletal and cardiac muscle are rich in this enzyme. Variations in CPK values can be related to sex, age and physical activity. They are elevated in the presence of muscle damage that could result from trauma, infarction, muscular dystrophies or inflammation. Elevated CPK values do not reveal what the underlying muscle pathology is. Muscle diseases may be associated with abnormalities of the muscle fiber itself or with neurogenic diseases resulting in secondary damage to muscle fibers. High increased CPK values are usually associated with myogenic disease.

V-3-L-12. SERUM PHOSPHORUS (INORGANIC PHOSPHORUS)

The level of inorganic phosphorus in the plasma can be influenced by the parathyroid glands, intestinal absorption, renal function, bone metabolism, nutrition, and ionized serum calcium levels.

Hyperphosphatemia can occur in renal failure with phosphorus retention, hypoparathyroidism with an excessive tubular reabsorption of phosphorus in the absence of adequate levels of parathormone, and with excessive vitamin D intake.

Hypophosphatemia can occur in inadequate intake of phosphorus, primary hyperparathyroidism due to the elimination of larger amounts of phosphorus in the urine, and after insulin administration.

V-3-L-13. SERUM SODIUM AND CHLORIDE

Chloride is the principal inorganic anion of the extracellular fluid. It is important in the maintenance of acid-base balance. When chloride in the form of hydrochloric acid or ammonium chloride is lost, alkalosis follows; when chloride is retained or ingested, acidosis follows.

Sodium and chloride ions provide the greatest part of the osmotically active solute in the plasma and can greatly influence the distribution of the water. The shift of sodium ions into cells or a loss of sodium from the body produces a decrease of extracellular fluid that greatly affects circulation, renal function, and the nervous system.

Increases in sodium may occur in dehydration or a primary water deficit, hyperadrenocorticoidism and central nervous system trauma or disease.

Decreased serum sodium levels can be seen in adrenal insufficiency, inadequate sodium intake, renal insufficiency, as a physiologic response to burns or trauma, losses from the gastrointestinal tract as in diarrhea or intestinal obstruction, water intoxication, and uncontrolled diabetes mellitus.

Elevated serum chloride levels can be seen in renal insufficiency, dehydration, overtreatment with saline solutions, congestion and edema associated with cirrhosis of the liver, and carbon dioxide deficit as occurs with hyperventilation.

Decreased serum chloride levels can be seen in gastrointestinal disease producing vomiting and diarrhea, in renal insufficiency with salt deprivation, in overtreatment with certain diuretics, in diabetic acidosis, in adrenal insufficiency, and in hypoventilation as occurs in pneumonia, emphysema, and pulmonary edema, resulting in respiratory acidosis.

V–3–L–14. SERUM POTASSIUM

Potassium represents the major cation of intracellular fluid. The concentration of potassium in the extracellular fluid normally varies over a narrow range from 3.5 to 5.0 mEq. per liter.

The potassium concentration in blood plasma determines the state of neuromuscular and muscular irritability. Elevated or decreased concentrations of potassium can affect the contraction of both skeletal and cardiac musculature.

Hyperkalemia is often associated with impaired renal excretion of potassium. Potassium excretion is largely accomplished by tubular secretion, not glomerular filtration; therefore, hyperkalemia does not occur until late in the course of renal disease with marked alteration in glomerular filtration and existing uremia. Metabolic acidosis contributes to the development of severe hyperkalemia, as does adrenal insufficiency.

Hypokalemia can result from excessive loss of potassium associated with protracted vomiting or diarrhea. Alkalosis results in the migration of potassium ions from the extracellular to intracellular fluid and increased urinary loss of potassium. Urinary loss of potassium occurs by secretion in the distal tubules. Excessive potassium is lost in hyperadrenocorticism and in renal tubular acidosis.

V–3–L–15. SERUM CHOLESTEROL (see Section V-4)

V–3–L–16. BLOOD GLUCOSE

If determinations of blood glucose levels are to be delayed for more than one hour, sodium fluoride, 3 mg./ml. should be added to the specimen.

The glucose level in the blood is maintained within a relatively narrow physiologic limit. A number of factors control blood glucose levels including hepatic gluconeogenesis and glycogenolysis, renal excretion and reabsorption, removal of glucose by the tissues, effects of hormonal processes on tissue metabolism, and the intestinal absorption of glucose.

The major hormone affecting blood glucose levels is insulin. Insulin can act to accelerate glucose oxidation, inhibit gluconeogenesis in the liver, accelerate the conversion of glucose to fat, increase liver glycogen formation, and inhibit the formation of ketones.

Elevated blood glucose levels (hyperglycemia) can occur in diabetes mellitus, hyperthyroidism, hyperadrenocorticoidism, hyperpituitarism, anoxia (because of the instability of liver glycogen in oxygen deficiency), production of epinephrine, certain physiologic conditions (digestion, exposure to cold, following general anesthesia), the administration of glucose-containing fluids, and acute pancreatic necrosis.

Decreased blood glucose levels (hypoglycemia) may occur in hyperinsulinism from a tumor of the pancreas (Islet cell adenoma), or from an overdose of exogenous insulin; following severe exertion; starvation; adrenal insufficiency; hypopituitarism; hepatic insufficiency; and in a functional hypoglycemic, von Gierke-like syndrome.

V–3–L–17. ALKALINE PHOSPHATASE (see Section V-4)

Alkaline phosphatase is present in high concentrations in bone, intestinal mucosa, renal tubule cells, and in the bile. The alkaline phosphatase in serum consists of a mixture of isoenzymes which can be separated by electrophoresis. Significant increases in alkaline phosphatase can be observed in both intrahepatic cholestasis and extrahepatic bile duct obstruction. In the cat, serum alkaline phosphatase can be cleared by the kidneys very rapidly, and severe liver disease with biliary obstruction seldom results in elevated levels of serum alkaline phosphatase.

Serum alkaline phosphatase may be increased in bone diseases, with increased osteoblastic and osteoclastic changes such as secondary hyperparathyroidism; obstruction of bile ducts (not in cats); certain bone tumors such as osteogenic sarcomas; and hyperadrenocorticism.

V–3–L–18. SGPT AND SGOT (see Section V-4)

V–3–L–19. SERUM LDH

Assay of total serum LDH, because of its ubiquitous origins and consequent difficulties encountered in interpretation of altered levels, has not been utilized widely as a diagnostic aid in veterinary medicine. Analysis of LDH isoenzymes, however, provides more specific diagnostic information. In normal canine serum, 5 isoenzymes of LDH are demonstrable, with $LDH_1 > LDH_3 > LDH_4 > LDH_2 > LDH_5$. This distribution may be altered following damage to tissues. The nature of the alteration provides a more accurate indication of the organs involved than does assay of total serum LDH.

LDH isoenzyme analysis provides a reliable and fairly specific aid to the diagnosis of active myocardial damage in the dog. There is a rapid rise and fall in the activity of LDH_1 and LDH_2 following experimentally induced myocardial damage in the dog. The presence of increased activity of these isoenzymes in serum provides good supportive evidence of recent or continuing myocardial damage. Conversely, the absence of elevated activity of these isoenzymes suggests that myocardial damage is not the cause of the problem, or is no longer active, or is proceeding at such a low level as not to be reflected in the serum.

Because of the abundance of LDH (LDH_1 and LDH_2) in erythrocytes, samples for analysis should be free of hemolysis; otherwise pronounced alterations in LDH activity are observed.

Increases in both total LDH and LDH isoenzymes have also been observed in dogs with neoplasia. The isoenzyme patterns observed in these cases vary, but the major increases have been observed in the isoenzymes of intermediate and slow electrophoretic mobility.

With liver disease and skeletal muscle damage, assay of LDH isoenzymes does not appear to offer any advantage over the more commonly assayed enzymes.

V–3–L–20. PROTEIN-BOUND IODINE (PBI)

The major portion of the iodine present in the body is in the plasma in an organic combination with protein. Thyroid hormone is normally the only organic iodine compound present in the blood in significant concentrations. Measurement of protein-bound iodine is, therefore, an indirect means of measuring circulating thyroxin.

The following factors are important when considering a PBI determination:

1. The test should be performed by a laboratory that routinely does PBI tests.

2. Any contamination of the serum with exogenous iodine will affect the test results.

3. Animals whose blood is to be analyzed for protein-bound iodine should not have received any form of iodine therapy from four to 24 weeks preceding the test.

4. New disposable syringes and blood collecting vials should be used in the test.

Because of a multiplicity of influencing factors, PBI determinations in small animals should be evaluated with great care (see Section V-2-C).

V–3–L–21. SERUM LIPASE

Normally, a low concentration of this fat-splitting enzyme is present in the blood. In the presence of acute pancreatitis, pancreatic lipase is released into the circulation in elevated amounts. Serum lipase procedures require a titration with either a pH meter or an indicated dye, as well as the use of an unstable substrate. A long incubation time is helpful. For these reasons, the test is usually performed by a commercial laboratory.

References

Additional information can be found in the following sources:

Coles, E. H.: Veterinary Clinical Pathology, 2nd ed. Philadelphia, W. B. Saunders Co., 1975.
Kaneko, J. J., and Cornelius, C. E. (eds.): Clinical Biochemistry of Domestic Animals, 2nd ed. New York, Academic Press, 1971.
Krook, L.: Metabolic skeletal disease. Lecture notes, New York State Veterinary College, 1973.
Medway, W., Prier, J. E., and Wilkinson, J. S. (eds.): Veterinary Clinical Pathology. Baltimore, Williams and Wilkins, 1969.

V–4. LIVER FUNCTION TESTS

The liver has many varied functions and no one laboratory test can be used as an indication of normal or abnormal liver function. Because of its tremendous size and regeneration capability, a large portion of the liver (80 per cent) may be injured before alterations in liver function are noticed. Repeated liver function tests are frequently needed to follow the course of liver diseases. The use of a limited battery of tests is indicated to obtain a liver profile to help determine what anatomical units of the liver are diseased.

Liver function tests are employed to determine the presence of liver disease, determine the type of disease present, and determine the extent of damage and the prognosis in liver disease. Liver function tests cannot be used alone, but should be correlated with clinical signs and possibly liver biopsy (see Section IV-9) to develop an overall picture.

LIVER EXCRETION TESTS

Bile Pigment Formation

1. Bile pigments result from the breakdown of hemoglobin, produced when erythrocytes are destroyed.

2. Heme is converted to biliverdin and then to free bilirubin (unconjugated by the reticuloendothelial system).

3. The free bilirubin is conjugated in the smooth endoplasmic reticulum of the liver to bilirubin glucuronide.

4. Conjugated bilirubin is secreted by the bile ducts, stored in the gallbladder, and excreted in the small intestine.

Increased Bile Pigment Formation

Increases in bile pigment can result in the production of clinical jaundice. Excess bile pigment may be produced by:

1. Increased destruction of erythrocytes, producing elevated amounts of hemoglobin, or

2. Decreased excretion or retention of conjugated bilirubin diglucuronide due to cellular disease of the liver, blockage of the excretory ducts of the liver, or both.

Measurement of Increased Bilirubin Levels

The icterus index is based on a comparison of the color of the patient's serum or plasma to potassium dichromate solutions of different concentrations. This test gives only a rough index of the amount of elevation of plasma bilirubin.

van den Bergh Reaction

In the plasma, bilirubin exists in the conjugated water-soluble form and reacts quickly (directly) with a diazo reagent, and in a nonconjugated form that is not water-soluble and reacts slowly (indirectly) with diazo reagents. Elevated levels of indirectly acting bilirubin indicate increased erythrocyte breakdown, resulting in high levels of unconjugated or free bilirubin. Elevated levels of bilirubin that react directly indicate hepatocellular damage or obstructive disease of the liver. The low renal threshold in the dog for bilirubin conjugates produces low serum levels of bilirubin in intrahepatic and obstructive disease.

Urine Bilirubin

Only the conjugated form of bilirubin can be present in the urine. The renal threshold for urine bilirubin is low in the dog so that levels of a trace to 1+ may normally be present in the urine. A 2+ to 3+ bilirubin reaction in the urine of a dog with a normal urine volume and a specific gravity between 1.020 and 1.035 indicates hyperbilirubinemia due to hepatocellular or obstructive disease.

Urine Urobilinogen

Urobilinogen is normally formed from bilirubin by the reaction of bacteria on bilirubin in the bowel. Most urobilinogen is excreted in the feces but a small portion is taken up by the portal circulation, returned to the liver, or finally excreted by the kidneys into the urine (Fig. 76).

Increased urine urobilinogen can result from impaired liver function, or from "overloading" of the liver because of increased bilirubin production in hemolytic jaundice. In hemolytic anemias, greater amounts of urinary urobilinogen are associated with both an increased amount of circulating bile pigments and secondary hepatic insufficiency.

Decreased or absent urobilinogen production can result from a delay in running the test, by a complete obstruction of the biliary passages, decreased destruction of erythrocytes, changes in the intestinal flora due to intestinal disease or excessive treatment with antibiotics, or a dilution of the urine such as may occur with polydypsia and polyuria, e.g., chronic interstitial nephritis.

Increased levels of bilirubin, producing icterus with an absence of urobilinogen in the urine, is indicative of obstructive jaundice (Table 62).

Fecal Urobilinogen (Stercobilinogen)

Stercobilinogen contributes to the normal brown color of the feces. Increased amounts of stercobilinogen produce a dark orange stool

Text continues on page 526.

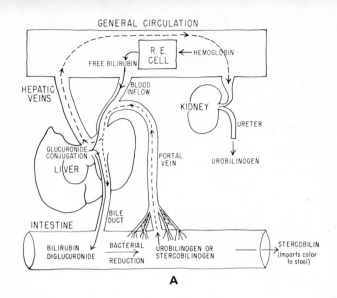

A

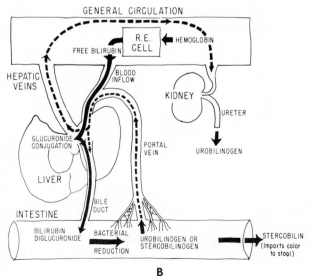

B

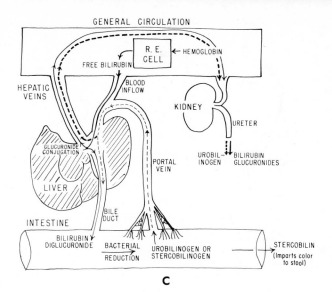

C

Figure 76. *A,* The normal enterohepatic circulation of bile pigments.

B, Hemolytic crisis. Observe the increase in the quantity of free bilirubin in the serum (unable to pass the renal filter), stercobilin in the stool (imparts a darker color to the stool), and urinary urobilinogen. Increased urinary urobilinogen may be due partly to the increased quantity of bile pigments metabolized owing to erythrocyte hemolysis. If secondary liver damage is extensive from hemosiderosis or bile pigment overload, some bilirubin glucuronide may be regurgitated and lost to the urine (not in diagram).

C, Hepatocellular pathology. Observe the presence of bilirubin glucuronide and increased amounts of urobilinogen in the urine. Increased urinary urobilinogen is due to the inability of the altered hepatic cells to quantitatively reexcrete this pigment into the bile. Free bilirubin may also be elevated in the serum owing to a decreased hepatic uptake of the pigment.

Legend continues on following page.

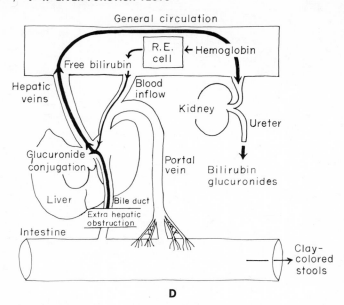

D

Figure 76. *Continued. D,* Extrahepatic obstruction. Observe regurgitation to the serum and subsequently the increased urinary excretion of bilirubin diglucuronide conjugated in the liver. Urinary urobilinogen and fecal stercobilin are absent. (From Kaneko, J. J., and Cornelius, C. E. (eds.): Clinical Biochemistry of Domestic Animals, 2nd ed., pp. 172–175. New York, Academic Press, 1971.)

whereas decreased amounts produce a light gray or clay-colored stool. Increased amounts of stercobilinogen occur when blood destruction is increased. Decreased amounts or the absence of stercobilinogen occurs in obstruction of the biliary passages or alterations in the intestinal flora by disease or antibiotics.

Sulfobromophthalein Excretion (BSP Test)

The uptake, conjugation and excretion by the liver of foreign dyes measures both the biochemical integrity of hepatic cells and hepatic blood flow.

BSP dye is removed from the vascular system by the reticuloendothe-

TABLE 62. DIFFERENTIAL DIAGNOSIS OF JAUNDICE

| | Blood | | Urine | | Feces |
Icterus	Anemia	van den Bergh	Bilirubin	Urobilinogen	Color
Increased production or deficient conjugation (hemolytic disease)	Present	Indirect elevated	+	4+	Dark
Impaired secretion into biliary passage (hepatocellular damage)	Absent usually	Direct elevated	2+ to 4+	2+ to 4+	Normal
Impaired excretion (extrahepatic obstruction)	Absent	Direct elevated	4+	0 to 1+	Clay-colored

lial and parenchymal cells of the liver. It is a satisfactory means of testing the excretory capabilities of the liver when no jaundice is present. Competition for hepatic uptake between foreign dyes such as BSP and bilirubin exists; thus, interpretation of this testing procedure is difficult in cases of hyperbilirubinemia. Any abnormalities in circulation time will also affect the results of the test.

Abnormal BSP retention in the vascular system can be produced in hepatic necrosis, hepatic fibrosis, hepatic lipoidosis, lymphosarcoma, cardiovascular disease, portal obstruction, and anemia.

Another dye that has been used in excretion tests is indocyanine green (ICG). It has certain advantages over BSP (Cornelius), and its removal rate is exponential for the first 15 minutes after injection.

EVALUATION OF SYNTHESIS IN THE LIVER
Protein Metabolism

Albumin, prothrombin, fibrinogen, and small amounts of globulin are all formed in the liver. Serum proteins can be affected both quantitatively and qualitatively in liver disease; however, changes in serum proteins are not specific for liver disease. In some diseases of the liver, especially chronic diseases, the level of serum albumin is decreased, which lowers the total serum protein and may reverse the A/G ratio. In many liver diseases, however, there is a compensatory rise in serum globulin in an attempt to maintain the serum protein level. In obstructive jaundice, the level of serum albumin is lowered late in the course of the disease after secondary liver damage has taken place. In cirrhosis or fibrosis of the liver, serum albumin is lowered but the level of serum albumin is dependent on the extent of damage to the liver.

Prothrombin Concentration

The synthesis of prothrombin is a function of the liver. A low prothrombin concentration may result from inadequate absorption of vitamin K in the intestinal tract because of an absence of bile, inability of a damaged liver to convert vitamin K to prothrombin, and ingestion of poisons such as warfarin.

In low prothrombin levels with evidence of clinical jaundice 5 to 10 mg. of vitamin K_1 may be given intramuscularly and the prothrombin time rechecked in 12 to 24 hours. If the prothrombin time has returned to between 85 and 90 per cent of normal the liver cells still retain their capacity to synthesize prothrombin. If a poor response to vitamin K administration is seen, then severe hepatocellular disease probably exists.

Cholesterol and Cholosterol Esters

The liver is involved in lipid metabolism including the esterification and excretion of cholesterol. Cholesterol is secreted with the bile and it is also metabolized in the liver to cholic acid. The ratio of free cholesterol to cholesterol esters is important in liver disease. The formation of cholesterol esters is depressed in both acute and chronic liver disease, thus changing the ratio of cholesterol ester to total cholesterol (normal is 60/100). High total serum cholesterol levels have been reported in diabetes mellitus, fatty degeneration of the liver, hypothyroidism (highly variable), and hyperadrenocorticoidism.

DETOXIFICATION IN THE LIVER
Uric Acid

Uric acid is converted to allantoin in the liver by uricase except in man, monkey, and the Dalmatian dog. In liver disease the amount of uric acid in the blood may be elevated. This test is extremely variable in the results produced in the dog and cat with liver disease.

EVALUATION OF ENZYME ACTIVITY

Increases in the concentration of enzymes in the blood associated with liver disease may be associated with the escape of enzymes from damaged hepatic parenchymal cells with necrosis or altered membrane permeability or altered biliary secretion, as occurs with obstructive jaundice.

Serum Alkaline Phosphatase

Serum alkaline phosphatase is a result of osteoblastic and osteoclastic (mainly osteoblastic) activity, and some of it is excreted in the bile. Elevations of serum alkaline phosphatase may indicate biliary duct obstruction. Bone diseases such as rickets and secondary nutritional hyperparathyroidism may also affect the alkaline phosphatase levels. The kidney of the cat is able to excrete alkaline phosphatase so that this test is invalid in obstructive disease in this animal.

Alkaline phosphatase levels can be measured by numerous procedures and reported in various units. Knowledge of the type of test used and its normal values is important in interpreting results.

Serum Transaminase

Serum glutamic oxaloacetic transaminase (SGOT) is found in high levels in the liver, the myocardium, and skeletal muscles. Serum glutamic-pyruvic transaminase (SGPT) is found in large concentrations in the liver of the dog and cat. These enzymes are involved in the transfer of NH_2 groups from amino to keto acids and provide for the metabolism of amino acids in the Krebs cycle. Destruction of liver cells can release these enzymes, which results in an increase in their concentration in the plasma.

Increased SGPT in the dog and cat is usually specific for hepatic necrosis. SGPT values of 10 to 50 units are considered normal, values of 50 to 400 units indicate moderate liver necrosis, and severe necrosis is indicated by values of more than 400 units.

The simultaneous use of BSP and SGPT is of value in differentiating advanced fibrosis from liver necrosis. In fibrosis the BSP excretion is decreased and the SGPT is normal, whereas in necrosis the opposite usually occurs.

SGOT is not specific for liver necrosis. Pathologic conditions involving the cardiac or skeletal muscles that produce necrosis will also elevate the SGOT.

Other serum enzyme tests of value in liver disease are being studied.

LIVER BIOPSY (see Section IV-9)

References

Additional information can be found in the following sources:

Hoe, C. M., and O'Shea, J. D.: The correlation of biochemistry and histopathology in kidney disease in the dog. Vet. Rec. 77:210, 1965.

Kaneko, J. J., and Cornelius, C. E. (eds.): Clinical Biochemistry of Domestic Animals, 2nd ed., Vol. I. New York, Academic Press, 1971.

Medway, W., Prier, J. E., and Wilkinson, J. S. (eds.): Textbook of Veterinary Clinical Pathology. Baltimore, Williams and Wilkins, 1969.

Osborne, C. A., Stevens, J. B., and Perman, V.: V. Needle biopsy of the liver. JAVMA 155:1605–1620, 1969.

Schiff, L.: Diseases of the Liver, 3rd ed. Philadelphia, J. B. Lippincott Co., 1969.

V–5. ANTIMICROBIAL SENSITIVITY TESTING

This in vitro test is classically performed using a pure culture growth of the infecting agent obtained by culture isolation from the primary specimen (see Section IV-4). The test serves to indicate organism susceptibility or resistance to specific antimicrobial agents. A response showing resistance should eliminate that agent from therapeutic consideration; however, a test showing susceptibility may not always guarantee similar results in vitro. In general, the following holds true: If the test shows resistance, the organism is not likely to respond to therapy with the antibiotic. If the test response is intermediate, the organism is susceptible if dosage is high or the antibiotic is concentrated in the urine. If the test shows susceptibility, the organism is susceptible to ordinary dosage. The tests, properly performed, do serve as a useful guide.

The test is not indicated:

1. When organisms (such as streptococcus) are of unvarying susceptibility.

2. When the number of organisms as determined by culture is deemed to be insignificant for infection.

3. When the primary specimen yields a mixture of infecting organisms so that uncertainty is created as to which, if any, is the etiologic agent. Interpretation of tests run on such samples is difficult and unreliable.

The test is indicated:

1. When body defenses may be defective and the utmost antimicrobial efficacy is necessary.

2. When the antibiotic such as Streptomycin allows the organisms to develop resistance easily.

3. When infections are caused by bacterial species that commonly have many strains of differing antibiotic susceptibility. Among bacteria that commonly show variable strains are E. coli, Staphylococcus, Proteus, and Pseudomonas.

The antimicrobial paper disc method is practical for small office laboratories. In carefully performed tests the following points should be emphasized:

1. Use Mueller-Hinton medium for the tests. (Sulfonamides often will not give satisfactory zones on media that contain blood.)

2. The size of the inoculum should be such as to produce a dense but not confluent plate growth. A heavy inoculum is better than a light inoculum. It can be applied from either a nutrient broth pure culture after the primary growth has been obtained or more rapidly by direct swab primary inoculation.

3. The method of inoculation should provide the most uniform distribution possible. Horizontal and vertical right angle spreading is a good method.

4. Single antibiotic discs (not ring-spoke discs) can be applied to the agar surface immediately and tapped into place for firm contact.

5. Once a package of sensitivity discs is opened it should be stored in the refrigerator and the discs either used or discarded within one month.

6. Select discs pertinent to the type of infection usually encountered in the organ system involved. For example, urinary tract infections are rarely caused by gram positive organisms (Staphylococcus or Streptococcus) whereas respiratory infections rarely are caused by gram negative organisms. Use only high level discs for urinary infections because the kidney hyperconcentrates the antibiotic. Urine levels, not serum levels, are crucial.

7. Veterinary clinicians usually select drugs from the following list for sensitivity tests: penicillin, erythromycin, tylosin chloramphenicol, tetracycline, streptomycin, neomycin, polymixin, nitrofurantoin, and sulfonamide. Occasionally one may add ampicillin, oxacillin, lincomycin, kanamycin, gentamicin and cephaloridine.

8. Drug sensitivity extrapolation must be done carefully. Results from methicillin may apply to any of the penicillinase-resistant penicillins; similarly. tetracycline and sulfonamide tests may hold for others of their groups. Polymyxin and colistin too are similar, and neomycin and kanamycin often cross-react.

9. After placement of the discs the plate is turned upside down and incubated at 35 to 37°C. for 18 hours. (It may be read with magnification after five to six hours.)

10. The zones of inhibition should be measured as diameters from zone edge to zone edge. Sulfonamides may give a soft inner zone of partial growth. Use the outer definite zone for measuring the diameter of inhibition.

11. *Do not compare the inhibition zone size of various antibiotics for determination of relative therapeutic merit.* For example, a polymyxin zone of 12 mm. may be just as effective as chloramphenicol at 18 mm. (Table 63).

12. Report organism as resistant if there is no inhibition of growth around the disc. Do not expect good therapeutic results with such an antibiotic.

13. Report organisms as susceptible if a clear zone of inhibition of significant size is evident around the disc. In vivo results do not always conform to in vitro tests, however.

TABLE 63. INTERPRETATIVE CHART OF ZONE SIZE
(Bauer-Kirby Method)

Therapeutic Agent	Test Disc	Inhibition Zone Diameter (mm.)		
		Resistant	Inter-mediate Suscep-tibility	Suscep-tible
Cephalexin		14 or less	15–17	18 or more
Cephaloridine	Cephalo-	14 or less	15–17	18 or more
Cephalothin	thin*	14 or less	15–17	18 or more
Cephaloglycin†	30 μg.	14 or less	—	15 or more
Chloramphenicol	30 μg.	12 or less	13–17	18 or more
Colistin	10 μg.	8 or less	9–10	11 or more
Erythromycin	15 μg.	13 or less	14–17	18 or more
Gentamicin‡	10 μg.	—	—	13 or more
Kanamycin	30 μg.	13 or less	14–17	18 or more
Nitrofurantoin†	300 μg.	14 or less	15–16	17 or more
Polymyxin B	300§	8 or less	9–11	12 or more
Streptomycin	10 μg.	11 or less	12–14	15 or more
Sulfonamides†	300 μg.	12 or less	13–18	17 or more
Tetracycline	30 μg.	14 or less	15–18	19 or more
Vancomycin	30 μg.	9 or less	10–11	12 or more
Ampicillin	10 μg.			
Gram (−) organisms;				
enterococci		11 or less	12–13	14 or more
Staphylococci		20 or less	21–28	29 or more
Hemophilus sp.‡		—	—	20 or more
Carbenicillin	50 μg.			
Pseudomonas sp.		12 or less	13–14	15 or more
E. coli; Proteus sp.		17 or less	18–22	23 or more
Penicillin G	10§			
Staphylococci		20 or less	21–28	29 or more
Other organisms		11 or less	12–21¶	22 or more

*A recent simplification in the single-disc method makes it possible to determine susceptibility to structurally related antibiotics with similar activity spectra by testing against only one member of the antibiotic family. Thus, susceptibility to the four cephalosporins is determined by one test disc containing 30 μg. cephalothin.

†Urinary tract infection only.

‡Tentative standards.

§Units.

¶Includes organisms which may cause systemic infections treatable by high doses.

From Bauer, A. W., et al.: Antibiotic susceptibility testing by a standardized single disk method. Amer. J. Clin. Path. *45*:493, 1966.

14. Disc potency, diffusion of the agent, and other factors mentioned modify the size of the zone of inhibition.

One of the difficulties of interpretation is caused by the inability to balance antibacterial concentration in the disc with that which can be obtained in the tissue at the infection site. For estimation of the effect of individual agents, the following list may be useful as a guide.

The appendix contains three tables that may be helpful.

1. Etiologic Agents in Typical Clinical Infections (Table 126).

2. Antimicrobial Agents for Treatment of Infection (Tables 126 and 127).

3. Most Effective pH for Optimal Antibacterial Activity (Table 128).

References

Additional information may be found in the following sources:

Bauer, A. W., et al.: Antibiotic susceptibility testing by a standardized single disk method. Amer. J. Clin. Path. *45*:493, 1966.

Wick, W. E., et al.: Laboratory testing of bacterial susceptibility to antibiotics. Lilly Research Laboratories, Indianapolis, Indiana.

V–6. MYCOLOGY

Woods light fluorescence of affected hair and skin may be observed in the majority of infections due to *M. canis,* a common dermatophyte of small animals. A similar response often is observed with *M. audouini* and *M. distortum,* rare animal dermatophytes. Not all specimens of these fungi fluoresce. When they do, the typical fluorescence is a yellow-green color. Other colors of fluorescence (purple, blue) may be due to medications, mineral oil, scales, or mineral particles. Fluorescing hair and skin make excellent samples for culture, and the distribution of these areas may indicate foci of infection not otherwise apparent.

Potassium hydroxide, 10 per cent, for digestion of hair and scale preparations may clear the sample of debris so that fungal mycelia can be observed more easily. Unless the fungous growth is abundant the test may be negative, and even if mycelia are observed, one cannot make valid conclusions about the pathogenicity of the organism. A positive test does help confirm suspicions and is a mandate for cultures and further identification.

Fungous cultures (see Section IV-5) afford the only accurate way to identify pathogenic organisms, and positive laboratory reports provide a definitive diagnosis.

1. The great majority (99 per cent [superficial mycoses]) of dermatomycoses of small animals are caused by *Microsporum canis,* or *gypseum,* or *Trichophyton mentagrophytes.* Although uncommon, all of the following should be considered pathogenic to dogs and cats: *M. distortum, M. audouini, M. vanbreuseghernii, T. equinum, T. verrucosum, T. gallinae,* and *T. rubrum.*

2. *Candida albicans,* a yeast, causes a mycosis of intermediate depth (moniliasis) that may affect skin and mocous membranes. It often is an opportunist associated with moist or macerated skin or mucous membrane, and the clinician should search carefully for another etiologic agent. Candida albicans and Pityrosporum canis are yeasts commonly found in otitis externa, but they may be present as secondary invaders.

3. Deep mycoses are usually associated with ulcerative or fistulous lesions and cultures may be made from exudates or tissues from these areas.

TABLE 64. DERMATOPHYTE IDENTIFICATION

	Gross Colony	**Macroconidia**
M. canis	White cottony surface; lemon yellow reverse. DTM (agar) made red	Spindle-shaped, thick-walled. 6 to 12 cells with terminal knob.
M. gypseum	Cinnamon brown flacculent surface. Buff reverse. DTM (agar) made red	Elliptical, thin, slightly rough walled. 3 to 6 cells
Trichophyton mentagrophytes	White colony with flat powdery surface. Light beige or red reverse. DTM (agar) made red	Smooth thin-walled clavate paddle or pencil-shaped; 2 to 6 cells. Many tightly wound spirals. Microconidia in grape-like terminal clusters
Yeasts	Gross colony	Microscopic
Candida albicans	On Sabouraud with chloramphenicol, white, soft, smooth, shiny colonies. Grow at 37° C.	Round, oval, budding cells. Old colonies have pseudohyphae and a few true mycelia chlamydospores formed
Pityrosporum canis	Grows at 37° C. but not at 25° C.	Bottle-shaped budding cells

TABLE 65. RELATIVE FREQUENCY OF OCCURRENCE OF DERMATOPHYTES IN CERTAIN HOSTS

Organism	Cat	Dog	Rodent	Monkey
M. canis	Usual*	Frequent*	Occasional*	Frequent*
M. gypseum	Occasional	Frequent*	Frequent	Occasional
T. mentagrophytes	Occasional*	Frequent*	Usual*	Frequent
M. distortum	Reported	Reported	–	Reported
M. audouini	–	Reported†	–	Reported
M. persicolor	–	Reported	–	–
M. cookei	–	Reported	Reported	Reported
M. vanbreuseghemii	Reported	Reported†	Reported	Reported
T. (M.?) gallinae	–	Reported	–	Reported
T. ajelloi	–	Questionable†	–	–
T. simii	–	Reported	–	Frequent (India)
T. equinum	–	Reported	–	–
T. verrucosum	Reported	Reported	–	–
T. megnini	–	Reported	–	–
T. rubrum	–	Reported	–	Reported
T. violaceum	Reported	–	–	–
E. floccosum	–	Reported	–	–

There are reports of *T. schoenleinii* infections in animals and birds where this fungus is common.

*Indicates similar findings at Purdue SAC.

†Indicates cases in our records or isolate from sample submitted for identification.

From Blakemore, J. C.: Dermatomycosis. *In* Kirk, R. W. (ed.): Current Veterinary Therapy V. Philadelphia, W. B. Saunders Co., 1974.

Other mycotic infections may produce granulomatous lesions of the lungs, liver, kidneys, and other internal organs. They may be diagnosed by culture or histologic examination of biopsy specimens. Some of the deep mycoses that should be considered in small animals include aspergillosis, maduromycosis, coccidioidomycosis, cryptococcosis, blastomycosis, sporotrichosis, and histoplasmosis.

References

Additional information can be found in the following sources:

Animal Ringworm in Public Health. United States Department of Health, Education and Welfare, Publication 727. Washington, 1960.

Rebell, G., Toplin, D., and Blank, H.: Dermatophytes, Their Recognition and Identification, 2nd ed. Dermatology Foundation of Miami. 1020 Northwest 16th St., Miami, Florida 33136, 1970.

Wilson, J. W., and Plunkett, O. A.: Fungous Diseases of Man. Berkeley, University of California Press, 1965.

V–7. INTERNAL PARASITES OF DOGS AND CATS

V–7–A. Ancylostomiasis (Ancylostoma caninum, Ancylostoma braziliense, Uncinaria stenocephala)

The life cycle of all three species of hookworms are similar and infections may be acquired by ingestion or by penetration of the skin by the larvae. Transplacental infection of the fetus and colostral transmission to newborn pups can also occur with *Ancylostoma caninum*. Adult worms live in the small intestine where growth and maturation after the ingestion of infective ova require from 18 to 21 days. Females lay large quantities of eggs that are passed in the feces and, under the proper conditions, hatch in 48 to 72 hrs. The larvae develop to the infective state within five to seven days.

Distribution

Ancylostomiasis occurs throughout the United States but is more prevalent in the southern states. A temperate climate and adequate rainfall are conducive to growth of hookworm population.

Clinical Picture

The clinical picture in hookworm disease is dependent upon the virulence of the species of hookworm involved, the degree of exposure to infective larvae, and the degree of resistance of the host, including immunological resistance.

These parasites are bloodsuckers. The major signs are associated with blood loss and gastrointestinal irritation. Weakness, unfitness, anemia, diarrhea, bloody or tarry stools, anorexia, depression, and death may occur. Larvae may wander through other internal organs, such as the liver and lungs, producing secondary signs of hepatitis and pneumonia. Infection of young puppies with hookworms *in utero* or after birth may produce a peracute syndrome with rapid blood loss, anemia, shock and death. Prenatal infection does not become patent until the eleventh postnatal day; therefore, fecal examination of puppies with peracute hookworm disease may be negative.

Transmission to Man

Infective larvae can penetrate the skin of man causing cutaneous larval migrans (creeping eruption). Hookworm larvae may cause visceral larval migrans with the invasion of vital organs such as liver, heart, and brain.

Diagnosis

A diagnosis can be made by demonstrating eggs or larvae in the feces. In puppies prenatally or neonatally infected with hookworms, severe clinical disease may occur during the prepatent period and diagnosis must be based on signs of the disease.

Chemotherapy

Disophenol (D.N.P.), 3.5 mg./lb., should be administered subcutaneously, or N-butyl chloride orally, 1 ml. for puppies under three months of age and dogs weighing 5 pounds or less. Maximum dose is 5 ml. for dogs of 40 pounds or more. Follow the directions of the manufacturer when administering N-butyl chloride. Fast dog for 12 hours before and give a laxative four hours following administration. Repeat treatment in two weeks. Supportive treatment such as blood and high protein diet together with antibiotics to control secondary infections is indicated. Dichlorvos is also effective (see Table 67).

Control

The clinical picture depends on the number of parasites present, the immunity, and the condition of the host. Control consists of trying to prevent exposure to large numbers of parasites. Concrete floor pens with adequate drainage should be used if possible. Sodium borate, 10 lb./100 sq. ft. may be applied to gravel runs. (This chemical will destroy nearby vegetation.)

V–7–B. Ascariasis (Toxocara canis, Toxocara cati, Toxascaris leonina)

The pattern of migration of these three helminths is variable. In the dog, *Toxocara canis,* and in the cat, *Toxocara cati* follow a tracheal migration route. Second stage larvae hatch in the stomach after ingestion, penetrate the bowel wall, enter the portal blood stream, wander in the hepatic parenchyma, enter the post cava and arrive in the lungs, breaking out of the capillaries to the alveoli and migrating up the bronchial tree and trachea to the pharynx, where they are swallowed. Following a moult in the stomach wall, the parasite matures in the small intestine.

If the Toxocara larvae hatch in numerous foreign hosts, the pattern of migration is altered, resulting in somatic migration.

Toxascaris leonina follows a mucosal migration in both dogs and cats. The second and third moults occur in the intestinal wall and the fourth stage larvae enter the lumen of the gut to mature.

Toxocara canis infections in puppies less than one month of age are produced by migration of second stage larvae from the bitch to the pups *in utero*.

Signs

Signs of Ascariasis are emaciation, dull harsh coat, restlessness, abdominal distention, diarrhea or constipation, and respiratory distress.

Heavy prenatal *Toxocara* infections can produce abdominal cramps and distention in young puppies. Obstruction of the intestinal tract may occur or the severely affected puppy may be predisposed to intussusception.

Diagnosis

Diagnosis is based on finding ova in the stool or the passage of adult ascarids in the stool or vomitus.

Transmission to Man

Toxocara larvae have been implicated in an increasing number of cases of visceral larval migrans infestations in the liver and eyes of young children. It is the responsibility of the veterinarian to keep pets as free as possible of Toxocara and inform pet owners that children should avoid contact with parasite-laden feces.

Chemotherapy

Administer piperazine, 50 mg./lb. and Dichlorvos as directed.

V–7–C. Trichuriasis (Whipworms, Trichuris vulpis)

This parasite inhabits the large bowel and cecum. Eggs are passed in the stool and require a higher temperature for embryonation than do ascarid eggs. The infective eggs are ingested by the host, hatch in the small intestine where the larvae develop in the jejunal glands, and then migrate posteriorly where they mature.

Signs

Signs depend on the numbers of parasites present and include intermittent diarrhea, loss of weight, emaciation, anemia, abdominal pain, flatulence, and "flank sucking." Many animals with light infections may show no signs.

Diagnosis

A diagnosis is based on finding eggs in the feces.

Chemotherapy

Administer Milibis, 100 mg./lb. daily for five days orally. Because trichuris larvae take three months to develop and may be more resistant to treatment than adults, repeated medication may be required, along with good sanitation measures to prevent reinfection.

V–7–D. Strongyloidosis (Strongyloides stercoralis)

This parasite lives in the mucosae of the anterior half of the small intestine in dogs, cats, foxes and man. The parasitic worms are all females and the eggs develop parthenogenetically. The eggs develop rapidly and hatch before evacuation in the feces. Some of the larvae develop into infective larvae, whereas others develop into free-living males and females. Infective larvae may enter by the oral route or may penetrate the skin. Larvae migrate by way of the circulation and lungs, going to the intestine as fourth stage larvae. Progeny may be shed in the feces seven to 20 days after infection.

Signs

Geographical strains of Strongyloides differ greatly in their virulence and infectiousness for hosts.

Signs include diarrhea, which usually contains blood, loss of weight, anorexia, listlessness, and bronchopneumonia.

Diagnosis

A diagnosis is based on recovery of the characteristic infective larvae in the feces after incubation in sterile sand for 48 hours. Examination of fresh fecal smears is also helpful.

Transmission to Man

Strongyloidiasis in man is a chronic debilitating disease. Man and dog can readily infect each other, therefore, caution should be used in handling infected dogs. Infected dogs should be isolated and extreme care should be taken to avoid human contamination.

Chemotherapy

Administer orally Thiabendazole, 25 mg./lb., for three consecutive days. Monthly fecal examinations should be made for one year following infection and therapy.

V–7–E. Tapeworms

In the United States, the vast majority of dogs and cats are domesticated and eat prepared, cooked foods, therefore, cestode parasitism in both man and animals is not a major problem. Exceptions to this general statement can be found with infections in dogs of *Dipylidium caninum* in which the intermediate host is the flea, and *Taenia pisiformis* in which the natural reservoir is the rabbit. Cats frequently harbor *Taenia taeniaeformis,* the larval stage of which is found in rats and mice (Table 66).

Treatment

Administer a single dose of Yomesan, 70 mg./lb., after fasting animal. It is more effective in cats than in dogs. Bunamidine HCl (Scoloban), 20 mg./lb., is also effective. A fasting period of 18 hours is necessary before medicating.

V–7–F. Lungworms

The metastrongyloid nematodes *Aelurostrongylus abstrusus* and *Capillaria aerophilia* are parasites that reproduce in the air passages and pulmonary vessels or parenchyma of the lungs.

Metastrongyloid parasites of dogs and cats require a mollusc as an intermediate host. Adult Aelurostrongylus worms live in the terminal respiratory bronchioles, alveolar ducts and small branches of the pulmonary arteries. Eggs are forced into the alveolar ducts and alveoli. The first stage larvae escape into the airways and are coughed up and swallowed, thus passing into the feces. The first stage larvae can survive in moist soil for up to five and a half months, in live molluscs for five months and in dead molluscs for three weeks. Various transport hosts (amphibians, birds, reptiles and rodents) may eat infected molluscs and serve as a source of infection when eaten by cats and dogs. When ingested, the infective, third stage larvae penetrate the mucosa of the esophagus,

Text continues on page 548.

TABLE 66. CESTODES FOR DOGS AND CATS

Name	Definitive Host	Intermediate Host	Remarks
Dipylidium caninum	Dog, cat, wolf, fox, other animals	Fleas and biting lice.	Proglottids are shaped like cucumber seeds. Probably the most common tapeworm of dogs
Taenia taeniaeformis	Cat, dog, fox, and other animals	Various rats, mice, and other rodents	This is a common tapeworm of cats
Taenia pisiformis	Dog, cat, fox, wolf, and other animals	Rabbits and hares, rarely squirrels and rodents	Common in hunting dogs and farm dogs who eat rabbits
Taenia hydatigenia	Dog, wolf, rarely cat	Domestic and wild cloven-hoofed animals, rarely rodents	More frequently found in farm dogs
Diphyllobothrium species	Man, dog, cat, and other fish eating animals	Found encysted in organs and free in body cavity of various fish	Found in northern United States and Canada
Echinococcus granulosus	Dog, wolf, fox, and other wild carnivores	Sheep, goats, cattle, swine, horses, deer, moose, and some rodents. Occasionally man and other animals	Public health significance is important.
Multiceps multiceps	Dog, fox, and coyote	Sheep, goats, and other ruminants	Found rarely in western North America

TABLE 67. SPECTRUM, DOSAGES, REPEAT TREATMENTS, AND POSSIBLE TOXICITIES OF CURRENT INTERNAL PARASITICIDES*

Drug	Stomach worm (Physaloptera spp.)	Ascarid (Toxascaris and Toxocara spp.)	Hook worm (Unicinaria and Ancylostoma spp.)	Whipworm (Trichuris spp.)	Tapeworm (Dipylidium and Taenia spp.)	Threadworm (Strongyloides spp.)	Coccidia (Eimeria and Isospora spp.)	Trichomonas
Diethylcarbamazine (caricide)*	+	+						
Piperazine (piperate, Antepar)*	+	+						
Dichlorvos (Task)		+	+	+				
Vincofos (vingard)		+	+	+	+			
Styrid-caricide†		+	+					
Vermiplex*‡		+	+					

*Chart developed by Dr. Danny Scott, D.V.M.

TABLE 67. SPECTRUM, DOSAGES, REPEAT TREATMENTS,
AND POSSIBLE TOXICITIES OF CURRENT
INTERNAL PARASITICIDES (*Continued*)

Fast	Purge	Dose	Repeat	Toxicities
	+	25 mg./lb.	3 weeks	Vomition and diarrhea; check for heartworms first
	+	50 mg./lb.	3 weeks	Vomition and diarrhea
	+	12 to 15 mg./lb.		Vomition (must then wait 14 days before retreating); diarrhea; intussusception; RBC and plasma cholinesterase for 1 to 2 weeks. Cannot use for few days before and after exposure to other cholinesterase inhibitors and cholinesterase inhibitor-potentiating drugs (phenothiazine tranquilizers, muscle relaxants, etc.). Check for heartworms first. Dog only.
	+	7 to 9 mg./lb.		As for dichlorvos; not for use in dog less than 3 months old.
		1 cc./20 lb.	Daily	Anorexia, vomition and diarrhea; check for heartworms first, dog only
12 hr. before and 4 hr. after	+	Coded capsules	3 weeks	Vomition and diarrhea

Table continues on following pages.

TABLE 67. SPECTRUM, DOSAGES, REPEAT TREATMENTS, AND POSSIBLE TOXICITIES OF CURRENT INTERNAL PARASITICIDES (*Continued*)

Drug	Stomach worm (Physaloptera spp.)	Ascarid (Toxascaris and Toxocara spp.)	Hookworm (Unicinaria and Ancylostoma spp.)	Whipworm (Trichuris spp.)	Tapeworm (Dipylidium and Taenia spp.)	Threadworm (Strongyloides spp.)	Coccidia (Eimeria and Isospora spp.)	Trichomonas
Disophenol (DNP)*			+					
Thenium closylate (canopar)			+					
Glycobiarsol (Milibis-V)*				+				
Niclosamide (Yomesan)*					+			
Bunamidine (scolaban)*§					+			
Thiabendazole (omnizole, Mintezol)*						+		+
Metronidazole (Flagyl)*							+	+
Quinacrine (Atabrine)							+	
Sulfadimethoxine (Bactrovet)*						+		

TABLE 67. SPECTRUM, DOSAGES, REPEAT TREATMENTS, AND POSSIBLE TOXICITIES OF CURRENT INTERNAL PARASITICIDES (Continued)

Fast	Purge	Dose	Repeat	Toxicities
		0.1 cc./lb. subcutaneously	3 weeks	Stings; stains coat yellow; hyperthermia (heat stroke) syndrome if overdosed 3 or 4 times.
		½ tablet for <10 lb., 1 tablet for > 10 lb.	3 weeks	Dog only
		100 mg./lb. for 5 days	3 months	Dog only
	+	1 tablet/7 lb.	3 weeks	Vomition and diarrhea
24 hr. before and 3 hr. after	+	½ tablet/cat; 1 tablet/9 lb. dog	3 weeks	Vomition and diarrhea
		25 mg./lb. for 3 days	Once a month till 2 or 3 negative fecals	Anorexia and vomition
		30 mg./lb. for 5 days		Transient neutropenia; contra-indicated when active CNS disease present
	+	50 to 100 mg. b.i.d. for 3 days	3 days	Skin and urine discoloration; retinal damage; cholinesterase inhibitor
		10 mg./lb. for 7 days		

*Preferred drugs (on basis of efficacy and safety).

†Styryl pyridinium-diethylcarbamazine, for ascarid, hookworm, and heartworm prevention.

‡Diphenthane—70 and methylbenzene.

§Drug of choice for *Echinococcus granulosus,* at 25 to 50 mg./kg., two doses at 48 hour interval.

stomach and small intestine, travelling to the bloodstream and lymphatics and finally to the lungs. The prepatent period is 34 to 42 days.

The life cycle of *Capillaria aerophilia* may be direct or may involve earthworms as facultative intermediate hosts. The life cycle is similar to that described for Aelurostrongylus.

Clinical Picture

Most cats affected with Aelurostrongylus exhibit few clinical disturbances. When severe infestations or debilitation occur, signs of illness may include a chronic cough with gradually increasing dyspnea, anorexia and fever. Occasionally, sneezing and oculonasal discharge may be present. The most dangerous period is six to 13 weeks after infection, when large numbers of eggs and larvae are produced.

Diagnosis

Fecal examination is the most practical diagnostic technique. The first stage larvae have a characteristic notched or S-shaped tail and appear in the feces. The Baerman apparatus is the most accurate way of finding larvae in the feces. Fecal examination will not reveal early infections (less than five to six weeks) when adult parasites are not yet mature, nor late infections when eggs are no longer produced.

Chemotherapy

Various chemotherapeutic agents have been used to treat Aelurostrongylus infections. Although data is limited, it appears that the oral administration of L-tetramisole (Tramisol, American Cyanamid Co.) at a dosage of 45 mg./kg./day every other day for five treatments is effective in eliminating larvae from the feces and controlling clinical signs. Atropine sulfate is used as a premedicant to avoid excessive salivation. It is important to remember that the disease is self-limiting, even in those cases showing clinical signs.

Control

Prevention of Aelurostrongylus infection requires preventing cats from catching molluscs or transport hosts. This is extremely difficult.

In *Capillaria aerophilia* infection, placing animals in wire bottom pens or on sanitized concrete runs will prevent reoccurrence of infestation.

V–7–G. Spirocerca lupi

The life cycle of *Spirocerca lupi* requires passage through coprophagous beetles and a range of facultative paratenic hosts, which can include lizards, chickens and mice. Dogs and cats may ingest infected insects or paratenic hosts that feed on insects or crustaceans. When infected larvae are ingested by a dog, they migrate in the adventitia of the visceral arteries and aorta to the walls of the esophagus and stomach. The degree of clinical signs present in spirocerca infection depends on the degree of trauma and functional obstruction caused by the migrating larvae. Spirocerca infection may produce signs of clinical disease characterized by vomiting, anorexia, dysphagia, aortic aneurysm, esophageal neoplasms and secondary pulmonary osteoarthropathy.

V–7–H. Dirofilariasis (Heartworm Disease)

Heartworm disease is endemic in the eastern and southern United States and its distribution is gradually spreading north and west. Any area that has a high mosquito population may have to deal with this disease. Furthermore, the transient nature of today's life style and the rapid modes of transportation allow frequent movement of families and pets.

Mosquito vectors feed on the muzzle, eyes, and perineum of dogs. If a dog carries microfilariae, they are ingested by the mosquito along with

TABLE 68. DIFFERENTIAL CHARACTERISTICS OF DIPETALONEMA AND DIROFILARIA MICROFILARIAE*

Criteria†	Dipetalonema reconditum	Dirofilaria immitis
Length	$<300\ \mu$ avg. 278μ (258–300)	$>300\ \mu$ avg. 318μ (300–345)
Width	avg. $5\ \mu$(4.5–5.4)	avg. $6.5\ \mu$ (6–7)
Anterior end	blunt	tapered
Numbers	few	many
Activity	move rapidly across field	undulate in one place

*From Sawyer, T. K., Weinstein, P. P., and Block, J.: Canine filariasis—The influence of the method of treatment on measurements of microfilaria in blood samples. Amer. J. Vet. Res. *24*:395–401, 1963.

†Important: All of these criteria must be used collectively in diagnosis.

the blood. After a two-week maturation, the larvae are infective (third stage), and dwell in the mouth parts of the mosquito. When the mosquito feeds again, these infective larvae are injected into the subcutaneous tissues of the victim. They live there for two to two and a half months, then invade the venous system. Young adult heartworms can reach the right ventricle in eight to 10 weeks postinfection. They are not capable of releasing microfilariae into the blood until six to seven months postinfection. Adult heartworms can live five years, and microfilaria can live for two to three years in the bloodstream.

Diagnosis

History

A suggestive history of exposure to an endemic heartworm area should prompt a laboratory check.

Symptoms

The animal may be asymptomatic. The diagnosis is generally made during a routine blood check. However, possible symptoms include loss of stamina, weight loss and poor physical condition, soft, moist cough (especially on exertion) and ascites. The dog may stand with elbows abducted, and syncope, seizures and anemia may occur. There may be acute vena caval or liver failure syndrome, in which signs develop over 12 to 24 hours. The dog displays weakness, collapse, anorexia and hemoglobinuria. Death occurs in 12 to 72 hours. Usually no ascites is present.

Physical Examination

Heart murmurs are usually absent. A split-second heart sound may be present due to the pulmonary hypertension that develops. Signs of right heart failure such as venous engorgement, jugular pulse, or ascites may be present.

Electrocardiography

The electrocardiogram often is normal with heartworm disease. Abnormalities may occur in the form of a moderate right axis deviation. Occasionally severe changes are seen. The lead CV_6LU has sometimes been helpful. The presence of an S wave deeper than 0.7 mv. would establish right ventricular hypertrophy.

Radiography

Radiographs are very helpful, especially when the disease has progressed. Right ventricular enlargement and a bulge in the area of the pulmonary artery may be seen on the dorsoventral view. The pulmonary arteries may be large. Rather than tapering to a fine point like a normal pulmonary artery, it tends to end abruptly. This plus the presence of diffuse patchy densities in the lung fields are evidence of pulmonary embolization.

Radiographs may make the diagnosis when EKG and blood tests are negative. Any animal that has right ventricular enlargement on x-ray should have its blood checked for microfilariae, and an EKG should be obtained.

Clinical Pathology

The diagnosis is made by finding microfilariae of *Dirofilaria immitis* in the bloodstream. They must be differentiated from the microfilariae of *Dipetalonema spp*. A number of different tests have been advocated for the detection of microfilaria, including the direct wet smear, membrane filtration test, capillary sedimentation test, saponin lysis test and modified Knotts test. The most reliable test is still the modified Knotts procedure.

The presence of eosinophilia may be associated with heartworm disease, but it is a nonspecific finding. Any animal with an unexplained eosinophilia should have a blood check, a chest x-ray and an EKG.

Dirofilariasis without microfilaremia can occur. This could be associated with previous contact with microfilaria and development of circulating antibody to *Dirofilaria immitis*. In this instance, evidence of adult Dirofilaria infection, such as the radiographic, cardiac, pulmonary parenchymal and vascular changes along with persistent eosinophilia may be helpful in recognizing the disease.

Treatment

Heartworm disease can be treated medically or surgically. Because of the drawbacks of surgery, and the success of medical therapy, most dogs are treated medically. Occasionally surgery is done when large numbers of adult Dirofilaria are present. This is difficult to determine. The number of microfilariae present in the peripheral circulation does not correspond with the number of adult microfilariae that may be present.

Medical Treatment

1. A CBC, BUN, urinalysis, and SGPT are taken. If any of these are abnormal, appropriate supportive therapy such as fluids, B vitamins, vitamin C, lipotrophic agents, antibiotics and steroids has been advocated. If the dog is in heart failure he should be digitalized prior to treatment.

2. Sodium caparsolate (1 per cent) is administered 1 ml./10 lb. of body weight twice a day for two days. The irritant action of this drug mandates a

TABLE 69. EFFECT OF CHEMICAL AGENTS ON DEVELOPMENTAL STAGES OF DIROFILARIA IMMITIS*

| Developmental Stage | Location | Chemotherapeutic Agents | | | | |
		Anti-monials	Diethyl-carbama-zine	Arsenicals	Dithi-azanine	Organo-phosphates
Microfilaria	Blood	+++	++	—	+++	++
Developing larvae	Adipose subserosa subcutaneous tissue	+	+++	+	—	?
Adult worm	Heart and pulmonary artery	+	—	+++	—	—

*From Levine, B. G.: Dirofilariasis, *In* Kirk, R. W. (ed.): Current Veterinary Therapy V. W. B. Saunders Co., 1974.

perfect intravenous injection. No drug can go perivascularly. The animal is hospitalized or kept at cage rest for 10 to 14 days after treatment. The drug kills the adult heartworms over a one- to three-week period. Exercise is restricted four to six weeks or more depending on the severity of the case.

Complications are drug toxicity or thromboembolism in the lungs from dead worms. Signs of drug toxicity include bilirubinuria, vomiting, icterus and dehydration.

3. At present dithiazanine iodide is the only drug available for use as a microfilaricide. Tetramazol is presently under investigation, and organophosphates were used but are not approved now. Dizan is given 2.5 mg./lb. three times a day for two days. If the blood test is still positive, the dosage is increased to 5 mg./lb. three times a day for three more days or until the blood test is negative. Dizan is started six to eight weeks after the caparsolate therapy.

4. Diethylcarbamazine (Caracide, Cyanamid) is used as a preventive agent. It is not a microfilaricide. It is effective against the third stage infective larvae. Caracide should *not* be used in dogs that test microfilaria positive because of a high percentage of allergic reactions in those dogs.

Caracide is given 2.5 mg./lb. three times daily. It should be begun 30 days before and continued for at least 60 days after leaving an endemic heartworm area. In endemic areas it is given year-round. Parasiticidal agents (Styrid) are also available to add to the dog's food to simplify prophylaxis.

References

Additional information can be found in the following sources:

Sawyer, T. K., Weinstein, P. P., and Block, J.: Canine filariasis—the influence of the method of treatment on measurements of microfilariae in blood samples. Amer. J. Vet. Res. *24*:395–401, 1963.

Stein, F. J., and Lawton, E. W.: Comparison of methods for diagnosis and differentiation of canine filariasis. JAVMA *163*:140–141, 1973.

Wong, M. M.: Dirofilariasis without circulating microfilariae: a problem in diagnosis. JAVMA *163*:133–139, 1973.

V–7–I. Coccidiosis

Isospora bigemina, Isopora rivolta and *Isospora felis* are the three common types of organisms causing coccidiosis in the United States.

Coccidiosis usually affects young dogs and cats, especially those from kennels, pet shops, catteries or other places where large numbers of animals are kept together. The disease is characterized by anorexia, diarrhea (frequently hemorrhagic), and loss of weight.

Diagnosis is based on finding oocysts in the feces coupled with the clinical history. Other intestinal parasites and systemic diseases such as distemper may complicate the diagnosis.

Infection of the host results from ingestion of infective oocysts. The coccidia undergo repeated cycles of asexual multiplication (schizogony) which finally terminate in formation of sexually differentiated gametes that combine to form zygotes. At this stage a protective covering is formed (oocyst.) Sporulation (sporogony) may occur in the intestinal tract or after the oocyst is eliminated in the feces. In the genus Isospora there are two sporocysts, each containing four sporozoites.

Diagnosis

Diagnosis is based on finding oocysts in the feces coupled with the clinical history. The diarrhea may precede a heavy outpouring of oocysts by a few days and may continue even after oocyst levels become low. It is, therefore, not always possible to confirm a clinical diagnosis of coccidiosis by finding oocysts in the feces. Other intestinal parasites and systemic diseases such as distemper may complicate the picture too.

Treatment

There is no good treatment for coccidiosis in dogs and cats once the signs of disease have appeared. Prophylaxis of clinical coccidiosis depends upon good sanitation and controlling the natural intake of sporulated oocysts by young animals. With good hygiene and sanitation, coccidiosis is a self-limiting disease. Treatment of patients with coccidiosis should be aimed at controlling the diarrhea, reducing the population of coccidial organisms, correcting fluid and electrolyte imbalances, and establishing good principles of animal hygiene and sanitation. Intestinal sulfonamides, neomycin, Furacin, tetracycline, and chloramphenicol have all been used to help control secondary infections and reduce the population of coccidial organisms.

References

Additional information can be found in the following sources:

Georgi, J. R.: Parasitology for Veterinarians. 2nd ed. Philadelphia, W. B. Saunders Co., 1975.

Merck Veterinary Manual, 4th edition. Rahway, New Jersey. Merck Company, 1973.

Soulsby, E. J. L.: Helminths, Arthropods and Protozoa of Domesticated Animals (Monnig), 6th ed. Baltimore, Williams and Wilkins, 1968.

V–7–J. Toxoplasmosis

Toxoplasma is an intestinal coccidian of cats. Cats, especially kittens under six months of age, can become infected and shed toxoplasma oocysts after eating mice, rats, birds or meat containing toxoplasma cysts. The prepatent period to the shedding of oocysts is three to five days after the ingestion of mice or meat containing toxoplasma cysts and 20 to 34 days after the ingestion of oocysts. Oocysts are shed by infected cats for one to five weeks during primary infection and in reduced numbers or not at all following reinfection. The oocysts are not infectious until sporulation, which requires one to five days (or longer, depending on environmental temperature and oxygenation). Under favorable circumstances, oocysts remain infectious for several months to a year or longer. Toxoplasmosis in man and other animals can result from the oral ingestion of sporulated oocysts.

The oocysts of toxoplasma develop two sporocysts and four sporozoites. *Isospora felis* and *Isospora rivolta* are the two common coccidian parasites found in young cats. The oocysts of *Isospora felis* measure 40 by 30 microns and *Isospora rivolta* 25 by 20 microns. Oocysts of toxoplasma are much smaller: 10 by 12 microns, or about twice the size of a red blood cell.

Standard techniques of fecal flotation at 1.15 specific gravity will concentrate the oocysts in the supernatant. Stools should be examined while fresh to detect oocysts in the feces.

It would appear from serologic evidence that man and animals can suffer from asymptomatic infections with Toxoplasma organisms. Toxoplasma antibodies have been found in varying percentages of cats, depending on the types of populations tested. Forty to 60 per cent of cats in the Kansas-Iowa area had Toxoplasma antibodies and reports indicate that 24 to 57 per cent of dogs in the United States have Toxoplasma antibodies.

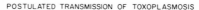
POSTULATED TRANSMISSION OF TOXOPLASMOSIS

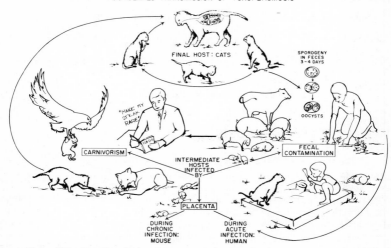

Figure 77. Postulated life cycle of *Toxoplasma*. Cats and certain other felines are shown as final hosts, and other animals and humans as intermediate hosts. Flies and cockroaches can serve as transport hosts. At right, infection with oocysts is shown. At left, transmission by carnivorism is indicated. Below, the transplacental route of transmission is indicated. (Modified from Frenkel, J. K.: Toxoplasmosis. *In* Marcial-Rojas, R. A. (ed.): Pathology of Protozoa and Helminthic Diseases. © 1971 The Williams and Wilkins Company, Baltimore.)

Clinically, symptomatic toxoplasmosis may involve many organs. Following oral ingestion of oocysts, the gastrointestinal tract is infected, and then there can be hematogenous and lymphogenous dissemination of the organism to other organs, including liver, lungs, lymph nodes, eyes, central nervous system and muscle.

Confirmation of Toxoplasma infection can be based on serologic evidence or isolation of Toxoplasma organisms by inoculating tissues into mice. Serologic examination should consist of paired sera examination taken one or two weeks apart. Sera can be examined by the Sabin-Feldman dye test, the indirect fluorescent antibody test or the agglutination test. A rise of three to fourfold in titer is presumptive evidence of an active Toxoplasma infection.

Material suspected of harboring Toxoplasma organisms can be injected intraperitoneally into mice. The procedures for detection of infected mice and recovery of organisms have been described.

Treatment

Sulfadiazine and pyrimethamine interfere in sequential steps with the biosynthesis of dihydrofolate and act synergistically against Toxoplasma. The toxic side effects can be prevented and alleviated with yeast and folinic acid. The shedding of oocysts by kittens can be nearly eliminated by treating with sulfadiazine, 120 mg./kg./day, or with 60 mg./kg./day of sulfadiazine together with 0.5 mg./kg./day of pyrimethamine. Cats passing oocysts in the stool should be handled according to the precautions discussed next.

Prevention of Infection by Toxoplasma

Animals are infected with Toxoplasma in the cyst stage from eating infected meat, in the oocyst stage from cats and soil, or from tachyzoites transplacentally. Feeding dried, cooked, or canned food to a cat that's kept indoors and has no opportunity to hunt mice or birds eliminates the risk of acquiring toxoplasmosis. Meat that has been frozen is less infectious, but may still harbor Toxoplasma cysts. Litter pans should be cleaned daily with boiling water or dry heat. Cat feces should be burned or flushed down a toilet. A pregnant woman should wear plastic gloves to clean the litter pan. The following points are important in the control of toxoplasmosis:

1. Do not feed cats raw meat products.

2. Control flies, cockroaches and other coprophagous animals that can serve as hosts of Toxoplasma.

3. Avoid contact with soil and sand that can be contaminated by cat feces.

4. Wash hands after handling cats or their excrement.

5. The presence of antibody against Toxoplasma does not mean that a cat is presently infected or in need of treatment. There is no need to get rid of the cat. In fact, immune cats are safer pets than nonimmune ones, since on reinfection they shed few oocysts or none at all.

References

Additional information can be found in the following sources:

Frenkel, J. K.: Toxoplasmosis. In Kirk, R. W. (ed.): Current Veterinary Therapy V. Philadelphia, W. B. Saunders Co., 1974.

Frenkel, J. K., and Dubey, J. P.: Toxoplasmosis and its prevention in cats and man. J. Infec. Dis., 126:664–673, 1972.

Krogstad, D. J., Juranek, D. D., and Walls, K. W.: Toxoplasmosis, with comments on risk of infection from cats. Ann. Intern. Med. 77:773–778, 1972.

V-8. FECAL SAMPLE COLLECTION AND EXAMINATION

COLLECTION

Fresh fecal samples are always desirable. Two to 4 ounce closed containers are best suited for fecal collections. Fecal samples can be picked up with disposable wooden tongue blades after the animal defecates, or taken directly from the rectum. An enema may be administered, but soapy or oily enemas should not be used, as they interfere with good examinations of the stool. Material left on thermometers usually is not adequate for fecal examinations except in a few heavy parasitic infestations. If samples must be kept for a few hours to several days, refrigeration or chemical fixation should be used.

GROSS EXAMINATION

Examine stool for adult worms or tapeworm segments. Note the presence of blood, mucus, fat, or other undigested material. Characterize the odor of the stool. Note the amount of stool passed and whether it is formed or unformed. The longer the total gastrointestinal passage time, the firmer the feces. If the stool is formed, note its shape and diameter.

Color

Feces are usually brown in color from the pigments urobilin and stercobilin derived from bacterial action on bilirubin. A dark brown to black tarry stool indicates that the animal is on a high meat diet or that there are blood pigments in the stool from upper gastrointestinal bleeding. Excessive amounts of bilirubin may produce a darker orange-brown stool. A grayish white, clay-colored stool is associated with biliary obstruction and pancreatic acinar insufficiency. A light brown or tan-colored stool is frequently seen in nursing puppies or dogs on a diet high in milk. A green stool may be seen in dogs with unchanged bilirubin in the stool. Fresh red blood in the stool indicates recent bleeding into the colon or rectum.

Mucus

Normal stools contain only a small amount of mucus, which may not be easily observed. Excess mucus in the stool is a sign of lower bowel disease and is associated with acute and chronic inflammatory disease of the terminal ileum, cecum and colon.

MICROSCOPIC EXAMINATION OF THE FECES

1. *Smear technique.* This technique is used when small quantities of material are available or when the fecal examination must be completed in a short period of time. This procedure involves mixing a small amount of fecal material in a drop or two of saline placed on a slide and examining it microscopically.

2. *Qualitative concentration methods.* This is the routine method for parasite examination. The concentration of parasite ova or oocysts may be determined in a number of ways. All the methods depend on mixing the fecal sample with a material whose specific gravity is heavier than most of the parasitic ova or oocysts, yet is lighter than the fecal debris. Solutions of sodium chloride, sucrose, glycerine, zinc sulfate or magnesium sulfate may be used to float the parasitic ova. Sugar flotation, although satisfactory for most parasitic ova, will not float the ova of tapeworms and flukes. Tapeworms are most easily diagnosed by gross examination of the feces for the typical segments. Fluke eggs can be found using the technique of Demnis, Stone, and Swanson (Benbrook) or the technique of Joy (described by Farrell).

3. *Methods for protozoa examinations.* The protozoan parasites, Trichomonas, Giardia, and Balantidium, disappear rapidly from fecal samples. In order to identify these parasites, the stool must be either examined or placed in a fecal fixative immediately after removal from the rectum. Wet smears are satisfactory in some cases of protozoan infections if the feces can be examined immediately and the infection is heavy. A second technique involving fixed feces provides the advantages of concentration and delayed examination. Prepare PAF fixative: phenol crystals (white), 20.0 gm.: normal saline (0.85 per cent), 825.0 ml.; ethanol (95 per cent), 125.0 ml.; formaldehyde solution, 50.0 ml. (23 ml. of liquified phenol may be substituted for the crystals). Cover the fresh feces with the PAF fixative and allow them to stand at room temperature for one hour or longer. Strain the fixed sample through gauze and then centrifuge the collective fluid at 1000 rpm for two or three minutes. Decant the excess fluid and wash and centrifuge the sediment twice with normal saline. Stain several drops of the sediment with thionin or azure A to allow for easy identification. If concentration is not desired, directly examine the sediment from the fixed feces.

4. *Methods for Strongyloides examination.* The rhabditiform larvae of *Strongyloides stercoralis* can be found in smears prepared from fresh feces. These larvae can be easily confused with other larval parasites and can be definitively identified by incubating the fecal specimen for 24 hours at room temperature or by culturing the feces on sterile sand for 48 hours. The infective filariform larvae will develop and can be identified by the esophageal length (one-third of total body length). A Baermann apparatus may also be utilized for examination of the larvae.

5. The feces should also be examined for the presence of undigested muscle (creatorrhea), fat (steatorrhea) or starch (amylorrhea) and for the presence or absence of pancreatic proteolytic enzymes. Fat droplets are demonstrated with a Sudan III stain. Muscle fibers are seen microscopically in direct fecal smears. One drop of Lugol's solution will turn undigested starch blue. Fecal trypsin can be identified by using the film strip digestion test or the more accurate gelatine tube test.

References

Additional information can be found in the following sources:

Adam, K. M. G., Paul, J., and Zaman, V.: Medical and Veterinary Protozoology: An Illustrated Guide. London, Churchill Livingstone, 1971.

Benbrook, E. A., and Sloss, M. W.: Veterinary Clinical Parasitology, 3rd ed. Ames, Iowa, State University Press, 1961.

Buckner, R. G., and Ewing, S. A.: Trichomoniasis. *In* Kirk, R. W. (ed.): Current Veterinary Therapy V. Philadelphia, W. B. Saunders Co., 1974.

Georgi, J. R.: Intestinal helminths. *In* Kirk, R. W. (ed.): Current Veterinary Therapy V. Philadelphia, W. B. Saunders Co., 1974.

V–8–A. Specific Tests for Evaluation of Gastrointestinal Function

FECAL FAT

The presence of excessive amounts of fat in the feces (steatorrhea) can be a prominent sign of a severe gastrointestinal disturbance, such as malabsorption. The normal dog excretes 3 to 5 gm. of fat in the stool per day and is not greatly affected by normal dietary intake of fat.

1. Demonstration of steatorrhea can be done by staining a fresh stool with a lipophilic stain such as Sudan III and examining under the microscope.

2. To perform a gross fat absorption test, draw a heparinized blood sample from a fasted animal and separate the plasma. Feed a meal enriched with corn oil (1 mg./lb.) or peanut oil 0.5 to 2.0 gm./kg. Take a second blood sample two hours after ingestion of the fat meal and compare plasma turbidity between pre- and post-fat ingestion samples. In the normal situation, the second plasma sample shows increased turbidity because of neutral fat droplets or chylomicrons. If both plasma samples are clear, either pancreatic exocrine function is inadequate or the intestine is not absorbing nutrients properly. Pancreatic exocrine insufficiency can be eliminated by repeating the test but predigesting the fat meal with pancreatic extracts. If the second sample of plasma still remains clear, a diagnosis of malabsorption should be considered.

3. For a 24-hour fecal fat excretion test, the animal should be placed on a constant diet for 48 hours. All stool should be collected for 24 hours and sent to laboratory for total fecal fat. Normal values are 3 to 5 gm. of fat in the stool per day. Steatorrhea is present when the total fecal fat exceeds 7 gm. per day.

4. The D-xylose absorption test measures the ability of the proximal jejunum to absorb five-carbon sugar. Fast the patient for 24 hours and empty the bladder prior to the administration of D-xylose. Administer 25 gm. of D-xylose in 200 cc. of warm water by stomach tube. Collect all urine for the next five hours; the bladder must be rinsed on final collection. Eight to 12 gm. of D-xylose should be present in the urine after five hours. Low levels of D-xylose can indicate a malabsorption problem. Kidney function must be normal for the accurate interpretation of this test.

5. The oral glucose tolerance test measures the ability of the proximal jejunum to absorb a six-carbon sugar, and the ability of the beta cells of the pancreas to supply insulin to permit normal glucose metabolism. Fast the dog for 12 hours and draw a fasting blood sample for baseline blood sugar. Administer 4 gm./kg. of dextrose in canned meat. Take blood samples at 30 minutes, one hour, two hours, and three hours. Normal dog blood sugar levels at the end of one hour are 120 to 140 mg. per cent, with a return to fasting level in two or three hours. A flat curve suggests glucose malabsorption and an abnormally elevated curve which persists over several hours may indicate insulin deficiency.

6. The oral vitamin A absorption test measures the ability of the intestine to digest and absorb lipids. Administer to the fasted dog 300,000 units of vitamin A (White's cod liver oil concentrate drops). Collect heparinized blood samples prior to the administration and after two, four, six, eight and 24 hours. Normal dogs show a two or threefold increase in vitamin A levels over fasting. A flat curve may indicate a lack of bile, pancreatic enzymes, malabsorption or disease of the ileum.

7. Another test is oral administration of ^{131}I-labeled triolein. On the day before the test, administer 0.3 cc. of Lugol's iodine in a capsule orally to block the thyroidal uptake of ^{131}I label. On the day of the test administer 20 microcuries of ^{131}I triolein. Collect blood samples over two, four, six, eight and 10 hours. Normal dogs show 8 to 15 per cent absorption after a 10-hour period.

8. Oral administration of ^{131}I-labeled oleic acid is similar to the test as described for triolein, substituting I_{131} oleic acid. Normal values are 10 to 15 per cent absorption in 10 hours.

Performance of the ^{131}I triolein and oleic acid tests in sequence aids in differentiating steatorrhea. In steatorrhea associated with a lack of pancreatic lipase, absorption of oleic acid will be normal; however, absorption of triolein, which requires lipolysis, will be reduced. The absorption of both compounds is reduced in malabsorption syndrome. Absorption of oleic acid may also be reduced in long-standing cases of pancreatic insufficiency.

References

Additional information can be found in the following sources:

Brobst, D. F., and Funk, A.: Simplified test of fat absorption in dogs. JAVMA *161*:1412–1417, 1972.

Hill, F. W. G.: Methods available for the study of digestion and absorption in dogs. Vet. Ann., pp. 94–103, 1970.

Kirk, R. W.: Symposium on physical diagnosis in small animals. Vet. Clin. North Amer. Vol. 1, No. 1, January, 1971.

Palminteri, A.: Symposium on gastrointestinal medicine and surgery. Vet. Clin. North Amer. Vol. 2, No. 1, January, 1972.

Tennant, B. C., and Ewing, G. O.: Gastrointestinal function. *In* Kaneko, J. J., and Cornelius, C. E. (eds.): Clinical Biochemistry of Domestic Animals, 2nd ed., Vol. II. New York, Academic Press, 1971.

V–9. PUNCTURE FLUIDS EXAMINATION

All serous cavities and tissue spaces of the body contain a small amount of fluid. Under normal circumstances, this consists of a low-protein blood filtrate. Abnormal amounts of fluids in body cavities are termed effusions. Aspirates of these fluids are studied in an attempt to classify the origin of these fluids as transudative (a noninflammatory accumulation of fluid associated with a physiochemical disturbance) or exudative (an accumulation of fluid associated with an inflammatory response).

PHYSICAL CHARACTERISTICS

1. Measure the volume of fluid removed.
2. Evaluate fluid for color and transparency.
   a. A pinkish to reddish color usually indicates the presence of erythrocytes.
   b. A yellowish color is imparted by excessive bilirubin, a high protein content, or degenerated erythrocytes.
   c. A milky white color may indicate chyle. If the cloudiness of the fluid is caused by the presence of chylomicrons, the fluid will clear upon adding ether and shaking.
   d. A thick, creamy fluid usually indicates the presence of a large number of leukocytes.

3. Note if the fluid coagulates. The ability to clot is dependent on the amount of fibrin present. Exudates may show rapid coagulation whereas transudates usually do not coagulate. Lysis of the clot may occur in exudates and may not be demonstrated.

4. Determine the specific gravity of the fluid. In general, the specific gravity is closely correlated with the protein content of the fluid. Transudates usually have a specific gravity less than, and exudates a specific gravity more than 1.017, although no hard line can be drawn at that point.

5. Smell the fluid for odor. Puncture fluids are usually odorless unless contaminated by putrefying bacterial organisms such as *E. coli* from the intestinal tract, or urine from a ruptured bladder.

CHEMICAL EXAMINATION
Seromucin Test

This test can be used to help distinguish a transudate from an exudate. Exudates are usually seromucin positive and transudates seromucin negative.

Total Proteins

Exudates usually have a high protein content (more than 3 gm./100 ml.) whereas transudates usually have a lower total protein content.

Urea Nitrogen

Urea nitrogen determinations can be used in determining the presence of nitrogenous material within the abdominal cavity in such conditions as rupture of the bladder, or in evaluating the efficiency of fluid that has been used in peritoneal dialysis.

MICROSCOPIC EXAMINATION

Total Cell Counts

Transudates usually have a low total cell count, frequently between 100 and 500 cells/cubic mm. Exudates usually have elevated cell counts that may exceed 50,000/cubic mm. Large numbers of erythrocytes may be seen if a vessel was damaged while a paracentesis was being performed.

Differential Smear

Large numbers of neutrophils indicate a purulent exudate and one should look for a causative organism. Lymphocytes indicate a chronic exudative or viral reaction. Very young, bizarrely shaped lymphocytes may point to tumor formation. If an allergy or parasitic problem is causing the formation of an exudate, eosinophils may be found. If a tumor is suspected, examination of cells by a competent cytologist may prove very helpful in making a diagnosis. Smears should be fixed while still wet with a commercial fixative such as Spraycyte (Clay Adams Co.). These smears can be stained by the method of Papanicolaou or Sano and examined. Both veterinary schools and hospitals have pathologists trained in the field of exfoliative cytology.

BACTERIOLOGIC EXAMINATION

1. Prepare a new methylene blue or Gram stain of aspirated material.
2. Culture (see Sections IV-4 and IV-5).
3. Animal inoculations may be indicated.

TRANSUDATES VERSUS EXUDATES

Unfortunately, many times no hard line can be drawn between a transudate and an exudate. Many conditions can alter the normal characteristics of a transudate, resulting in a "modified transudate." Such condi-

TABLE 70. PROPERTIES OF TRANSUDATES AND EXUDATES

	Transudate	**Exudate**
Appearance	Clear, serous, or light yellow	Cloudy and turbid
Specific gravity	Below 1.017	Above 1.017
Coagulation	Negative	May be positive
Seromucin	Negative	Usually positive
Types of cells	Usually a few endothelial and red blood cells	Heavy cell population, neutrophils or lymphocytes
Bacteria	Usually absent	May be present
Protein	Less than 3 gm./100 ml.	Greater than 3 gm./100 ml.

tions as hepatic obstruction, chylothorax and congestive heart failure can produce greatly altered transudates, making it difficult to distinguish between a ''modified transudate'' and an exudate. In addition, both transudates and exudates may be present in one disease process. It is helpful to keep in mind the underlying mechanisms of the formation of each type of fluid and relate this to the disease process in the animal.

References

Additional information can be found in the following sources:

Medway, W.: Textbook of Veterinary Clinical Pathology. Baltimore, Williams and Wilkins Co., 1969.

Perman, V.: Transudates and exudates. *In* Kaneko, J. J., and Cornelius, C. E. (eds.): Clinical Biochemistry of Domestic Animals, 2nd ed., Vol. II. New York, Academic Press, 1971.

Perman, V., Osborne, C. A., and Stevens, J. B.: Laboratory evaluation of abnormal body fluids. Clin. North Amer., Vol. 4, No. 2, pp. 255–268, May, 1974.

Roszel, J. F.: Exfoliative cytology in the diagnosis of malignant canine neoplasms. Vet. Scope *I*: 1967.

Stevens, J. B., Perman, V., and Osborne, C. A.: Biopsy sample management, staining, and examination. Vet. Clin. North Amer. Vol. 4, No. 2, pp. 233–253, May, 1974.

V–10. SYNOVIAL FLUID

Synovial fluid is a protein dialysate of plasma that contains mucin produced by the synovial cells.

Synovial fluid can be obtained by arthrocentesis (the aseptic aspiration of a joint cavity). Routines for performing arthrocentesis have been described (Hardy).

Examination of Synovial Fluid

1. The physical characteristics should be noted including color, turbidity, viscosity, clot formation, and quantity.

2. A determination of the total cell count and a differential count should be performed.

3. A total protein estimation should be made.

4. Bacteriologic examination including culture should be performed. Cell counts made in dogs with aspirates from the carpal, elbow, shoulder, hip, stifle, and hock joints showed that from 0 to 2900 cells with a mean of 430 cells/cu. mm. could be found (Sawyer).

The cell count of normal synovial fluid should contain less than 10 per cent polymorphonuclear leukocytes (polymorphs). The following mean per cent values have been reported for the dog: monocytes 39.72, lymphocytes 44.16, clasmatocytes 4.20, polymorphs 1.38 (Sawyer).

In traumatic osteoarthritis clasmatocytes were found to be increased in number.

In traumatic or degenerate joint lesions, there may be an increase in the nonmucin protein content of the joint fluid because of the degeneration or change in permeability of blood vessels. Mucin concentration is usually decreased in infectious arthritis but stays normal in traumatic or degenerative joint lesions.

Polyarthritis associated with systemic lupus has been described in the dog and L. E. cells have been located in the synovial fluid.

When joint effusions of unknown etiology are present, it can be advantageous to obtain a synovial membrane biopsy. The technique for this has been described (Hardy).

Normal joint fluid should be sterile when cultured (see Section IV-4).

References

Additional information can be found in the following sources:

Hardy, R. M., and Wallace, L. J.: Arthrocentesis and synovial membrane biopsy. Vet. Clin. North Amer., Vol. 4, No. 2, pp. 449–462, May, 1974.

Perman, V., and Cornelius, C. E.: Synovial fluid. *In* Kaneko, J. J., and Cornelius, C. E. (eds.): Clinical Biochemistry of Domestic Animals, 2nd ed., Vol. II. New York, Academic Press, 1971.

Sawyer, D. C.: Synovial fluid analysis in canine joints. JAVMA *143*:609–612, 1963.

V-11.   URINALYSIS

PHYSICAL EXAMINATION

Collection

Use a clean, transparent container. Do not collect the first part of the urine stream, but then collect 2 or 3 ounces of an early morning sample. This is most likely to be concentrated and to contain constitutents of diagnostic significance.

A fresh sample is desirable, so present it promptly for laboratory evaluation (especially culture), or refrigerate it for adequate preservation for several hours.

Short-term preservation of casts and cellular elements can be effected by acidification of the urine. If urine is alkaline, add 0.1 normal hydrochloric acid a drop at a time until pH is on acid side. To prevent microbial growth in a urine sample, add one drop of 40 per cent formalin per 30 ml. of urine, or thymol, 5 to 10 cc.

Volume

Normal urine volume is variable and dependent on diet, fluid intake, environmental factors, body size and weight and exercise. A normal dog will produce 12 to 20 ml. of urine/lb./24 hours (see Section II–18).

Color and Appearance

Normal urine is usually yellow to amber in color (due to urochrome pigments) and is clear.

1. A very pale yellow colorless urine indicates a very dilute urine such as may occur in diabetes insipidus, chronic interstitial nephritis, pyometra, or excessive fluid intake.

2. A dark yellow to orange urine usually indicates a concentrated urine such as occurs in dehydration, fever, or reduced fluid intake.

3. A cloudy appearing urine usually indicates crystalluria or the

presence of a high cell content as may occur with an infection of the urinary tract.

4. An orange urine may indicate excessive amounts of urobilinogen or the presence of the metabolic end products of agents such as Azo gantrisin.

5. A red urine may indicate hemorrhage, food pigments, or the presence of dyes such as phenolsulphonphthalein.

6. Greenish urine may indicate increased levels of bilirubin. Greenish blue urine can be produced by such drugs as dithiazanine iodide and methylene blue.

Transparency

Urine is usually clear upon being voided. Highly concentrated urine or urine with a high crystal or cell count may be cloudy. If the urine is allowed to stand after being collected, precipitates of crystals form and the urine becomes cloudy. The cause of urine turbidity is best evaluated by sediment examination.

Reaction (pH)

The pH of the urine usually depends on the diet and metabolism of the animal. The urine of the dog and cat is normally acid (pH 6 to 7).

1. Increased acidity of the urine can be produced by an all-meat diet, fever, metabolic and respiratory acidosis, prolonged vigorous exercise, or the administration of acidifying drugs such as ammonium chloride, ascorbic acid, or DL-methionine.

2. An alkaline urine can be produced by urinary retention, cystitis (especially those infections caused by Proteus that split urea to form ammonia), metabolic and respiratory alkalosis, or treatment with drugs such as sodium bicarbonate or sodium lactate.

Odor

Abnormal urine odors are significant only in freshly voided specimens. An odor of ammonia is the most common abnormal odor of urine; it can occur if urea has been degraded by urea-splitting bacteria, as may occur in cystitis, or in states of metabolic acidosis. A putrid odor to the urine indicates degradation of large quantities of protein. Ketonuria may impart a fruity odor to the urine.

Specific Gravity

1. Urine specific gravity may range from 1.001 to 1.060 in normal dogs and from 1.001 to 1.080 in normal cats. The range of 1.015 to 1.045 is more commonly found. If the specific gravity is 1.025, one can assume that the distal tubules and collecting ducts are competent, that at least 30 per cent of the nephrons are functional, and that the hypothalamo-neurohypophyseal system is intact. Patients with an elevated BUN and a urine concentration of greater than 1.025 have either prerenal uremia or primary glomerular disease. Patients with prerenal uremia should re-establish normal renal function by restoring vascular volume and perfusion pressure. Patients with primary glomerular disease have a persistent proteinuria and no definable cause of poor renal perfusion.

The kidneys have a very large reserve capacity and impairment of concentrating ability of the kidney is not detectable until at least two-thirds of the total population of nephrons are nonfunctional. The loss of the ability to concentrate and dilute urine may develop gradually. Urine with a specific gravity of 1.007 to 1.017 from a clinically dehydrated or azotemic patient is indicative of primary renal failure.

2. Random sample specific gravities are unreliable. Repeated tests are much more valuable, especially in the animal whose urine has a low specific gravity. A lowered specific gravity may be associated with polyuria. It occurs in chronic interstitial nephritis, diabetes insipidus, pyometra, advanced uremia, adrenocorticohyperplasia, and pyelonephritis. It may be produced by excessive increase in fluid intake (polydipsia) or by the reabsorption of edema fluid.

With kidney tubule damage, such as occurs in chronic interstitial nephritis, the specific gravity of the urine may be fixed at 1.010 ± 0.002. This is the specific gravity of the glomerular filtrate and indicates an inability of the renal tubules to dilute or concentrate the filtrate (isosthenuria).

Urine concentration tests may be performed on animals with a low specific gravity urine. Posterior pituitary extract can be given to animals suspected of having diabetes insipidus. Withholding water for 12 to 18 hours can also be used as a concentration test; however, this is dangerous in animals suspected of having chronic interstitial nephritis or uremia.

3. An increased specific gravity can be seen in cystitis, acute nephritis (in the oliguric phase), diabetes mellitus, reduction in fluid intake, fever, and dehydration from any cause.

Osmolality

Osmolality is the measure of osmotic pressure of a fluid dependent on the number of particles of solute per unit volume of solvent. Osmolality is measured by determining the freezing point depression of a solution. The osmotic concentration of plasma, interstitial fluid, trancellular fluid and intracellular fluid is about 300 mOsm per kg. of water. The osmotic concentration of urine is variable and is dependent on the fluid and electrolyte balance of the body. In normally hydrated dogs and cats, urine osmolality is usually 500 to 1200 mOsm per kg. The ratio of urine osmolality to plasma osmolality has been used as an index of renal function:

1. A U/P Osm ratio above one indicates that the kidneys are capable of concentrating urine above the concentration of plasma. If the animal is deprived of water for 24 hours, the normal canine U/P Osm ratio is three or higher.

2. A U/P Osm ratio of one indicates that water and solute are being excreted in a state which is iso-osmotic with plasma.

3. A U/P Osm ratio below one indicates that the kidneys are capable of absorbing solute in excess of water.

V–11–A. Chemical Examination of the Urine

Protein

Protein in the urine of normal patients cannot be demonstrated by normal qualitative methods. If the glomerular membrane is damaged or if bleeding occurs anywhere in the urogenital tract protein may be found in the urine. Albumin is the first protein to leak through a damaged glomerular membrane, followed by alpha, beta, and gamma globulin, and fibrinogen.

Proteins may appear in the urine under certain physiologic conditions, such as excessive muscular activity, convulsions, consumption of a large amount of protein in the diet, or emotional and physical stress.

Abnormal levels of proteins in the urine may be produced by prerenal, extraurinary or urinary disorders. Prerenal proteins should, by definition, arise from nonrenal sources, and may be found in hemoglobinuria, myoglobinuria or multiple myeloma.

Extraurinary cause of proteinuria include metastatic neoplastic disease, altered circulation associated with embolic phenomena and increased abdominal pressure with resultant altered blood flow to kidneys. Nonrenal causes of increased urinary proteins can include inflammation of the lower urinary tract, hematuria, or contamination of the urine from genital tract infection.

Elevated amounts of protein in the urine can be found in kidney diseases such as nephritis, amyloidosis, pyelonephritis and glomerular disease.

Persistent proteinuria in the absence of hematuria or pyuria indicates the presence of generalized glomerular disease.

Bence-Jones protein, a low molecular weight thermosensitive urinary protein, may be found in the urine if multiple myeloma is present.

Glucose

Normal urine does not contain glucose, for the glucose that has been filtered at the glomerular membrane has been reabsorbed in the proximal convoluted tubules. If the glucose level in the blood exceeds 175 mg./100 ml. of blood, glucose will appear in the urine. A few dogs have a low renal threshold for glucose and may produce urine that constantly contains small amounts of glucose.

Elevated levels of glucose in the urine (fasted sample) may be present in:

1. Emotional glycosuria induced by fear, excitement, or violent exercise in which the level of epinephrine is increased and glucocorticoids are mobilized.

2. General anesthesia, which promotes a rapid release of glucose from storage compartments in the liver.

3. Diabetes mellitus.

4. Hyperthyroidism, because of the rapid uptake of glucose from the gastrointestinal tract.

5. Acute pancreatic necrosis.

6. Hyperpituitarism.

7. Overactivity of the adrenal cortex.

8. Nephritis due to damage of the resorptive capabilities of the proximal convoluted tubules.

9. Primary renal glycosuria caused by a renal tubular enzymatic defect.

10. Animals given drugs such as glucocorticoids or glucose solutions, or those ingesting excessive amounts of carbohydrates in the diet.

The administration of certain drugs will produce a false-positive reaction for glycosuria when tested by a method depending on the reduction of copper. Some of these are antibiotics such as streptomycin, Aureomycin, Terramycin, Chloromycetin, penicillin; and chemicals such as lactose, pentose, ascorbic acid, morphine, salicylates, chloral hydrate, and formaldehyde.

Ketone Bodies

The ketone bodies are acetone, acetoacetic acid and betahydroxybutyric acid. If these substances are found to be increased, ketosis is present. Any decrease in carbohydrate utilization results in increased fatty acid oxidation and increased ketone formation. Conditions such as starvation, diabetes mellitus, pyrexia, low-carbohydrate, high-fat diets, and hypoglycemic syndromes can produce ketonuria. Young animals tend to develop ketonuria with starvation more rapidly than do older animals. Ketone bodies have a diuretic action and contribute to the polyuria seen with diabetes mellitus.

Bile Pigments (See Section V-4)

Urobilinogen

Tests for urobilinogen must be performed on fresh urine samples, for the oxidation of urobilinogen produces urobilin, which turns the urine brown. Urobilinogen is formed by the action of bacteria in the intestinal tract upon bilirubin. Some of the urobilinogen is excreted in the feces; some is reabsorbed and returned to the liver by the portal circulation where it is excreted into the bile. However, some of the reabsorbed urobilinogen is circulated to the kidneys and excreted in the urine. Urobilinogen in dilutions of 1:32 to 1:64 may normally be found in canine and feline urine.

1. Decreased amounts of urobilinogen are usually found in obstructive jaundice, disease of the intestinal tract impairing absorption, in overtreatment with oral antibiotics that change the normal intestinal bacterial flora, or chronic interstitial nephritis, resulting in a polyuria with a low specific gravity and dilution of the urine.

2. Increased amounts of urobilinogen can be found in hepatitis, cirrhosis of the liver, or hemolytic jaundice.

Substances that interfere with the test for urobilinogen are indole, bile and nitrates, sulfonamides, procaine, and formalin.

Indican

Indole is formed by the putrefying action of bacterial organisms on protein (tryptophan). Indole from the intestinal tract is absorbed by the blood and oxidized in the liver to indoxyl, which combines with potassium sulfate to form indican.

Indican is usually absent or present only in very small amounts in the urine of normal cats and dogs. Conditions producing an increased putrefaction of protein within the intestinal tract can produce elevated levels of indican in the urine. These conditions include constipation, intestinal obstruction, enteritis, gastritis, and high protein diet. The putrefaction of proteins elsewhere in the body such as in abscesses or peritonitis can also cause an elevation of urinary indican. Therefore, the significance of indican in the urine is of little value in making a conclusive diagnosis.

Chlorides

Urine chloride content varies greatly with diet, acid-base balance, water balance, endocrine function and the amounts of other electrolytes present within the body. Only 24 hour urine collections are of value in determining urine chlorides. Urine chloride values are of real significance only in a complete study of acid-base balance.

1. Decreased urine chloride values can be seen in animals given salt-free diets, fasting animals, and those with symptoms of excessive vomiting and diarrhea, congestive heart failure, or ascites.

2. Increased urine chlorides can be seen in animals with increased salt intake, Addison's disease (where low mineralocorticoid levels lead to an inability to conserve salt), and in some forms of diuretic therapy.

Calcium

Twenty four hour urine samples are needed for calcium determinations. Repeated urinary calcium determinations are usually needed to interpret the results adequately.

1. Decreased urinary calcium levels can be seen in patients with canine puerperal tetany, or in hypoparathyroidism.

2 .Increased urinary calcium levels may be present in patients with nutritional secondary hyperparathyroidism, hypervitaminosis D, hyperthyroidism, or those given calcium-containing solutions.

Creatine and Creatinine

Twenty four hour urine samples are needed. Creatine is an important part in the makeup of muscle, brain, and blood where, in the form of creatine phosphate, it functions as a high energy substance. Normally, small amounts of creatinine can be found in the urine. In cachectic states, starvation, febrile diseases, and muscular diseases (where there is muscle wasting) the urinary levels of creatine may be elevated. Urinary creatinine levels, however, may be reduced in muscle disease where there is muscle wasting. This occurs because the formation of creatinine occurs in the muscle, and damage to muscle (resulting in wasting) reduces creatinine formation.

17-Ketogenic Steroids

Twenty-four hour urine samples are needed. The range of 17-ketogenic steroids has been stated as 2.13 to 6.98 mg./24 hours, with a mean value of 3.54 mg./24 hours (Siegal). The measurement of 17-ketogenic steroids is a valuable procedure in assessment of the pituitary adrenal axis and in hyper- and hypoadrenocorticoidism (see Section V-2-A). Many clinicians prefer the simpler method of measuring plasma cortisol for this information.

Blood

Hematuria, or the presence of blood in the urine, may be associated with metabolic, infectious, toxic, neoplastic or traumatic disorders. Free hemoglobin in urine is associated with hemolytic disease. Myoglobin reacts with most tests for hemoglobin and is present because of muscle injury that can be associated with trauma, abnormal metabolism, toxic or altered circulation.

Hematuria can be found in conditions such as nephritis, urolithiasis, cystitis, cystic calculi, prostatitis, pyelonephritis, neoplasms of the kidney, prostate or bladder, during estrus in females and in thrombocytopenia.

Hemoglobinuria may be produced in babesiasis, hemolytic disease of the newborn, autoimmune, hemolytic anemia, incompatible blood transfusions, severe burns, chemical toxins and numerous plant poisonings.

Confirmation of a positive occult blood test for hematuria depends on sediment examination of the urine.

V–11–B. Microscopic Examination of the Urine

Normal urine contains very little sediment. Centrifuge the fresh urine sample (at 1000 RPM) to concentrate the sediment. Examine and note the amount, color, and consistency of the sediment. A red sediment indicates the presence of erythrocytes, a white sediment indicates the presence of crystals or cellular debris, and a yellow tinge may indicate bile pigments. Resuspend and stain the urine sediment (new methylene blue or Sternheimer-Malbin stain) for further examination if necessary. Interpret sediment findings in the light of urine specific gravity. Additionally, it is important to know whether the sample was obtained by catheterization or was a "catch" sample.

Organized Sediment

Epithelial Cells

All urine contains a few epithelial cells. The number may be increased because of catheterization procedures. Large squamous cells come from the urethral or vaginal epithelium. These cells may be increased in vaginitis. Transitional epithelial cells originate from the renal pelvis, ureters, urinary bladder and urethra. Transitional epithelial cells are increased in cystitis, pyelonephritis, calcium formation, ureteritis, prostatitis, and urethritis. Round or polyhedral epithelial cells come from the epithelium of the kidney tubules and may be increased in nephritis. Tumors of the bladder may exfoliate tumor cells into the urine.

Erythrocytes (Hematuria)

Erythrocytes may appear in the urine because of inflammation, necrosis, trauma, shock, infarction, congestion, calculi formation, clotting defects, parasites, and poisons such as mercury, arsenic, or thallium. Erythrocytes are crenated in concentrated urine and swollen in dilute urine.

Leukocytes (Pyuria)

Increased numbers of leukocytes usually indicate an inflammatory process within the genitourinary tract. Such conditions as cystitis, urethritis, pyelonephritis, nephritis, prostatitis, vaginitis, metritis, or balanitis may produce pyuria. If the origin of leukocytes cannot be determined after examining the sediment from a "catch" sample of urine, then a sample should be obtained by catherization or cystocentesis.

Bacteria

Normal, freshly voided urine should be sterile. Urine that is not fresh or that has been contaminated during collection will contain bacteria. Bacteriuria is only significant if the urine sample was taken aseptically. Infections of the urinary or genital tract may produce large numbers of bacteria together with erythrocytes and leukocytes. A count of $> 10,000$

bacteria/ml. of freshly collected and cultured urine is significant. Urine sediment containing bacteria should be stained by Gram's method and the sediment should be cultured (see Section IV-4).

Parasites

The eggs of *Dioctophyma renale* (dog and mink) and *Capillaria plica* (dog, cat, and fox) may be found in the urine. The urine sample also may be contaminated by feces containing parasite ova.

Spermatozoa

Spermatozoa may be seen frequently in the urine of male dogs, but has no clinical significance.

Casts

Casts are structures formed in the renal tubules, principally the distal collecting tubules. They are formed by a combination of protein and mucopolysaccharide and denote the leakage of protein through damaged glomeruli or tubular cells. Casts are more frequently seen in concentrated, acidic urine in degenerative or inflammatory diseases of the kidney. Casts are formed in the loops of Henle, distal convoluted tubules and collecting ducts.

Different types of casts will have different clinical significance:

1. Hyaline casts are formed from protein and are soluble in alkaline urine. A few hyaline casts may be found in normal sediment but increased numbers usually are indicative of renal irritation.

2. Granular casts are a form of hyaline casts that contain granules consisting of degenerating tubular epithelial cells. These casts indicate a degeneration of tubular cells and are usually indicative of nephritis.

3. Epithelial casts are produced by exfoliated cells of the tubular epithelium. They denote degeneration and necrosis of tubular epithelial cells.

4. Waxy casts indicate severe kidney damage—usually acute nephritis, renal degeneration, or amyloidosis—and the finding of these casts indicates an unfavorable prognosis.

5. Fatty casts will stain orange or red with Sudan III stain. These casts are produced in degenerative diseases of the kidneys with the deposition of lipid material in the tubules.

6. Blood casts indicate glomerulonephritis or hemorrhage within the nephron of the kidney.

7. Leukocyte casts indicate inflammation within the kidney tubules (as in acute nephritis).

TABLE 71. CANINE UROLITHS

Classification on Mineral Content	Phosphate	Urate	Cystine	Oxalate
Composition	Mg^{++}, NH_4, Ca^{++} PO_4^{--}	NH_4 urate	Amino acid cystine	Calcium oxalate
Percentage of all uroliths	60 to 90	10	5	10
Radiographic appearance	Opaque	Translucent	Translucent	Opaque
Sex predilection	F	M	M	—
Site predilection	Bladder	Urethra	Urethra	Urethra
Physical appearance	Yellow-white, hard; crush to chalk-like powder	Yellow, brittle; concentric laminations	Creamy, yellow, smooth; easily crushed	White, hard, brittle, with sharp crystals on surface
Optimum urine pH	<6.0*	7.0†	>7.5‡	—

*If uroliths are pure phosphate calculi.
†Use of allopurinol is very helpful in controlling urate calculi.
‡D-Penicillamine (Cuprimine) is effective in controlling cystine calculi.

Mucus

Mucus threads within the urine indicate irritation of the genitourinary tract. Mucus is produced by genital secretions, and is a normal occurrence.

Unorganized Urinary Sediment

The presence and amount of crystals in the urine are dependent on the concentration and pH of the urine. Chemical analysis of the crystals is important, since many of them have a mixed composition.

Acid urine may contain amorphous urates (more so in Dalmatians), uric acid, and calcium oxalate crystals. Triple phosphate crystals may be found in slightly acid or alkaline urine.

Alkaline urine may contain triple and amorphous phosphate crystals.

Cystinuria is a metabolic disorder found frequently in male Dachshunds, Labrador Retrievers, Irish Terriers, Cairn Terriers, Cocker Spaniels, Boxers, Poodles, Scottish Terriers, Corgis, and Shelties.

V–12.   RENAL FUNCTION TESTS

Precise and specific renal function tests are impractical for use in everyday veterinary practice. There are several tests, however, that are useful in estimating renal function and in detecting kidney disease. However, even these methods do not provide a specific diagnosis—that depends on results of renal biopsy, urography, pyelography, or renal angiography. The tests that can be useful to the clinician for measuring renal function are urinalysis, the urine specific gravity, the plasma creatinine, and the creatinine clearance, the 15 minute urine phenolsulfonphthalein excretion test, and the 60 minute plasma phenolsulfonphthalein test.

URINALYSIS

Its interpretation is covered more fully in Section V-11. The evaluation of proteinuria is important. The qualitative test will not detect concentrations less than 20 mg./100 ml. and with large urine volumes, dilution may mask serious proteinuria. Protein losses in urine greater than 300 mg./24 hours need study to find the cause. It may be renal parenchymal damage or an extra-renal problem such as fever, congestive heart failure, jaundice, stress, or excessive physical exertion.

The urine sediment deserves special study too. The presence of leukocytes reflects infection whereas erythrocytes indicate renal or extra-renal damage. Red blood cell casts, although rare in dogs, are indicative of bleeding within the nephron. Other cellular and sediment findings may be important clues to a difficult diagnosis.

PRACTICAL MEASUREMENTS OF TUBULAR FUNCTION
Urine Specific Gravity

A specific gravity of 1.025 or greater in a routine urinalysis indicates that the kidneys can concentrate urine normally. If a urine sample from a *dehydrated* patient is low (1.008 to 1.012) it indicates that the kidneys cannot concentrate. In either case a concentration test is not necessary.

Evaluation of antidiuretic hormone (ADH) production and tubular function can be made by withholding water for 18 to 24 hours and evaluating the resulting urine (see Section V-2-B).

Phenolsulfonphthalein Urine Test (PSP)

Because this dye is about 85 per cent protein-bound, only a small amount is filtered by the glomeruli. The rest is excreted by the tubules and thus is used to estimate effectively tubular function in dogs. It also gives an estimate of renal plasma flow (not as accurately as PAH clearance, however) since 50 to 60 per cent of PSP is removed normally with the first pass through the kidneys. With a prolonged test period even a severely damaged kidney may excrete normal amounts of dye. Thus the amount excreted in the first 15 minutes is used as an indication of renal plasma flow. The total amount excreted over one hour may be helpful in evaluating tubular function (normally 50 to 60 per cent). Excretion of less than 25 per cent of the 6 mg. test dose in 15 minutes is evidence of severe renal damage.

The method is as follows: The patient must be well hydrated. The bladder is emptied and a catheter left in situ. Six mg. of PSP is given intravenously. All urine is collected for 15 minutes and measured for PSP (alkalinize with NaOH and use colorimeter). All urine is collected for 60 minutes and measured for PSP.

Sixty Minute Plasma Phenolsulfonphthalein Concentration Test

PSP dye can be used to evaluate renal function. It is especially useful in the evaluation of function before evidence of extensive kidney disease

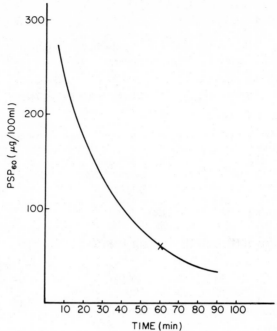

Figure 78. Typical plasma disappearance curve for PSP in the dog after intravenous injection of 1 mg. PSP/kg. of body weight. (From Kaufmann, C. F., and Kirk, R. W.: The sixty-minute plasma phenolsulfonphthalein concentration as a test of renal function in the dog. JAAHA 9: 67, 1973.)

is established by other diagnostic criteria, such as the blood urea nitrogen test or serum creatinine determination. This test is not specific for any particular renal function, but rather indicates tubular excretion and glomeruli function.

A pretest heparinized blood sample of 4 ml. is obtained and then PSP dye, 1 mg./kg. of body weight, is injected intravenously. A 4 ml. heparinized blood sample is withdrawn exactly 60 minutes after injection.

The normal range of PSP_{60} is less than 80 μg./100 ml. for all dogs. A value of 120 or greater is indicative of functional problems, and values between 80 and 120 μg./100 ml. can indicate renal disease.

The total amount of PSP excreted by the kidney in a given period of time is dependent upon how much PSP is delivered to the kidney by the circulation. The PSP_{60} is elevated in cases of renal tubular dysfunction, glomerular disease or conditions that affect renal plasma flow.

Reference

Additional material can be found in the following source:

Kaufmann, C. F., and Kirk, R. W.: The sixty-minute plasma phenolsulfonphthalein concentration as a test of renal function in the dog. JAAHA 9:66-70, 1973.

PRACTICAL MEASUREMENTS OF GLOMERULAR FILTRATION

1. Creatinine clearance gives a reliable estimation of glomerular filtration rate (GFR) in the dog. (It is better than the urea clearance test.) One needs to have a high urine flow and quantitative values for serum or plasma creatinine and urine creatinine/minute. Normal GFR in Beagle dogs is 95 ml./min./sq. m. of body surface.

2. A simple serum creatinine is more reliable than the blood urea nitrogen as an indicator of overall renal function, although both are insensitive to change until renal function is reduced to 40 per cent of normal (Best). In most cases, BUN will be elevated earlier than the creatinine. Plasma creatinine, as opposed to urea nitrogen, is not affected by protein intake, caloric balance, or liver function. It is influenced only by muscle mass, which is usually constant. Plasma creatinine is normally less than 1 mg./100 ml. and its level can be used for prognostic purposes. A range of 2.0 to 4.0 mg./100 ml. indicates renal disease with at least 60 per cent of nephrons being nonfunctional. A range of 4.0 to 7.0 is very serious, even more nephrons being damaged. A value above 7.0 mg. creatinine usually signifies a hopeless case. When more than 75 per cent of the nephrons are destroyed, the kidneys usually cannot sustain life.

References

Additional information can be found in the following sources:

Best, A. N.: How to evaluate kidney function. Philadelphia, Smith, Kline, and French Laboratories, February, 1966.

Ewald, B. H.: Renal function tests in normal beagle dogs. Amer. J. Vet. Res. 124:741-749, May, 1967.

Kaneko, J. J., and Cornelius, C. E.: Clinical Biochemistry of Domestic Animals, 2nd ed., Vol. II. New York, Academic Press, 1971.

Osborne, C. A., Low, D. G., and Finco, D. R.: Canine and Feline Urology. Philadelphia, W. B. Saunders Co., 1972.

Stevens, J. B., and Osborne, C. A.: Urinalysis: Indications, methodology, and interpretation. Proceedings 41st meeting AAHA, pp. 359–403, 1974.

Sunderman, F. W., and Sunderman, F. W., Jr.: Laboratory Diagnosis of Kidney Diseases. St. Louis, Warren H. Green, Inc., 1970.

VI

CHARTS AND TABLES

VI–1. TABLES OF WEIGHTS AND MEASURES

TABLE 72. METRIC SYSTEM

Weight

1000	grams	=	kilogram	(kg.)*
100	grams	=	hectogram	(hg.)
10	grams	=	decagram	(dkg.)
1.0	gram*	=		(gm.)
0.1	gram	=	decigram	(dg.)
0.01	gram	=	centigram	(cg.)
0.001	gram	=	milligram	(mg.)*
0.000001	gram	=	microgram	$\begin{cases} (\mu g.) \\ (\gamma) \end{cases}$

Volume

1000	cubic centimeters	=	liter	(l.)*
100	cubic centimeters	=	deciliter	(dl.)
10	cubic centimeters	=	centiliter	(cl.)
1.0	cubic centimeter*	=	milliliter	(ml., cc.)
0.001	cubic centimeter	=	$\begin{cases} \text{microliter} \\ \text{cubic millimeter} \end{cases}$	$(\mu l.)$ (cu. mm.)

*Commonly employed units.

TABLE 73. APOTHECARIES' SYSTEM

Weight			
1	grain*	=	(gr.)
20	grains	=	1 scruple	(Ə)
60	grains	=	1 dram	(ʒ)*
480	grains (8 drams)	=	1 ounce, Troy	(ʒ)*
5760	grains (12 ounces)	=	1 pound, Troy	(lb.)

Volume			
1	minim*	=	(min., ℔)
60	minims	=	fluid dram (fl. dr., ʒ)*
480	minims (8 fl. drams)	=	fluidounce (fl. oz., ʒ)*
7680	minims (16 fl. oz.)	=	pint	(pt., O)
32	fluid ounces	=	quart	(qt.)

*Commonly employed units.

TABLE 74. HOUSEHOLD MEASURES

| MEASURE | APPROXIMATE EQUIVALENTS | |
	Metric	*Apothecaries'*
1 drop	1/20 ml.	1 minim
1 teaspoon	5 ml.	1 + dram
1 dessertspoon	8 ml.	2 drams
1 tablespoon	15 ml.	½ ounce
1 wineglass	60 ml.	2 ounces
1 glass	250 ml.	8 ounces

TABLE 75. CONVERSION FACTORS

1 milligram	= 1/65	grain	(1/60)
1 gram	= 15.43	grains	(15)
1 kilogram	= 2.20	pounds	[avoirdupois]
	2.68	pounds	[Troy]
1 milliliter	= 16.23	minims	(15)
1 liter	= 1.06	quarts	(1 +)
	33.80	fluidounces	(34)
1 grain	= 0.065	gm.	(60 mg.)
1 dram	= 3.9	gm.	(4)
1 ounce	= 31.1	gm.	(30 +)
1 minim	= 0.062	ml.	(0.06)
1 fluid dram	= 3.7	ml.	(4)
1 fluidounce	= 29.57	ml.	(30)
1 pint	= 473.2	ml.	(500 —)
1 quart	= 946.4	ml.	(1000 —)

Figures in parentheses are commonly employed approximate values.

TABLE 76. APPROXIMATE CONVERSIONS — POUNDS TO KILOGRAMS

Pounds	Kilograms
11	5
22	10
33	15
44	20
55	25
66	30
88	40
110	50
132	60
154	70
176	80
198	90
220	100
242	110

TABLE 77. CONVERSION FACTORS—METRIC TO APOTHECARIES*

METRIC	APOTHECARIES
1 milligram (mg.)	$\frac{1}{64}$ grain
64.79 milligrams	1 grain (65 mg.)
1 gram	15.43 grains (15 grains)
1 cubic centimeter (cc.)	16 minims
3.888 cubic centimeters or grams	1 dram (4 cc. or grams)
31.103 cubic centimeters or grams	1 ounce (30 cc. or grams)
473.167 cubic centimeters	1 pint (500 cc.)

*Approved *approximate* dose equivalents are enclosed in parentheses. Use *exact* equivalents in calculations.

TABLE 78. WEIGHTS*

METRIC	APOTHECARIES	METRIC	APOTHECARIES
0.0001 gram—0.1 mg.	$\frac{1}{640}$ grain ($\frac{1}{600}$ grain)	0.057 gram —57 mg.	$\frac{7}{8}$ grain
0.0002 gram—0.2 mg.	$\frac{1}{320}$ grain ($\frac{1}{300}$ grain)	0.06 gram —60 mg.	$\frac{9}{10}$ grain (1 grain)
0.0003 gram—0.3 mg.	$\frac{1}{210}$ grain ($\frac{1}{200}$ grain)	0.065 gram —65 mg.	1 grain (60 mg.)
0.0004 gram—0.4 mg.	$\frac{1}{150}$ grain	0.07 gram —70 mg.	$1\frac{1}{20}$ grains
0.0005 gram—0.5 mg.	$\frac{1}{120}$ grain	0.08 gram —80 mg.	$1\frac{1}{5}$ grains
0.0006 gram—0.6 mg.	$\frac{1}{100}$ grain	0.09 gram —90 mg.	$1\frac{1}{3}$ grains
0.0007 gram—0.7 mg.	$\frac{1}{90}$ grain	0.097 gram —97 mg.	$1\frac{1}{2}$ grains (0.1 gram)
0.0008 gram—0.8 mg.	$\frac{1}{80}$ grain	0.12 gram —120 mg.	2 grains
0.0009 gram—0.9 mg.	$\frac{1}{75}$ grain	0.2 gram —200 mg.	3 grains
0.001 gram—1 mg.	$\frac{1}{64}$ grain ($\frac{1}{60}$ grain)	0.24 gram —240 mg.	4 grains (0.25 gram)
0.0011 gram—1.1 mg.	$\frac{1}{60}$ grain	0.3 gram —300 mg.	$4\frac{1}{2}$ grains
0.0013 gram—1.3 mg.	$\frac{1}{50}$ grain (1.2 mg.)	0.33 gram —330 gm.	5 grains (0.3 gram)
0.0014 gram—1.4 mg.	$\frac{1}{48}$ grain	0.4 gram —400 mg.	6 grains
0.0016 gram—1.6 mg.	$\frac{1}{40}$ grain (1.5 mg.)	0.45 gram —450 mg.	7 grains
0.0018 gram—1.8 mg.	$\frac{1}{36}$ grain	0.5 gram —500 mg.	$7\frac{1}{2}$ grains
0.0020 gram—2 mg.	$\frac{1}{32}$ grain ($\frac{1}{30}$ grain)	0.53 gram —530 mg.	8 grains
0.0022 gram—2.2 mg.	$\frac{1}{30}$ grain	0.6 gram —600 mg.	9 grains
0.0026 gram—2.6 mg.	$\frac{1}{25}$ grain	0.65 gram —650 mg.	10 grains (0.6 gram)
0.003 gram—3 mg.	$\frac{1}{20}$ grain	0.73 gram —730 mg.	11 grains
0.004 gram—4 mg.	$\frac{1}{16}$ grain ($\frac{1}{15}$ grain)	0.80 gram —800 mg.	12 grains (0.75 gram)
0.005 gram—5 mg.	$\frac{1}{12}$ grain	0.86 gram —860 mg.	13 grains
0.006 gram—6 mg.	$\frac{1}{10}$ grain	0.93 gram —930 mg.	14 grains
0.007 gram—7 mg.	$\frac{1}{9}$ grain	1. gram —1000 mg.	15 grains
0.008 gram—8 mg.	$\frac{1}{8}$ grain	1.06 grams—1060 mg.	16 grains
0.009 gram—9 mg.	$\frac{1}{7}$ grain	1.13 grams—1130 mg.	17 grains
0.01 gram—10 mg.	$\frac{1}{6}$ grain	1.18 grams—1180 mg.	18 grains
0.013 gram—13 mg.	$\frac{1}{5}$ grain (12 mg.)	1.26 grams—1260 mg.	19 grains
0.016 gram—16 mg.	$\frac{1}{4}$ grain (15 mg.)	1.30 grams—1300 mg.	20 grains
0.02 gram—20 mg.	$\frac{1}{3}$ grain	1.50 grams—1500 mg.	22 grains
0.025 gram—25 mg.	$\frac{3}{8}$ grain	2 grams—2000 mg.	30 grains ($\frac{1}{2}$ dram)
0.03 gram—30 mg.	$\frac{2}{5}$ grain	4 grams	—1 dram (60 grains)
0.032 gram—32 mg.	$\frac{1}{2}$ grain (30 mg.)	5 grams	—75 grains
0.04 gram—40 mg.	$\frac{3}{5}$ grain ($\frac{2}{3}$ grain)	8 grams	—2 drams (7.5 grams)
0.043 gram—43 mg.	$\frac{2}{3}$ grain (40 mg.)	10 grams	—$2\frac{1}{2}$ drams
0.05 gram—50 mg.	$\frac{3}{4}$ grain	15 grams	—4 drams
		30 grams	—1 ounce

*Approved *approximate* dose equivalents are enclosed in parentheses. Use *exact* equivalents in calculations.

TABLE 79. LIQUID MEASURES*

METRIC	APOTHECARIES	METRIC	APOTHECARIES
0.03 cubic centimeter — ½ minim		8 cubic centimeters—2	fluid drams
0.05 cubic centimeter — ¾ minim		10 cubic centimeters—2½	fluid drams
0.06 cubic centimeter —1 minim		15 cubic centimeters—4	fluid drams
0.1 cubic centimeter —1½ minims		20 cubic centimeters—5½	fluid drams
0.2 cubic centimeter —3 minims		25 cubic centimeters— ⅚	fluid ounce
0.25 cubic centimeter —4 minims		30 cubic centimeters—1	fluid ounce
0.3 cubic centimeter —5 minims		50 cubic centimeters—1¾	fluid ounces
0.5 cubic centimeter —8 minims		60 cubic centimeters—2	fluid ounces
0.6 cubic centimeter —10 minims		100 cubic centimeters—3½	fluid ounces
0.75 cubic centimeter —12 minims		120 cubic centimeters—4	fluid ounces
1 cubic centimeter —15 minims		200 cubic centimeters—7	fluid ounces
2 cubic centimeters—30 minims		250 cubic centimeters—8	fluid ounces
3 cubic centimeters—45 minims		360 cubic centimeters—12	fluid ounces
4 cubic centimeters—1 fluid dram		500 cubic centimeters—1	pint
5 cubic centimeters—1¼ fluid drams		1000 cubic centimeters—1	quart

*Note: A cubic centimeter (cc.) is the approximate equivalent of a milliliter (ml.). The terms are used interchangeably in general medicine.

From Conn, H. F. (ed.): Current Therapy 1974. Philadelphia, W. B. Saunders Co., 1974.

VI–1–A. Tables for Making Percentage Solutions

The U.S.P. XVI specifies: "The term *per cent* used in prescriptions without qualification means, for mixtures of solids, per cent weight in weight; for solutions or suspensions of solids in liquids, per cent weight in volume; for solutions of liquids in liquids, per cent volume in volume; and for solutions of gases in liquids, per cent weight in volume."

TABLE 80. MAKING WEIGHT IN VOLUME PERCENTAGE SOLUTIONS

The following table gives the proportion of material to be used with solvent q.s. to make the volume at top of the column. Multiples or fractions of these volumes may be calculated from these figures.

STRENGTH OF SOLUTION	Dissolve the weight specified below in distilled water q.s. to make 100 cc.	Dissolve the weight specified below in distilled water q.s. to make 500 cc.	Dissolve the weight specified below in distilled water q.s. to make 1 fl. oz.	Dissolve the weight specified below in distilled water q.s. to make 1 pint
0.25 per cent	0.25 gm.	1.25 gm.	1.14 grs.	18¼ grs.
0.5 per cent	0.5 gm.	2.5 gm.	2.28 grs.	36½ grs.
1 per cent	1 gm.	5 gm.	4.56 grs.	73 grs.
2 per cent	2 gm.	10 gm.	9.13 grs.	146 grs.
3 per cent	3 gm.	15 gm.	13.7 grs.	219 grs.
4 per cent	4 gm.	20 gm.	18.26 grs.	292 grs.
5 per cent	5 gm.	25 gm.	22.8 grs.	365 grs.
6 per cent	6 gm.	30 gm.	27.38 grs.	437 grs.
8 per cent	8 gm.	40 gm.	36.5 grs.	583 grs.
10 per cent	10 gm.	50 gm.	45.6 grs.	729 grs.
12.5 per cent	12.5 gm.	62.5 gm.	57 grs.	913 grs.
15 per cent	15 gm.	75 gm.	68.5 grs.	1095 grs.
16⅔ per cent	16.6 gm.	83.3 gm.	76 grs.	1217 grs.
20 per cent	20 gm.	100 gm.	91.28 grs.	1460 grs.
25 per cent	25 gm.	125 gm.	114 grs.	1825 grs.
30 per cent	30 gm.	150 gm.	137 grs.	2187 grs.
33⅓ per cent	33.3 gm.	166.6 gm.	152 grs.	2433 grs.
50 per cent	50 gm.	250.0 gm.	228 grs.	3500 grs.

437.5 grains = 1 Avoirdupois ounce; 480 grains = 1 Apothecaries' ounce.

TABLE 81. MAKING WEIGHT IN WEIGHT PERCENTAGE SOLUTION

Given are proportions of material and solvent weight in weight used for making solutions of 1 fluid ounce, 1 pint, 100 cc., and 500 cc. Multiples or fractions of these volumes may be calculated from these figures. For exactness, use the amount of water shown. If slight variations are unobjectionable the material is dissolved in enough water to make the volume given at the top of the column.

STRENGTH OF SOLUTION	APPROXIMATE AMOUNT OF SOLUTION							
	100 cc.		500 cc.		1 Fluid Ounce		1 pint	
	Material	Distilled Water	Material	Distilled Water	Material	Distilled Water	Material	Distilled Water
1:5000	0.02 gm.	100 cc.	0.1 gm.	500 cc.	$\frac{1}{10}$ gr.	500 grs.	1½ grs.	7498 grs.
1:2000	0.05 gm.	100 cc.	0.25 gm.	500 cc.	¼ gr.	500 grs.	3¾ grs.	7496 grs.
1:1000	0.1 gm.	100 cc.	0.5 gm.	500 cc.	½ gr.	500 grs.	7½ grs.	7492 grs.
1:500	0.2 gm.	100 cc.	1 gm.	499 cc.	1 gr.	499 grs.	15 grs.	7485 grs.
1:200	0.5 gm.	100 cc.	2.5 gm.	497.5 cc.	$2\frac{3}{10}$ grs.	458 grs.	37 grs.	7363 grs.
1 per cent	1 gm.	99 cc.	5 gm.	495 cc.	$4\frac{3}{5}$ grs.	455 grs.	74 grs.	7326 grs.
2 per cent	2.02 gm.	99.1 cc.	10.1 gm.	495.5 cc.	9¼ grs.	452 grs.	148 grs.	7252 grs.
3 per cent	3.05 gm.	98.5 cc.	15.25 gm.	492.5 cc.	14 grs.	453 grs.	224 grs.	7243 grs.
4 per cent	4.08 gm.	98 cc.	20.4 gm.	490 cc.	19 grs.	456 grs.	300 grs.	7200 grs.
5 per cent	5.13 gm.	97.5 cc.	25.6 gm.	487.5 cc.	24 grs.	456 grs.	380 grs.	7220 grs.
6 per cent	6.2 gm.	96.9 cc.	31 gm.	484.5 cc.	29 grs.	454 grs.	455 grs.	7136 grs.
8 per cent	8.33 gm.	95.8 cc.	41.7 gm.	479 cc.	39 grs.	448 grs.	612 grs.	7044 grs.
10 per cent	10.5 gm.	94.8 cc.	52.6 gm.	474 cc.	48 grs.	432 grs.	772 grs.	6952 grs.
12½ per cent	13.3 gm.	93.1 cc.	66.5 gm.	465.5 cc.	62 grs.	427 grs.	976 grs.	6832 grs.
15 per cent	16.13 gm.	91.4 cc.	80.6 gm.	457 cc.	75 grs.	425 grs.	1188 grs.	6732 grs.
16⅔ per cent	18.11 gm.	90.6 cc.	90.6 gm.	453 cc.	84 grs.	420 grs.	1336 grs.	6682 grs.
20 per cent	22.12 gm.	88.5 cc.	110.6 gm.	442.5 cc.	102 grs.	408 grs.	1634 grs.	6538 grs.
25 per cent	28.4 gm.	85.2 cc.	142 gm.	426 cc.	132 grs.	396 grs.	2104 grs.	6312 grs.
30 per cent	35.04 gm.	81.8 cc.	175.2 gm.	409 cc.	165 grs.	385 grs.	2625 grs.	6125 grs.
33⅓ per cent	39.5 gm.	79 cc.	197.6 gm.	395 cc.	185 grs.	370 grs.	2954 grs.	5908 grs.
50 per cent	64.5 gm.	64.5 cc.	322.5 gm.	322.5 cc.	295 grs.	295 grs.	4720 grs.	4720 grs.

TABLE 82.   COMMON ABBREVIATIONS USED IN PRESCRIPTION WRITING

ā	before	n.r.	not to be renewed
aa	of each	O.	pint
ad lib.	freely as wanted	o.d.	daily
aq.	water	pil.	pill
b.i.d.	twice a day	p.r.n.	according to circumstances
C.	gallon	pv.	powder
c̄	with	q.i.d.	four times a day
cap.	capsule	q.s.	as much as needed
div.	divide	q. 3 h.	every three hours
dos.	dose	s.i.d.	once a day
eq. pts.	equal parts	Sig. or S.	write on the label
ft.	make	sol.	solution
h.	hour	s.o.s.	if necessary
haust.	drench	s̄s	half
M.	mix	stat.	immediately
no.	number	tab.	tablet
		t.i.d.	three times a day

TABLE 83. COMPARISON CHART OF FAHRENHEIT AND CENTIGRADE THERMOMETRIC READINGS*

Cent. Deg.	Fahr. Deg.	Cent. Deg.	Fahr. Deg.	Cent. Deg.	Fahr. Deg.	Cent. Deg.	Fahr. Deg.
−40	−40.0	−4	24.8	32	89.6	68	154.4
−39	−38.2	−3	26.6	33	91.4	69	156.2
−38	−36.4	−2	28.4	34	93.2	70	158.0
−37	−34.6	−1	30.2	35	95.0	71	159.8
−36	−32.8	0	32.0	36	96.8	72	161.6
−35	−31.0	+1	33.8	37	98.6	73	163.4
−34	−29.2	2	35.6	38	100.4	74	165.2
−33	−27.4	3	37.4	39	102.2	75	167.0
−32	−25.6	4	39.2	40	104.0	76	168.8
−31	−23.8	5	41.0	41	105.8	77	170.6
−30	−22.0	6	42.8	42	107.6	78	172.4
−29	−20.2	7	44.6	43	109.4	79	174.2
−28	−18.4	8	46.4	44	111.2	80	176.0
−27	−16.6	9	48.2	45	113.0	81	177.8
−26	−14.8	10	50.0	46	114.8	82	179.6
−25	−13.0	11	51.8	47	116.6	83	181.4
−24	−11.2	12	53.6	48	118.4	84	183.2
−23	−9.4	13	55.4	49	120.2	85	185.0
−22	−7.6	14	57.2	50	122.0	86	186.8
−21	−5.8	15	59.0	51	123.8	87	188.6
−20	−4.0	16	60.8	52	125.6	88	190.4
−19	−2.2	17	62.6	53	127.4	89	192.2
−18	−0.4	18	64.4	54	129.2	90	194.0
−17	+1.4	19	66.2	55	131.0	91	195.8
−16	3.2	20	68.0	56	132.8	92	197.6
−15	5.0	21	69.8	57	134.6	93	199.4
−14	6.8	22	71.6	58	136.4	94	201.2
−13	8.6	23	73.4	59	138.2	95	203.0
−12	10.4	24	75.2	60	140.0	96	204.8
−11	12.2	25	77.0	61	141.8	97	206.6
−10	14.0	26	78.8	62	143.6	98	208.4
−9	15.8	27	80.6	63	145.4	99	210.2
−8	17.6	28	82.4	64	147.2	100	212.0
−7	19.4	29	84.2	65	149.0	101	213.8
−6	21.2	30	86.0	66	150.8	102	215.6
−5	23.0	31	87.8	67	152.6	103	217.4
						104	219.2

*From Catalogue 65, Hospital and Surgical Equipment. V. Mueller, Chicago.

TABLE 84. CONVERSION TABLE FOR STANDARD FRENCH (CHARRIERE) GAUGE*

The standard French, or Charriere, Scale (abbreviated F. or Fr.) is generally used in the size calibration of catheters and other tubular instruments. It is based on the metric system, with each unit being approximately 0.33 mm., and a difference of 0.33 mm. in diameter between consecutive sizes. Example: 27F. indicates a diameter of 9 mm.; 30F. a diameter of 10 mm.

A convenient conversion table from the French Scale to the English and American Scales sometimes used for certain instruments is given below.

1mm.				2mm.			3mm.			4mm.			5mm.
•	•	•	●	●	●	●	●	●	●	●	●	●	●
3	4	5	6	7	8	9	10	11	12	13	14	15

16	17	18	19	20	22	24	26	28	30	32	34
		6mm.				8mm.			10mm.		

38	36		45	40
	12mm.		15mm.	

Table continues on following page.

TABLE 84. CONVERSION TABLE FOR STANDARD FRENCH (CHARRIERE) GAUGE* *(Continued)*

French	English	American	French	English	American
1	–	–	–	9	11
–	–	1	17	–	–
2	–	–	18	10	12
3	–	2	19	–	–
–	1	–	–	11	13
4	–	–	20	–	–
–	–	3	21	12	14
5	–	–	22	–	–
6	2	4	–	13	15
7	–	–	23	–	–
–	3	5	24	14	16
8	–	–	25	–	–
9	4	6	–	15	17

TABLE 84.   CONVERSION TABLE FOR STANDARD FRENCH (CHARRIERE) GAUGE* *(Continued)*

French	English	American	French	English	American
10	5	—	26	—	—
—	—	7	27	16	18
11	6	—	28	—	—
12	—	8	—	17	19
13	—	—	29	—	—
—	7	9	30	18	20
14	—	—	32	—	21
15	8	10	33	19	22
16	—	—	35	—	23

*From Catalogue 65, Hospital and Surgical Equipment. V. Mueller, Chicago.

VI-2. A ROSTER OF NORMAL VALUES*

TABLE 85. NORMAL BLOOD VALUES (BENTINCK-SMITH)

		Dog		Cat	
			Average		Average
Erythrocytes (millions/cu. mm.)		5.5–8.5	6.8	5.5–10.0	7.5
Hemoglobin (gm./100 ml.)		12.0–18.0	14.9	8.0–14.0	12.0
P.C.V. (cc./100 cc.)		37.0–55.0	45.5	24.0–45.0	37.0
M.C.V. cu. μ		66–77.0	69.8	40–55	45
M.C.H. $\mu\mu$ gm.		19.5–24.5	22.8	13.0–17.0	15.0
M.C.H.C.		31.0–34.0	33.0	31–35	33
Thrombocytes (cu. mm.)		$2.0–9.0 \times 10^5$	4.7	$3–7 \times 10^5$	4.5
Icterus index		2–5	Less than 5.0	2–5	
Specific gravity		1.054–1.062	1.057		1.054
Osmotic pressure serum colloids		240–330 mm. H_2O	300	230–470 mm. H_2O	310
Reticulocytes (% of total RBC)		0.0–1.5	0.4	0.0–1.0	0.2
RBC Diameter μ		6.7–7.2	7.0	5.5–6.3	5.8
Resistance to hypotonic saline	Min.	0.40–0.50	0.46	0.66–0.72	0.68
	Max.	0.32–0.42	0.33	0.46–0.54	0.5
M:E ratio		0.75–2.5 :	1.0	3.4:1.0	
Leukocytes/cu. mm.		6–18,000	11,000	8–25,000	17,000
Band neutrophil (%)		0–3	0.8	0–3	0.5
Neutrophil (%)		60–77	70.0	35–75	59
Lymphocyte (%)		12–30	20.0	20–55	32
Monocyte (%)		3–10	5.2	1–4	3
Eosinophil (%)		2–10	4.0	2–12	5.5
Basophil		rare	rare	rare	0

TABLE 86. ABSOLUTE NUMBER OF EACH LEUKOCYTE TYPE IN THE DOG PER CU. MM. (BENTINCK-SMITH)

(Mean and Standard Deviation)

Age	Number of Dogs	Total Leukocyte Count	Band Neutrophils	Mature Neutrophils	Lymphocytes	Monocytes	Eosinophils
1–6 mo.	14	11,000 ± 2,300	50 ± 70	6,400 ± 1,200	3,400 ± 1,200	650 ± 350	450 ± 300
6–12 mo.	21	12,000 ± 3,200	70 ± 80	7,700 ± 2,250	2,700 ± 1,200	750 ± 300	750 ± 400
1–2 yr.	17	11,300 ± 2,800	50 ± 90	7,200 ± 2,400	2,800 ± 950	750 ± 250	500 ± 300
2 yr.	18	11,000 ± 2,250	100 ± 150	7,000 ± 2,000	2,500 ± 850	800 ± 300	500 ± 300
All ages	76*	11,500 ± 2,800	70 ± 100	7,300 ± 2,200	2,800 ± 1,000	750 ± 300	550 ± 350

* Included are six animals of unstated ages.

TABLE 87. ABSOLUTE NUMBER OF EACH LEUKOCYTE TYPE IN THE CAT PER CU. MM. (BENTINCK-SMITH)

(Mean and 2 Standard Deviations)

Age	Number of Cats	Total Leukocyte Count	Band Neutrophils	Mature Neutrophils	Lymphocytes	Monocytes	Eosinophils
Adult	24	5500–19,500	100 (0–300)	7500 (2500–12,500)	4000 (1500–7000)	350 (0–850)	650 (0–1500)

*The tables in Section VI–2 are taken from Kirk, R. W. (ed.): Current Veterinary Therapy V. Philadelphia, W. B. Saunders Co., 1974.

TABLE 88. NORMAL BLOOD VALUES IN OTHER MAMMALS

SPECIES	RBC CELLS/cu. mm. $\times 10^6$	Hb gm./100 ml.	PCV %	MCV cu. μ	MCH $\mu\mu$gm.	MCHC %	TOTAL PROTEIN PLASMA gm./100 ml.	IC- TERUS INDEX	THROMBO- CYTES/cu. mm. $\times 10^5$
Monkey (*Macaca mulatta*)	5.57 ±0.73	11.72 ±3.02	37 ±6.75					7	
Rabbit	4–7 6	8–15 12	30–50 40				6.2		7.43 2.18
Guin Pig	4–7 6	11–17 14	35–45 40				4.7		2–9
Hamster	7.5 ±0.5	17.6 ±1.0	47.4 ±2.4						2.97–9.52 ±3.38–0.89
Rat	7–10 9	12–18 15	35–45 40	60.4 ±3.0	19.1 ±0.8	31.8 ±1.6	6.0		8.38 ±0.58
Mouse	7–11 9	10–20 15	35.45 40						2.46–3.39
Mink	8.9–10.4 9.68	9.5–15.6 11.9	41–57	56.4– 82 68	18.3– 24 20	27.8– 35 29			1.94–3.80 3.50
Chinchilla	5.6–8.4 6.93	11.8–14.6 13.2							
Kinkajou	6.52	10.9	36	55	17	30			
Opossum	4	10.1	31.9	79	26	32			2.5
Skunk	10.0	15.1	51.4	54	16	30			
Woodchuck	7.33	13.9	48	66	19	30			

TABLE 88.   NORMAL BLOOD VALUES IN OTHER MAMMALS
(Continued)

WBC CELLS/cu. mm. ×10³	NEUTRO-PHILS	EOSINOPHILS	MONOCYTES	LYMPHO-CYTES	OSMOT-IC FRA-GILITY	COMMENT AND REFERENCES
15.15 ±5.98	35.79% ±16.70%	2.63% ±2.37%	0.717% ±0.379%	60.52% ±17.26%		Wintrobe, Krise.
6–12 9	2000–6000 4000 Amphophil*	0–500 200	100–1000 500	200–500 300	Max. 0.5 Min. 0.3	Archer, Albritton, Pintor, Perk. * Amphophils vary in size of granule and degree of acido-philia. Eosinophil larger gran-ules densely packed.
7–14 10	2000–6000 4000	200–2000 500	200–2000 500	3000–8000 * 5000	Max. 0.52 Min. 0.32	* Foa-Kurloff body is a large red to purple body in cytoplasm of the lymphocyte. Archer, Al-britton, Perk.
8.56 ±1.54	29% ±11%	0.68%	2.43%	67.9% ±11.9%	Max. 0.4 Min. 0.3	Stewart, Schalm, Schermer, Perk.
5–23 14	1000–5000 3000	0–1000 200	0–1000 500	7000–13,000 10,000	Max. 5.0 Min. 3.0	Archer, Hulse, Albritton, Perk·
4–12 8	500–4000 2000	0–500 200	0–1000 500	3000–9000 6000	Min. 0.50 Max. 0.30	Archer, Copley and Robb, Rus-sell, Green.
3.8–10.2 6.38	18.5–69.0% 41.7%	2.5–16.0% 7.2%	0–5.5% 1.1%	22.5–57.5% 43.5%		Kennedy, Kubin.
5.4–15.6 9.3	39–54% 45%	0–5% 2%	0–5% 1%	45–60% 51%		Newberne.
	32%	15%		53%		Wintrobe—one animal.
12	39%	4.7%	9.3%	46%		Basophil 1%—Wintrobe—four animals.
16	48%	7%	3.0%	42%		Wintrobe—two animals.
15.7	70.2	1.7	0.7%	26.2%		Basophil 0.4%—Wintrobe—three animals.

TABLE 89. BLOOD OR PLASMA CHEMICAL COMPOSITION (BENTINCK-SMITH)

(mg./100 ml.)

	Dog	Cat
Nitrogenous Constituents, Nonprotein		
Nonprotein nitrogen	20–36 (B)	30–48 (B)
Urea nitrogen	10–20 (B)	20–30 (B)
Urea = 2.14 × urea nitrogen		
Creatinine	1–2 (B)	1–2 (B)
Uric acid	0–1.0 (B) Values greater than 1.0 in the Dalmatian.	1.0–1.9 (B)
Allantoin	0.8–1.35 (B) 0.57–0.64 (P) Dalmatian	
Amino acids	7–8 mg. (B) Amino Acid Nitrogen 4.2–7.6 (B)	
Protein Constituents		
Total proteins	5.3–7.5 gm./100 ml. (P)	5.4–7.0 gm./100 ml. (P)
Albumin	3.0–4.8 gm./100 ml. (P)	1.7–2.8 gm./100 ml. (P)
Globulin	1.3–3.2 gm./100 ml. (P)	2.4–4.8 gm./100 ml. (P)
Albumin globulin ratio	1.5–2.3	0.6–0.7
Fibrinogen	0.3–0.5 gm./100 ml. (P)	0.2–0.4 gm./100 ml. (P)

(B) = Blood
(P) = Plasma
(S) = Serum

TABLE 90. ELECTROPHORETIC ANALYSIS OF PLASMA PROTEINS IN VERONAL CITRATE BUFFER (BENTINCK-SMITH)

(pH 8.6; ionic strength 0.1%)

	Dog	Cat
Albumin	39.6	41.4
Alpha$_1$ globulin	16.9	8.1
Alpha$_2$ globulin	8.0	20.2
Alpha$_3$ globulin		4.7
Beta globulin	13.0	8.7
Fibrinogen	13.3	5.2
Gamma Globulin	9.3	12.5

Carbohydrates		
Glucose	60–100 mg./100 ml. (B)	77–118 mg./100 ml. (B)

Organic Acids
Lactic   2–13 (B) 12.6–36 (P) mg./100 ml.
Citric   1.7–3.9 (P) mg./100 ml.
Pyruvate   0.1–0.2 (B) mEq./L.

(B) = Blood
(P) = Plasma

TABLE 91. BLOOD, PLASMA, SERUM CONSTITUENTS CHEMICAL COMPOSITION (BENTINCK-SMITH)

(mg./100 ml.)	Dog	Cat
Lipids		
Total cholesterol	140–210 (S)	75–151 (S)
Cholesterol esters	84–168 (S)	45–120 (S)
Free cholesterol	28–84 (S)	15–60 (S)
Total lipids	47–725 (P)	145–607 (P)
Electrolytes		
Calcium	9–11.5 (S)	9–11 (S) (Krook)
Inorganic phosphorus	2.5–5 (S)	4.5–8.1 (S)
Sodium	137–149 mEq./L. (S)	147–156 mEq./L. (S)
Potassium	3.7–5.8 mEq./L. (P)	4.0–4.5 mEq./L. (P)
Magnesium	1.4–2.4 mEq./L. (S)	2.2 mEq./L. (S)
Chloride	99–100 mEq./L. (P)	117–123 mEq./L. (P)
Sulfate	2.0 mEq./L. (P)	
Carbon dioxide combining power	18–24 mEq./L. (P)	18 mEq./L. (P)
pH	7.31–7.42	7.24–7.4

Normal Blood Gases pO_2: $\begin{cases} \text{85–95 mm. Hg (arterial) standard temperature and pressure} \\ \text{40–60 mm. Hg (venous) standard temperature and pressure} \end{cases}$

$pCO_2 \begin{cases} 29\text{--}36 \text{ mm. Hg (arterial) standard temperature and pressure} \\ 29\text{--}42 \text{ mm. Hg (venous) standard temperature and pressure} \end{cases}$

Enzymes

Alkaline phosphatase   3–6 Bodansky Units/100 ml. (S)   0–7.1 Bodansky Units/100 ml. (S)

Lipase   Less than 1 Sigma Tietz Unit /ml. (S)

Amylase   423–562 Somogyi units/100 ml. (S)

     Occasionally 1000 Somogyi units/100 ml. (S) (Egdahl)

Transaminase

SGOT   Below 23 Sigma Frankel Units   Below 19 Sigma Frankel Units

SGPT   Below 22 Sigma Frankel Units   Below 16 Sigma Frankel Units

Miscellaneous

Bilirubin   0.1–1.0 (S)   0.1–1 (S)

17 Hydroxycorticosteroids   3–10 μg./100 ml. (P)

Protein-bound iodine   2.5–7.0 μg./100 ml. (S)

     lower limit 2.6 μg./100 ml. (S) (Kaneko)

Thyroid uptake of radioiodine[131] I   11–40% 72 hours postinjection

Sulfobromophthalein Retention test   5 mg./kg. dose = 0–10% after 30 minutes

(B) = Blood

(P) = Plasma

(S) = Serum

*Editor's Note: These values are guidelines only and should approximate values found in normal dogs in a hospital environment. However, variations in technique of collection and handling samples may cause marked deviation.

TABLE 92. BLOOD HEMOSTATIC DYNAMICS (BENTINCK-SMITH)

	Dog	Cat
Bleeding time		
Dorsum of nose	2–4 min.	
Lip	85–110 sec.	
Ear	2.5–3 min.	
Abdomen	1–2 min.	
		3 min.
Coagulation time		
Glass	6–7.5 min.	
Silicone	28–40 min.	
Prothrombin time	6–9 sec. (puppies show prolonged values up to 55 sec. until the age of 2 days)	
Prothrombin levels	350 units	319 units
Factor V	158–203 units	123–170 units

TABLE 93. NORMAL URINE VALUES (BENTINCK-SMITH)

(mg./kg. of body weight per day except where indicated)

	Dog	Cat
Specific gravity	1.018–1.060	1.018–1.040
Volume	24–41 ml./kg. body wt./day	22–30 ml./kg. body wt./day
Calcium	1–3	0.20–0.45
Magnesium	1.7–3.0	0.13 mEq./kg./day
Phosphorus	20–30	
Phosphate		
Potassium	40–100	36 mEq./kg./day
Sulfate total	30–50	

Sulfur total S	25–40	
Ethereal S	1.3–3.5	
Neutral S	5–10	
Allantoin	35–45	80
Creatine	10–50	
Creatinine	30–80	12–20
Urea	800–4000	300–500
Uric acid	0.2–13.0	4.5
Nitrogen		
Total nitrogen	500–1100	250–800
Ammonia	60	30–60
	(0.2–3.7 mEq./kg. body wt./day) proportional to pH	
17 Ketosteroids	0.040–0.100	
Bicarbonate	0.05–3.2 mEq./kg. body wt./day	
Chloride	0–10.3 mEq./kg. body wt./day	
Sodium	0.04–13 mEq./kg. body wt./day	
Phosphate	0–1.04 mEq./kg. body wt./day	
Indican	Absent to a trace	Absent to a trace
Bilirubin	No reliable quantitative data	No reliable quantitative data
	1–2+ reaction Harrison spot test	1–2+ reaction Harrison spot test
Urobilinogen	Less than 1:32 Wallace & Diamond test	Less than 1:32 Wallace & Diamond test
pH	5.0–7.0	5.0–7.0

TABLE 94. URINE ELECTROLYTE REABSORPTION RATE IN THE DOG (BENTINCK-SMITH)

(mm./min./100 ml. glomerular filtrate)

Bicarbonate	2.08–3.00
Calcium	0.10–0.12
Chloride	11.0–11.8
	10.24–13.0 under conditions of acidosis with NaCl loading
Phosphate	0.135–0.155
Potassium	0.308–0.512 (net reabsorption) pentobarbital anesthesia
Sodium	12.4–14.4 three subjects given 50 ml. 0.9% NaCl/kg. body wt.
Sulfate	0.080–0.205

TABLE 95. RENAL FUNCTION IN THE DOG (BENTINCK-SMITH)

Renal plasma flow ml./min./sq. m. body surface	134–398
Effective renal blood flow ml./min./sq. m. body surface	480
Glomerular filtration rate ml./min./sq. m. body surface	45.8–122.2
Filtration fraction %	0.213–0.421
Urea clearance ml./min. sq. m. body surface	28.2–83.0
p-Aminohippurate Tm. mg./min./sq. m. body surface	15.5–22.7
Glucose Tm. mg./min./sq. m. body surface	302.6
Diodrast Tm. mg./min./sq. m. body surface	20 (13–48)

TABLE 96. WATER BALANCE DATA (BENTINCK-SMITH)

Water Balance Resting State (Body weight values in grams. Others are gm./100 gm. of body weight per day.)

	Dog	Cat
Body weight	18,600	2900
Water turnover	6.0	8.4
Water intake	4.6	7.2
Food and water	1.4	1.2
Metabolic water	1.9	4.1
Urine output	4.1	4.3
Other, sweat, lungs and incorporation into new protein		

Body Water and Plasma Volume	Dog, Adult Lean	Cat, Adult
Total body water ml./kg.	700 (619–756)	580
Extracellular body water ml./kg.	320 (239–408)	288
Plasma volume ml./kg.	52.7 (35.0–70.4)	46.6 (32.2–56.4)

TABLE 97. CEREBROSPINAL FLUID (BENTINCK-SMITH)

(mg./100 ml. except where indicated)

	Dog	Cat
Quantity	0.9–16 ml.	0.5–2.5 ml.
Aspect	clear, colorless	clear, colorless
Pressure	24–172 mm. H_2O	100 mm. H_2O (under ether anesthesia)
Specific gravity	1.003–1.012	
Freezing point depression	− 0.61°C to 0.63°C	
Alkali reserve	48.5–68.6 vol. %	
Cells/cu. mm.	1–8 lymphocytes occasional endothelial cell	0–1 lymphocytes
Calcium		5.2
Chloride	761–883 as NaCl	670–723 as NaCl
Sugar	61–116	85
Phosphorus	2.8–3.5	
Magnesium	2.6–3.8	
Nonprotein nitrogen	below 40	
Total protein	11–55	
Albumin	16.5–37.5	8.3–16.6
Globulin	5.5–16.5	
Pandy test	negative	negative

TABLE 98. CANINE SEMEN (BENTINCK-SMITH)

Collection by hand manipulation with a teaser (125 ejaculates)

	Mean	Standard Deviation	Range
Volume	5 ml.	4.3	0.5–20.4
% Motile sperm	75	7.5	30–90
pH	6.72	0.19	6.49–7.10
Conc./cu. mm.	148	84.6	27.2–388.8
Motile sperm per ejaculate	396×10^6	243.0	56–1086
% Normal sperm	86	14.7	34–97
Total sperm per ejaculate $\times 10^6$	528	321.0	94–1428

Mean volumes of 3 fractions 65 ejaculates

	ml.	Range	pH	Average pH Whole Ejaculate
1st Fraction	0.8	0.25–2.0	6.37	6.75
2nd Fraction	0.6	0.4–2.0	6.10	
3rd Fraction	4.0	1.0–16.3	7.20	5.8–6.9

TABLE 99. CANINE SYNOVIA (BENTINCK-SMITH)

Knee	
pH 7.29–7.37	
Volume 0–0.3 ml.	
Leukocytes, total	327–1450 cells/cu. mm.
Polymorphonuclear	1.7 (0–7) %
Clasmatocytes	6.5 (0–20) %
Lymphocytes	15.7 (2–36) %
Monocytes	68.5 (56–90) %
Synovial cells	4.8 (1–9) %
Unclassified phagocytes	3.4 (0–14) %
Nitrogen, mucin	(43–58) gm./100 ml.

TABLE 100. DIGESTIVE SECRETIONS OF THE CAT (BENTINCK-SMITH)

	Gastric Juice	Bile (Gallbladder)	Pancreas	Duodenum
Specific Gravity				1.009
pH				8.7–8.9
Fixed base		26.1–31.8 mEq./L.		
Calcium	1.7–5.3 mEq./L.†	4.6–5.1 mEq./L.	4.6–5.1 mEq./L.	
Chloride	155.5–165.7 mEq./L.†	0–20 mEq./L.	67–93 mEq./L.	
Phosphorus	0.16–0.55 mg./100 ml.†			
Potassium	11.5–13.6 mEq./L.†			
Sodium	12.17–55.65 mEq./L.†			
Hydrochloric acid				
Total	127.5–154.7 mEq./L.			
Free	97.25–122.20 mEq./L. *			

*Sham feeding
†Food stimulation

TABLE 101. DIGESTIVE SECRETIONS OF THE DOG (BENTINCK-SMITH)

	Gastric Juice	Bile (Gallbladder)	Pancreas	Duodenum	Jejunum	Ileum
Specific gravity	1,002–1,004		1,004–1,031	1.009		
pH	1.4–4.5	5.18–6.97	7.1–8.2	8.4	6.83	7.61–8.66
Bicarbonate			93–143 mEq./L.		5.2–30 mEq./L.	69.8–114.0 mEq./L.
Calcium	.95–3.30 mEq./L.	26.1 mEq./L.	1.8–2.0 mEq./L.		1.6–5.4 mEq./L.	5.0–5.5 mEq./L.
Chloride	98–143 mEq./L.		71–106 mEq./L.		141–153 mEq./L.	68.1–87.9 mEq./L.
Magnesium	0.5 mg./100 ml.		0.2–1.4 mEq./L.		0.2–1.9 mEq./L.	
Phosphate	0.25 mg./100 ml.		0.7–3.6 mEq./L.		1.2–7.9 mEq./L.	0.5–0.7 mEq./L.
Total phosphorus		82–280 mg./100 ml.				
potassium	10.3–22 mEq./L.*		2.5–7.0 mEq./L.		4.2–10.2 mEq./L.	4.7–6.8 mEq./L.
Sodium	46.3–79.0 mEq./L.*		149–162 mEq./L.		126–192 mEq./L.	146–156 mEq./L.
Hydrochloric acid Av. Total 32 (0–50 mEq./L.)* Free 151 (0–168 mEq./L.)†						
Acids	0.3–19.7 gm./ml.					

*Sham feeding
†Food stimulation

TABLE 102. BLOOD VALUES AND SOME VALUES OF CHEMICAL CONSTITUENTS OF SERUM (SCHUCHMAN)

	Rats	Mice	Hamsters	Guinea Pigs	Rabbits	Mongolian Gerbil
SGPT (Sigma-Frankel units)	25-42	32-41	22-36	10-25	14-27	—
Alkaline phosphatase (Bodansky units)	4.1-8.6	2.4-4.0	2-3.5	1.5-8.1	2.1-3.2	—
BUN (mg./100 ml.)	10-20	8-30	10-40	8-20	5-30	18-24
Sodium (mEq./liter)	144	114-154	106-185	120-155	100-145	144-158
Potassium (mEq./liter)	5.9	3.0-9.6	2.3-9.8	6.5-8.2	3.0-7.0	3.8-5.2
Bilirubin total (mg./100 ml.)	—	0.18-0.54	0.3-0.4	0.24-0.30	0.15-0.20	—
Blood glucose (mg./100 ml.)	50-115	108-192	32.6-118.4	60-125	50-140	69-119
RBC $\times 10^6$	7.2-9.6	9.3-10.5	4-9.3	4.5-7	3.2-7.5	8.3-9.3
Hemoglobin (gm./100 mL.)	14.8	12-14.9	9.7-16.8	11-15	10-15	10-16
Hematocrit (per cent)	40-50	35-50	40-52	35-50	35-45	35-45
WBC $\times 10^3$	8-14	8-14	7-15	5-12	8-10	9-14
Segmented	30	26	16-28	42	30-50	10-20
Nonsegmented	0	0	8	0	0	0
Lymphocyte	65-77	55-80	64-78	45-81	30-50	70-89
Eosinophil	1	3	1	5	1	1
Monocyte	4	5	2	8	9	0
Basophil	0	0	0	2	0	0

*These are values found in healthy-appearing animals and can be used as guides but should not be interpreted as physiologic normals for the species listed.

613

TABLE 103. USEFUL INFORMATION (SCHUCHMAN)

	Hamster	Rabbit	Mouse	Rat	Gerbil	Guinea Pig
Weight at birth	2 gm.	100 gm.	1.5 gm.	5.5 gm.	3 gm.	100 gm.
Puberty	(F) 28–31 days (M) 45 days (best to breed 70 days)	4–9 months	35 days	50–60 days	(F) 3–5 months (M) 10–12 weeks	(F) 20–30 days (M) 70 days
Duration of estrus cycle°	4 days	15–16 days	4 days	4 days	4 days	16 days
Gestation	16 days	28–36 days	19–21 days	21–23 days	24 days	62–72 days
Separation of adults during parturition and weaning	Yes	Yes	No	No	No (mates for life)	No
Number per litter	4 to 10	7	10	8–10	1–12	1–4
Eyes open	15 days	10 days	11–14 days	14–17 days	16–20 days	Prior to birth
Wean at	25 days	42–56 days	21 days	21 days	21 days	14–21 days or 160 gm.
Postpartum estrus	Within 24 hours	14 days	Within 24–48 hours	Within 24–48 hours	Within 24–72 hours	Within 24 hours
Breeding life	11–18 months	1–3 years (maximum 6 years)	12–18 months	14 months	15–20 months	3–4 years

Adult weight	(F) 120 gm. (M) 108 gm.	(F) 4 kg. (M) 4.3 kg.	(F) 30 gm. (M) 30 gm.	(F) 300 gm. (M) 500 gm.	(F) 75 gm. (M) 85 gm.	(F) 850 gm. (M) 1000 gm.
Life span	2–3 years	5–7 years	3–3½ years	3 years	4 years	4–5 years
Body temperature (°F.)	97–101	101–103.2	96.4–100	99.5–100.6	100.8	100.4–102.5
Daily adult water consumption	8–12 ml./day	80 ml./kg. body weight	3–3.5 ml./day	20–30 ml./day	4 ml./day	10 ml./100 gm. body weight
Daily adult food consumption (varies with age and condition)	7–12 gm./day	150–100 gm./day	2.5–4 gm./day	20–40 gm./day	10–15 gm./day	30–35 gm./day
Diet	Commercial rat, mouse or hamster chow supplemented with kale,† cabbage,† apples, milk	Commercial rabbit pellets, greens in moderation	Commercial mouse chow	Commercial rat or mouse chow	Commercial mouse or rat chow (lowest fat possible), sunflower seeds	Commercial guinea pig chow, good quality hay, kale, cabbage, fruits (cannot rely on vitamin C levels of commercial ration)
Room temperature (°F.)	65–75	62–68	70–80	76–78	65–80	65–75
Humidity (per cent)	50	50	50	50	less than 50	50

*All species listed are seasonal polyestrus.
†Better source of vitamin C than lettuce.

TABLE 104. NORMAL BLOOD VALUES FOR BUDGERIGARS (LEONARD)

	Leonard's Data		Gallagher's Data	
		Average		*Average*
Erythrocytes (millions/cu. mm.)	3.44–7.52	5.48	3.60–5.40	4.50
Hemoglobin (gm./100 ml.)	13.0–18.0	15.5	14.0–19.4	16.7
Packed cell volume (ml./100 ml.)	42.9–59.1	51	41.2–65.2	53.2
Mean corpuscular volume (cu. μ)	65.2–121.0	93.1	91.9–139.3	115.6
Mean corpuscular hemoglobin ($\mu\mu$ gm.)	21.4–35.8	28.6	29.1–44.1	36.6
Mean corpuscular hemoglobin concentration	25.2–36.0	30.6	27.7–34.9	31.3
Thrombocytes (cu. mm.)	–	–	7610–51,290	29,450
Reticulocytes (percentage of total red blood cells)	–	–	3.1–10.3	6.7
Leukocytes (number/cu. mm.)	1922–5684	3803	0–8320	4000
Heterophils (percentage)	18.1–100	61.3	39.2–89.6	64.4
Lymphocytes (percentage)	0–57.9	21.9	3.6–55.2	29.4
Monocytes (percentage)	0–10.6	3.4	0–7.5	3.0
Basophils (percentage)	0–30	13.3	0–7.7	3.2

VI-3. TABLES OF NORMAL PHYSIOLOGICAL DATA

TABLE 105. NOMOGRAM FOR THE ESTIMATION OF SURFACE AREA OF THE DOG*

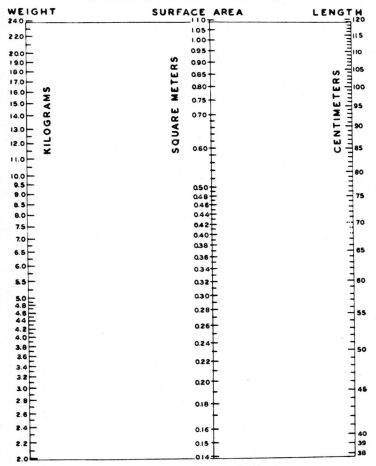

*Length = Nose to anus measured along abdomen.

From Smith, H. W.: Principles of Renal Physiology, 3rd ed. New York, Oxford University Press, 1957.

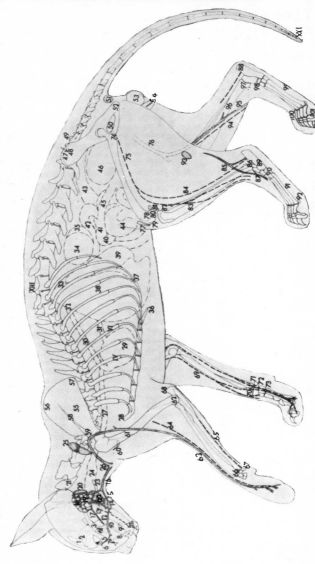

Figure 79. Anatomy of the living cat. (From Sis, R. F., and Getty, R.: Anatomy of the living cat. Vet. Med., 63:147, February, 1968.)

HEAD AND NECK

1. Frontal sinus
2. Zygomatic process of frontal bone
3. Temporal process of zygomatic bone
4. Zygomatic gland
5. V. angularis oculi
6. Dorsal recess of nasal cavity
7. Infraorbital foramen and nerve
8. Root of canine tooth
9. First premolar
10. Third premolar
11. Mental foramen and nerve
12. Facial vein
13. Mandibular foramen and mandibular alveolar nerve on medial side of ramus of mandible
14. Mandibular lymph node
15. Transverse vein
16. External jugular vein
17. Parotid duct
18. External acoustic meatus
19. Parotid gland
20. Caudal parotid lymph node
21. Wing of atlas
22. Mandibular gland
23. Thyrohyoid bone
24. Larynx
25. Dorsal superficial cervical lymph node
26. Ventral superficial cervical lymph node

TRUNK

IV. Fourth rib
VI. Sixth rib
XIII. Spine of T13
27. Trachea
28. Manubrium sterni
29. Heart
30. Aorta
31. Posterior vena cava
32. Diaphragm
33. Diaphragmatic line of pleural reflection
34. Right kidney
35. Left kidney
36. Xiphoid process
37. Costal arch
38. Liver
39. Stomach
40. Transverse colon
41. Ascending colon
42. Duodenum
43. Descending colon
44. Small intestine
45. Ileum
46. Bladder
47. Crest of ilium
48. Lumbosacral aperture
49. Sacrum
50. Obturator foramen
51. Anal sac
52. Tuber ischiadicum
53. Testis
54. Os penis
XXI. Twenty-first coccygeal vertebra

FORELIMB

55. Scapula
56. Cranial angle
57. Caudal angle
58. Spine
59. Acromion
60. Clavicle
61. Deltoid tuberosity
62. Lateral epicondyle of humerus
63. Cephalic vein
64. Superficial branch of radial nerve
65. Ulnar nerve
66. Styloid process of ulna
67. Accessory carpal bone
68. Olecranon
69. Median nerve
70. Subcutaneous surface of radius
71. Antebrachiocarpal articulation
72. Intercarpal articulation
73. Carpometacarpal articulation

HINDLIMB

74. Trochanter major
75. Ischiatic nerve
76. Femoral vein
77. Patella
78. Lateral epicondyle
79. Femoral trochlea
80. Lateral condyles
81. Fabella
82. Head of fibula
83. Peroneal (Fibular) nerve
84. Tibial nerve
85. Lateral saphenous vein (V. saphena parva)
86. Lateral malleolus
87. Trochlea of talus (tibial tarsal bone)
88. Calcaneal tuber
89. Calcaneus (fibular tarsal bone)
90. Fourth tarsal
91. Metatarsal V
92. Plantar sesamoid
93. Popliteal lymph node
94. Saphenous nerve
95. Saphenous vein (V. saphena magna)
96. Medial margin of tibia
97. Medial malleolus
98. Central tarsal
99. Metatarsal II
100. Proximal phalanx
101. Middle phalanx
102. Distal phalanx

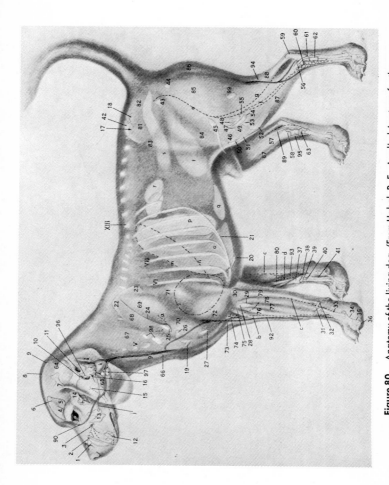

Figure 80. Anatomy of the living dog. (From Habel, R. E.: Applied Anatomy for the Veterinary Student, 2nd ed. Ithaca, N. Y., published by the author, 1963.)

Skeleton, Joints, Ligaments: 1, incisive bone; 2, root of canine tooth; 3, infraorbital for. and n.; 4, zygomatic proc.; 5, frontal sinus; 6, frontal crest; 7, scutiform cart.; 8, sagittal crest; 9, external occipital protuberance; 10, temporomandibular joint; 11, external acoustic meatus; 12, mental for. and n. on the mandible ventral to premolars 1 and 2; 13, premolar 4; 14, zygomatic arch; 15, mandibular for. and mandibular alveolar n. on the med. side of ramus of mandible; 16, angular proc. of mandible; I, wing of atlas; V, transverse proc. of C 5; VI, 6th rib; VIII, 8th rib; XIII, spine of T 13; 17, lumbosacral space; 18, crest of sacrum; 19, manubrium sterni; 20, xiphoid proc.; 21, costal arch.

C. Forelimb: 22, cran. angle of scapula; 23, caud. angle of scapula; 24, spine of scapula; 25, acromion; 26, greater tubercle of humerus; 27, deltoid tuberosity; 28, lat. epicondyle of humerus; 29, lat. collat. lig. of elbow; 30, olecranon; 31, styloid proc. of ulna; 32, accessory carpal bone; 33, 5th metacarpal bone; 34, P I; 35, P II; 36, P III; 37, subcutaneous surface of radius; 38, radiocarpal joint; 39, midcarpal joint; 40, carpometacarpal joint; 41, 2nd metacarpal bone; 42, cran. dors. iliac spine; 43, trochanter major; 44, tuber ischiadicum; 45, os penis; 46, femoral trochlea; 47, epicondyle of femur; 48, fabella; 49, lat. condyle of femur; 50, patella; 51, patellar lig.; 52, tibial tuberosity; 53, lat. condyle of tibia; 54, lat. collat. lig. of stifle; 55, head of fibula; 56, lat. malleolus; 57, subcutaneous surface of tibia; 58, med. malleolus; 59, tuber calcanei; 60, trochlea of tibial tarsal bone; 61, lat. tarsal ligament; 62, fourth tarsal bone; 63, central tarsal bone. **Muscles and Tendons:** 64, temporalis; 65, masseter; 66, sternocephalicus; 67, brachiocephalicus; 68, supraspinatus; 69, infraspinatus; 70, deltoideus; 71, triceps, long head; 72, triceps, lat. head; 73, biceps brachii; 74, brachialis; 75, extensor carpi radialis; 76, extensor dig. communis; 77, extensor dig. lat.; 78, extensor carpi ulnaris; 79, flexor carpi ulnaris; 80, flexor carpi radialis; 81, gluteus med.; 82, gluteus supf.; 83, sartorius; 84, quadriceps femoris; 85, biceps femoris; 86, semitendinosus; 87, tibialis cranialis; 88, gastrocnemius; 89, deep flexor tendon. **Blood Vessels and Lymph Nodes:** 90, v. angularis oculi; 91, jugular v.; 92, cephalic v.; 93, ulnar a.; 94, lat. saphenous v.; 95, a. dorsalis pedis; 96, parotid ln.; 97, mandibular ln.; 98, supf. cervical ln.; 99, popliteal ln. **Nerves:** a, suprascapular; b, supf. br. of radial; c, ulnar; d, median; e, sciatic; f, peroneal; g, tibial. **Internal Organs:** h, zygomatic gland; i, parotid gland; j, parotid duct; k, mandibular gland; l, heart (radiograph); m, diaphragm (radiograph); n, basal border of lung (percussion); o, liver (percussion); p, stomach (radiograph, 24-hour fast, barium meal); q, spleen (radiographic section of ventral end); r, left kidney (radiograph); s, descending colon (radiograph); t, bladder (radiograph).

TABLE 106. 63 DAY PERPETUAL GESTATION

	1	2	3	4	5	6	7	8	9	10	11	12	13	14	15	16	17	18	19	20	21	22	23	24	25	26	27	28	29	30	31
Conception—Jan.	1	2	3	4	5	6	7	8	9	10	11	12	13	14	15	16	17	18	19	20	21	22	23	24	25	26	27	28	29	30	31
Due—March (April)	5	6	7	8	9	10	11	12	13	14	15	16	17	18	19	20	21	22	23	24	25	26	27	28	29	30	31	1	2	3	4
Conception—Feb.	1	2	3	4	5	6	7	8	9	10	11	12	13	14	15	16	17	18	19	20	21	22	23	24	25	26	27	28			
Due—April (May)	5	6	7	8	9	10	11	12	13	14	15	16	17	18	19	20	21	22	23	24	25	26	27	28	29	30	1	2			
Conception—Mar.	1	2	3	4	5	6	7	8	9	10	11	12	13	14	15	16	17	18	19	20	21	22	23	24	25	26	27	28	29	30	31
Due—May (June)	3	4	5	6	7	8	9	10	11	12	13	14	15	16	17	18	19	20	21	22	23	24	25	26	27	28	29	30	31	1	2
Conception—Apr.	1	2	3	4	5	6	7	8	9	10	11	12	13	14	15	16	17	18	19	20	21	22	23	24	25	26	27	28	29	30	
Due—June (July)	3	4	5	6	7	8	9	10	11	12	13	14	15	16	17	18	19	20	21	22	23	24	25	26	27	28	29	30	1	2	
Conception—May	1	2	3	4	5	6	7	8	9	10	11	12	13	14	15	16	17	18	19	20	21	22	23	24	25	26	27	28	29	30	31
Due—July (August)	3	4	5	6	7	8	9	10	11	12	13	14	15	16	17	18	19	20	21	22	23	24	25	26	27	28	29	30	31	1	2
Conception—June	1	2	3	4	5	6	7	8	9	10	11	12	13	14	15	16	17	18	19	20	21	22	23	24	25	26	27	28	29	30	
Due—August (Sept.)	3	4	5	6	7	8	9	10	11	12	13	14	15	16	17	18	19	20	21	22	23	24	25	26	27	28	29	30	31	1	
Conception—July	1	2	3	4	5	6	7	8	9	10	11	12	13	14	15	16	17	18	19	20	21	22	23	24	25	26	27	28	29	30	31
Due—September (Oct.)	2	3	4	5	6	7	8	9	10	11	12	13	14	15	16	17	18	19	20	21	22	23	24	25	26	27	28	29	30	1	2
Conception—Aug.	1	2	3	4	5	6	7	8	9	10	11	12	13	14	15	16	17	18	19	20	21	22	23	24	25	26	27	28	29	30	31
Due—October (Nov.)	3	4	5	6	7	8	9	10	11	12	13	14	15	16	17	18	19	20	21	22	23	24	25	26	27	28	29	30	31	1	2
Conception—Sept.	1	2	3	4	5	6	7	8	9	10	11	12	13	14	15	16	17	18	19	20	21	22	23	24	25	26	27	28	29	30	
Due—November (Dec.)	3	4	5	6	7	8	9	10	11	12	13	14	15	16	17	18	19	20	21	22	23	24	25	26	27	28	29	30	1	2	
Conception—Oct.	1	2	3	4	5	6	7	8	9	10	11	12	13	14	15	16	17	18	19	20	21	22	23	24	25	26	27	28	29	30	31
Due—December (Jan.)	3	4	5	6	7	8	9	10	11	12	13	14	15	16	17	18	19	20	21	22	23	24	25	26	27	28	29	30	31	1	2
Conception—Nov.	1	2	3	4	5	6	7	8	9	10	11	12	13	14	15	16	17	18	19	20	21	22	23	24	25	26	27	28	29	30	
Due—January (Feb.)	3	4	5	6	7	8	9	10	11	12	13	14	15	16	17	18	19	20	21	22	23	24	25	26	27	28	29	30	31	1	
Conception—Dec.	1	2	3	4	5	6	7	8	9	10	11	12	13	14	15	16	17	18	19	20	21	22	23	24	25	26	27	28	29	30	31
Due—February (March)	2	3	4	5	6	7	8	9	10	11	12	13	14	15	16	17	18	19	20	21	22	23	24	25	26	27	28	1	2	3	4

TABLE 107. LONGEVITY — LIFE CYCLE DATA

SPECIES	SCIENTIFIC NAME	PERIOD OF GESTATION IN DAYS	LIFE SPAN IN YEARS	BREEDING SEASON
Cat	*Felis domesticus*	63	9–10	Throughout year {(In North) Jan.–Sept.
Chinchilla	*Chinchilla laniger*	105–111	2–3	Throughout year
Dog	*Canis familiaris*	63	10–14	Throughout year
Ferret	*Mustela furo*	40–42	10–11	Spring
Fox	*Vulpes fulva*	60–63	7–10	Winter
Guinea pig	*Cavia cobaia*	63	4–5	Throughout year
Hamster, common	*Cricetus cricetus*	20	2–3	Spring
Hamster, golden	*Cricetus auratus*	16	2–3	Throughout year
Kinkajou	*Potos falvus*	—	20–22	Rare
Mink	*Mustela vison*	40–42	10–11	Spring
Mouse	*Mus musculus*	20–23	3–3½	Throughout year
Rabbit	*Lepus caniculus*	30	5–7	Throughout year
Raccoon	*Procyon lotor*	63	12–14	Feb.–March
Rat	*Rattus norvegicus*	21	2–3	Throughout year
Skunk	*Mephitis* spp.	62	7–8	Feb.–March

TABLE 107. LONGEVITY — LIFE CYCLE DATA (CONT'D)

PRIMATES	AGE OF PUBERTY	GESTATION	LIFE SPAN	MENSTRUAL CYCLE	OVULATION
Old World Monkeys					
Chimpanzee	9 years	236 days	near 40 years	35 days	16th day
Gorilla					
Green guenon		7 months	16 years	31 days	
Mangebey monkey		164–200 days		30 days	
Rhesus macaque	3 years	146–180 days	20–30 years	28 days	13th day
Pigtail macaque		210 days	19 years		
New World Monkeys					
Capuchin	2½ years	6 months	8–20 years	None visible	
Common marmoset (twins common)	1 year	140–150 days	12½ years	24–27 days	
Spider monkey		139 days	12 years		
Squirrel monkey		139 days?	9–15 years		
Woolly monkey	2½ years	139 days	12 years		

TABLE 108. SOCIALIZATION PROCESSES IN THE DOG*

AGE IN WEEKS	1	2	3	4	5	6	7	8	9	10	11	12	13	14	15
Behavior		Neonatal and transitional periods		Onset of socialization period			Weaning		Play. Exploration. Dominant-subordinate relationships						
Relationships		Maternal feeding and shelter			Interaction with peers and environment										
Processes		Nurture			Approach behavior Unstable learning				Avoidance behavior Stable learning				Socialization complete		
Variables		Early experience				Prenatal influences and genetic factors									
Dog-human relations		Too "human dependent"				Optimum age for socialization with both dog and man							Too "dog attached"		

*From Fox, M. W.: Canine Pediatrics. Springfield, Ill., Charles C Thomas, 1966.

TABLE 109. TIME OF EPIPHYSEAL FUSION OF BONES AS SHOWN BY RADIOGRAPHS.*

Tuber Scapulae	4½-6 months
Humeral head and tubercles	10-12 months
Condyles and medial epicondyle of humerus	8 months
Radius	
Proximal epiphysis	9-11 months
Distal epiphysis	10-12 months
Ulna	
Olecranon	8-10 months
Distal epiphysis	10-12 months
Epiphysis of accessory carpal bone	4½ months
Distal epiphysis of the metacarpal bones and proximal epiphysis of first and second phalanges.	6-7 months
Fusion of the ilium, ischium, pubis, and os acetabuli	5-6 months
Proximal end of femur	9-11 months
Distal epiphysis of femur	9-12 months
Epiphysis of tibial tuberosity	
Fuses with proximal epiphysis	6-9 months
Fuses with shaft of tibia	10-14 months
Proximal articular epiphysis of tibia	10-14 months
Proximal articular epiphysis of fibula	9-11 months
Distal epiphysis of tibia	9-11 months
Distal epiphysis of fibula	8-13 months
Epiphysis of tuber calcanei	
With fibular tarsal bone	6 months

*The data in this table were derived from Greyhounds and large mongrels. (Chapman[1] has shown that fusion may occur in purebred Beagles approximately 2 months earlier for all bones.)

From Habel, R. E.: Applied Anatomy, 5th ed. Ithaca, N. Y., published by the author, 1965.

[1]Chapman, W. L., Appearance of Ossification Centers and Epiphyseal Closures as Determined by Radiographic Techniques. J. A. V. M. A. *147,* No. 2, July 15, 1965.

VI–3–A. Canine and Feline Growth Curves†

Figures 82 through 86 show the "normal" relationship between age and weight for five breeds of dogs. Figure 87 shows growth curves for cats.

†From *Your Dog's Growth Book,* W. K. Kellogg Co., Battle Creek, Michigan. Fifteen breeds as marked. "Normal" rate-of-growth curves arrived at as indicated for cocker spaniels and German shepherds are compared with textbook growth-rate standard curve for human infant. From Horswell, L. A.: What can be learned by charting the growth of puppies. American Kennel Gazette, November-December, 1937.

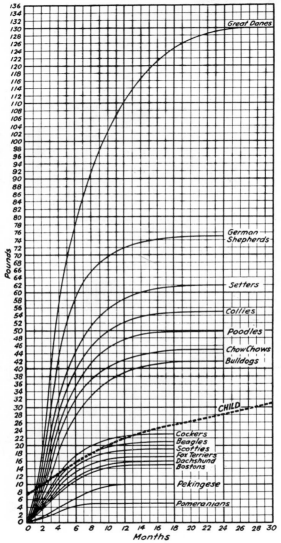

Figure 81.

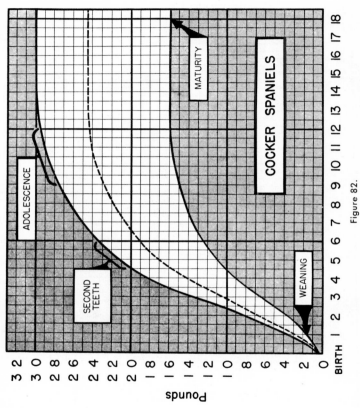

Figure 82.

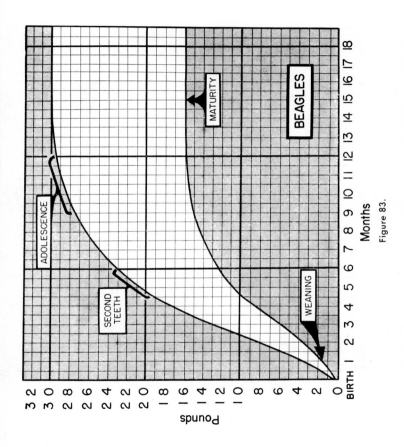

Figure 83.

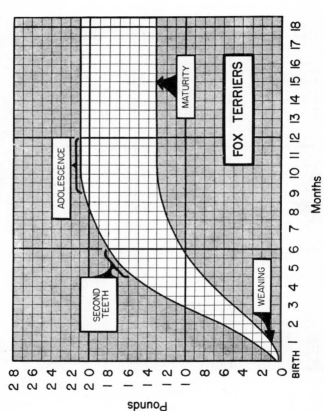

Months

Figure 84.

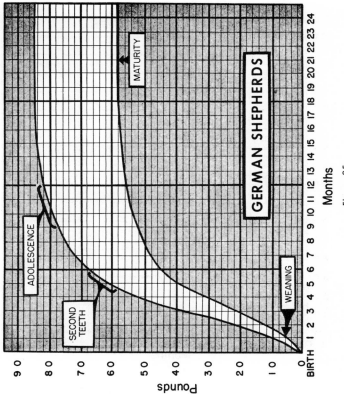

GERMAN SHEPHERDS

Months

Figure 85.

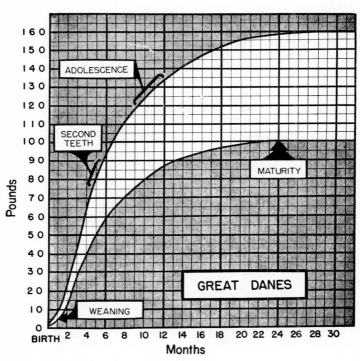

Figure 86.

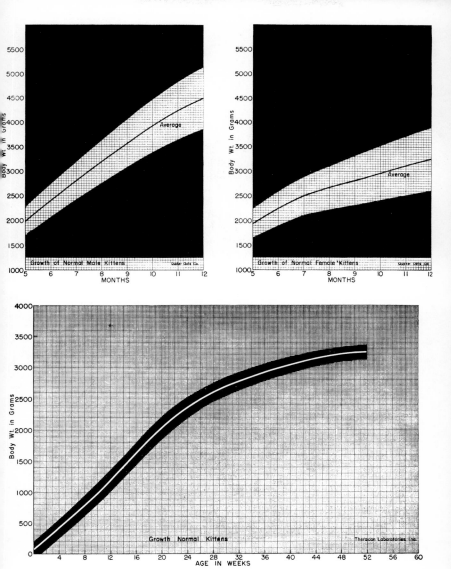

Figure 87. Feline growth charts.

633

VI-3-B. Guidelines for Tail Docking

The natural tail of most spaniels begins to taper in width at about one-third of length. This should be the guide point for docking. The part remaining should be of equal thickness from root to tip.

The guides for terriers are approximate. The tip of the tail when docked should be on an even plane with the skull. Consideration must be given to the size of the pup, relative proportion of length of back and neck, and length and thickness of tail. Tails which are relatively short, stubby and thick should be docked less than those which are long and thin. It is better to leave a tail too long than too short.

Be certain sufficient skin is left to adequately cover the transected tail without tension. Sutures are desirable.

Consult breeders, judges and professional handlers to augment information on breed standards. For breeds not shown on the chart, be certain owner is aware of breed standards. Some breeds should not be docked, and some breeds have naturally short tails.

TABLE 110. GUIDELINES FOR TAIL-DOCKING*

Breed	Amount of Tail to Leave on Dog
Affenpinscher	One-third
Airedale terrier	Three-quarters
Australian terrier	Two-fifths
Boston terrier**	One-third
Bouvier des Flandres	about ½ in.††
Boxer	½ to ¾ in.††
Brussels griffon	One-fourth
Doberman pinscher	2 vertebrae (approx.)
English toy spaniel	One-third
Fox terrier	Two-thirds
Fox terrier, toy (Amertoy)	½ in.††
Griffon (wirehaired pointing)	One-third
Irish terrier	Three-quarters
Kerry blue terrier	One-half
Lakeland terrier	Two-thirds

TABLE 110. GUIDELINES FOR TAIL-DOCKING* *(Continued)*

Breed	Amount of Tail to Leave on Dog
Norwich terrier	One-fourth
Old English sheepdog†	1 vertebra
Pinscher (miniature)	One-fourth
Pointer (German shorthaired)	Two-fifths
Pointer (German wirehaired)	Two-fifths
Poodle (all)	From one-third to one-half
Rottweiler†	1 vertebra
Schipperke	1 vertebra
Schnauzer (giant)	3 vertebrae (approx.)
Schnauzer (miniature)	One-fourth
Schnauzer (standard)	2 vertebrae (approx.)
Sealyham terrier	One-half
Silky terrier	One-third
Spaniel (Brittany)	3 vertebrae
Spaniel (Clumber)	One-third
Spaniel (Cocker)	One-third
Spaniel (English cocker)	One-third
Spaniel (English springer)	One-third
Spaniel (field)	One-third
Spaniel (Sussex)	One-third
Spaniel (Welsh springer)	One-half
Viszla	Two-thirds
Weimaraner	Three-fifths
Welsch Corgi (Pembroke)†	1 vertebra
Welsh Terrier	Two-thirds
West H. W. T.	Not cut
Wheaten Terrier (soft-coated)	One-fourth
Yorkshire terrier	One-third

*From J.A.V.M.A., January 1, 1968.

†Usually tailless; if pups are born with tails, dock so as to leave one vertebra.

**Owner should be notified that docking disqualifies the Boston terrier, Cardigan Corgi and W.H.W.T. for showing.

††When docked at one week of age.

VI-3-C. Nutrient Requirements of Dogs

TABLE 111. NUTRIENT REQUIREMENTS OF DOGS
(PERCENTAGE OR AMOUNT PER KILOGRAM OF FOOD)

		Dry Basis	Dry Type	Semi-moist	Canned or Wet
Moisture level (%):		0	10	25	75
Dry-matter basis (%):		100	90	75	25
Nutrient			*Requirement*		
Protein	%	22.0	20.0	16.5	5.5
Fat	%	5.5	5.0	4.0	2.0
Linoleic or					
arachidonic acid	%	1.6	1.4	1.2	0.4
Minerals					
Calcium	%	1.1	1.0	0.8	0.3
Phosphorus	%	0.9	0.8	0.7	0.25
Potassium	%	0.6	0.5	0.45	0.2
Sodium chloride	%	1.1	1.0	0.8	0.3
Magnesium	%	0.05	0.04	0.03	0.01

Iron	mg.	60.0	54.0	45.0	15.0
Copper	mg.	7.3	6.5	5.5	1.8
Cobalt°	mg.	2.4	2.2	1.8	0.61
Manganese	mg.	5.0	4.5	3.6	1.2
Zinc	mg.	20.0	18.0	15.0	5.0
Iodine	mg.	1.54	1.48	1.16	0.39
Vitamins					
Vitamin A	mg.	1.5†	1.4	1.2	0.4
Vitamin D	mg.	0.007†	0.006	0.005	0.002
Vitamin E	mg.	48.0	43.0	36.0	12.0
Vitamin B$_{12}$	mg.	0.02	0.02	0.017	0.006
Folic acid	mg.	0.18	0.17	0.13	0.04
Thiamine	mg.	0.73	0.65	0.55	0.18
Riboflavin	mg.	2.2	1.9	1.6	0.5
Pyridoxine	mg.	1.0	0.9	0.75	0.25
Pantothenic acid	mg.	2.2	1.9	1.6	0.54
Niacin	mg.	10.6	10.0	7.5	2.5
Choline	mg.	1200.0	1100.0	900.0	300.0
Vitamin K	mg.	1.4	1.3	1.1	0.4

*The requirement for cobalt is related to the need for vitamin B$_{12}$. See text.

†This amount of crystalline A corresponds to 5000 IU/kg. of feed. (One mg. of vitamin A alcohol = 3333 IU of vitamin A; 1 mg. of beta carotene = 1667 IU of vitamin A activity. For dogs, carotene is about one-half as valuable as vitamin A alcohol.)

‡This amount of pure vitamin D corresponds to 264 IU of vitamin D/kg. of feed.

From *Nutrient Requirements of Dogs*, Publ. ISBN 0–309–02043–3, Committee on Animal Nutrition. Agricultural Board. National Academy of Sciences–National Research Council, Washington, D.C. 1972.

TABLE 112. NUTRIENT REQUIREMENTS OF DOGS (AMOUNTS PER KILOGRAM OF BODY WEIGHT PER DAY)

Nutrient		Adult Maintenance	Growing Puppies
Protein	gm.	4.4	8.8
Fat	gm.	1.3	2.6
Minerals			
Calcium	mg.	200.0	400.0
Phosphorus	mg.	160.0	320.0
Potassium	mg.	220.0	220.0
Sodium chloride	mg.	330.0	530.0
Magnesium	mg.	11.0	22.0
Iron	mg.	1.30	1.30
Copper	mg.	0.17	0.17
Cobalt	mg.	0.055	0.055
Manganese	mg.	0.110	0.22
Zinc	mg.	0.110	0.22
Iodine	mg.	0.033	0.066
Vitamins			
Vitamin A	IU	99.0	198.0
Vitamin D	IU	6.6	20.0
Vitamin E			
(α-tocopherol)	mg.	2.0	2.2
Vitamin B_{12}	μg.	0.7	0.7
Folic acid	μg.	4.4	8.8
Thiamine	μg.	20.0	20.0
Riboflavin	μg.	44.0	88.0
Pyridoxine	μg.	22.0	55.0
Pantothenic acid	μg.	51.0	99.0
Niacin	μg.	242.0	397.0
Choline	mg.	25.0	55.0
Vitamin K	μg.	33.0	66.0

From *Nutrient Requirements of Dogs,* Publ. ISBN 0–309–02043–3, Committee on Animal Nutrition, Agricultural Board, National Academy of Sciences–National Research Council. Washington, D.C., 1972.

TABLE 113. ESTIMATED DAILY FOOD INTAKES REQUIRED BY DOGS OF VARIOUS SIZES

Weight of Dog		Requirements for Maintenance				Requirements for Growth			
		Air-Dry Food*		Canned Dog Food†		Air-Dry Food*		Canned Dog Food†	
kg.	lb.	gm./kg. of Body Weight	kg./Dog	gm./kg. of Body Weight	kg./Dog	gm./kg. of Body Weight	kg./Dog	gm./kg. of Body Weight	kg./Dog
2.3	5	40	0.09	134	0.31	80	0.18	268	0.62
4.5	10	33	0.15	113	0.51	66	0.30	225	1.01
6.8	15	28	0.19	95	0.65	56	0.38	212	1.44
9.1	20	27	0.25	90	0.82	54	0.49	178	1.62
13.6	30	25	0.34	88	1.17	50	0.68	172	2.33
22.7	50	25	0.57	84	1.91	50	1.13	167	3.79
31.8	70	25	0.79	84	2.67				
49.8	110	24	1.20	83	4.13				

*Air-dry foods contain 6 to 12 per cent of moisture. Calculations of the amounts of dry foods are based on energy supplied by food containing 90 per cent of dry matter, 77 per cent of protein plus carbohydrates, 5 per cent of fat, and 10 per cent of ash, fiber and other material. This supplies a calculated 1580 kcal./lb. (or 3480 kcal./kg.), of which 80 per cent is digestible. On this basis, digestible kcal. would be 1264/lb. (or 2784/kg.).

†Calculated on the basis of 25 per cent of dry matter and nutrient ratios the same as those stated in the preceding footnote. Total energy is calculated as 439 kcal./lb. and 966 kcal./kg. Available energy is calculated as 413 kcal. (85 per cent of the total) and 821 kcal./kg.

Note: The daily food intake for soft, moist diets depends on moisture level, acceptability and caloric content. Soft, moist products vary in moisture level.

From *Nutrient Requirements of Dogs,* Publ. ISBN 0-309-02043-3, Committee on Animal Nutrition. Agricultural Board, National Academy of Sciences–National Research Council, Washington, D.C., 1972.

TABLE 114. PROTEIN AND CALORIE REQUIREMENTS OF DOGS IN DIFFERENT PHYSIOLOGICAL STATES

Physiologic State	Protein Requirement (gm. Reference Protein/kg. Body Weight$^{0.73}$ Per Day)	Calorie Requirement (Cal./kg. Body Weight$^{0.73}$ Per Day)	Protein Value of Diet (NDp Cal. %)*
Weaning			
Start	8.3	280	12.0
Finish	6.7	280	10.0
Half grown	4.0	210	7.6
Adult	1.6	140	4.6
Pregnant	6.0	200	12.0
Lactating	13.0	500	10.0

Source: Payne (1965). Reprinted with permission, Pergamon Press, Ltd.
*Cal = kcal.
From *Nutrient Requirements of Dogs*, Publ. ISBN 0-309-02043-3, Committee on Animal Nutrition, Agricultural Board, National Academy of Sciences–National Research Council, Washington, D.C., 1972.

TABLE 115. PROTEIN, CALORIES AND SULFUR AMINO ACIDS IN SOME COMMON FOOD PRODUCTS

| | On a Dry Basis | | |
Product*	Dry Matter (%)	Protein (gm./100 gm. of food)	Kilocalories/gm.	Total Sulfur Amino Acids in Each Gram of Protein (mg.)
Barley, grain, (4)	89.0	13.0	3.3	34
Carrot, roots, fresh (4)	12.9	6.6	3.5	–
Corn, grits, cracked fine screened, (4)	88.2	9.0	3.8	32
Cattle, meat, lean (5)	37.5	75.0	4.4	43
Oats, cereal byproduct, mx 4% fiber, (4)	91.2	12.0	3.9	32
Pea, seeds, (5)	89.5	13.0	3.6	33
Potato, tubers, fresh, (4)	23.1	8.5	3.7	26
Rice, groats, polished, (4)	88.5	8.0	3.8	32
Cattle, milk, skimmed dehy, mx 8% moisture, (5)	94.3	36.0	3.6	37
Soybean, flour, solv-extd fine sift, mx 3% fiber, (5)	92.3	50.0	3.4	37
Wheat, grain, (4)	88.9	20.0	3.8	38
Chicken, eggs wo shells, raw, (5)	26.3	47.0	6.0	63
Reference protein	–	100.0	4.0	42

*NRC names.

From *Nutrient Requirements of Dogs,* Publ. ISBN 0-309-02043-3, Committee on Animal Nutrition, Agricultural Board, National Academy of Sciences–National Research Council, Washington, D.C., 1972.

TABLE 116. INEVITABLE NITROGEN LOSSES FROM DOGS

Method	Nitrogen (mg./kg. of Body Weight$^{0.73}$ Per Day)
Addition of endogenous losses	270*
Nitrogen equilibrium experiments	235†
Nitrogen equilibrium experiments	300‡
Mean value	268

Source: Payne (1965). Reprinted with permission, Pergamon Press, Ltd.
*Terroine and Sorg-Matter (1927).
†Allison et al. (1946).
‡Melnick and Cowgill (1937).
From *Nutrient Requirements of Dogs,* Publ. ISBN 0-309-02043-3, Committee on Animal Nutrition, Agricultural Board, National Academy of Sciences–National Research Council, Washington, D.C., 1972.

TABLE 117. AVERAGE WEIGHT GAINS OF MALE DOGS IN DIFFERENT STAGES OF GROWTH

Breed of Dog	Birth to Start of Weaning Period	Gain (gm./kg. of Body Weight$^{0.73}$ Per Day) Start of Weaning Period*	End of Weaning Period*	Half Grown	Average Mature Body Weight (kg.)
Great Dane	50	40	30	20	45.0
Beagle	43	35	25	16	12.0
Wirehaired fox terrier	40	45	35	18	5.1
Mean value	44	40	30	18	—

Source: Payne (1965). Reprinted with permission, Pergamon Press, Ltd.
*Two-week weaning period.
From *Nutrient Requirements of Dogs*, Publ. ISBN 0-309-02043-3, Committee on Animal Nutrition, Agricultural Board, National Academy of Sciences–National Research Council, Washington, D.C., 1972.

TABLE 118. SUBSTITUTES FOR MATERNAL MILK*

		% of Solids		
	% Solids	Fat	Protein	Carbohydrates
Esbilac (powder) Replaces bitch's milk	98.4	44.1	33.2	15.8
Liquid Esbilac Replaces bitch's milk	15.3	44.1	33.2	15.8
KMR (Formerly Tabbi-Lac) Replaces queen's milk	18.2	25.0	42.2	26.1
SPF-Lac Replaces sow's milk	15.2	36.6	33.0	24.8
Foal-Lac (Powder) Replaces mare's milk	94.9	14.4	20.2	56.6
Lam-O-Lac Replaces ewe's milk	91.2	40.8	30.4	24.0

*These commercial products are manufactured by Pet-Vet Products, Borden Chemical, Borden Inc., Norfolk, Virginia 23501

TABLE 119. COMPOSITION OF ANIMAL MILKS*

Common or Domesticated Animals

	% Solids	% of Solids		
		Fat	Protein	Carbohydrates
Mouse (muridae)	25.8	46.9	34.9	12.4
Rat (Muridae)	26.5	47.5	34.7	12.5
Guinea Pig (Caviidae)	17.9	30.6	47.8	16.4
Hamster (Cricetidae)	26.4	47.7	34.0	12.8
Rabbit (Leporidae)	30.5	34.2	51.0	6.4
Cat (Felidae)	18.2	25.0	42.2	26.1
Dog (Canidae)	24.0	44.1	33.2	15.8
Pig (Suidae)	20.0	36.6	33.0	24.8
Sheep (Bovidae)	20.5	41.9	27.9	26.3
Goat (Bovidae)	12.8	32.0	29.0	32.8
Cow (Bovidae)	11.9	29.9	25.6	38.7
Horse (Equidae)	10.9	14.4	20.2	56.6
Donkey (Equidae)	9.5	9.5	17.6	68.2

Zoo or Exotic Animals

	% Solids	% of Solids		
		Fat	Protein	Carbohydrates
Order Monotremata				
Echidna (Tachyglossidae)	34.5	56.9	32.7	8.1
Order Marsupialia				
Bennets Wallaby (Macropodidae)	13	35.3	30.8	34.6

Table continues on following page.

TABLE 119. COMPOSITION OF ANIMAL MILKS* *(Continued)*

| | Zoo or Exotic Animals | | | % of Solids | |
	% Solids	Fat	Protein	Protein	Carbohydrates
Red Kangaroo (Macropodidae)	13.3	30.0	24.3		35.3
Silver-grey phalanger (Phalangeridae)	20	30.5	46.0		16.0
Virginia Opossum (Didelphidae)	14.0	33.6	28.6		32.1
Order Insectivora					
Water shrew (Soricidae)	30.8	65.0	32.4		.3
Short tailed Shrew (Soricidae)	21.5	30.2	51.2		14.9
Hedgehog (Erinaceidae)	21.6	46.9	33.3		9.2
Order Primates					
Rhesus Macaque (Cercopithecidae)	12.2	31.9	17.2		48.4
Orangutan (Pongidae)	11.2	31.3	12.8		53.7
Chimpanzee (Pongidae)	12.1	30.5	9.9		57.9
Order Edentata					
Ant Eater (Myrmecophagidae)	32.1	62.3	34.2		.9
Order Rodentia					
Grey Squirrel (Sciuridae)	26.6	47.3	34.5		12.8
Beaver (Castoridae)	33.0	60.0	27.3		6.7
Porcupine (Erethizontidae)	29.7	44.4	41.8		6.0
Coypu (Capromyidae)	43.4	64.3	31.6		1.3
Order Cetacea					
Bottle-Nosed Dolphin (Delphinidae)	28.6	58.4	33.7		2.7
Dolphin (Delphinidae)	46.9	74.3	22.6		1.9
Spotted Dolphin (Delphinidae)	31.0	58.0	30.4		2.0

	Col 1	Col 2	Col 3	Col 4
Porpoise (Delphinidae)	77.8	77.8	20.2	2.3
Great Blue Whale (Balaenopteridae)	38.5	51.8	32.2	14.6
Humpback Whale (Balaenopteridae)	53.3	72.2	—	—
Fin Whale (Balaenopteridae)	48.3	77.0	—	—
Sei Whale (Balaenidae)	35.6	62.3	33.7	5.0
Baleen Whale (Balaenidae)	30.2	64.2	31.2	1.3
Order Carnivora				
Wolf (European) (Canidae)	23.4	41.0	39.3	14.5
Coyote (Canidae)	24.5	43.7	40.4	12.2
Jackal (Canidae)	24.7	42.5	40.5	12.1
Fox (Canidae)	18.1	34.8	34.5	25.2
Raccoon Dog (Canidae)	19.2	18.3	41.8	34.5
East African Hunting Dog (Canidae)	23.6	40.3	39.4	14.8
Brown Bear (Ursidae)	11.0	29.1	32.7	36.3
Grizzly Bear (Ursidae)	11.1	27.3	34.2	36.0
Polar Bear (Ursidae)	23.3	40.7	41.2	12.9
Raccoon (Procyonidae)	13.4	29.1	30.0	35.0
Mink (Mustelidae)	20.1	17.9	36.6	40.6
Otter (Mustelidae)	35.9	66.7	30.6	0.3
Lynx (European) (Felidae)	21.6	28.7	47.2	20.8
Puma (Felidae)	35.5	52.4	33.8	11.0
Leopard (Felidae)	22.5	29.0	49.3	18.7
Lion (Felidae)	35.5	53.2	35.2	7.6
Cheetah (Felidae)	23.7	40.0	39.7	14.8
Order Pinnipedia				
Hooded Seal (Phocidae)	50.1	80.1	13.2	4.0
Harp Seal (Phocidae)	53.9	79.1	19.4	1.5
Grey Seal (Phocidae)	67.7	78.5	16.5	3.8
California Sealion (Otariidae)	50.9	71.7	27.1	0.0

Table continues on following page.

TABLE 119. COMPOSITION OF ANIMAL MILKS* *(Continued)*

	Zoo or Exotic Animals			
		% of Solids		
	% Solids	Fat	Protein	Carbohydrates
Order Proboscidea				
Indian Elephant (Elephantidae)	16.9	39.6	20.1	37.8
Elephant (Elephantidae)	33.3	66.3	9.6	22.2
Order Perissodactyla				
Black Rhinocerous (Rhinocerotidae)	7.9	Trace	19.5	76.7
Zebra (Equidae)	13.8	34.8	21.7	38.4
Order Artiodactyla				
Wild Pig (Suidae)	17.0	30.0	41.8	21.8
Collared Peccary (Tayassuidae)	16.1	24.8	31.7	39.4
Hippopotamus (Hippopotamidae)	13.9	25.1	38.1	31.1
Bactrian Camel (Camelidae)	15.0	35.9	25.3	34.0
Arabian Camel (Camelidae)	13.6	32.9	25.7	36.4
Llama (Camelidae)	13.4	23.5	29.1	41.8

Giraffe (Giraffidae)	13.7	34.3	21.2	39.4
Okapi (Giraffidae)	18.4	10.7	53.9	27.9
Sika Deer (Cervidae)	36.2	52.4	34.3	9.3
Red Deer (Cervidae)	23.8	38.7	43.7	11.8
Virginia Deer (Cervidae)	23.1	34.6	46.1	12.3
Black-tailed Deer (Cervidae)	25.5	45.5	37.5	15.3
Moose (Cervidae)	19.5	28.7	46.7	16.9
Reindeer (Cervidae)	34.9	58.2	30.7	7.1
Water Buffalo (Bovidae)	17.2	42.9	20.9	31.4
Buffalo (Bovidae)	19.3	40.9	30.6	24.4
Philippine Carabao (Bovidae)	21.4	48.4	27.5	20.2
Bison (Bovidae)	13.1	13.0	36.6	43.5
Pronghorn Antelope (Antilocapridae)	25.2	51.6	27.3	15.9
Texas Antelope (Antilocapridae)	35.2	58.8	30.1	6.8
Impala (Bovidae)	35.0	58.2	30.9	6.8
Grant's Gazelle (Bovidae)	34.2	57.0	30.4	8.2
Thomson's Gazelle (Bovidae)	34.2	57.3	30.7	7.9
Palestine Gazelle (Bovidae)	36.2	52.4	34.3	9.1
Musk Ox (Bovidae)	21.7	50.6	24.4	16.6

*Figures for all species were obtained from literature and are subject to error. Data courtesy of Smith-Douglas Division, Borden Chemical, Borden Inc., Norfolk, Virginia 23501.

VI-4. IMMUNIZATION PROCEDURES

TABLE 120. MINIMAL DISEASE PREVENTION
RECOMMENDATIONS FOR DOGS*

Age	Recommendations
2–6 weeks	Orphan pups that did not receive colostrum can be vaccinated with canine tissue culture origin distemper-hepatitis vaccine.
6–8 weeks	Physical examination including fecal examination for internal parasites and complete blood count.
	Worming, if indicated.
	Instructions for proper feeding and care.
	Vaccination with measles-distemper combination modified live virus vaccine.
	Add modified live virus hepatitis vaccine if in endemic area. Optional.
10 weeks	Distemper-hepatitis MLV† vaccine if valuable dog with need for ultra care.
	Repeat worming if needed.
12–14 weeks	Repeat distemper-hepatitis MLV† vaccine.
	Repeat worming if needed.
4–6 months	Rabies vaccination with modified live virus vaccine or rabies inactivated virus vaccine (murine source).
	Repeat fecal exam and worm if indicated.
One year (and annually thereafter)	Distemper-hepatitis MLV† vaccine.
	Physical examination.
	Fecal examination and worm if indicated.
Every third year	Rabies vaccination (or as required by local ordinance).

*From Minimal disease prevention recommendations for dogs. *In* Kirk, R. W. (ed.): Current Veterinary Therapy V. Philadelphia, W. B. Saunders Co., 1974.

†Leptospirosis bacteria may be indicated with the distemper-hepatitis vaccination in areas where there is a great possibility of exposure to this disease.

TABLE 121. RABIES VACCINES*

Rabies Live-Virus Vaccines

1. Chicken embryo origin: low egg passage, Flury strain.
2. Cell culture origin: canine kidney, high egg passage, Flury strain.
3. Cell culture origin: procine kidney, ERA strain.
4. Cell culture origin: chicken embryo, low egg passage, Flury strain.

Age at First Vaccination	First Booster	Subsequent Boosters
3 to 4 months	At 1 year of age	Every 3 years†
Over 4 months	1 year after first vaccination	Every 3 years†

†Maximal interval; boosters may be given more frequently if desired.

*Editor's Note: A new rabies inactivated-virus vaccine has been prepared from the brains of infected mice younger than 12 days of age. It is said to be as potent and immunogenic as the modified live vaccines, and contains no encephalitogenic properties. It will not produce rabies in any animal and is said to be safe and effective for use in dogs, cats and any wild animals. It may produce longer lasting immunity but present requirements are for annual revaccination.

From Minimal disease prevention for dogs. *In* Kirk, R. W. (ed.): Current Veterinary Therapy V. Philadelphia, W. B. Saunders Co., 1974.

Table continues on following page.

TABLE 121. RABIES VACCINES* *(Continued)*

Rabies, Inactivated-Virus Vaccine

1. Cell culture origin: primary hamster kidney (fixed virus with adjuvant).
2. Cell culture origin: primary hamster kidney (fixed virus) without adjuvant.

Age at First Vaccination	First Booster	Subsequent Boosters
3 to 4 months	3 to 4 weeks after first vaccination	Every year thereafter
Over 4 months	3 to 4 weeks after first vaccination	Every year thereafter

3. Tissue origin: caprine neural tissue, fixed virus.

Age at First Vaccination	First Booster	Subsequent Boosters
3 to 4 months	1 year after first vaccination	Every year thereafter
Over 4 months	1 year after first vaccination	Every year thereafter

TABLE 122. VACCINATION PROCEDURES FOR CATS*

Feline panleukopenia:

1. Antiserum (hyperimmune and normal).
   Passive protection only.
   For use in orphan and high risk kittens.
   Prophylactically: 1 to 2 ml./lb.
   Therapeutically: 1 to 4 ml./lb.
   Active immunization carried out 21 to 30 days later.

2. Modified live-virus vaccine (72 hours until protection).
   Started at 9 to 10 weeks of age.
   Second dose advised between 12 and 16 weeks.
   Contraindicated in kittens under four weeks and in pregnant cats.
   Boosters recommended annually.
   If cat older than 12 weeks, one vaccination adequate.

3. Inactivated vaccines (6 days before protection).
   Tissue culture origin recommended.
   Started at 9 to 10 weeks of age.
   Second dose between 12 and 16 weeks.
   Safe in pregnant cats and orphan kittens (start about four weeks).
   Boosters recommended annually.

*See editor's note for Table 121.

From Minimal disease prevention for cats. *In* Kirk, R. W. (ed.): Current Veterinary Therapy V. Philadelphia, W. B. Saunders Co., 1974.

Table continues on following page.

TABLE 122. VACCINATION PROCEDURES FOR CATS* *(Continued)*

Rabies:
1. Modified live virus
   Tissue culture origin.
   Approximately one month before protection.
   Annual boosters recommended although titer duration probably as long as in dog.
   Usually vaccinate at five to six months; can administer as early as three months.
2. Inactivated tissue culture.
   Two doses at 30-day intervals (Hamster TCO; Murine Nervous TO, one dose.
   Annual booster.

Feline pneumonitis:
Modified live virus: chick embryo origin.
Generally not recommended: virus of vaccine usually does not produce a good antibody response.

VI–4–A. *Immunization Procedures for Exotic Pets*

TABLE 123. SPECIES SUSCEPTIBLE TO CANINE DISTEMPER VIRUS AND FELINE PANLEUKOPENIA VIRUS.*

Family	Distemper	Panleukopenia
Canidae		
dogs, coyote, fox, jackel, wolf, dingo, cape hunting dog, etc.	+	−
Felidae		
tiger, leopard, lion, ocelot, margay, bobcat, mountain lion, jaguar, cheetah, lynx, jungle cat, golden cat, etc.	−	+
Procyonidae		
lesser panda, raccoon, coatimundi, kinkajou	+	Raccoon Coatimundi Lesser panda (?) Kinkajou (?)
Viverridae		
binturong, foussa, linsang, mongoose, civit, genet	Binturong Civit Others (?)	Binturong Others (?)
Ursidae		
bears	+	+(?)
Hyaenidae		
hyenas	+	−
Mustelidae		
ferret, mink, otter, skunk, wolverine, badger, martin, sable, gnison, fisher	+	All but ferret

*Extracted and assembled from reports by Drs. P. S. Chaffee, C. Sedgwick and L. Griner (American Association of Zoo Veterinarians) and Norden News, Spring, 1970, Norden Laboratories, Lincoln, Nebraska. Used by permission of Dr. Wilbur B. Amand, New York State Veterinary College, Cornell University, Ithaca, N.Y.

VI–4–B. *Immunization of Wild Animal "Pets" Against Common Diseases*

As with domestic animals, there is no unanimity of opinion as to the proper method(s) which should be used in immunizing wild animals. The following information represents current approaches to the problem.

Family Canidae. Coyote, fox, jackel, wolf, dingo, cape hunting dog, etc.

Canine distemper–infectious canine hepatitis: Administer modified live virus vaccine (MLV) as for domestic dog. Revaccinate annually and prior to anticipated possible exposure if six months have elapsed since last vaccination.

Leptospirosis: Leptospira canicola–icterohemorrhagiae bacterin. Use according to the manufacturers' recommendations for domestic dogs. Begin at time of initial distemper-hepatitis vaccine. Repeat every six months where risk of exposure is high.

Rabies: Inactivated nervous tissue vaccine (phenolized, ovine or caprine origin) or inactivated virus tissue culture vaccine (hamster origin). Use according to manufacturers' recommendations. Begin vaccination at three to six months of age; revaccinate annually.

Family Felidae. Tiger, leopard, lion, cheetah, jaguar, lynx, ocelot, margay, bobcat, mountain lion, jungle cat, golden cat, etc.

Feline panleukopenia: Wild *Felidae* appear to be exquisitely susceptible to the feline panleukopenia virus. Proper and adequate vaccination is a *must!*

Vaccinate with killed virus vaccine or (preferably) a modified live virus (MLV) vaccine. Begin vaccination when eight to 10 wks. of age and repeat two or three times at two-week intervals. Revaccinate adults at six to 12 month intervals. Use manufacturer's recommendations (note: some individuals prefer to administer two doses per injection to the large adult cats).

Pneumonitis: The use of MLV pneumonitis vaccine is definitely an *elective procedure* and cannot be recommended as a routine procedure for the individual cat. Pneumonitis vaccine might best be administered to wild *Felidae* with anticipated exposure to other domestic or wild *Felidae* (such as cat shows, etc.). In this situation the vaccine should be administered 10 to 14 days prior to anticipated exposure.

Rabies: Inactivated nervous tissue vaccine (phenolized, caprine, ovine) or inactivated virus tissue culture vaccine (hamster origin). Vaccinate kittens at three to six months of age; repeat annually in adults. Follow manufacturers' recommendations.

Family Procyonidae. Lesser panda, raccoon, coatimundi, kinkajou.

Canine distemper: Killed virus vaccine or MLV vaccine may be administered according to the manufacturers' recommendations. Adults should be revaccinated annually.

Infectious canine hepatitis: Limited data available; inapparent infection may occur in raccoons. No recommendations.

Feline panleukopenia: Although proven cases have only been reported in the raccoon and the coatimundi, the current trend is to vaccinate all captive members of the family *Procyonidae*. Killed virus vaccine or MLV vaccine may be used according to the manufacturers' recommendations. Adults should be revaccinated every six to 12 months.

Leptospirosis: Leptospira canicola-icterohemorrhagiae bacterin. Vaccinate as per family *Canidae*.

Pneumonitis: Elective procedure as per family *Felidae*.

Rabies: Inactivated nervous tissue vaccine (phenolized, ovine or caprine origin). Initial vaccine may be given at three to six months of age. Adults should be revaccinated yearly.

Family Viverridae. Binturong, foussa, linsang, mongoose, civit.

Canine distemper: Cases of proven canine distemper have been reported in the binturong and civit. It is suggested that all captive *Viverridae* be vaccinated for canine distemper as per the family *Canidae*.

Infectious canine hepatitis: No data available.

Feline panleukopenia: Cases are poorly documented, but it has been recommended that at least the binturong if not all captive *Viverridae* be vaccinated for feline panleukopenia as per the family *Felidae*.

Rabies: Vaccinate as per the family *Canidae* and *Felidae* (inactivated nervous tissue vaccine, phenolized).

Family Ursidae. Bears.

Canine distemper: Although several species of bears are reported to be susceptible to canine distemper, bears are not routinely vaccinated at zoos. Nevertheless, it might be advisable to vaccinate individual pet bears where the risk of exposure is high. Killed virus vaccine or MLV vaccine as per family *Canidae*.

Infectious canine hepatitis: Infection of bears with ICH has been described but not confirmed. No recommendations.

Feline panleukopenia: Cases of panleukopenia (not verified by virus isolation) have been reported in young bear cubs. No recommendations can be given at this time as to the advisability of vaccinating bears for feline panleukopenia.

Rabies: No data available.

Family Hyaenidae. Hyenas.

Canine distemper: All species of hyena are susceptible and should be vaccinated for canine distemper as per family *Canidae*.

Infectious canine hepatitis: No data available.

Rabies: As per family *Canidae*.

Family Mustelidae. Ferret, mink, otter, skunk, wolverine, badger, martin, sable, gnison, fisher.

Canine distemper: Certainly the mink, ferret and skunk are susceptible, and probably all captive *Mustelidae* should be vaccinated for canine distemper using a MLV vaccine as per family *Canidae*.

Infectious canine hepatitis: Limited data available. No recommendations.

Viral enteritis (may be variant of feline panleukopenia): Mink only. Autogenous or commercial mink enteritis formalized vaccine or killed feline panleukopenia virus vaccine. Kits, six to eight weeks of age; adults should be revaccinated annually. Follow manufacturers' recommendations.

Feline panleukopenia: It has been suggested that all *Mustelidae* except the ferret are susceptible to feline panleukopenia and should receive vaccine as per the family *Felidae.* Mink should receive either killed panleukopenia vaccine or formalized mink enteritis vaccine. They need not receive both.

Botulism (mink and ferret): *Clostridium botulinum* type C toxoid. Kits can be vaccinated at 10 to 12 weeks of age; adults should be revaccinated yearly.

Rabies: Inactivated nervous tissue vaccine (phenolized, ovine or caprine origin). Vaccinate as per family *Felidae.*

Order Marsupialia, Family Didelphidae. Opossum.

The opossum is highly resistant to infection by canine distemper and rabies and probably does not need to be vaccinated for these diseases.

Order Primates. Subhuman.

Poliomyelitis (apes only—gorilla, orang-utan, chimpanzee and gibbon): Live oral polio virus vaccine. Adults, one 12 month booster with trivalent vaccine. Initial dose, a child's dose of trivalent vaccine administered twice at six- to eight-week intervals.

Rabies: Depends on likelihood of exposure. Inactivated nervous tissue vaccine or the newer tissue culture vaccines (duck embryo). MLV rabies vaccine should be avoided. Revaccinate annually or as per manufacturers' recommendations.

Tuberculosis (immunization *not* recommended): Susceptible nonhuman primates should be subjected to periodic tuberculin tests and either eliminated or vigorously treated with appropriate medication if found to be positive. Test procedure (WHO recommendations): Koch's Old Tuberculin (full strength). 0.1 cc. *intradermally* in the upper eyelid. Read test at 24, 48 and 72 hours postinjection; positive test is characterized by swelling and erythema with closure of the eye. Should have three successive negative tests at two-week intervals.

Measles, smallpox, etc.: Vaccination of primates (especially apes) against the common childhood diseases is an elective procedure and depends upon the degree of exposure to which the primate may be subjected. Consult with a pediatrician on the choice of immunizing agent(s).

Hepatitis: Where the possibility of disease exists or where there is known exposure to a hepatitis patient, gamma globulin may be administered prophylactically.

Order Rodentia. Mouse, rat, hamster, gerbil, guinea pig, squirrel.

Rabies: Vaccination is not recommended for these animals if maintained caged; where risk of exposure is high an inactivated nervous tissue vaccine may be used and repeated annually.

Ectromelia (mice and rats): Routine vaccination is not recommended, since this viral disease does not appear to be a problem in the U.S.

Order Lagamorpha. Rabbit and hare.
See Order *Rodentia* (above).

VI–4–C. *Shipping Regulations for Small Animals**

Interstate Regulations

For the exact requirements regarding the entry of dogs and cats into the various states of the United States and Puerto Rico, inquiry should be made to the State Veterinarian in the state of destination.

Under most circumstances, no animal that is affected with or has recently been exposed to any infectious, contagious or communicable disease or that originates from a rabies quarantined area shall be shipped or, in any manner, transported or moved into any state until written permission for such entry is first obtained from the State Veterinarian or chief animal health official of the state to which the animal is to be transported.

Common carriers will usually not accept dogs or cats for interstate movement without health certificates; thus it would seem advisable, even if not specifically required, that such certificates be issued by the accredited practicing veterinarian in the state of origin.

International Regulations

Travelers from the United States to foreign countries on vacations and duty assignments frequently desire to take their pets with them.

*From Kirk, R. W. (ed.): Current Veterinary Therapy V. Philadelphia, W. B. Saunders Co., 1974.

Similarly, persons returning from abroad need to make arrangements for the reentry of their pets and for animals acquired in other countries. For both importations and exportations, there are usually health requirements with which one must comply.

MOVEMENT INTO FOREIGN COUNTRIES

There are no United States regulations governing the movement of dogs and cats to any foreign country. The regulations that must be complied with are those of the receiving country. These regulations are many, varied and subject to change. If pets are to be moved to any foreign country except Canada, the owner should obtain from the nearest consulate of the country of destination that country's regulations governing the import of pets and procedural instructions, such as the number of copies to be furnished, an indication of whether the health certificate must be validated by the consulate or whether certified copies of the pedigree or photograph of the pet must accompany the health certificate.

Dogs from the United States may be imported into Canada through any Canadian customs port of entry when accompanied by a certificate signed by a veterinarian licensed in Canada or the United States. The certificate must show that the dog has been vaccinated against rabies during the preceding 12 months.

IMPORTATION OR REENTRY OF DOGS INTO THE UNITED STATES

The entry of dogs into the United States from all foreign countries is under the jurisdiction of the Public Health Service of the United States Department of Health, Education and Welfare. An excerpt from the United States Public Health Service regulations regarding importation of dogs is quoted:

Vaccination for rabies shall be accomplished with nerve tissue vaccine more than one month but not more than 12 months before the dog's arrival, or with chicken embryo vaccine more than one month but not more than 36 months before arrival.

VI–5. HEREDITARY DEFECTS OF DOGS

TABLE 124. HEREDITARY DEFECTS OF DOGS*

Breed	Mode†	Disease
	?	Trembling
	?	Cerebellar hypoplasia
Alaskan malamute	R?	Dwarfism
	?	Renal hypoplasia
Antarctic sledge dog	XR	Hemophilia A (Factor VIII deficiency)
Basenji	R?	Non-spherocytic hemolytic anemia (pyruvate kinase deficiency)
	D?	Persistent pupillary membrane
	?	Inguinal and midline hernias
	—	Colibacillosis
Basset	XR?	Cervical vertebral deformity
	D	Achondroplasia, limbs
Beagle	R	Factor VII deficiency
	—	Hemophilia A (Factor VIII deficiency)
	R?	Brachyury (short tail)
	?	Intervertebral disc degeneration
	P?	Otocephaly
	P	Valvular pulmonic stenosis
	?	Incomplete right bundle branch block
	P?	Cleft lip and palate
	?	Hypercholesterolemia
	D?	Cataract
	?	Atopic dermatitis
	—	Distemper
	?	Renal hypoplasia
Boxer	?	Intervertebral disc degeneration
	P	Subaortic stenosis
	?	Atrial septal defect
	?	Gingival hyperplasia
	—	Mast cell tumors
	—	Aortic and carotid body tumors
Brussels griffon	?	Short skull
Bulldog	R?	Brachyury (short tail)
	?	Short skull
	P	Valvular pulmonic stenosis (English bulldog)
	?	Congenital Anasarca (English bulldog)
	P?	Cleft lip and palate (English bulldog)
	?	Hydrocephalus (English bulldog)
Cardigan	?	Primary retinal dystrophy–central or macular type
Chihuahua	XR	Hemophilia A (Factor VIII deficiency)
	P	Valvular pulmonic stenosis

*From Patterson, D. F.: A catalogue of hereditary diseases of the dog. *In* Kirk, R. W. (ed.): Current Veterinary Therapy V. Philadelphia, W. B. Saunders Co., 1974.

Table continues on following page.

TABLE 124. HEREDITARY DEFECTS OF DOGS* *(Continued)*

Breed	Mode†	Disease
Collie	R	Cyclic neutropenia (grey collie syndrome)
	–	Hemophilia A (Factor VIII deficiency)
	P	Patent ductus arteriosus
	?	Deafness (cochlear degeneration)
	R	"Collie eye anomaly"
	ID	Heterochromia iridis ("walleye")
	?	Optic nerve hypoplasia
	?	Primary retinal dystrophy—central or macular type (border collie)
	?	Inguinal and midline hernias
Dachshund	D	Achondroplasia, limbs
	?	Intervertebral disc degeneration
	?	Over and undershot jaw (long-haired dachshund)
	P?	Cleft lip and palate
	?	Diabetes mellitus
	ID	Heterochromia iridis ("walleye")
	XR?	Cystine stones (cystinuria)
	?	Renal hypoplasia
Dalmatian	R	Uric acid stones
	?	Deafness (cochlear degeneration)
	?	Atopic dermatitis
Doberman pinscher	?	Polyostotic fibrous dysplasia
	?	His bundle degeneration
	?	Renal hypoplasia
Elkhound	?	Osteogenesis imperfecta
	R	Primary retinal dystrophy—peripheral type
	?	Renal hypoplasia
Foxhound	?	Vertebral osteochondrosis
	?	Deafness (cochlear degeneration)
German shepherd	XR	Hemophilia A (Factor VIII deficiency)
	P	Hip dysplasia
	P?	Ununited anconeal process
	P	Subaortic stenosis
	P	Persistent right aortic arch
	?	Esophageal achalasia
	D	Cataract
	?	Conjunctival dermoid cyst
	P?	Behavioral abnormalities
	XR?	Cystine stones (cystinuria)
German shorthair pointer	R?	Familial amaurotic idiocy
Great Dane	ID	Heterochromia iridis ("walleye")
	P	Stockard's paralysis
	XR?	Cystine stones (cystinuria)
Greyhound	XR	Hemophilia A (Factor VIII deficiency)
	R	Short spine
	?	Esophageal achalasia

TABLE 124. HEREDITARY DEFECTS OF DOGS* *(Continued)*

Breed	Mode†	Disease
Keeshond	P	Conus septum defects
	R?	Epilepsy
Mexican hairless	D	Hairlessness
Newfoundland	P	Subaortic stenosis
Pekingese	?	Intervertebral disc degeneration
	?	Short skull
Pomeranian	P	Patent ductus arteriosus
	?	Tracheal collapse
Poodle	R?	Achondroplasia (miniature poodle)
	?	Epiphyseal dysplasia (miniature poodle)
	?	Osteogenesis imperfecta
	P	Patent ductus arteriosus
	R	Primary retinal dystrophy—peripheral type (miniature and toy poodles)
	?	Cerebrospinal demyelination (miniature poodle)
	R?	Epilepsy
	P?	Behavioral abnormalities
	?	Tracheal collapse (toy poodle)
	?	Ectodermal defect (miniature poodle)
	XR?	Cystine stones (cystinuria)
Retriever	XR	Hemophilia A (Factor VIII deficiency) (Labrador retriever)
	?	Craniomandibular osteopathy (Labrador retriever)
	P?	Ununited anconeal process (Labrador retriever)
	P?	Primary retinal dystrophy—central or macular type (Labrador and golden retrievers)
	XR?	Cystine stones (cystinuria) (Labrador retriever)
Rhodesian ridgeback	?	Dermoid sinus
St. Bernard	P	Stockard's paralysis
Setter	XR	Hemophilia A (Factor VIII deficiency) (Irish setter)
	XR	Carpal subluxation (Irish setter)
	P	Persistent right aortic arch (Irish setter)
	R	Primary retinal dystrophy—peripheral type (Irish setter)
	R?	Neuronal ceroid-lipofuscinosis (English setter)
Shetland sheepdog	XR	Hemophilia A (Factor VIII deficiency)
	R?	Cataract (old English sheepdog)
	ID	Heterochromia iridis ("walleye")
Shiba-Inu (Japan)	R	Short spine
Shih-Tzu	P?	Cleft lip and palate
Spaniel	R?	Anury (taillessness) (cocker spaniel)
	R?	Brachyury (short tail) (cocker spaniel)
	R?	Cranioschisis (cocker spaniel)
	?	Intervertebral disc degeneration (cocker spaniel)
	?	Over and undershot jaw (cocker spaniel)
	P?	Ununited anconeal process (cocker spaniel)
	P	Patent ductus arteriosus (cocker spaniel)

Table continues on following page.

TABLE 124. HEREDITARY DEFECTS OF DOGS* *(Continued)*

Breed	Mode†	Disease
	P?	Cleft lip and palate (cocker spaniel)
	—	Glaucoma (cocker spaniel)
	—	Primary retinal dystrophy—peripheral type (cocker spaniel)
	?	Primary retinal dystrophy—central or macular type (English springer spaniel)
	?	Hydrocephalus (cocker spaniel)
	P?	Behavioral abnormalities (cocker spaniel)
	?	Inguinal and midline hernias (cocker spaniel)
	—	Skin neoplasms, generally
	?	Renal hypoplasia
	D	Cutaneous asthenia (springer)
Terriers	XR	Hemophilia B (Factor IX deficiency) (cairn terrier)
	?	Craniomandibular osteopathy (West Highland white, Scottish, and cairn terriers)
	?	Osteogenesis imperfecta (Bedlington terrier)
	P	Valvular pulmonic stenosis (Fox terrier)
	P?	Cleft lip and palate (Staffordshire terrier)
	?	Esophageal achalasia (wirehair fox terrier)
	?	Goiter (fox terrier)
	?	Glaucoma (wirehaired fox terrier)
	?	Lens luxation (fox and Sealyham terriers)
	R?	Retinal dysplasia (Sealyham terrier)
	R	Retinal dysplasia (Bedlington terrier)
	R?	Ataxia (Fox terrier—Sweden)
	R	Krabbe's leukodystrophy (cairn and West Highland white terriers)
	R	Scottie cramp (Scottish terrier)
	?	Inguinal and midline hernias (bull terrier)
	?	Laryngeal malformations (Skye terrier)
	?	Atopic dermatitis (Scottish and wirehaired fox terriers)
	—	Pituitary tumors (Boston terrier)
	—	Hair follicle tumors (Kerry blue terrier)
	—	Mast cell tumors (Boston terrier)
	—	Aortic and carotid body tumors (Boston terrier)
	XR?	Cystine stones (cystinuria) (Irish terrier)
Tervueren shepherd (Netherlands)	?	"Fits" (epilepsy?)
Vizsla	XR	Hemophilia A (Factor VIII deficiency)
Weimaraner	XR	Hemophilia A (Factor VIII deficiency)
	?	Syringomyelia
Welsh corgi	?	Primary retinal dystrophy—both types
	XR?	Cystine stones (cystinuria)
Miscellaneous		
All breeds	D	Blood group incompatibility
Mixed breeds	?	Cartilaginous exostoses

TABLE 124. HEREDITARY DEFECTS OF DOGS* *(Continued)*

Breed	Mode†	Disease
Many breeds	D?	Polydactyly (rear dew claws)
Most breeds	Sex-limited R?	Cryptorchidism
Small breeds	?	Legg-Calve-Perthes disease
Toy breeds	?	Patellar luxation
	?	Tracheal collapse
	?	Von Gierke-like syndrome (glycogen storage disease)
Giant breeds	−	Osteosarcoma
Hairless breeds	D	Hairlessness
Brachycephalic breeds	?	Elongated soft palate
White dogs, various breeds	?	Deafness (cochlear degeneration)
Breeds with red or black coat color	−	Melanoma
Not given	R	Glossopharyngeal defect
Purebred vs. mixed	−	Neonatal death, generally

†R: autosomal recessive
D: autosomal dominant
XR: X-linked recessive
XD: X-linked dominant
ID: incomplete dominant
P: polygenic
?: unknown or unproven
−: no information

VI–6. DRUG THERAPY

TABLE 125. INSULIN PREPARATIONS AVAILABLE

Type of Insulin	Appearance	Time Required to Take Effect (hrs.)*	Maximum Action (hrs.)	Duration of Effect (hrs.)
Regular (crystalline)	Solution	1/4	4 to 6	6 to 8
Semilente	Amorphous	1/2	4 to 6	12 to 16
Globin	Solution	2 to 3	6 to 10	12 to 18
NPH	Crystalline	3	8 to 12	18 to 24
Lente	30 per cent amorphous 70 per cent crystalline	8 to 12	8 to 12	18 to 28
P21	Amorphous	3 to 4	14 to 20	24 to 36
Ultra lente	Crystalline	3 to 4	16 to 18	30 to 36

*After subcutaneous injection.

TABLE 126. USE OF ANTIMICROBIAL AGENTS FOR TREATMENT OF INFECTIONS

Organism	Disease	Drug of Choice	Alternative Drug
Staphylococcus aureus	Pyoderma, endocarditis, osteomyelitis, soft tissue infections	Penicillin G sensitive: Penicillin G Penicillin G resistant: Methicillin, oxacillin, lincomycin	Ampicillin, cephaloridine chloramphenicol, erythromycin, lincomycin, nafcillin, novobiocin, oxacillin
Enterococcus	Urinary infection, abscesses, bacteremia	Penicillin G plus streptomycin	Ampicillin, erythromycin plus streptomycin
Hemolytic streptococcus	Urinary infections, otitis, soft tissue infections, upper respiratory infections	Penicillin G	Ampicillin, cephaloridine, lincomycin, sulfonamides
Escherichia coli	Urinary infections	Nitrofurantoin,‡ sulfonamide, ampicillin	Cephaloridine, chloramphenicol, tetracycline
	Other infections	Ampicillin, chloramphenicol, tetracycline	Kanamycin,‡ neomycin,‡ polymyxin B‡
Proteus mirabilis	Urinary and soft tissue infections	Ampicillin, chloramphenicol, furadantin	Cephaloridine, gentamicin‡ kanamycin, streptomycin,
Pseudomonas aeruginosa	Urinary and soft tissue infections, burns	Gentamicin,‡ polymyxin B‡	Carbenicillin, chloramphenicol
Klebsiella, Aerobacter	Respiratory and urinary infections	Gentamicin	Chloramphenicol or kanamycin
Salmonella	Gastroenteritis	Chloramphenicol	Ampicillin, nitrofurans

Table continues on following page.

TABLE 126. USE OF ANTIMICROBIAL AGENTS FOR TREATMENT OF INFECTIONS *(Continued)*

Organism	Disease	Drug of Choice	Alternative Drug
Brucella	Abortions from *Brucella canis*	Tetracycline plus streptomycin	—
Pasteurella multocida	Abscesses, snuffles	Penicillin G°	Tetracycline
Bacillus anthracis	Anthrax	Penicillin G	Erythromycin, tetracycline
Fusobacterium (Vincent)	Ulcerative stomatitis	Penicillin G	Tetracycline
Clostridium tetani	Tetanus	Penicillin G°	Tetracycline
Other clostridia	Gas gangrene	Penicillin G°	Tetracycline
Mycobacterium tuberculosis	Tuberculosis	Isoniazid with streptomycin or *p*-aminosalicylic acid	—
Bordetella bronchiseptica	Respiratory infections	Tetracycline	Chloramphenicol
Leptospira	Leptospirosis	Penicillin G with streptomycin	Tetracycline
Haemobartonella	Haemobartonellosis	Thiacetarsamide	Tetracycline
Rickettsia	Salmon disease	Tetracycline	Chloramphenicol
Psittacosis and ornithosis	Pneumonia	Tetracycline	Chloramphenicol
Mycoplasma	PPLO infections (pneumonia)	Tetracycline	Chloramphenicol, nitrofurantoin
Toxoplasma	Toxoplasmosis	Pyrimethamine with sulfonamide	—

Coccidia	Coccidiosis	Trisulfapyrimidines with phthalylsulfathiazole	Tetracycline
Giardia lamblia	Giardiasis (enteritis)	Metronidazole, quinacrine	Furazolidone
Trichomonas caninus	Trichomonad enteritis	Glycobiarsol	—
Nocardia	Nocardiosis	Sulfonamide*	Chloramphenicol, tetracycline
Actinomyces	Actinomycosis	Penicillin G*	—
Blastomyces	Blastomycosis	Amphotericin B‡	Sulfonamide, nystatin
Candida, Coccidioides, Histoplasma, Cryptococcus, Mucor, Aspergillus	Pneumonia, skin and soft tissue lesions, bone lesions, disseminated disease	Amphotericin B‡	—
Microsporon, Trichophyton, Epidermophyton	Skin, hair and nail bed infections	Griseofulvin	—
Pityrosporon	Skin and ear infections	2 per cent "tame" iodine or 25 per cent glyceryl triacetate applied topically	—

*Large dosage.
†For effect in urine.
‡Toxic effects possible with parenteral dosage.
From Antibiotic therapy. *In* Kirk, R. W. (ed.): Current Veterinary Therapy V. Philadelphia, W. B. Saunders Co., 1974.

TABLE 127. DOSAGES AND ROUTES AND SCHEDULES OF ADMINISTRATION OF SELECTED ANTIMICROBIAL DRUGS IN DOGS AND CATS*

Drug	Dosage	Route	Repeat Dose
Amphotericin B	0.12 to 0.75 mg./lb.	IV, IP	2 to 3 times per week
Cephalexin	15 mg./lb.	Oral	12 hours
Cephaloridine	5 mg./lb.	SC, IM	12 hours
Chloramphenicol	10 to 25 mg./lb.	Oral	8 hours
	3 mg./lb.	IM, IV	12 hours
Colistimethate	0.5 mg./lb.	IM	6 hours
Erythromycin	5 mg./lb.	Oral	8 hours
Gentamicin	2 mg./lb.	IM	12 hours for two days, then once every 24 hours
Glycobiarsol (Milibis V)	100 mg./lb. for five days	Oral	24 hours
Griseofulvin	10 mg./lb.	Oral	Once daily for six weeks with fat meal, or
	70 mg./lb.	Oral	Once weekly for six weeks with fat meal
Hetacillin (Ampicillin)	5 to 10 mg./lb.	Oral	8 to 12 hours
Kanamycin	3 mg./lb.	IM	12 hours
Lincomycin	7 mg./lb.	Oral	8 hours
	5 mg./lb.	IM	12 hours
Metronidazole (Flagyl)	30 mg./lb.	Oral	24 hours
Neomycin	10 mg./lb.	Oral	6 hours (not absorbed)
	5 mg./lb.	IM, IV	12 hours
Nitrofurantoin	1.5 mg./lb.	IV	12 hours
	2 mg./lb.	Oral	8 hours (with food)
Novobiocin	5 mg./lb.	Oral	8 hours
Nystatin	100,000 U	Oral	6 hours

Penicillins			
Ampicillin	13 mg./lb.	IM, IV	8 hours
Methicillin	10 mg./lb.	IM, IV	6 hours
Nafcillin	10 mg./lb.	IM	12 hours
	5 mg./lb.	Oral	6 hours
Oxacillin	5 mg./lb.	Oral, IM, IV	6 hours
Penicillin G, Na or K	10,000 units/lb.	Oral	6 hours (not with food)
	10,000 units/lb.	IV, IM	4 to 6 hours
Penicillin G, procaine	10,000 units/lb.	IM	24 hours
Polymyxin B	1.0 mg./lb.	IM	12 hours
Pyrimethamine	0.5 mg./lb.	Oral	48 hours
Quinacrine (Atabrine)	50 to 100 mg./dog; give three days; skip three days and repeat	Oral	24 hours
Streptomycin	5 mg./lb.	IM	12 hours
Sulfonamides			
Sulfadimethoxine	10 mg./lb.	Oral, IV	24 hours
Sulfamerzine, sulfamethazine	25 mg./lb.	Oral, IV	12 hours
Sulfisoxazole	20 mg./lb.	Oral	8 hours
Sulfonamides, enteric			
Phthalylsulfathiazole	50 mg./lb.	Oral	12 hours (not absorbed)
Tetracyclines	8 mg./lb.	Oral	8 hours
	3 mg./lb.	IV, IM	12 hours
Thiacetarsamide	1.0 mg./lb. for two days	IV	12 hours
Tylosin	5 mg./lb.	Oral	8 hours
	3 mg./lb.	IM, IV	12 hours

*From Antibiotic therapy. *In* Kirk, R. W. (ed.): Current Veterinary Therapy V. Philadelphia, W. B. Saunders Co., 1974.

TABLE 128. MOST EFFECTIVE pH FOR OPTIMAL ANTIBACTERIAL ACTIVITY

Antimicrobial Drug	pH	5.5	6.0	6.5	7.0	7.5	8.0
x Ampicillin		+	+	+			
Cephalothin*			+	+	+	+	+
x Chloramphenicol*				+	+	+	+
x Colistin						+	+
Erythromycin†							+
Gentamicin						+	+
x Kanamycin						+	+
Lincomycin						+	
Methenamine mandelate			+				
x Neomycin†		+				+	+
x Nitrofurantoin†		+	+				
Novobiocin			+				
x Oxacillin			+				
x Penicillin G			+	+			
x Polymyxin*							+ (best)
x Streptomycin†						+	+
Sulfonamides* (pH not important except as it affects solubility)			+	+	+	+	+
Tetracycline*			+	+	+		
x Oxytetracycline*		+	+	+			
Chlortetracycline†			+				

*The pH is not important. Effectiveness of the drug is not highly dependent on pH, but (+) indicates optimal range.
†The pH is very important. Effectiveness of the drug is highly dependent on pH; (+) indicates optimal range.
ˣEspecially useful in urinary infusions.

672

TABLE 129. COMMON URINARY ACIDIFIERS AND THEIR DOSAGE RECOMMENDATIONS*

Drug	Dosage (Approximate)	Manufacturer
DL-Methionine (Odor-Trol)	(200 mg. tablets) 1 tablet/15 lb. of body weight twice daily	Haver-Lockhart Labs., Shawnee, Kansas 66201
Ammonium chloride	200 mg./kg./day in divided dosages	Eli-Lilly & Co., Indianapolis, Indiana
Ascorbic acid	250 to 500 mg. four times daily, initially	Available as U.S.P. product from many sources
Acid phosphates (pHos-Phaid)	(250 or 500 mg. tablets) 1 to 2 tablets twice daily/15 to 30 lb. of body weight	Fort Dodge Labs., Inc., Fort Dodge, Iowa 50501
Ethelenediamine dihydrochloride (Chlor-Ethamine)	(100 mg. tablets) 1 tablet three times daily for cats	Pitman-Moore Inc., Washington Crossing, New Jersey 08560
Mandelic acid (Mandelamine)	0.250 gm. tablets or suspension (250 mg./teaspoon) 1 tablet/30 lb. of body weight four times daily	Warner-Chilcott Labs., Morris Plains, New Jersey 07950

*From Urinary acidifiers and clinical applications. *In* Kirk, R. W. (ed.): Current Veterinary Therapy V. Philadelphia, W. B. Saunders Co., 1974.

TABLE 130. CHARACTERISTICS OF THE STAGES OF ANESTHESIA WITHOUT PREMEDICATION*

Stages of Anesthesia		Depression of Central Nervous System	Nerves Depressed	Mucous Membrane Color (1)	Pupil Size (2)	Eyeball Activity (3)	Muscle Tone
I Analgesia (stage of voluntary movement)		Sensory cortex		Normal ――― Flushed		Voluntary	
II Delirium (stage of involuntary movement)		Motor cortex ――― Decerebrate rigidity (4)		Flushed		++++	
III (Surgical)	Plane 1	Midbrain	III	Flushed ――― Normal		+	
	Plane 2	Spinal cord (increased depression)	V ― X	Normal		Fixed	
	Plane 3	Spinal cord (increased depression)	VI	Normal ――― Pale		3rd eyelid relaxed	
	Plane 4	Spinal cord (severe depression)		Pale			
IV Paralysis (death follows)		Medullary paralysis		Pale and cyanotic			None

*From Lumb, W. V.: Small Animal Anesthesia. Philadelphia, Lea & Febiger, 1963.

TABLE 130. CHARACTERISTICS OF THE STAGES OF ANESTHESIA WITHOUT PREMEDICATION* *(Continued)*

Respiration	Pulse and Blood Pressure (B.P.)	Reflexes						Miscellaneous
		Lid	Corneal	Skin	Swallowing	Cough	Pedal	
Rapid and irregular	Rapid pulse and elevated B.P.	+	+	+	+	+	+	—— Pain abolished
Very irregular (erratic)	Rapid pulse and elevated B.P.	+	+	+	+	+	+	Unconscious —— Swallowing, emesis, may occur
Slow and regular	Normal pulse and normal B.P.	+ ---- −	+	−	−	+	−	
Slow and regular	Normal pulse and normal B.P.	−	+ to − ---- −	−	−	−	−	
Delayed thoracic —— Chiefly abdominal	Rapid pulse and fall in B.P. (5)	−	−	−	−	−	−	Smooth muscle depressed —— Pedal reflex absent (6)
Abdominal (shallow)	Rapid, weak pulse and fall in B.P.	−	−	−	−	−	−	Anal reflex present
None (diaphragm paralyzed)	Shock level	−	−	−	−	−	−	Anal and bladder sphincters relaxing

1. Cyanosis occurs in any stage of oxygen want.

2. Pupil size in the etherized dog is so inconsistent that it is not a reliable sign.

3. Nystagmus is not prominent in the dog as it is in some other species.

4. Decerebrate rigidity (extension of the limbs) is frequently observed in the dog just before entering Stage III. Relaxation occurs on entering Plane 1.

5. It has been estimated that 15 minutes in Plane 3 is as shock-producing as 2 hours in Plane 2.

6. Pedal reflex activity is abolished with ether in Plane 1, but may persist as long as Plane 3 when barbiturate anesthesia is employed.

TABLE 131. INDICATIONS AND CONTRAINDICATIONS FOR SOME COMMON ANESTHETIC AGENTS*

Physical Condition or Reason for Anesthesia	Pentobarbital	Thiamylal	Thiopental	Halothane	Methoxyflurane	Ether	Morphine-Apomorphine	Infiltration, Field, or Nerve Block	Epidural	Tranquilizer
Animals under 3–6 weeks of age	No	With caution		X	X	X	No	X	No	With caution
Aged animals	No	X	X	X	X	X	X	X	X	X
Brachycephalic dogs	Only if necessary. Intubation essential	X	X	X	X	X	X	X	X	X
Cesarean section	Not advisable	X		X	X	X	X	+ Tranquilizer X	X	+ Another agent X
Febrile animals	Only if necessary	X	X	X	X	If necessary	X	X	X	X
Ruminants	No	With caution—intubation essential					No	X	X	X
Equine	With caution in foals	Induction only	X		X	X	No	X	X	X
Swine	X	X	X		X	X	No	X	X	With extreme caution
Shock	No	With extreme caution					No	X	No	With extreme caution
Uremia	No	Use only when absolutely necessary		X			No	X	X	With caution
Cardiac disease Compensated	Only if necessary	X	X			X	X	X	X	X
Cardiac disease Uncompensated	No	Use only when absolutely necessary					No	X	No	When absolutely necessary. Reduce dose
Respiratory disease	No	X	X	Suitable in conditions where lung irritation is not important			No	X	X	When necessary. Reduce dose
Hepatic disease	No	Use only when absolutely necessary				No	No	X	X	When necessary. Reduce dose

X = Generally suitable for use.

*From Lumb, W. V., and Jones, E. W.: Veterinary Anesthesia. Philadelphia, Lea and Febiger, 1973.

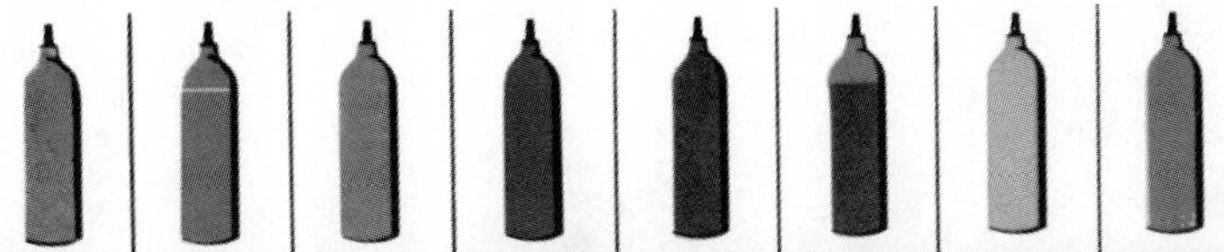

Size	Gray CO_2	Gray and Green CO_2-O_2	Orange $(CH_2)_3$	Red C_2H_4	Brown He	Brown-Green He-O_2	Blue N_2O	Green O_2	Cylinder Dimensions	Weight of Empty Cylinder (lbs.)
G	3200 gals.	1400 gals.		2800 gals.	1100 gals.	1126 gals.	3655 gals.	1400 gals.	$8\frac{1}{2} \times 55''$	100
M		800 gals.		1600 gals.			2000 gals.	800 gals.	$7 \times 47''$	66
E		165 gals.		330 gals.			420 gals.	165 gals.	$4\frac{1}{4} \times 29\frac{3}{4}''$	15
D	250 gals.	95 gals.	230 gals.	200 gals.	80 gals.	82 gals.	250 gals.	95 gals.	$4\frac{1}{4} \times 20\frac{1}{4}''$	$10\frac{1}{4}$
B		40 gals.		100 gals.			100 gals.	40 gals.	$3\frac{1}{4} \times 16\frac{1}{2}''$	$5\frac{3}{4}$
A	50 gals.	20 gals.		40 gals.	15 gals.	15 gals.	50 gals.	20 gals.	$3 \times 10\frac{3}{4}''$	$2\frac{1}{2}$
†DD			230 gals.						$3\frac{3}{4} \times 23\frac{1}{4}''$	$8\frac{3}{4}$
†BB			100 gals.						$2\frac{3}{4} \times 19\frac{3}{4}''$	4
†AA			40 gals.						$2\frac{3}{4} \times 11''$	3

† Cyclopropane cylinders may be chrome plated and bear orange labels.

Figure 88. Net contents of cylinders for all gases. (Courtesy of Ohio Medical Products (Division of Airco, Inc.), PO. Box 1319, Madison Wisconsin 53701.)

TABLE 132. MEDICATIONS APPROPRIATE FOR PARENTERAL TREATMENT OF CAGE BIRDS*

Drug	Strength	Manufacturer	Suggested Dosage	
			Vol./gm. Body Weight	Vol./30-gm. Parakeet
Vitamins and Amino Acid Preparations				
B₁₂	100 μg./ml.	U.S.P.	0.0002–0.0067 ml.	0.006–0.1 ml.
Bejectal with vitamin C		Abbott Lab.	0.00017–0.00034 ml.	0.005–0.01 ml.
Vitamin A	100,000 units/ml.	U.S.P.	0.00034 ml.	0.01 ml.
Vi-Syneral		U.S. Vitamin & Pharmaceutical Corp.	0.00017–0.00034 ml.	0.005–0.01 ml.
Vitamin C	100 mg./ml.	U.S.P.	0.00034 ml.	0.01 ml.
Synkavite	5 mg./ml.	Roche Lab.		0.01 ml.
Injacom with vitamin D₃	As supplied	Roche Lab.	0.00034 ml.	0.01–0.03 ml.
Antibiotics and sulfonamides				
Chloromycetin Succinate	100 mg./ml.	Parke Davis & Co.	0.00034–0.0005 ml.	0.01–0.015 ml.
Tylocine	50 mg./ml.	Corvel, Inc.	0.00034–0.00068 ml.	0.01–0.02 ml.
Bactrovet	100 mg./ml.	Pitman-Moore Co.	0.00024 ml.	0.007 ml.
Symbio	80 mg./ml.	Warren-Teed Co.	0.00034–0.00068 ml.	0.01–0.02 ml.
Erythromycin	50 mg./ml.	Abbott Lab.	0.00009 ml.	0.005–0.01 ml.

Penicillin G, potassium	Diluted 500,000 units/ml.		0.00034-0.00068 ml.	0.01-0.02 ml. (5000-10,000 units)
Spectinomycin	100 mg./ml.	Diamond Labs.	0.00034-0.00068 ml.	0.01-0.02 ml.
Lincocin	100 mg./ml.	Upjohn	0.00034-0.00068 ml.	0.01-0.02 ml.
Gentocin	50 mg./ml.	Schering Corp.	0.00034 ml.	0.01 ml.
Hormones				
Stilbestrol	25 mg./ml.	U.S.P.	0.0001-0.00034 ml.	0.003-01. ml.
Testosterone	25 mg./ml.	U.S.P.	0.00034 ml.	0.01 ml.
Azium	1 mg./ml.	Schering Corp.	0.0002-0.00068 ml.	0.006-0.02 ml.
ACTH	40 units/ml.	Armour Corp.	0.00034-0.00068 ml.	0.001-0.02 ml.
Winstrol V	50 mg./ml.	Winthrop Lab.		0.01-0.03 ml.
Vetalog	2 mg./ml.	Squibb		0.005-0.01 ml.
Miscellaneous				
Nembutal	60 mg./ml.	Abbott Lab.	0.00083 ml.	0.025 ml.
Equi-Thesin	As supplied	Jensen-Salsbery Lab., Inc.	0.0022-0.0025 ml.	0.066 ml.
Jenotone	25 mg./ml.	Jensen-Salsbery Lab., Inc.	0.0004 ml.	0.012 ml.
Saline and 5% dextrose				
Sodium iodide	20% solution	U.S.P.		0.01-0.03 ml.

*From Physical examination procedures for parenteral treatment of cage birds. *In* Kirk, R. W. (ed.): Current Veterinary Therapy V. Philadelphia, W. B. Saunders Co., 1974.

TABLE 133. PARENTERAL ANTIBIOTICS FOR USE IN REPTILES*

Drug	Manufacturer	Route of Administration	Frequency of Administration	Recommended Dosage	Remarks/Precautions
Ampicillin trihydrate (Polyflex)	Bristol Lab.	Intramuscular; subcutaneous	Once daily; twice daily	3–6 mg./kg.	
Benzathine penicillin with procaine penicillin (Flocillin)	Bristol Lab.	Intramuscular	Varies with species and ambient temperature	10,000 units total penicillin activity/kg. 24–72 hours	
Chloramphenicol (Chloromycetin Succinate)	Parke-Davis	Intravenous; intramuscular; subcutaneous	Twice daily; four times daily	10–15 mg./kg. in divided doses	Should not be used in presence of impaired renal or hepatic function or dehydration
Gentamycin sulfate (Gentocin)	Schering Corp.	Intramuscular; subcutaneous	Twice daily first day; once daily thereafter	4 mg./kg. first day twice daily; once daily next 2–6 days	Should not be used in presence of impaired renal or hepatic function or dehydration
Kanamycin sulfate (Kantrex)	Bristol Lab.	Intravenous; intramuscular; intraperitoneal; also as a wound-flushing agent	Twice daily; once daily	10–15 mg./kg. in divided doses	Should not be used in presence of impaired renal or hepatic function or dehydration
Lincomycin (Lincocin)	Upjohn Co.	Intramuscular	Twice daily; once daily	6 mg./kg.	Should not be used in presence of impaired renal or hepatic function or dehydration

Drug	Manufacturer	Route	Frequency	Dosage	Remarks
Neomycin sulfate with polymyxin sulfate (Daribiotic)	Beecham-Massengill	Intramuscular; intravenous; local wound-flushing agent	Twice daily; once daily	10 mg./kg.	Should not be used in presence of impaired renal or hepatic function or dehydration
Oxytetracycline hydrochloride (Liquamycin), injectable and intramuscular	Pfizer	Intravenous; intramuscular, respectively	Once daily	6–10 mg./kg.	May produce some local inflammation at injection site
Potassium penicillin G, buffered, U.S.P.	Squibb	Intramuscular; intraperitoneal; local wound-flushing agent	Varies widely	20,000–80,000 units/kg.	May cause cardiac arrest at high and rapid uptake dosages due to K^+ ion
Streptomycin sulfate, injectable, U.S.P.	Squibb	Intramuscular	Twice daily	10 mg./kg.	Should not be used in presence of impaired renal or hepatic function or dehydration
Sulfadimethoxine (Symbio)	Affiliated Lab.	Intravenous; intramuscular	Once daily	30 mg./kg. first day; 15 mg./kg. second to fourth day	Should not be used in presence of impaired renal or hepatic function or dehydration; hydration must be maintained

*From Bacterial diseases of captive reptiles. In Kirk, R. W. (ed.): Current Veterinary Therapy V. Philadelphia, W. B. Saunders Co., 1974.

TABLE 134. ANTHELMINTICS FOR EXOTIC AND ZOO ANIMALS*

Animal Group	Product	Dosage
Monotremata	Thiabendazole (TBZ)	25–50 mg./lb. (active ingredient)
	Piperazine (Pip.)	50 mg./lb. (base)
Marsupialia	TBZ	
	Pip.	
	Task	(active ingredient 12–15 mg./lb.) in divided doses
	D.N.P.	0.1 ml./lb. subcutaneously
	Scoloban	100 mg./10 lb.
	Yomesan	500 mg./7 lb. (1 tablet)
Chiroptera	Pip.	25–50 mg./lb.
	TBZ	50 mg./lb.
Primates	TBZ	25–100 mg./lb.
	Pip.	40–50 mg./lb.
	D.N.P.	0.1 ml./lb.
	Dizan	5–10 mg./lb. daily for 3–10 days
	Task	7–8 mg./lb. daily for 2–3 days
	Levamisole	4–8 mg./lb.
Edentata and Philodota	TBZ	25–50 mg./lb.
	Pip.	40–50 mg./lb.
Lagomorpha and Rodentia	TBZ	50–125 mg./lb.
	Pip.	40–50 mg./lb. single dose

	TBZ	Mice: 50 mg. in 7 ml. drinking H_2O for 10 days
		Rats and Hamsters: 300 mg. in 50 ml. H_2O for 10 days
		Rabbits and Guinea Pigs: 40–50 mg./lb. single dose
Pinnipedia	TBZ	25–50 mg./lb.
	Pip.	40–50 mg./lb.
	Task (Atgard V)	12–15 mg./lb. (3 to 4 divided doses)
	Scoloban	100 mg./10 lb.
	Levamisole	5–10 mg./lb. orally or by injection
Probascidea	TBZ	20 gm./1000 lb. (Equizole)
"Hoofed Stock"	TBZ	Zebra: 50–60 mg./kg.
		Ruminants: 50–100 mg./kg.
		All-Low Level Feeding: 10 lb. omnizole crumbles/100 lb. of feed for 1–3 days, 10 days off; then 1 lb. omnizole crumbles/100 lb. of feed, 10 days on, 10 days off, etc.
	Task (Atgard V;	Ruminants: 8–10 mg./kg. daily for 5 days or 5 gm./1000 lb. (5 mg./lb.) in a single dose; repeat in 1 week
	(Equigard)	Zebra: 40 mg./kg. (20 mg./lb.)
	Levamisole	As directed on package (3–4 mg./lb.)
Carnivora	TBZ	25–50 mg./lb.
	Pip.	40–50 mg./lb. (repeat)
	D.N.P.	0.1 ml./lb.
	Dizan	5–10 mg./lb. for 5–7 days

Table continues on following page.

TABLE 134. ANTHELMINTICS FOR EXOTIC AND ZOO ANIMALS* (Continued)

Animal Group	Product	Dosage
Aves	Canopar Scoloban°	25 mg./kg. (active ingredient) 100 mg./8–10 lb. (on empty stomach) Do not exceed 800 mg.°
	Task (Atgard V)	12–15 mg./lb. (active ingredient) in 3–5 divided doses
	Levamisole	5–10 mg./lb.
	TBZ	125–250 mg./lb. single oral dose for large birds (0.125–0.25 mg./gm. small caged birds); can lower dosage and give low level for 5–12 days
	Pip.	100–250 mg./lb. single dose or 6–10 gm./gal. of drinking H₂O for 1–4 days (0.3–0.5 mg./gm. single dose in caged birds)
	Scoloban	10 mg./lb.
	Levamisole	20 mg./lb.
Reptiles†	Pip.	40–50 mg./lb. (given in food animal or per stomach tube)
	TBZ	50–100 mg./lb. (as Pip.)
	Task	6–8 mg./lb. daily for 2 doses (not recommended)
	Scoloban	10–25 mg./lb.
	Levamisole	10–15 mg./lb.

*From Soifer, F. K.: Anthelmintics for exotic and zoo animals. *In* Kirk, R. W. (ed.): Current Veterinary Therapy V. Philadelphia, W. B. Saunders Co., 1974.

†Vermifuges should be administered to turtles at half the measured body weight to allow for the shell.

TABLE 135. DRUG DOSAGES

Name of Drug	Dog	Cat
Acepromazine	0.05 to 0.25 mg./lb., I.V., I.M., or SQ	0.05 to 0.10 mg./lb., I.M. or SQ
Acetazolamide	5 mg./lb. q6h, P.O.	Same
Acetylsalicylic Acid (aspirin)	0.1 to 2.0 gm. q4 to 6h, P.O. (may cause g.i. irritation)	Not recommended
ACTH	1 U/lb./day, I.M. (therapeutic) or 40 U/dog, I.M. (response test), post sample in 2 hours	Same
Aldactone (Spirinolactone)	1 to 2 mg./lb. divided b.i.d.	Same
Alevaire	50 to 60 ml./hr. for 30 to 60 min. q12h (nebulization)	Same
Allopurinol (Zyloprim)	2.5 to 5.0 mg./lb. divided b.i.d., P.O.	Not recommended
Aminophylline	5 mg./lb. q8h, P.O., I.M. or I.V.	Same
Ammonium chloride	50 mg./lb. q12h, P.O.	10 mg./lb. q12h, P.O.
Amphetamine	2 mg./lb., I.V., or I.M.	Same
Amphotericin B	0.1 to 0.2 mg./lb., dilute in 5% dextrose to 0.1 mg./ml.; give over 2 hr. period I.V., 2 to 3 times/week; or, over 30 min. period I.P., every other day, for 60 to 90 days. Total dose 5 to 10 mg./lb.	Not recommended
Ampicillin	10 mg./lb. q8h, P.O., I.M., or I.V.	Same
Apomorphine	20 μg./lb., I.V.	Not recommended
Amprolium	50 to 100 mg./lb./day in food or water for 7 to 10 days; or 0.4 mg./20 lb., I.V. rapid injection	Not recommended
Aqua-B (vitamin B complex)	0.5 to 2.0 ml., I.V., I.M., or SQ q24h	0.5 to 1.0 ml., I.V., I.M., or SQ q24h

Table continues on following page.

TABLE 135. DRUG DOSAGES *(Continued)*

Name of Drug	Dog	Cat
Aquamephyton (vitamin K₁)	5 to 20 mg., I.V., I.M., or SQ q12h	1 to 5 mg., I.V., I.M., or SQ q 12h
Arecoline hydrobromide	7.5 mg./10 lb., P.O., after 12-hr. fast	Not for use in cats
Ascorbic acid (vitamin C)	100 to 500 mg./day (maintenance) or 100 to 500 mg. q8h (urine acidifier)	100 mg./day (maintenance) or 100 mg. q8h (urine)
Atropine	0.05 mg./lb., I.V., I.M., or SQ q6h; 1% solution in eye	Same, topically in eye (causes salivation)
Azulfidine	30 mg./lb. q8h, P.O.	Not recommended
BAL	2 mg./lb., I.M. q4h until recovered	Not recommended
Benzyl benzoate	Topically	Not recommended
Bethanecol	5 to 25 mg. q8h, P.O.	2.5 to 5.0 mg. q8h, P.O.
Bismuth (milk of)	5 to 10 ml. q4h, P.O.	2.5 to 5.0 ml. q4h, P.O.
Bismuth (subnitrate, subgallate, or subcarbonate)	0.3 to 3.0 gm. q4h, P.O.	Same
Blood	10 ml./lb. or to effect, I.V. or I.P.	Same
Brewer's yeast	0.1 gm./1.0 lb., o.d., P.O.	Same
Bunamidine (Scolaban)	20 mg./lb., P.O. after 18-hr. fast	Same
Caffeine	0.1 to 0.5 gm., I.M.	Not recommended
Calcium	240 mg./lb./day, P.O.	60 mg./lb./day, P.O.
Calcium carbonate	1 to 4 gm./day, P.O.	Same
Calcium EDTA	50 mg./lb., diluted to 10 mg./ml. in 5% dextrose, and given SQ in 4 divided doses; continue for 5 days	Same
Calcium gluconate (10% solution)	10 to 30 ml., I.V., *slowly*	5 to 15 ml., I.V., *slowly*
Calcium lactate	0.5 to 2.0 gm., P.O.	0.2 to 0.5 gm., P.O.
Canex	0.3% rotenone in oil, topically	Same
Canine distemper-hepatitis vaccine	1 vial SQ at 8, 12, and 16 weeks of age; annual booster	Not for use in cats

Drug	Dosage	Cats
Canopar	½ tab. b.i.d., P.O., up to 10-lb. dog; 1 tab., o.d. for greater than 10 lb.; repeat in 3 weeks	Not for use in cats
Cardioquin	5 to 10 mg./lb. q8 to 12h, P.O.	Same
Centrine	½ to 2½ tabs q8 to 12h, P.O.	Not recommended
Cephalexin	15 mg./lb. orally q12h	Same
Cephaloridine (Loridine)	5 mg./lb. q12h, I.M. or SQ	Same
Charcoal (activated)	2 heaping tabs. in 200 ml. tap water, P.O., for 30-lb. dog	Same
Cheracol	5 ml. q4h, P.O.	3 ml. q4h, P.O.
Chloramphenicol	10 to 25 mg./lb. q8h, P.O., I.V., or SQ; 1% ointment topically	Same
Chlordane	0.5% solution on dog or premises	Not recommended
Chlorethamine	0.2 to 1.0 gm. q8h, P.O.	100 mg. q8h, P.O.
Chlorpheniramine	4 to 8 mg. q12h, P.O.	2 mg. q12h, P.O.
Chlorpromazine (thorazine)	0.5 to 1.0 mg./lb. q12h, I.V. or I.M.; 1-2 mg./lb. q8h, P.O.; 0.25 mg./lb. as ∝ = blocker in shock	Same
Chlorthiazide (Diuril)	10 to 20 mg./lb. q12h, P.O.	Same
Codeine	1 mg./lb. q6h, SQ (pain) or 5 mg./dose q6h, P.O. (cough)	Not recommended
Cod liver oil	1 tsp./20 lb., o.d., P.O.	Same
Colistimethate (Coly-mycin)	0.5 mg./lb. q6h, I.M.	Not recommended
Coramine	¼ to 1 ml./15 lb., SQ, I.M., or I.V.	Same
Cyclophosphamide (Cytoxan)	50 mg./m² BSA, o.d., P.O., every other day	12.5 mg./cat o.d., P.O., every other day
Cyclothiazide	0.5 to 1.0 mg., o.d., P.O.	Not recommended
Darbazine	¼ ml. q12h, SQ (up to 4 lb.) ½ to 1 ml. q12h, SQ (5 to 14 lb.) 2 to 3 ml. q12h, SQ (15 to 30 lb.) 3 to 4 ml. q12h, SQ (30 to 45 lb.) 4 to 5 ml. q12h, SQ (45 to 60 lb.) 6 ml. q12h, SQ (over 60 lb.)	Same

Table continues on following page.

TABLE 135. DRUG DOSAGES (Continued)

Name of Drug	Dog	Cat
Daribiotic	0.5 to 1.0 ml. q12h, I.M. (small dog, 0.25 ml. q12h)	0.25 ml. q12h
Delta Albaplex	1 to 2 tab/day P.O. (5 to 15 lb.) 1 tab q12h 2 to 4 tab/day P.O. (15 to 30 lb.) 4 to 6 tab/day P.O. (30 to 60 lb.) 6 to 8 tab/day P.O. (over 60 lb.)	1 tab q12h
Desoxycorticosterone acetate (DOCA)	1 to 5 mg., I.M., q24h	0.5 to 1.0 mg., I.M., q24h
Desoxycorticosterone pivalate	Each 25 mg. releases 1 mg. DOCA/day for 1 month, I.M.	Same
Dexamethasone (Azuin)	0.25 to 2.0 mg., o.d., P.O., or I.M.: 2 to 5 mg./lb., I.V., for shock	0.1 to 0.5 mg., o.d., P.O. or I.M.: 2 to 5 mg./lb., I.V., for shock
Dextran	10 ml./lb. (to effect), I.V.	Same
Dextrose solutions (5% in water, saline, or Ringer's solution)	20 to 25 ml./lb., I.V., SQ, or I.P., q24h	Same
D.F.P. (Floropryl)	0.1% solution for eyes, topically	Same
Diathal	0.03 ml./lb. q12h, I.M.	Use with caution on cats, pups, and toy breeds
Diazepam (valium)	2.5 to 20 mg., I.V. or P.O.	2.5 to 5.0 mg., I.V. or P.O.
Dichlorphenamide	For 30-lb. dog, 50 mg. t.i.d. orally	10 to 25 mg. t.i.d.
Dichlorvos (TASK)	12 to 15 mg./lb., P.O. (see manufacturer's recommendations); repeat in 3 weeks	Not recommended
Diethyl carbamazine (Caricide)	15 to 30 mg./lb., P.O. (vermifuge) or 2.5 mg./lb./day (heartworm prevention)	5 to 10 mg./lb., P.O.
Diethylstilbestrol	0.1 to 1.0 mg./day P.O., or 1 mg./lb. up to 25 mg. total, I.M. (repositol) once	0.05 to 0.10 mg./day, P.O. (caution)

Digoxin	0.05 to 0.10 mg./lb. in 4 equal doses over 48-hr. period (digitalization); mainte-nance dose: $^1/_6$ of total digitalization dose or about 0.01 mg./lb.	Same
Dihydrocodeinone	5 mg. q6h, P.O.	Not recommended
Dihydrostreptomycin (Streptomycin)	5 mg./lb. q8 to 12 h, I.M. or SQ	Same
Dimenhydrinate (Dramamine)	25 to 50 mg. q8h, P.O.	12.5 mg. q8h, P.O.
Diphenhydramine (Benadryl)	1 mg./lb. q12h, P.O., or 5 to 50 mg. q12h, I.V.	Not recommended
Diphenthane 70	100 mg./lb., P.O., after 12-hr. fast; re-peat in 3 weeks	Same
Diphenylhydantoin (Dilantin)	3 mg./lb. q8 to 12h, P.O.	Not recommended
Diphenylthiocarbazone	30 mg./lb. q8h, P.O., for 5 days *beyond* recovery	Not recommended
Disophenol (D.N.P.)	3.5 mg./lb., SQ; repeat in 3 weeks	Not recommended
Dithiazanine (Dizan)	2 to 3 mg./lb., o.d., P.O., for 7 to 10 days (microfilariae)	10 mg., o.d., P.O., for 4 to 5 days (lungworm)
Domeboro's solution	1 to 2 tabs./pint of water; apply topically q4h	Same
Doxapram	2.5 to 5.0 mg./lb., I.V.	Same
D-penicillamine	15 mg./lb. divided b.i.d., P.O.	Not recommended
Drocarbil (Nemural)	2 mg./lb. P.O. after light meal; repeat in 3 weeks (caution)	Same (caution)
Ephedrine	5 to 15 mg., P.O.	2 to 5 mg., P.O.
Epinephrine (1:1000 solution)	0.1 to 0.5 ml., SQ, I.M., I.V., or I.C.	0.1 to 0.2 ml., SQ, I.M., I.V., or I.C.
Erythromycin	5 to 10 mg./lb. q8h, P.O.	Same
Estradiol (E.C.P.) cyclo-pentylproprionate	0.25 to 2.0 mg., I.M., *once*	0.25 mg., I.M., *once*

Table continues on following page.

TABLE 135. DRUG DOSAGES (*Continued*)

Name of Drug	Dog	Cat
Ether	0.5 to 4.0 ml. (induce 8%; maintain 4% to effect)	Same
Ethoxzolamide (Cardrase)	2 mg./lb. q12h, P.O.	Same
Feline panleukopenia antiserum	Not for use in dogs	1 to 5 ml., SQ (prevention) or 5 to 10 ml., SQ (exposure)
Feline panleukopenia vaccine	Not for use in dogs	1 vial SQ at 8, 12, and 16 weeks of age; annual booster
Ferrous sulfate	100 to 300 mg./day, P.O.	50 to 100 mg./day, P.O.
Fludrocortisone (Florinef)	0.2 to 0.8 mg., o.d., P.O.	0.1 to 0.2 mg., o.d. P.O.
Flumethasone (Flucort)	0.0625 to 0.25 mg./day, I.V., I.M., or SQ; or 0.03 to 0.25 mg./day, P.O.	0.03 to 0.125 mg./day, I.V., I.M., SQ, or P.O.
9-Fluoroprednisolone (Predef)	1 mg., o.d., I.M.	0.5 mg., o.d., I.M.
Folic acid	5 mg./day, P.O.	2.5 mg./day, P.O.
Fulvidex	Topically in ear	Same
Furadex	1 to 2 mg./lb. q8 to 12 h, P.O.	Same
Furosemide (Lasix)	1 to 2 mg./lb. q8 to 12h, P.O.; no more than 40 to 50 mg. *total I.V.* to *any dog,* q12h	1 to 2 mg./lb. q8 to 12h, P.O.; 5 to 10 mg. total I.V. q8 to 12h
Gentamicin	2 mg./lb., I.M. or SQ, q12h for 2 days, then q24h for 5 days	Same
Globulon	0.2 ml./lb., SQ	Not recommended
Glycerin	0.3 ml./lb., P.O., q8h	Same
Glycobiarsol (Milibis-V)	100 mg./lb., o.d., for 5 days; repeat in 3 months	Not recommended
Goodwinol	Topically for Demodex, o.d. for 4 to 6 weeks	Same

Griseofulvin (Fulvicin)	10 mg./lb., o.d., for 6 weeks, or 70 mg./lb. once a week, or 100 mg./lb. every 10 days; prophylaxis: 100 mg./lb. once; teratogenic	Same
Halothane	Induce 3%; maintain 0.5 to 1.0%	Same
Heparin	0.5 mg./lb., I.V.	Same
Hetacillin	5 to 10 mg./lb., P.O., q12h	50 to 100 mg., P.O., q12h
Hydrochlorothiazide (Hydrodiuril)	1 to 2 mg./lb. q12h. P.O.	Same
Hydrocortisone	2 mg./lb. q12h, P.O.	Same
Hydrocortisone sodium succinate	10 to 20 mg./lb., I.V., for shock	Same
Hydrogen peroxide (3%)	5 to 10 ml. q15min., P.O., until emesis	Same
Initol	15 ml./lb., P.O. (nutrition) or 1 ml./lb., P.O. (plasma turbidity test)	11 ml./lb., P.O.
Innovar Vet	1 ml./15 to 20 lb., I.M., or 1 ml./25 to 60 lb., I.V.	Not recommended
Insulin (regular)	1.U/lb., I.V., q2 to 6h (ketoacidosis), modified to effect	3 to 5U, SQ, q6h, modified to effect
Insulin (intermediate)	¼ to ½ U/lb., SQ, q24h, modified as needed	3 to 5 U, SQ, q24h, modified as needed
Iron dextran	5 mg./lb., I.M., weekly in divided doses	Same
Isuprel	0.1 to 0.2 mg. q6h, I.M. or SQ; 15 to 30 mg. q4h, P.O.; 1 mg. in 200 ml. 5% dextrose to effect, I.V.; elixir 0.2 ml. q8h, P.O.	Same
Jenotone	1 mg./lb. q12h, I.M. or SQ	Same
Kanamycin	3 mg./lb. q12h, I.M. or SQ	Same
Kaobiotic	1 tab/9 lb./day in 2 or 3 divided doses	Same
Kaopectate	½ to 1 ml./lb. q2 to 6h, P.O.	Same
Ketamine	Not recommended	5 to 15 mg./lb., I.M.
Lactated Ringer's solution	20 to 25 ml./lb./day, I.V., SQ, or I.P.	Same

Table continues on following page.

TABLE 135. DRUG DOSAGES (*Continued*)

Name of Drug	Dog	Cat
Led-o-san	Topically	Same
Levamisole (L-Tetramisole)	5 mg./lb., o.d., P.O. for 6 to 10 days (microfilariae)	10 to 20 mg./lb., o.d., P.O., every other day for 5 to 6 treatments (lungworm)
Lidocaine (without epinephrine)	2 to 4 mg./lb., I.V., over 2-min. period; follow with 2 mg./ml. slow drip in 5% dextrose	Same
Lime sulfur (1:16 to 1:40 solution)	Topically	Same
Lincomycin	5 to 10 mg./lb. q8h, P.O., or q12h, I.M.	Same
Lindane	0.025 to 0.1% aqueous solution topically	Not recommended
Mandelic acid (Mandelamine)	0.25 mg./30 lb. q8h	Not recommended
Mannitol hexanitrate	15 to 30 mg., P.O.	Same
Mannitol (20% solution)	0.5 to 1.0 gm./lb., I.V., q6h	Same
Maxidex	Topically in eyes q2 to 8h	Same
Maxitrol	Topically in eyes q2 to 8h	Same
Measles vaccine	1 vial, SQ, between 4 and 12 weeks of age	Not recommended
Meclizine (Bonine)	25 mg., o.d., P.O.	12.5 mg., o.d., P.O.
Melatonin	1 to 2 mg., SQ, o.d., for 3 days; repeat monthly as needed	Not recommended
Meperidine (Demerol)	5 to 7 mg./lb., SQ, as needed	1-2 mg./lb., SQ, as needed
Mercuhydrin	1 mg./lb., I.M., SQ, or I.V.	Same
Methenamine mandelate	5 mg./lb. q6h, P.O., or to effect	Not recommended
Methetharimide	6 mg./lb., I.V.	Same
Methicillin	10 mg./lb. q6h, I.M. or I.V.	Same
d-L-Methionine	0.2 to 1.0 gm. q8h, P.O.	0.2 gm. q8h, P.O.
Methischol	1 cap/30 lb. q8h, P.O.	1 cap q12h, P.O.

Methotrexate	2.5 to 5.0 mg./m² BSA, o.d., P.O., for 4 days; may repeat at 3-week intervals as needed	Not recommended
Methoxyflurane	Induce 2 to 3%; maintain 0.5%	Same
Methylprednisolone	0.5 mg./lb., o.d., P.O., or once weekly (depo), I.M.	Same
Metrazol	5 mg./lb., I.V., or 100 mg., P.O.	3 mg./lb., I.V.
Metronidazole (Flagyl)	30 mg./lb., o.d., P.O. for 5 days	Not recommended
Metropine	0.5 to 1.0 mg. q8h, P.O.	Not recommended
Metropectin	2 to 4 tab q8h, P.O.	Not recommended
Milk of magnesia	5 to 30 ml., P.O.	5 to 15 ml., P.O.
Mineral oil	5 to 15 ml., P.O.	2 to 6 ml., P.O. (caution)
Mitox	Topically in ears, o.d., for 5 to 7 days; then once a week for 5 to 7 weeks	Same
Morphine	1 to 2 mg./lb., I.M. or SQ	0.1 mg./lb., I.M. or SQ
Nalorphine	0.5 mg./lb., I.V., I.M., or SQ	Not recommended
n-Butyl chloride	0.2 ml./lb. after 12-hr. fast	Not recommended
Neo-darbazine	1 cap q12h, P.O. (10 to 20 lb.); 2 cap q12h, P.O. (20 to 30 lb.) (spansule #1) 1 cap q12h, P.O. (30 to 60 lb.); 2 cap q12h, P.O. (over 60 lb.) (spansule #3)	Same
Neomycin	10 mg./lb. q6h, P.O., or 5 mg./lb. q12h, I.M. or I.V.	Same
Neostigmine	1 to 2 mg., I.M., as needed; 5 to 15 mg., P.O., as needed	Not recommended
Nitrofurazone (0.2% ointment or solution)	Topically	Topically
Nitrofurantoin	1 to 2 mg./lb. q8h, P.O. with food	Same
Nitrofurantoin sodium	1.5 mg./lb. q12h, I.M. (max. 10 days)	Not recommended
Novobiocin	5 mg./lb. q8h, P.O.	Same
Octin	½ to 1 ml., I.M.; 1 tab q8 to 12h, P.O.	¼ to ½ ml., I.M., or ½ to 1 tab. q12h, P.O.

Table continues on following page.

TABLE 135. DRUG DOSAGES (Continued)

Name of Drug	Dog	Cat
o.p'-DDD	25 mg./lb., o.d., P.O., to effect (approx. 5 to 10 days); then once every 2 weeks	Not recommended
Ouabain	0.02 mg./lb. total dose, I.V.; give ½ dose stat, then ⅛ dose q30 min.; maintenance: ¼ of total q3h	Same
Oxacillin	5 mg./lb. q6h, P.O., I.M., or I.V.	Same
Oxymorphone (Numorphan)	0.2 mg./lb., I.V.	Same
Oxytocin	5 to 10 U, I.M. or I.V.; repeat q15 to 30 min.	0.5 to 3.0 U, I.M. or I.V.
2-PAM	20 mg./lb., I.V., over 2-min. period, q12h as needed (*can* go I.M. or SQ)	Not recommended
Pancreatin	2 to 10 tab with food	1 to 2 tab with food
Paregoric	3 to 5 ml. q6h, P.O.	Not recommended
Penicillin G (Procaine)	20,000 U/lb., I.M. or SQ, q24h	Same
Penicillin G (Sodium)	20,000 U/lb., I.V. or I.M., q6h, or 80 to 100,000 U/lb., P.O., q6h	Same
Phenobarbital	1 mg./lb. q12h, P.O., or 3 mg./lb., I.M. or I.V.	2 to 3 mg./lb. q12h, P.O.
Phenylbutazone (Butazolidin)	20 mg./lb. q8h, P.O.	5 to 7 mg./lb. q12h, P.O.
Phthalofyne (Whipcide)	90 mg./lb., P.O., after 24-hr. fast; repeat in 3 months	Not recommended
Piperazine	50 to 100 mg./lb., P.O.; repeat in 3 weeks	Same
Pitressin (ADH)	10 U, I.V. or I.M. (aqueous); or 0.5 to 1.0 ml., I.M., every other day (oil)	Not recommended
Polymyxin B	1 mg./lb. q12h, I.M.	Not recommended
Potassium chloride	1 to 3 gm./day, P.O., or I.V.; maximum 10 mEq./hr. and 40 mEq./day/dog	0.2 gm./day, P.O.
Prednisolone	0.25 to 1.0 mg./lb., P.O. or I.M., divided b.i.d	Same

Prednisone	0.25 to 1.0 mg./lb., P.O. or I.M., divided b.i.d.	Same
Primidone	25 mg./lb., divided b.i.d., P.O.	Not recommended
Probanthine	7.5 to 30 mg. q8 to 12h, P.O.	Not recommended
Procainamide	½ to 2 cap q4 to 6h, P.O., or 100 to 500 mg., I.V. or I.M., q2h	Same
Promazine (Sparine)	1-2 mg./lb., I.M.	Same
Propiopromazine (Tranvet)	0.2 mg./lb., I.V. or I.M.	Not recommended
Propranolol	10 to 40 mg. q8h, P.O., or 1 to 3 mg., I.V. *slowly*	5 to 10 mg. q8h, P.O. or 0.5 to 1.0 mg., I.V. *slowly*
Prussian blue	0.2 gm./lb./day orally, subdivided into 3 doses	Not recommended
Psymod	0.5 to 2.0 mg./10 lb., I.V., I.M., sq, or P.O.	Same
Pyrimethamine	1 mg./lb./day, P.O., for 3 days; then 0.5 mg./lb. every other day	Same
Quadrinal	¼ to ½ tab q4 to 6h, P.O.	¼ tab q4 to 6h, P.O.
Quibron	1 to 3 cap q8h; elixir 5 ml./30 lb. q8h, P.O.	½ cap q8h; elixir 2 ml. q8h, P.O.
Quinacrine (Atabrine)	50 to 100 mg. q12h, P.O., for 3 days; repeat in 3 days	Not recommended
Quinidine	5 to 10 mg./lb., P.O., q6 to 8h	Same
Quinaglute	5 to 10 mg./lb., P.O., q12h	Same
Rabies vaccine (C.E.O.)	1 vial, I.M. (as per state regulation)	Not recommended
Rabies vaccine (T.C.O.)	1 vial, I.M. (as per state regulation)	Same
Renzol	1 tab/20 lb., P.O., q8h	Same
Respireze	1 tab q6 to 8h (up to 25 lb.) or 2 tab q6 to 8h (over 25 lb.), P.O.	Not recommended
Rheomacrodex	100 to 500 ml., I.V.	50 to 100 ml., I.V.
Riboflavin	10 to 20 mg./day, P.O.	5 to 10 mg./day, P.O.
Ringer's solution	20 to 25 ml./lb./day, I.V., I.P., or SQ	Same

Table continues on following page.

TABLE 135. DRUG DOSAGES (Continued)

Name of Drug	Dog	Cat
Rompun	0.5 to 2.0 mg./lb., SQ, I.M., or I.V.	Same
Ronnel (Ectoral)	35 mg./lb. P.O., divided b.i.d., or as 1 to 2% aqueous solution topically	Not recommended
Sodium bicarbonate	25 mg./lb., P.O., q8 to 12h	Same
Sodium chloride (0.9% solution)	20 to 25 ml./lb./day, I.V., I.P., or SQ	Same
Sodium dioctyl sulfosuccinate	100 to 300 mg. q12h, P.O.	100 mg. q12 to 24h, P.O.
Sodium iodide (20% solution)	1 ml./10 lb. q8 to 12h, P.O. or I.V.	Same
Sodium levothyroxine	0.1 to 0.6 mg., o.d., P.O., or 0.05 to 0.3 mg. b.i.d., P.O.	0.05 to 0.1 mg., o.d., P.O.
Sodium sulfate	1 tsp./10 lb., P.O.	Same
Stanozolol (Winstrol-v)	½ to 2 tab q12h, P.O.	½ tab q12h, P.O.
Sulfadimethoxine	10 mg./lb., o.d., P.O. or I.V.	Same
Sulfamerazine	25 mg./lb. q12h, P.O. or I.V.	Same
Sulfamethazine	25 mg./lb. q12h, P.O. or I.V.	Same
Sulfathalidine	50 mg./lb. q12h, P.O.	Same
Sulfisoxazole	20 mg./lb. q8h, P.O.	Same
Styrid-caricide	1 ml./20 lb., o.d., P.O. (heartworm prevention)	Not recommended
Tannalbin	1 to 3 gm. q8h, P.O.	Not recommended
Tansal (5% tannic acid, 5% salicylic acid, and 70% alcohol)	Topically q8h	Same
Temaril-P	1 cap, o.d., P.O. (up to 10 lb.) 2 cap, o.d., P.O. (11 to 20 lb.) 4 cap, o.d., P.O. (21 to 40 lb.) 6 cap, o.d., P.O. (over 40 lb.)	Same

Drug		
Testosterone	1 mg./lb., o.d., every 2 to 3 days, P.O. (up to 30 mg. total); or 1 mg./lb., up to 30 mg. total. I.M. every 10 days (repositol)	Same
Tetracycline (or oxytetracycline. chlortetracycline)	8 to 10 mg./lb. q8h, P.O., or 3 mg./lb. q12h, I.V.	Same
Thiabendazole	25 to 50 mg./lb., o.d., P.O.	Not recommended
Thiacetarsamide (Caparsolate or Filicide)	0.1 ml./lb., I.V., b.i.d. for 2 days	0.05 ml./lb., I.V., once on day 1; skip a day; repeat on day 3
Thiamine	10 to 100 mg./day, P.O.	5 to 30 mg./day, P.O.
Thyroid (dessicated)	5 mg./lb. day, P.O.	Same
Tolnaftate (sodium)	Topically, o.d.	Same
Toluene (methyl benzene)	100 mg./lb., P.O.	Same
Tresaderm	Topically q12h	Same
Triacetyloleandomycin	25 mg./lb., P.O., divided q8h	Not recommended
Triamcinolone	0.25 to 2 mg., o.d., P.O., or I.M.	0.1 mg., o.d., P.O., or I.M.
Tripelennamine	0.5 mg./lb. q12h, P.O., or 1 ml./40 lb., I.M.	Same
TSH	5 to 10 U, I.V. post sample in 4 hours; I.M. or SQ sample in 12 hours	5 U, I.M. or SQ
Tylosin	5 mg./lb. q8 to 12h, P.O., or 1 mg./lb., I.M. or I.V.	Same
Vigojex	1 ml./25 lb., I.M., every 10 to 21 days	Same
Vigoral	1 to 3 tab, o.d., P.O.	½ to 1 tab, o.d., P.O.
Vincristine	0.5 mg./m² BSA, I.V., once a week as needed	0.1 mg., I.V., once a week as needed
Vi-sorbin	1 to 3 tsp., P.O., daily	½ tsp., P.O., daily
Vitamin A	200 U/lb./day, P.O., for 10 days	Same
Vitamin B₁₂	100 to 200 μg./day	50 to 100 μg./day
Vitamin D	15 U/lb./day, P.O., for 10 days	Same
Vitamin E	500 mg./day, P.O.	100 mg./day, P.O.
Vitamin K (Menadione)	1 mg./lb./day, I.M., for 10 days	Same
Yomesan	70 mg./lb., P.O.; repeat in 3 weeks	Same

INDEX

Page numbers in *italics* refer to illustrations. Page numbers followed by the letter "t" refer to tables.

Normal values of laboratory data vary widely, depending on the patient's sex, breed and age, and on the laboratory. The values in these tables are approximations for use as guidelines only.

These tables are normal data from clinical laboratory sheets used at the N.Y.S. Veterinary College, Cornell University.

Routine Chemistry

GENERAL	DOG	CAT
Bilirubin, total (mg./dl.)	0.07–0.61	0.15–0.20
direct (mg./dl.)	0.0–0.14	–
indirect (mg./dl.)	0.07–0.61	–
BSP (% ret.) at 30 min.	5.0	–
Cholesterol (mg./dl.)	125–250	75–151
Creatinine (mg./dl.)	1–2	1–2
Glucose (mg./dl.)	60–100	64–118
Iron (μg./dl.)	94–122	68–215
TIBC (μg./dl.)	280–340	170–400
PSP (μg./dl.) plasma clearance at 60 min.	60–100	–
Urea N. (mg./dl.)	10–20	20–30
Uric acid (mg./dl.)	0–1.0	1.0–1.9
GOT (SF U.)	<50	<50
GPT (SF U.)	<50	<50
CPK (IU)	0–70	10–60
LDH (BB U.)	<600	
Alk. Phos. (S U.)	<5	<5
Lipase (ST U.)	<1	<1
Amylase (Som. U.)	<800	<800
Proteins total, serum (gm./dl.)	5.4–7.1	5.4–7.8
Fibrinogen (mg./dl.)	300–600	300–600
A:G	0.8–1.7	0.4–1.7
Albumin (gm./dl.)	2.3–3.2	2.1–3.3
Globulin (gm./dl.)	2.7–4.4	2.6–5.1
ACID – BASE		
pH (units)	7.31–7.42	7.24–7.40
pCO_2 (mm. Hg)	29–42	29–42
Base excess (mEq./l.)	±2.5	±2.5
Bicarbonate (mEq./l.)	17–24	17–24
ELECTROLYTES		
Sodium (mEq./l.)	140–155	147–156
Potassium (mEq./l.)	3.7–5.8	4.0–4.5
Chloride (mEq./l.)	105–115	117–123
Osmolality (mOsm./l.)	280–305	280–305
Calcium (mg./dl.)	8.4–11.2	7.0–10.0
Phosphorus (mg./dl.)	2.5–5.0	4–7
Magnesium (mg./dl.)	1.8–2.4	2–3
SPECIAL CHEMISTRY		
δ-ALA (μg./dl.)	<500	–
Blood lead (μg./dl.)	0–20	–
T-4 (μg./dl.)	2.0–6.0	1.5–4.0
Cortisol (μg./dl.)	5–10	–